D0702192

Nurse's Rapid Reference

Wolters Kluwer | Lippincott Williams & Wilkins
Health

Philadelphia · Baltimore · New York · London
Buenos Aires · Hong Kong · Sydney · Tokyo

Staff

EXECUTIVE PUBLISHER
Judith A. Schilling McCann, RN, MSN

EDITORIAL DIRECTOR
David Moreau

CLINICAL DIRECTOR
Joan M. Robinson, RN, MSN

ART DIRECTOR
Elaine Kasmer

SENIOR MANAGING EDITOR
Jaime Stockslager Buss, MSPH, ELS

CLINICAL PROJECT MANAGER
Kate Stout, RN, MSN, CCRN

EDITORS
Sid Karpoff, Liz Schaeffer

COPY EDITORS
Kristin Baum, Karl Schaeffer

DESIGNER
Debra Moloshok

DIGITAL COMPOSITION SERVICES
Diane Paluba (manager),
Joyce Rossi Biletz, Donald G. Knauss,
Donna S. Morris

ASSOCIATE MANUFACTURING MANAGER
Beth J. Welsh

EDITORIAL ASSISTANTS
Karen J. Kirk, Jeri O'Shea, Linda K. Ruhf

DESIGN ASSISTANT
Kate Zulak

INDEXER
Judy Young

NRR010408

LIBRARY OF CONGRESS
CATALOGING-IN-PUBLICATION DATA
Nurse's rapid reference.
    p. ; cm.
Includes bibliographical references and index.
1. Nursing—Handbooks, manuals, etc. I.
Lippincott Williams & Wilkins.
[DNLM: 1. Nursing Process—Handbooks. 2.
Nursing Care—Handbooks. WY 49 N974273
2008]
  RT51.N854 2008
  610.73—dc22
ISBN-13: 978-0-7817-8742-0 (alk. paper)
ISBN-10: 0-7817-8742-4 (alk. paper) 2007049038

Contents

Contributors
and consultants

Karen Balich-Reitz, RN, MS
Staff Nurse
MacNeal Hospital – Good Samaritan
Berwyn, Ill.

Helen C. Ballestas, RN, MSN, CRRN
Faculty, Nursing Department
New York Institute of Technology
Old Westbury

Kimberly R. Blount, MSN, CRNP, CS
Assistant Professor of Nursing
Gannon University
Villa Maria School of Nursing
Erie, Pa.

Julie A. Calvery, RN, MS
Instructor
University of Arkansas
Fort Smith

Lillian Craig, RN, MSN, FNP-C
Adjunct Faculty
Oklahoma Panhandle State University
Goodwell

Laurie Donaghy, RN, CEN
Staff Nurse
Frankford Hospital
Philadelphia

Kathy C. Flamm, RN, MSN, ANP-C
Adult Nurse Practitioner
Gateway Medical Internal Medicine
West Chester, Pa.

Joyce A. Harvey, RN
Registered Nurse, Step-down Unit
University of Pittsburgh Medical Center – Passavant

Sharon L. G. Lee, RN, MS, APRN, CCRN, CEN, FNP-C
Assistant Professor
BryanLGH College of Health Sciences
Lincoln, Nebr.

Carol T. Lemay, RN
Clinical Consultant
Brattleboro, Vt.

Patricia Lemelle-Wright, RN, MS
Staff Nurse
University of Chicago Hospital
Clinical Instructor
Malcolm X College
Moraine Valley Community College
Chicago, Ill.

Valerie D. Lyttle, RN, BSN, CEN
Patient Care Manager
Auburn (Wash.) Regional Medical Center

Lauren R. Roach, LPN, HCSD
Clinical Support Nurse
Good Samaritan Home Care Services, LLC
Vincennes, Ind.

Darlene K. Shaffer, RN
Clinical Consultant
Altoona, Pa.

Wendy Wolsleger, RN, BSN
Staff Nurse
Mercy Regional Medical Center
Durango, Colo.

I   *Disorders*

Acute pyelonephritis

Overview

Acute pyelonephritis, also called *acute infective tubulointerstitial nephritis*, is a bacterial infection of the renal parenchyma that affects one or both kidneys. With treatment, extensive permanent damage is rare. This disorder is more common in women than in men.

CAUSES
◆ Bacterial infection of the kidneys
◆ *Escherichia coli*
◆ Microorganisms (the same as those that cause lower urinary tract infection [UTI])

RISK FACTORS
◆ Renal procedures that use instrumentation such as cystoscopy
◆ Hematogenic infection such as septicemia
◆ Sexual activity in women
◆ Pregnancy
◆ Neurogenic bladder
◆ Obstructive disease
◆ Renal diseases
◆ Structural abnormalities
◆ Lower UTI
◆ Inadequate feminine hygiene

PATHOPHYSIOLOGY
◆ Infection spreads from the bladder to the ureters to the kidneys, commonly through vesicoureteral reflux.
◆ Vesicoureteral reflux may result from congenital weakness at the junction of the ureter and bladder.
◆ Bacteria refluxed to intrarenal tissues may create colonies of infection within 24 to 48 hours.
◆ Female anatomy allows for higher incidence of infection.

COMPLICATIONS
◆ Renal calculi
◆ Renal failure
◆ Renal abscess
◆ Multisystem infection
◆ Septic shock
◆ Chronic pyelonephritis

Assessment

HISTORY
◆ Pain over one or both kidneys, occasionally suprapubic
◆ Urinary urgency and frequency
◆ Burning during urination
◆ Dysuria, nocturia, hematuria
◆ Anorexia, vomiting, diarrhea
◆ Fatigue, malaise, weakness
◆ Symptoms that develop rapidly over a few hours or a few days
◆ Chills, rigors

PHYSICAL FINDINGS
◆ Mild to moderate suprapubic pain
◆ Pain on flank palpation (costovertebral angle tenderness)
◆ Cloudy urine
◆ Ammonia-like or fishy odor to urine
◆ If fever is present, temperature of 102° F (38.9° C) or higher
◆ Shaking chills
◆ Negative pelvic examination findings

DIAGNOSTIC TEST RESULTS
◆ *Urinalysis, culture, and sensitivity testing:* pyuria, significant bacteriuria, low specific gravity and osmolality, and slightly alkaline urine pH, or proteinuria, glycosuria, and ketonuria (less frequent)
◆ *White blood cell count, neutrophil count, and erythrocyte sedimentation rate:* increased
◆ *Kidney-ureter-bladder radiography:* calculi, tumors, or cysts in the kidneys or urinary tract
◆ *Excretory urography:* asymmetrical kidneys, possibly indicating a high frequency of infection

Treatment

- Identification and correction of predisposing factors for infection, such as obstruction or calculi
- Short courses of therapy for uncomplicated infections
- Rest periods as needed
- Increased fluid intake

MEDICATIONS

- 14-day course of antibiotics (I.V. or oral fluoroquinolone is drug of choice)
- Urinary analgesics such as phenazopyridine (Azo-Standard)
- Antipyretics as needed

Nursing interventions

- Give prescribed drugs as ordered and evaluate the patient's response to treatment.
- Monitor the patient's vital signs and renal function studies.
- Record intake and output and encourage increased fluids.
- Note the patient's pattern of urination and urine characteristics.
- Obtain daily weight.

PATIENT TEACHING

- Explain the disorder, diagnostic testing, and treatment plan.
- Teach about about the administration, dosage, and possible adverse effects of prescribed medications.
- Stress avoiding bacterial contamination by following hygienic toileting practices, such as women wiping the perineum from front to back after bowel movements.
- Describe the proper technique for collecting a clean-catch urine specimen.
- Encourage routine checkups for patients with a history of recurrent UTIs.
- Review the signs and symptoms of recurrent infection.

Acute respiratory distress syndrome

Overview

Acute respiratory distress syndrome (ARDS) is a four-stage syndrome that can rapidly progress to intractable and fatal hypoxemia. It's a severe form of alveolar or acute lung injury involving noncardiogenic pulmonary edema and may be difficult to recognize. Hypoxemia is a hallmark sign of the disorder, even with increased supplemental oxygen. Patients with three concurrent causes have an 85% probability of developing ARDS. Little or no permanent lung damage occurs in those who recover.

CAUSES
- Acute miliary tuberculosis
- Anaphylaxis
- Aspiration of gastric contents
- Diffuse pneumonia (especially viral)
- Drug overdose
- Gestational hypertension
- Hemodialysis
- Idiosyncratic drug reaction
- Indirect or direct lung trauma (most common)
- Inhalation of noxious gases
- Leukemia
- Massive blood transfusion
- Near drowning
- Oxygen toxicity
- Pancreatitis
- Delayed coronary artery bypass grafting
- Thrombotic thrombocytopenic purpura
- Uremia
- Venous air embolism

PATHOPHYSIOLOGY
- Increased permeability of the alveolocapillary membranes allows fluid to accumulate in the lung interstitium, alveolar spaces, and small airways, causing the lung to stiffen.
- Ventilation is impaired, reducing oxygenation of pulmonary capillary blood.
- Elevated capillary pressure increases interstitial and alveolar edema.
- Alveolar closing pressure exceeds pulmonary pressures, leading to closure and collapse of the alveoli.

COMPLICATIONS
- Metabolic acidosis
- Respiratory acidosis
- Cardiac arrest
- Multiple organ dysfunction syndrome

Assessment

HISTORY
- One or more causative factors
- Dyspnea, especially on exertion

PHYSICAL FINDINGS
Stage I
- Shortness of breath, especially on exertion
- Normal to increased respiratory and pulse rates
- Diminished breath sounds

Stage II
- Respiratory distress
- Use of accessory muscles for respiration
- Pallor, anxiety, and restlessness
- Dry cough with thick, frothy sputum
- Bloody, sticky secretions
- Cool, clammy skin
- Tachycardia, tachypnea
- Elevated blood pressure
- Basilar crackles

Stage III
- Respiratory rate more than 30 breaths/minute
- Tachycardia with arrhythmias
- Labile blood pressure
- Productive cough
- Pale, cyanotic skin
- Crackles, rhonchi possible

Stage IV
- Acute respiratory failure with severe hypoxia
- Deteriorating mental status (may become comatose)

- Pale, cyanotic skin
- Lack of spontaneous respirations
- Bradycardia with arrhythmias
- Hypotension
- Metabolic and respiratory acidosis

- *Initial arterial blood gas (ABG) analysis:* partial pressure of arterial oxygen (Pao_2) less than 60 mm Hg and a partial pressure of arterial carbon dioxide ($Paco_2$) less than 35 mm Hg
- *Subsequent ABG analysis:* increased $Paco_2$ (more than 45 mm Hg), decreased bicarbonate levels (less than 22 mEq/L), and decreased Pao_2 despite oxygen therapy
- *Chest X-rays:* bilateral infiltrates (early stage); ground-glass appearance (later stages); "whiteouts" of both lung fields (later stages)
- *Gram stain, sputum culture and sensitivity, blood cultures:* infectious organisms
- *Toxicology tests:* drug ingestion with overdose
- *Serum amylase:* increased, pancreatitis
- *Pulmonary artery catheterization:* pulmonary artery wedge pressure between 12 and 18 mm Hg

Treatment

- Treatment of the underlying cause
- Correction of electrolyte and acid-base imbalances
- Fluid restriction
- Tube feedings or parenteral nutrition
- Bed rest during acute phase
- Prone positioning to improve lung perfusion
- Mechanical ventilation, if indicated

MEDICATIONS

- Humidified oxygen
- Bronchodilators
- Diuretics
- Sedatives (with mechanical ventilation)
- High-dose corticosteroids
- Vasopressors if hypotensive

- Antimicrobials if nonviral infection is identified

Nursing interventions

- Give prescribed drugs, as ordered, and evaluate the patient's response to treatment.
- Maintain a patent airway, perform tracheal suctioning as necessary.
- Reposition the patient every 2 hours; assess skin condition and provide skin care.
- Administer tube feedings or parenteral nutrition as ordered.
- Allow periods of uninterrupted sleep.
- Perform passive range-of-motion exercises.
- Provide emotional support to the patient and his family.
- Monitor vital signs and pulse oximetry.
- Monitor hemodynamic parameters.
- Record intake and output.
- Assess respiratory status (breath sounds, ABG results) every 2 hours or per the patient's clinical status.
- Check mechanical ventilator settings per unit protocol.
- Note sputum characteristics.
- Obtain daily weight.
- Monitor laboratory studies and report critical values.
- Watch for complications, such as cardiac arrhythmias, disseminated intravascular coagulation, GI bleeding, infection, malnutrition, and pneumothorax.

PATIENT TEACHING

- Explain the disorder, diagnostic testing, and treatment plan.
- Teach about the administration, dosage, and possible adverse effects of prescribed medications.
- Describe possible complications, such as GI bleeding, infection, and malnutrition, and when to notify the practitioner.
- Refer the patient to a pulmonary rehabilitation program if indicated.
- Provide information on how to contact the ARDS Clinical Network for more information and support.

Acute respiratory failure

Overview

Acute respiratory failure is the inability of the lungs to adequately maintain arterial oxygenation or eliminate carbon dioxide because of inadequate ventilation.

CAUSES

- Accumulated secretions secondary to cough suppression
- Airway irritants
- Any condition that increases the work of breathing and decreases the respiratory drive of patients with chronic obstructive pulmonary disease
- Bronchospasm
- Central nervous system depression
- Endocrine or metabolic disorders
- Gas exchange failure
- Heart failure
- Myocardial infarction (MI)
- Pulmonary emboli
- Respiratory tract infection
- Thoracic abnormalities
- Ventilatory failure

PATHOPHYSIOLOGY

- Hypercapnic respiratory failure primarily results from inadequate alveolar ventilation.
- Hypoxemic respiratory failure primarily results from inadequate exchange of oxygen between the alveoli and capillaries.
- Combined hypercapnic and hypoxemic respiratory failure is common.

COMPLICATIONS

- Tissue hypoxia
- Chronic respiratory acidosis
- Metabolic alkalosis
- Respiratory and cardiac arrest

Assessment

HISTORY

- Infection
- Accumulated pulmonary secretions secondary to cough suppression
- Trauma
- MI
- Heart failure
- Pulmonary emboli
- Exposure to irritants (smoke or fumes)
- Myxedema
- Metabolic acidosis

PHYSICAL FINDINGS

- Cyanosis of the oral mucosa, lips, nail beds
- Yawning, use of accessory muscles
- Pursed-lip breathing
- Nasal flaring
- Ashen skin
- Tachypnea
- Cold, clammy skin
- Asymmetrical chest movement
- Decreased tactile fremitus over obstructed bronchi or a pleural effusion
- Increased tactile fremitus over consolidated lung tissue
- Hyperresonance
- Diminished or absent breath sounds
- Wheezes (in asthma)
- Rhonchi (in bronchitis)
- Crackles (in pulmonary edema)

DIAGNOSTIC TEST RESULTS

- *Arterial blood gas (ABG) analysis:* hypercapnia and hypoxemia
- *Serum white blood cell count:* increased (in bacterial infections)
- *Serum hemoglobin and hematocrit:* decreased
- *Serum electrolytes:* hypokalemia and hypochloremia
- *Blood cultures, Gram stain, and sputum cultures:* pathogen present

Disorders

- *Chest X-rays:* underlying pulmonary diseases or conditions, such as emphysema, atelectasis, lesions, pneumothorax, infiltrates, and effusions
- *Electrocardiography*: arrhythmias, cor pulmonale, or myocardial ischemia
- *Pulse oximetry, arterial oxygen saturation:* decreased oxygen saturation levels

Treatment

- Mechanical ventilation
- High-frequency ventilation if the patient doesn't respond to conventional mechanical ventilation
- Fluid restriction with heart failure
- Bed rest (during acute phase)

MEDICATIONS
- Cautious oxygen therapy to increase partial pressure of arterial oxygen
- Diuretics
- Bronchodilators
- Corticosteroids
- Antacids
- Histamine-receptor antagonists as ordered
- Antibiotics
- Positive inotropic agents
- Vasopressors
- Sedatives (with mechanical ventilation)

Nursing interventions

- Assist with endotracheal intubation.
- Administer oxygen as ordered and monitor pulse oximetry and ABG values.
- Give prescribed drugs, as ordered, and evaluate the patient's response to treatment.
- Monitor vital signs, intake and output, and laboratory studies.
- Assess respiratory status per unit policy and clinical status.
- Continuously observe cardiac rate and rhythm.

- Perform postural drainage and chest physiotherapy and suction as needed.
- Encourage pursed-lip breathing and encourage the use of an incentive spirometer after the patient is extubated.
- Reposition the patient every 1 to 2 hours and provide skin care.
- Assist with or perform oral hygiene.
- Schedule care to provide frequent rest periods for the patient.
- Observe for improvement or deterioration in chest X-ray results.
- Observe and document sputum quality, consistency, and color.

For mechanical ventilation
- Suction the trachea after hyperoxygenation as needed.
- Secure the endotracheal (ET) tube per facility policy.
- Provide alternative communication means.
- Provide sedation as necessary.
- Check ventilator settings and alarms per facility protocol.
- Assess for complications of mechanical ventilation.
- Maintain ET tube position and patency.

PATIENT TEACHING
- Explain the disorder, diagnostic testing, and treatment plan.
- Teach about the administration, dosage, and possible adverse effects of prescribed medications.
- Describe possible complications, such as GI bleeding, infection, and malnutrition, and when to notify the practitioner.
- Refer the patient to a pulmonary rehabilitation program if indicated.
- Refer the patient to a smoking-cessation program, if applicable.
- Provide information on how to contact the National Lung Health Education Program for more information and support.

Disorders

Adrenal hypofunction

Overview

Primary adrenal hypofunction, or *adrenal insufficiency* (Addison's disease), originates within the adrenal gland and involves the decreased secretion of mineralocorticoids, glucocorticoids, and androgens. Secondary adrenal hypofunction originates outside the gland and is characterized by decreased glucocorticoid secretion. Adrenal crisis (also called *addisonian crisis*) is a critical deficiency of mineralocorticoids and glucocorticoids. It's a medical emergency that requires immediate, vigorous treatment.

CAUSES
◆ Impaired pituitary secretion of corticotropin
◆ Acute stress, sepsis, trauma, or surgery
◆ Omission of steroid therapy in patients with chronic adrenal insufficiency

PATHOPHYSIOLOGY
◆ Primary adrenal hypofunction results from the partial or complete destruction of the adrenal cortex.
◆ It manifests as a clinical syndrome in which the symptoms are associated with deficient production of the adrenocortical hormones cortisol, aldosterone, and androgen.
◆ High levels of corticotropin and corticotropin-releasing hormones result.
◆ Secondary adrenal hypofunction involves all zones of the cortex, causing deficiencies of the adrenocortical hormones, glucocorticoids, androgens, and mineralocorticoids.
◆ Cortisol deficiency causes decreased liver gluconeogenesis (the formation of glucose from molecules that aren't carbohydrates), which results in low blood glucose levels that can become dangerously low in patients who take insulin routinely.
◆ Aldosterone deficiency causes increased renal sodium loss and enhances potassium reabsorption.
◆ Hypotension results from sodium excretion.
◆ Low plasma volume and arteriolar pressure increase angiotensin II production.
◆ Androgen deficiency may decrease hair growth in axillary and pubic areas (less noticeable in men) as well as on the extremities of women.

COMPLICATIONS
◆ Hyperpyrexia
◆ Psychotic reactions
◆ Deficient or excessive steroid treatment
◆ Shock
◆ Profound hypoglycemia
◆ Ultimate vascular collapse, renal shutdown, coma, and death (if untreated)

Assessment

HISTORY
◆ Synthetic steroid use, adrenal surgery, or recent infection
◆ Muscle weakness
◆ Fatigue
◆ Weight loss
◆ Craving for salty food
◆ Decreased tolerance for stress
◆ GI disturbances
◆ Dehydration
◆ Amenorrhea (in women)
◆ Impotence (in men)

PHYSICAL FINDINGS
◆ Poor coordination
◆ Decreased axillary and pubic hair (in women)
◆ Bronze coloration of the skin and darkening of scars
◆ Areas of vitiligo
◆ Increased pigmentation of mucous membranes
◆ Weak, irregular pulse
◆ Hypotension

DIAGNOSTIC TEST RESULTS
◆ *Rapid corticotropin stimulation test:* elevated (primary disorder), low (secondary disorder)

◆ *Plasma cortisol level:* less than 10 mcg/dl in the morning, even lower in the evening
◆ *Serum sodium and fasting blood glucose levels:* decreased
◆ *Serum potassium, calcium, and blood urea nitrogen levels:* increased
◆ *Hematocrit:* elevated
◆ *Lymphocyte, eosinophil counts:* increased
◆ *Chest X-ray:* small heart
◆ *Abdominal computed tomography scan:* adrenal calcification (if the cause is infectious)

Treatment

◆ I.V. fluids
◆ Small, frequent, high-protein meals
◆ Periods of rest as needed

MEDICATIONS
◆ Lifelong corticosteroid replacement, usually with cortisone or hydrocortisone
◆ Oral fludrocortisone (Florinef)
◆ Hydrocortisone
◆ I.V. hydrocortisone replacement (for adrenal crisis)

Nursing interventions

◆ Monitor vital signs, cardiac rhythm, intake and output, daily weight, laboratory results, and capillary glucose levels.
◆ Observe for cushingoid signs such as fluid retention around the eyes and face.
◆ Check for petechiae.
◆ Assess for signs of shock (decreased level of consciousness and urine output).

PATIENT TEACHING
◆ Explain the disorder, diagnostic testing, and treatment plan.
◆ Teach about the administration, dosage, and possible adverse effects of prescribed medications.
◆ Teach about the symptoms of steroid overdose (swelling, weight gain) and steroid underdose (lethargy, weakness) and possible need for dosage to be increased during times of stress or illness

(when the patient has a cold, for example).
◆ Explain about the possibility of adrenal crisis being precipitated by infection, injury, or profuse sweating in hot weather.
◆ Stress the importance of carrying a medical identification card that states the patient is on steroid therapy. (The drug name and dosage should be included on the card.)
◆ Demonstrate how to give a hydrocortisone injection, and instruct the patient to keep an emergency kit containing hydrocortisone in a prepared syringe available for use in times of stress.
◆ Refer the patient to the National Adrenal Diseases Foundation for information and support.

Alcoholism

Overview

Alcoholism is a chronic disorder in which a patient can't control his intake of alcoholic beverages. It interferes with physical and mental health, social and familial relationships, and occupational responsibilities. Alcoholism affects all social and economic groups and occurs at all life cycle stages, beginning as early as elementary school age.

CAUSES
◆ Unknown

RISK FACTORS
◆ Being male
◆ Low socioeconomic status
◆ Family history
◆ Depression
◆ Anxiety
◆ History of other substance abuse disorders
◆ Peer pressure
◆ Stressful lifestyle

PATHOPHYSIOLOGY
◆ Alcohol is soluble in water and lipids and permeates all body tissues.
◆ The liver, which metabolizes 90% of absorbed alcohol, is the most severely affected organ, developing hepatic steatosis and hepatic fibrosis.
◆ Laënnec's cirrhosis develops after inflammatory response (alcoholic hepatitis) or, in the absence of inflammation, from direct activation of lipocytes (Ito cells).
◆ Lactic acidosis and excess uric acid are promoted. Gluconeogenesis, beta-oxidation of fatty acids, and the Krebs cycle are opposed, resulting in hypoglycemia and hyperlipidemia.
◆ Cell toxicity results from the reduction of mitochondrial oxygenation, depletion of deoxyribonucleic acid, and other actions.

COMPLICATIONS
◆ Cardiomyopathy
◆ Pneumonia
◆ Cirrhosis
◆ Esophageal varices
◆ Pancreatitis
◆ Alcoholic dementia
◆ Wernicke's encephalopathy
◆ Seizure disorder
◆ Depression
◆ Multiple substance abuse
◆ Suicide and homicide
◆ Death

Assessment

HISTORY
◆ Need for daily or episodic alcohol use for adequate function
◆ Inability to discontinue or reduce alcohol intake
◆ Episodes of anesthesia or amnesia during intoxication
◆ Episodes of violence during intoxication
◆ Alcohol interfering with social and familial relationships and occupational responsibilities
◆ Malaise, dyspepsia, mood swings or depression, and an increased incidence of infection
◆ Secretive behavior

PHYSICAL FINDINGS
◆ Poor personal hygiene
◆ Unusually high tolerance for sedatives and opioids
◆ Signs of nutritional deficiency
◆ Signs of injury
◆ Withdrawal signs and symptoms
◆ Major motor seizures

DIAGNOSTIC TEST RESULTS
◆ *Blood alcohol levels:* 0.10% weight/volume (200 mg/dl) or higher
◆ *Serum electrolyte levels:* abnormal
◆ *Serum ammonia levels:* increased
◆ *Serum amylase levels:* increased
◆ *Urine toxicology:* abuse of other drugs
◆ *Liver function study:* abnormal
◆ *CAGE screening test:* two affirmative results, indicating that the patient is seven times more likely to be alcohol dependent

◆ *Alcohol Use Disorders Identification Test*: score of 8 or greater, indicating alcohol dependency

◆ *Michigan Alcohol Screening Test:* score of 5 or greater, indicating alcohol dependency

OTHER CRITERIA

According to the *Diagnostic and Statistical Manual of Mental Disorders, Fourth Edition, Text Revision,* a diagnosis is confirmed when the patient exhibits at least three of these signs and symptoms:
◆ more alcohol ingested than intended
◆ persistent desire or efforts to diminish alcohol use
◆ excessive time spent obtaining alcohol
◆ frequent intoxication or withdrawal symptoms
◆ impairment of social, occupational, or recreational activities
◆ continued alcohol consumption despite knowledge of a social, psychological, or physical problem that's caused or exacerbated by alcohol use
◆ marked tolerance
◆ characteristic withdrawal symptoms
◆ use of alcohol to relieve or avoid withdrawal symptoms
◆ persistent symptoms for at least 1 month or recurrence over a longer time.

Treatment

Immediate
◆ Respiratory support
◆ Prevention of aspiration of vomitus
◆ Replacement of fluids
◆ Correction of hypothermia or acidosis
◆ Treatment of trauma, infection, or GI bleeding

Long-term
◆ Detoxification, rehabilitation, and aftercare program
◆ Individual, group, or family psychotherapy
◆ Ongoing participation in a support group
◆ Safety precautions, including preventing aspiration of vomitus

◆ Seizure precautions
◆ Well-balanced diet

MEDICATIONS
◆ I.V. glucose
◆ Anticonvulsants
◆ Antiemetics
◆ Antidiarrheals
◆ Sedatives, particularly benzodiazepines
◆ Naltrexone (Depade)
◆ Antipsychotics
◆ Daily oral disulfiram
◆ Vitamin supplements

Nursing interventions

◆ Ensure adequate airway, breathing and circulation.
◆ Provide safety measures.
◆ Institute seizure precautions.
◆ Give prescribed drugs and evaluate the patient's response.
◆ Orient the patient to reality.
◆ Maintain a calm environment, minimizing noise and shadows.
◆ Avoid restraints, unless necessary for protection.
◆ Monitor mental status, vital signs, intake and output, and nutritional and hydration status.

PATIENT TEACHING
◆ Explain the disorder, diagnostic testing, and treatment plan.
◆ Teach about the administration, dosage, and possible adverse effects of prescribed medications.
◆ Stress the importance of abstaining from alcohol and create a plan for relapse prevention.
◆ Refer the patient to a rehabilitation program.
◆ Refer the patient to support group services, such as Alcoholics Anonymous.
◆ Refer the patient to personal and family counseling.

Alzheimer's disease

Overview

Alzheimer's disease is a degenerative disorder of the cerebral cortex (especially the frontal lobe) that accounts for more than 50% of all dementia cases. There is no cure or definitive treatment. Because of the affects of Alzheimer's disease on the brain, the patient's history may need to be obtained from a family member or caregiver.

CAUSES
◆ Unknown
◆ Autosomal dominant inherited mutated gene

RISK FACTORS
◆ Neurochemical factors
◆ Risk factor gene (in late-onset Alzheimer's disease)
◆ Aging
◆ Family history
◆ Aluminum and manganese
◆ Trauma
◆ Slow-growing central nervous system viruses

PATHOPHYSIOLOGY
◆ Parts of the brain that control thought, memory, and language are initially involved.
◆ Brain damage is caused by amyloid, a genetic substance.
◆ Affected brain tissue exhibits three distinguishing features: neurofibrillary tangles, neuritic plaques, and granulovascular degeneration.

COMPLICATIONS
◆ Injury from violent behavior, wandering, or unsupervised activity
◆ Pneumonia and other infections
◆ Malnutrition and dehydration

Assessment

HISTORY
◆ Insidious, almost imperceptible, onset
◆ Forgetfulness and subtle memory loss, difficulty learning and remembering new information
◆ Loss of short-term memory but retention of long-term memory
◆ General deterioration in personal hygiene
◆ Inability to concentrate
◆ Tendency to perform repetitive actions and experience restlessness
◆ Personality changes (irritability, depression, paranoia, hostility, apathy, anxiety, fear)
◆ Nocturnal awakening
◆ Disorientation
◆ Suspicion and fear of imaginary people and situations
◆ Misperceptions about own environment
◆ Misidentification of objects and people (inability to recognize family and friends)
◆ Complaints of stolen or misplaced objects
◆ Labile emotions
◆ Mood swings, sudden angry outbursts, and sleep disturbances

PHYSICAL FINDINGS
◆ Impaired sense of smell (usually an early symptom)
◆ Impaired stereognosis
◆ Gait disorders
◆ Tremors
◆ Loss of recent memory
◆ Positive snout reflex
◆ Organic brain disease in adults
◆ Urinary or fecal incontinence
◆ Seizures

DIAGNOSTIC TEST RESULTS
◆ *Diagnosis by exclusion*: rules out other diseases
◆ *Autopsy:* positive diagnosis
◆ *Positron emission tomography:* metabolic activity in the cerebral cortex

- *Computed tomography:* excessive and progressive brain atrophy (rules out other neurologic problems)
- *Magnetic resonance imaging:* biochemical and anatomic changes; rules out intracranial lesions
- *Cerebral blood flow studies:* abnormalities in blood flow to the brain
- *Cerebrospinal fluid analysis:* chronic neurologic infection
- *EEG:* slowing of brain waves (in late stages of the disease)
- *Neuropsychological tests:* impaired cognitive ability and reasoning

Treatment

- Behavioral interventions focused on managing cognitive and behavioral changes (patient-centered or caregiver training)
- Well-balanced diet (may need to be monitored)
- Safe activities as tolerated (may need to be monitored)

MEDICATIONS
- Cerebral vasodilators
- Psychostimulators
- Antidepressants
- Anxiolytics
- Neurolytics
- Anticonvulsants (experimental)
- Anti-inflammatories (experimental)
- Anticholinesterase agents
- Vitamin E

Nursing interventions

- Provide familiar objects to help with orientation and behavior control.
- Protect the patient from injury.
- Provide rest periods.
- Be consistent and give simple step-by-step instructions.
- Provide an effective communication system.

- Use soft tones and a slow, calm manner when speaking to the patient.
- Encourage independence.
- Offer frequent toileting.
- Assist with hygiene and dressing.
- Provide an exercise program.
- Give prescribed drugs and evaluate the patient's response.
- Frequently remind the patient of the day and hour.
- Place familiar objects in the patient's reach and view.
- Monitor fluid intake and nutrition status.

PATIENT TEACHING
- Explain the disorder, diagnostic testing, and treatment plan to the patient and the family.
- Teach about the administration, dosage, and possible adverse effects of prescribed medications.
- Teach about assistive devices for dressing and grooming.
- Stress the importance of cutting food and providing finger foods, if indicated.
- Encourage the family to promote the patient's independence.
- Review home safety precautions.
- Refer the patient (and his family or caregivers) to the Alzheimer's Association, a local support group, or to social services for additional support.

Amyotrophic lateral sclerosis

Overview

Amyotrophic lateral sclerosis (ALS), also known as *Lou Gehrig disease,* is a chronic, rapidly progressive, and debilitating neurologic disease that's incurable and invariably fatal. It attacks neurons responsible for controlling involuntary movements and is characterized by weakness that begins in upper extremities and progressively involves the neck and throat, eventually leading to disability, respiratory failure, and death.

CAUSES
◆ Exact cause unknown
◆ Immune complexes such as those formed in autoimmune disorders
◆ Inherited autosomal dominant trait in 10% of patients
◆ Virus that creates metabolic disturbances in motor neurons

Precipitating factors causing acute deterioration
◆ Severe stress such as myocardial infarction
◆ Traumatic injury
◆ Viral infections
◆ Physical exhaustion

PATHOPHYSIOLOGY
◆ Excitatory neurotransmitter accumulates to toxic levels.
◆ Motor units no longer innervate.
◆ Progressive degeneration of axons causes loss of myelin.
◆ Upper and lower motor neurons progressively degenerate.
◆ Progressive degeneration of motor nuclei in the cerebral cortex and corticospinal tracts occurs.

COMPLICATIONS
◆ Respiratory tract infections and respiratory failure
◆ Complications of immobility
◆ Aspiration pneumonia
◆ Injury from fall

Assessment

HISTORY
◆ Mental function intact
◆ Family history of ALS
◆ Asymmetrical weakness first noticed in one limb
◆ Easy fatigue and easy cramping in the affected muscles

PHYSICAL FINDINGS
◆ Location of the affected motor neurons
◆ Fasciculations in the affected muscles
◆ Progressive weakness in muscles of the arms, legs, and trunk
◆ Brisk and overactive stretch reflexes
◆ Difficulty talking, chewing, swallowing, and breathing
◆ Shortness of breath and occasional drooling

DIAGNOSTIC TEST RESULTS
◆ *Cerebrospinal fluid protein:* increased
◆ *Muscle biopsy:* atrophic fibers
◆ *Electromyography:* electrical abnormalities of involved muscles

Treatment

◆ Rehabilitative measures
◆ Occupational and physical therapy
◆ Supportive measures
◆ Well-balanced diet; possibly tube feedings

MEDICATIONS
◆ Oxygen therapy
◆ Muscle relaxants
◆ Antidepressants
◆ Diphenhydramine (Benadryl) (for excessive salivation)
◆ Dantrolene (Dantrium)
◆ Baclofen (Lioresal)
◆ I.V. or intrathecal administration of thyrotropin-releasing hormone
◆ Riluzole (Rilutek) (slows progression)

Nursing interventions

◆ Provide emotional and psychological support.
◆ Promote the patient's independence.
◆ Reposition the patient every 2 hours and provide skin care.
◆ Give prescribed drugs.
◆ Provide airway and respiratory management.
◆ Monitor respiratory status.
◆ Note speech and swallowing ability.
◆ Maintain aspiration precautions.
◆ Monitor nutritional status and promote nutrition.
◆ Provide safety measures.
◆ Assess for complications.

PATIENT TEACHING
◆ Explain the disorder, diagnostic testing, and treatment plan.
◆ Teach about the administration, dosage, and possible adverse effects of prescribed medications.
◆ Explain a swallowing therapy regimen.
◆ Promote proper skin care.
◆ Demonstrate range-of-motion, deep-breathing, and coughing exercises.
◆ Stress safety measures in the home.
◆ Refer the patient to a local ALS support group.
◆ Refer the patient to a mental health counselor, if indicated.

Anaphylaxis

Overview

Anaphylaxis is a dramatic, acute atopic reaction to an allergen marked by sudden onset of rapidly progressive urticaria and respiratory distress. The sooner signs and symptoms appear after exposure to the antigen, the more severe the reaction. Severe reactions may initiate vascular collapse, leading to systemic shock and, possibly, death.

CAUSES
◆ Systemic exposure to sensitizing drugs, foods, insect venom, or other specific antigens

PATHOPHYSIOLOGY
◆ After initial exposure to an antigen, the immune system produces specific immunoglobulin (Ig) antibodies in the lymph nodes. Helper T cells enhance the process.
◆ The antibodies (IgE) then bind to membrane receptors located on mast cells and basophils.
◆ After the body reencounters the antigen, the IgE antibodies, or cross-linked IgE receptors, recognize the antigen as foreign, which activates the release of powerful chemical mediators.
◆ IgG or IgM enters into the reaction and activates the release of complement factors.

COMPLICATIONS
◆ Airway obstruction
◆ Respiratory failure
◆ Systemic vascular collapse
◆ Death

Assessment

HISTORY
◆ Immediately after exposure, complaints of a feeling of impending doom or fright and exhibition of apprehension, restlessness, cyanosis, cool and clammy skin, erythema, edema, tachypnea, weakness, sweating, sneezing, dyspnea, nasal pruritus, and urticaria
◆ Dyspnea and complaints of chest tightness

PHYSICAL FINDINGS
◆ Confusion
◆ Hives
◆ Hoarseness or stridor, wheezing
◆ Swelling in the throat possibly leading to occlusion
◆ Severe abdominal cramps, nausea, diarrhea
◆ Urinary urgency and incontinence
◆ Dizziness, drowsiness, headache, restlessness, and seizures
◆ Hypotension, shock; sometimes angina and cardiac arrhythmias
◆ Angioedema

DIAGNOSTIC TEST RESULTS
◆ *Allergen-specific skin test:* identifies allergen

Treatment

◆ Maintaining a patent airway
◆ Cardiopulmonary resuscitation, if cardiac arrest occurs
◆ Nothing by mouth until the patient is stable
◆ Bed rest until the patient is stable

MEDICATIONS
◆ Immediate injection of epinephrine 1:1,000 aqueous solution, 0.1 to 0.5 ml subcutaneously or I.V.
◆ Corticosteroids: methylprednisolone (Solu-Medrol)
◆ Histamine$_1$-receptor blocker: diphenhydramine (Benadryl) I.V.
◆ Volume expander infusions as needed
◆ Inhaled beta-agonist: Albuterol (Proventil)
◆ Vasopressors
◆ Aminophylline (Truphylline) I.V.
◆ Histamine$_2$-receptor blocker: cimetidine (Tagamet)

Nursing interventions

◆ Provide supplemental oxygen, and prepare to assist with insertion of an endotracheal tube if necessary.

◆ Continually reassure the patient, and explain all tests and treatments.

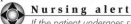 **Nursing alert**

If the patient undergoes skin or scratch testing, monitor for signs of a serious allergic response. Keep emergency resuscitation equipment readily available.

◆ Monitor vital signs, respiratory status, neurologic status, and response to treatment.

◆ Observe for complications.

PATIENT TEACHING

◆ Explain the disorder, diagnostic testing, and treatment plan.

◆ Teach about the administration, dosage, and possible adverse effects of prescribed medications.

◆ Explain the risk of delayed symptoms and importance of reporting them immediately.

◆ Stress avoidance of exposure to known allergens and the importance of carrying an anaphylaxis kit and learning to use it appropriately.

◆ Provide information on obtaining medical identification jewelry to identify the allergy to others.

Anemia, iron deficiency

Overview

Iron deficiency anemia, which is most prevalent among premenopausal women, infants, children, adolescents, alcoholics, and elderly people, is a decrease in total iron body content, leading to diminished erythropoiesis. It produces smaller (microcytic) cells with less color on staining (hypochromia). This condition can persist for years without producing signs or symptoms

CAUSES
◆ Blood loss secondary to drug-induced GI bleeding or as a result of heavy menses, hemorrhage from trauma, GI ulcers, malignant tumors, and varices
◆ Inadequate dietary intake of iron
◆ Intravascular hemolysis-induced hemoglobinuria or paroxysmal nocturnal hemoglobinuria
◆ Iron malabsorption
◆ Lead poisoning (in children)
◆ Mechanical erythrocyte trauma caused by a prosthetic heart valve or vena cava filter
◆ Pregnancy

PATHOPHYSIOLOGY
◆ Body stores of iron, including plasma iron, cause a decrease in total iron body content.
◆ Transferrin, which binds with and transports iron, also can decrease content levels.
◆ Insufficient body stores of iron lead to a depleted red blood cell (RBC) mass and a decreased hemoglobin (Hb) concentration, resulting in decreased oxygen-carrying capacity of the blood.

COMPLICATIONS
◆ Infection
◆ Organ and joint damage from overreplacement of oral or I.M. iron supplements
◆ Pneumonia

Assessment

HISTORY
◆ Fatigue
◆ Inability to concentrate
◆ Headache, shortness of breath (especially on exertion)
◆ Increased frequency of infections
◆ Pica
◆ Menorrhagia
◆ Dysphagia
◆ Vasomotor disturbances
◆ Numbness and tingling of the extremities
◆ Neuralgic pain

PHYSICAL FINDINGS
◆ Red, swollen, smooth, shiny, and tender tongue (glossitis)
◆ Eroded, tender, and swollen corners of the mouth (angular stomatitis)
◆ Spoon-shaped, brittle nails
◆ Tachycardia

DIAGNOSTIC TEST RESULTS
◆ *Serum Hb levels:* decreased (men, less than 12 g/dl; women, less than 10 g/dl)
◆ *Mean corpuscular Hb levels*: decreased (severe anemia)
◆ *Serum hematocrit*: decreased (men, less than 47 ml/dl; women, less than 42 ml/dl)
◆ *Serum iron levels:* decreased (high binding capacity)
◆ *Serum ferritin levels:* decreased
◆ *Serum RBC count:* decreased with microcytic and hypochromic cells; in early stages, may be normal, except in infants and children
◆ *Bone marrow staining studies:* depleted or absent iron stores, normoblastic hyperplasia
◆ *GI studies, such as guaiac stool tests, barium swallow and enema, endoscopy, and sigmoidoscopy:* confirms or rules out bleeding caused by iron deficiency

Treatment

- Based on underlying cause
- Nutritious, nonirritating diet
- Planned rest periods during activity
- Blood transfusion, if severe

MEDICATIONS

- Oral preparation of iron or a combination of iron and ascorbic acid
- I.M. iron (in rare cases)
- Total-dose I.V. infusions of supplemental iron (for pregnant and elderly patients with severe disease)

Nursing interventions

- Watch for signs or symptoms of decreased perfusion to vital organs.
- Provide oxygen therapy as necessary.
- Monitor vital signs and laboratory results.
- Assess the family's dietary habits for iron intake, noting food choices, childhood eating patterns, and cultural food preferences.
- Give prescribed analgesics for headache and other discomfort.
- Provide frequent rest periods.
- Monitor iron infusion rate carefully and observe for an allergic reaction.
- Use the Z-track injection method when administering iron I.M. to prevent skin discoloration, scarring, and irritating iron deposits in the skin.
- Provide nonirritating foods.

PATIENT TEACHING

- Explain the disorder, diagnostic testing, and treatment plan.
- Teach about the administration, dosage, and possible adverse effects of prescribed medications.
- Teach the dangers of lead poisoning, especially if the patient reports a history of pica.
- Stress the importance of continuing therapy, even after the patient begins to feel better.
- Advise the patient to drink a liquid iron supplement through a straw to avoid staining the teeth.
- Explain signs and symptoms of adverse effects of iron therapy (see *Recognizing iron overdose*).
- Explain the importance of compliance with prescribed treatment and follow-up care.

Recognizing iron overdose

Signs and symptoms of iron overdose include diarrhea, fever, severe stomach pain, nausea, and vomiting. If these signs and symptoms occur, notify the practitioner and give prescribed treatment, which may include chelation therapy, vigorous I.V. fluid replacement, gastric lavage, whole-bowel irrigation, and supplemental oxygen.

Anemia, sickle cell

Overview

Sickle cell anemia, which has no cure, is a congenital hemolytic disease that results from a defective hemoglobin (Hb) molecule (HbS) that causes red blood cells (RBCs) to become sickle shaped. Sickle-shaped cells impair circulation, resulting in chronic ill health (fatigue, dyspnea on exertion, swollen joints), periodic crises, long-term complications, and premature death. About 1 in 10 blacks carry the abnormal gene; if two such carriers have offspring, each child has a 1 in 4 chance of developing the disease.

Types of sickle cell crises include painful crisis (the most common type, appearing periodically after age 5), aplastic crisis, acute splenic sequestration crisis, and hemolytic crisis.

CAUSES
◆ Homozygous inheritance of the HbS-producing gene (defective Hb gene from each parent)

PATHOPHYSIOLOGY
◆ Abnormal HbS found in the patient's RBCs becomes insoluble whenever hypoxia occurs.
◆ RBCs become rigid, rough, and elongated, forming a crescent or sickle shape.
◆ Sickling can produce hemolysis (cell destruction).
◆ Altered cells accumulate in capillaries and smaller blood vessels, making the blood more viscous.
◆ Normal circulation is impaired, causing pain, tissue infarctions, and swelling.

COMPLICATIONS
◆ Chronic obstructive pulmonary disease
◆ Heart failure
◆ Retinopathy
◆ Nephropathy

Assessment

HISTORY
◆ Usually no signs or symptoms until after age 6 months
◆ Chronic fatigue
◆ Unexplained dyspnea or dyspnea on exertion
◆ Joint swelling
◆ Aching bones
◆ Chest pain
◆ Ischemic leg ulcers
◆ Increased susceptibility to infection
◆ Pulmonary infarctions and cardiomegaly

PHYSICAL FINDINGS
◆ Jaundice or pallor
◆ Small in stature for age
◆ Delayed growth and puberty
◆ Spiderlike body build (narrow shoulders and hips, long extremities, curved spine, and barrel chest) in adult
◆ Tachycardia
◆ Hepatomegaly and, in children, splenomegaly
◆ Systolic, diastolic murmurs
◆ Sleepiness, with difficulty awakening
◆ Hematuria
◆ Pale lips, tongue, palms, and nail beds
◆ Body temperature greater than 104° F (40° C) or a temperature of 100° F (37.8° C) that persists for 2 or more days

In painful crisis
◆ Severe abdominal, thoracic, muscle, or bone pain
◆ Possible increased jaundice, dark urine, and a low-grade fever

In aplastic crisis
◆ Pallor, lethargy, sleepiness, dyspnea, possible coma
◆ Markedly decreased bone marrow activity, and RBC hemolysis

In acute splenic sequestration crisis
◆ Lethargy and pallor
◆ Hypovolemic shock and death (if untreated)

In hemolytic crisis
♦ Liver congestion, hepatomegaly

DIAGNOSTIC TEST RESULTS
♦ *Stained blood smear:* sickle cells, HbS with Hb
♦ *RBC counts:* decreased
♦ *White blood cell and platelet counts:* elevated
♦ *Erythrocyte sedimentation rate:* decreased
♦ *Serum iron levels:* increased
♦ *RBC survival:* decreased
♦ *Reticulocyte count:* increased
♦ *Hb levels:* normal or low
♦ *Chest X-ray:* characteristic "Lincoln log" spinal deformity detected in lateral, leaving the vertebrae resembling logs forming the corner of a cabin
♦ *Ophthalmoscopic examination:* corkscrew-shaped or comma-shaped vessels in the conjunctivae

Treatment

♦ Avoidance of extreme temperatures
♦ Avoidance of stress
♦ Well-balanced diet with adequate amounts of folic acid–rich foods
♦ Adequate fluid intake
♦ Bed rest in crisis
♦ Blood cell exchange
♦ Blood transfusion, oxygen therapy, and large amounts of oral or I.V. fluids, in an acute sequestration crisis

MEDICATIONS
♦ Anti-infectives
♦ Analgesics
♦ Iron supplements
♦ Sedation and administration of analgesics during crisis

Nursing interventions

♦ Assess respiratory status and administer oxygen as needed.
♦ Administer blood transfusions or assist with blood cell exchange.

♦ Monitor vital signs, intake and output, and laboratory study results.
♦ Encourage adequate fluid intake and administer I.V. fluids as ordered.
♦ Apply warm compresses, warmed thermal blankets, and warming pads or mattresses to painful areas of the patient's body, unless he has neuropathy.
♦ Administer analgesics and antipyretics as necessary and evaluate effect.
♦ Give prescribed prophylactic antibiotics.
♦ Use strict sterile technique when performing treatments.
♦ Encourage bed rest, with the head of the bed elevated during crisis.

PATIENT TEACHING
♦ Explain the disorder, diagnostic testing, and treatment plan.
♦ Teach about the administration, dosage, and possible adverse effects of prescribed medications.
♦ Teach the patient about conditions that provoke hypoxia, such as strenuous exercise, use of vasoconstricting medications, cold temperatures, unpressurized aircraft, and high altitude.

 Nursing alert
Stress the importance of normal childhood immunizations, meticulous wound care, good oral hygiene, regular dental checkups, and a balanced diet as safeguards against infection.

♦ Describe the symptoms of vaso-occlusive crisis and when to seek medical care.
♦ Stress the need to inform all practitioners that the patient has this disease before undergoing any treatment, especially major surgery.
♦ Review dietary recommendations and the need to increase fluid intake.
♦ Stress the importance of follow-up care.
♦ Provide information about genetic counseling.
♦ Provide contact information for the Sickle Cell Disease Association.

Aneurysm, abdominal aortic

Overview

An abdominal aortic aneurysm is an abnormal dilation in the arterial wall of the aorta, commonly between the renal arteries and iliac branches. It can be fusiform (spindle-shaped), saccular (pouchlike), or dissecting. It's seven times more common in hypertensive men than in hypertensive women.

CAUSES
◆ Arteriosclerosis or atherosclerosis (in 95% of cases)
◆ Syphilis, other infections
◆ Trauma

PATHOPHYSIOLOGY
◆ Degenerative changes in the aorta's tunica media layer create a focal weakness from which the tunica intima and tunica adventitia layers stretch outward.
◆ Increasing blood pressure within the aorta progressively weakens vessel walls and enlarges the aneurysm.

COMPLICATIONS
◆ Hemorrhage
◆ Shock
◆ Dissection

Assessment

HISTORY
◆ Asymptomatic until aneurysm enlarges and compresses surrounding tissue
◆ Syncope (when aneurysm ruptures)
◆ Asymptomatic or abdominal pain (from bleeding into the peritoneum) when clot forms and bleeding stops

PHYSICAL FINDINGS
Intact aneurysm
◆ Gnawing, generalized, steady abdominal pain
◆ Lower back pain unaffected by movement
◆ Auscultation of a bruit or thrill in mid-epigastric area
◆ Gastric or abdominal fullness
◆ Sudden onset of severe abdominal pain or lumbar pain, with radiation to flank and groin
◆ Possible pulsating mass in the periumbilical area shouldn't be palpated

Ruptured aneurysm
◆ Severe, persistent abdominal and back pain (rupture into the peritoneal cavity)
◆ GI bleeding with massive hematemesis and melena (rupture into the duodenum)
◆ Mottled skin, poor distal perfusion
◆ Absent peripheral pulses distally
◆ Decreased level of consciousness
◆ Diaphoresis
◆ Hypotension
◆ Tachycardia
◆ Oliguria
◆ Distended abdomen
◆ Ecchymosis or hematoma in the abdominal, flank, or groin area
◆ Paraplegia resulting from reduced blood flow to the spine
◆ Systolic bruit over the aorta
◆ Tenderness over affected area

DIAGNOSTIC TEST RESULTS
◆ *Abdominal ultrasonography or echocardiography:* size, shape, and location of the aneurysm
◆ *Anteroposterior and lateral abdominal X-rays:* aortic calcification outlining mass, at least 75% of the time
◆ *Computed tomography scan:* visualization of aneurysm's effect on nearby organs
◆ *Aortography:* condition of vessels proximal and distal to the aneurysm and extent of aneurysm (to avoid underestimating aneurysm diameter from only showing flow channel, not surrounding clot)

Treatment

◆ Careful control of blood pressure
◆ Monitoring of aneurysm size
◆ Fluid and blood replacement
◆ Weight reduction if appropriate
◆ Low-fat diet

- Activity as tolerated
- Endovascular grafting or resection if aneurysm is large or produces symptoms
- Bypass procedures for poor perfusion distal to aneurysm
- Repair of ruptured aneurysm with a graft replacement

MEDICATIONS
- Beta-adrenergic blockers
- Antihypertensives
- Analgesics
- Antibiotics

Nursing interventions

For an intact aneurysm
- Before elective surgery, weigh the patient, insert an indwelling urinary catheter and an I.V. line, and assist with insertion of the arterial line and pulmonary artery catheter to monitor hemodynamic status.
- Give prescribed preventive antibiotics.
- Offer the patient and his family psychological support.
- Monitor cardiac rhythm, hemodynamics parameters, vital signs, intake and output, and pulse oximetry.

For a ruptured aneurysm
- Administer fluids and blood products as ordered.
- Give prescribed drugs.
- Prepare for surgery.

After surgery
- Assess peripheral pulses for graft failure or occlusion.
- Watch for signs of bleeding retroperitoneally from the graft site.
- Maintain blood pressure in prescribed range with fluids and medications.
- Assess the patient for severe back pain, which can indicate that the graft is tearing.
- Provide pulmonary toileting.
- Reposition every 2 hours and provide skin and wound care.
- Assess respiratory status and monitor arterial blood gas values.
- Check nasogastric tube for patency and the amount and type of drainage.

PATIENT TEACHING
- Explain the disorder, diagnostic testing, and treatment plan.
- Teach about the administration, dosage, and possible adverse effects of prescribed medications.
- Provide information on the surgical procedure and the expected postoperative care.
- Stress the importance of taking all medications as prescribed and carrying a list of medications at all times, in case of an emergency.
- Review physical activity restrictions and the need to follow them until the patient is medically cleared by the practitioner.
- If surgery wasn't performed, explain the need for regular examination and ultrasound checks to monitor the size of the aneurysm.

Aneurysm, intracranial

Overview

An intracranial aneurysm is a localized dilation in the wall of a cerebral artery. The most common form is the berry aneurysm, a saclike outpouching in a cerebral artery. Intracerebral aneurysms usually occur at an arterial junction in the circle of Willis, the circular anastomosis forming the major cerebral arteries at the base of the brain. They typically rupture and cause subarachnoid hemorrhage, which is life-threatening.

CAUSES
◆ Congenital defect, degenerative process, or a combination of the two
◆ Trauma

PATHOPHYSIOLOGY
◆ Blood flow exerts pressure against a congenitally weak arterial wall, stretching it like an overblown balloon and making it likely to rupture.
◆ Rupture is followed by a subarachnoid hemorrhage in which blood spills into the space normally occupied by cerebrospinal fluid.
◆ Blood spills into brain tissue, where a clot can cause potentially fatal increased intracranial pressure and brain tissue damage.

COMPLICATIONS
◆ Neurologic deficits
◆ Rebleeding
◆ Vasospasm
◆ Death

Assessment

HISTORY
◆ Headache
◆ Intermittent nausea
◆ Seizure
◆ Photophobia
◆ Blurred vision

PHYSICAL FINDINGS
◆ Ruptured intracranial aneurysm graded according to the patient's signs and symptoms (see *Determining severity of an intracranial aneurysm rupture*)
◆ Nuchal rigidity
◆ Back and leg pain
◆ Fever
◆ Restlessness
◆ Irritability
◆ Hemiparesis
◆ Hemisensory defects
◆ Dysphagia
◆ Visual defects (diplopia, ptosis, dilated pupil, and inability to rotate the eye caused by compression on the oculomotor nerve, if aneurysm is near the internal carotid artery)

DIAGNOSTIC TEST RESULTS
◆ *Computed tomography scan:* subarachnoid or ventricular bleeding, with blood in subarachnoid space and displaced midline structures
◆ *Magnetic resonance imaging:* cerebral blood flow void
◆ *Skull X-rays:* calcified wall of the aneurysm and areas of bone erosion
◆ *Cerebral angiography:* altered cerebral blood flow, vessel lumen dilation, and differences in arterial filling

Treatment

◆ Avoidance of coffee, other stimulants, and aspirin
◆ Bed rest in a quiet, darkened room with minimal stimulation
◆ Surgical repair by clipping, ligation, or wrapping (before or after rupture)

MEDICATIONS

◆ Analgesics
◆ Antihypertensive agents
◆ Sedatives
◆ Calcium channel blockers
◆ Corticosteroids
◆ Anticonvulsants
◆ Aminocaproic acid

Nursing interventions

◆ Establish and maintain a patent airway.
◆ Monitor vital signs, neurologic status, intake and output, and pulse oximetry.
◆ Monitor intracerebral pressure as indicated.
◆ Position the patient to promote pulmonary drainage and prevent upper airway obstruction.
◆ Initiate aneurysm precautions (bed rest in a quiet, darkened room, keeping the head of the bed flat or elevated less than 30 degrees, as ordered; limited visitation; avoidance of strenuous physical activity and straining with bowel movements; and restricted fluid intake).
◆ Assist with active range-of-motion (ROM) exercises; if the patient is paralyzed, perform regular passive ROM exercises.
◆ Assess the gag reflex and assist during meals if appropriate.
◆ Provide emotional support to the patient and his family.

PATIENT TEACHING

◆ Explain the disorder, diagnostic testing, and treatment plan.
◆ Teach about the administration, dosage, and possible adverse effects of prescribed medications.
◆ Provide information about the surgical procedure and expected postoperative care.
◆ Stress the importance of follow-up care.
◆ Describe signs and symptoms of complications.
◆ Refer the patient to a visiting nurse or a rehabilitation center if necessary.

Determining severity of an intracranial aneurysm rupture

The severity of symptoms varies from patient to patient, depending on the site and amount of bleeding. Five grades characterize a ruptured intracranial aneurysm:

◆ *Grade I:* minimal bleeding—The patient is alert with no neurologic deficit; he may have a slight headache and nuchal rigidity.
◆ *Grade II:* mild bleeding—The patient is alert, with a mild to severe headache and nuchal rigidity; he may have third-nerve palsy.
◆ *Grade III:* moderate bleeding—The patient is confused or drowsy, with nuchal rigidity and, possibly, a mild focal deficit.
◆ *Grade IV:* severe bleeding—The patient is stuporous, with nuchal rigidity and, possibly, mild to severe hemiparesis.
◆ *Grade V:* moribund (commonly fatal)—If the rupture is nonfatal, the patient is in a deep coma or decerebrate.

Ankylosing spondylitis

Overview

Ankylosing spondylitis, also called *rheumatoid spondylitis* or *Marie-Strümpell disease,* primarily affects sacroiliac, apophyseal, and costocervical joints and adjacent ligamentous or tendinous attachments to bone. A rheumatoid disease, it usually occurs as a primary disorder but may occur secondary to Reiter syndrome, psoriatic arthritis, or inflammatory bowel disease.

CAUSES
◆ Unknown
◆ Familial tendency
◆ Immune system activation by bacterial infection (causing initial inflammation)

PATHOPHYSIOLOGY
◆ Beginning in the sacroiliac joint, the condition gradually progresses to the lumbar, thoracic, and cervical spine.
◆ The large synovial joint is less frequently involved.
◆ Deterioration of bone and cartilage leads to fibrous tissue formation and the eventual fusion of the spine or peripheral joints.

COMPLICATIONS
◆ Atlantoaxial subluxation
◆ Deposits of amyloid material in the kidneys, which may lead to renal impairment or failure
◆ Respiratory compromise

Assessment

HISTORY
◆ Intermittent lower back pain most severe in the morning or after inactivity and relieved by exercise
◆ Mild fatigue, fever, anorexia, and weight loss
◆ Possible description of pain in shoulders, hips, knees, and ankles
◆ Pain over the symphysis pubis, which may lead to its being mistaken for pelvic inflammatory disease

PHYSICAL FINDINGS
◆ Stiffness or limited motion of the lumbar spine
◆ Pain and limited chest expansion
◆ Kyphosis
◆ Iritis
◆ Warmth, swelling, or tenderness of affected joints
◆ Possible sausage-shaped small joints, such as toes
◆ Aortic murmur caused by regurgitation
◆ Cardiomegaly
◆ Upper lobe pulmonary fibrosis, which mimics tuberculosis, that may reduce vital capacity to 70% or less of predicted volume

DIAGNOSTIC TEST RESULTS
(See *Diagnosing primary ankylosing spondylitis.*)
◆ *HLA typing test:* presence of human leukocyte antigen (HLA)-B27 in about 95% of patients with primary ankylosing spondylitis, up to 80% of patients with secondary disease
◆ *Serum rheumatoid factor test:* Absence of rheumatoid factor, which helps rule out rheumatoid arthritis, a disease with similar symptoms
◆ *Serum alkaline phosphate and creatine kinase test:* slightly elevated with active bone remodeling
◆ *Erythrocyte sedimentation rate:* elevated in active disease
◆ *Serum immunoglobulin A levels:* elevated
◆ *X-ray studies:* bilateral sacroiliac involvement (the hallmark of the disease), blurring of the joints' bony margins in early disease, patchy sclerosis with superficial bony erosions, eventual squaring of vertebral bodies, and "bamboo spine" with complete ankylosis

Treatment

- Good posture, stretching, deep-breathing exercises
- Braces and lightweight supports if appropriate
- Heat, warm showers, baths, ice
- Nerve stimulation
- Nutritious diet
- Activity as tolerated
- Hip replacement surgery in the case of severe hip involvement
- Spinal wedge osteotomy in the case of severe spinal involvement

MEDICATIONS
- Nonsteroidal anti-inflammatory drugs

Nursing interventions

- Assist with range-of-motion excercises.
- Offer support and reassurance.
- Give prescribed analgesics.
- Apply heat locally and massage as indicated.
- Pace periods of exercise and rest to help the patient achieve comfortable energy levels and lung oxygenation.
- Ensure proper body alignment and positioning.
- Involve other caregivers, such as a social worker, visiting nurse, and dietitian.
- Monitor mobility and comfort level.
- Assess respiratory status and heart sounds.

PATIENT TEACHING
- Explain the disorder, diagnostic testing, and treatment plan.
- Teach about the administration, dosage, and possible adverse effects of prescribed medications.
- Provide information about the surgical procedure and expected postoperative care.
- Stress the importance of follow-up care.

- Describe signs and symptoms of complications.
- Refer the patient to a visiting nurse or a rehabilitation center when necessary.
- Explain activity restrictions and recommendations.
- Review the importance of sleeping in a prone position on a hard mattress and avoiding using pillows under the neck or knees.
- Provide information on proper nutrition and weight maintenance.
- Refer the patient to physical therapy as needed.
- Refer the patient to the Spondylitis Association of America or the Arthritis Foundation for additional support and information.

Diagnosing primary ankylosing spondylitis

For a reliable diagnosis of primary ankylosing spondylitis, the patient must meet criterion 7 and any one of criteria 1 through 5, or any five of criteria 1 through 6 if the patient doesn't have criterion 7.

Seven criteria
1. Axial skeleton stiffness for at least 3 months that's relieved by exercise
2. Lumbar pain that persists at rest
3. Thoracic cage pain of at least 3 months' duration that persists at rest
4. Past or current iritis
5. Decreased lumbar range of motion
6. Decreased chest expansion (age-related)
7. Bilateral, symmetrical sacroiliitis demonstrated by radiographic studies

Overview

Anthrax is an acute bacterial infection occurring most commonly in herbivorous animals. Humans have greater natural resistance to anthrax than animals, but the potential exists for its use in bioterrorism and biological warfare. Human cases are classified as either agricultural or industrial, and they occur in three forms, based on transmission mode: cutaneous, inhalation (woolsorter's disease, the most commom form), and GI. Treatment is initiated as soon as exposure to anthrax is suspected.

CAUSES
◆ Bacterial infection with *Bacillus anthracis*

Human cases
◆ Contact with infected animals or contaminated animal products
◆ Ingestion
◆ Inhalation
◆ Insect bites

Agricultural cases
◆ Bites from contaminated or infected flies
◆ Consumption of contaminated meat
◆ Contact with animals that have anthrax

Industrial cases
◆ Infected animal hides, bones, goat's hair, or wool

RISK FACTORS
◆ Working in a laboratory or industrial setting (risk of occupational exposure)

PATHOPHYSIOLOGY
◆ *B. anthracis* is an encapsulated, chain-forming, aerobic, gram-positive rod that forms hardy oval spores that can survive for years under adverse conditions.
◆ An extracellular pathogen, the rod evades phagocytosis, invades the bloodstream, and multiplies rapidly.
◆ In cutaneous anthrax, spores enter the body through abraded or broken skin or by biting flies. Spores germinate within hours, the vegetative cells multiply, and anthrax toxin is produced.
◆ In inhalation anthrax, spores are deposited directly into the alveoli and phagocytized by macrophages; some are carried to and germinate in mediastinal nodes. This may result in overwhelming bacteremia, hemorrhagic mediastinitis, and secondary pneumonia.
◆ In GI anthrax, primary infection can be caused in the intestine by organisms that survive passage through the stomach causing acute inflammation of the intestinal tract.

COMPLICATIONS
◆ Septicemia
◆ Hemorrhagic mediastinitis
◆ Pneumonia
◆ Respiratory failure
◆ Hemorrhagic thoracic lymphadenitis
◆ Meningitis
◆ Death

Assessment

HISTORY
Cutaneous anthrax
◆ Contact with animals or animal products
◆ Painless ulcer
◆ Mild or no constitutional symptoms

Inhalational anthrax
◆ Initial prodromal flulike symptoms
◆ Malaise, dry cough
◆ Mild fever, chills
◆ Headache, myalgia
◆ Severe respiratory distress
◆ Chest pain

GI anthrax
◆ Nausea, vomiting
◆ Decreased appetite
◆ Fever
◆ Abdominal pain
◆ Vomiting blood
◆ Severe bloody diarrhea

Physical findings

Cutaneous anthrax
- Initially, a small, papular, pruritic lesion that resembles an insect bite
- Lesion that develops into a vesicle in 1 to 2 days
- Lesion that finally becomes a small, painless ulcer with a necrotic center, surrounded by nonpitting edema
- Smaller secondary vesicles that may surround some lesions
- Lesions that are generally located on exposed areas of the skin
- Painful, regional, nonspecific lymphadenitis

Inhalational anthrax
- Increasing fever
- Dyspnea, stridor
- Hypoxia, cyanosis
- Hypotension, shock

GI anthrax
- Fever
- Rapidly developing ascites

Diagnostic test results
- *Gram stain, direct fluorescent antibody staining, culture, and cerebrospinal fluid analysis:* presence of B. anthracis
- *Blood cultures:* presence of B. anthracis
- *Complete blood count:* polymorphonuclear leukocytosis (in severe disease)
- *Serum antibody tests:* presence of specific B. anthracis antibody
- *Chest X-ray:* symmetric mediastinal widening in hemorrhagic mediastinitis

Treatment
- Adequate fluid intake
- Activity as tolerated

Medications
- Antibiotics
- Oxygen as needed

Nursing interventions
- Give prescribed drugs.
- Maintain a patent airway and adequate ventilation.
- Assess respiratory status, neurologic status, and cardiovascular status.
- Report any case of anthrax in either livestock or humans to the local board of health.
- Maintain standard precautions.
- Encourage verbalization of fears and concerns.
- Provide adequate hydration and a well-balanced diet.
- Assist the patient in developing effective coping mechanisms.
- Provide adequate rest periods.
- Monitor vital signs, intake and output, and pulse oximetry.
- Evaluate skin lesions and provide wound care.
- Assess the patient's response to treatment and observe for complications.

Patient teaching
- Explain the disorder, diagnostic testing, and treatment plan.
- Teach about the administration, dosage, and possible adverse effects of prescribed medications.
- Discuss when to notify the practitioner of potential complications.

Aortic stenosis

Overview

Aortic stenosis, which is classified as either acquired or rheumatic, is the narrowing of the aortic valve that affects blood flow in the heart. Symptoms may not appear until ages 50 to 70, even though stenosis may have been present since childhood.

CAUSES
◆ Atherosclerosis
◆ Congenital aortic bicuspid valve
◆ Idiopathic fibrosis and calcification
◆ Rheumatic fever

RISK FACTORS
◆ Diabetes mellitus
◆ Hypercholesterolemia

PATHOPHYSIOLOGY
◆ Stenosis of the aortic valve impedes forward blood flow.
◆ The left ventricle requires greater pressure to open the aortic valve.
◆ Added workload increases myocardial oxygen demands.
◆ Diminished cardiac output reduces coronary artery blood flow.
◆ Left ventricular hypertrophy and failure result.

COMPLICATIONS
◆ Left-sided heart failure
◆ Right-sided heart failure
◆ Infective endocarditis
◆ Cardiac arrhythmias, especially atrial fibrillation
◆ Left ventricular hypertrophy
◆ Sudden death

Assessment

HISTORY
◆ May be asymptomatic
◆ Dyspnea on exertion
◆ Angina
◆ Exertional syncope
◆ Fatigue
◆ Palpitations
◆ Paroxysmal nocturnal dyspnea

PHYSICAL FINDINGS
◆ Small, sustained arterial pulses that rise slowly
◆ Distinct lag between carotid artery pulse and apical pulse
◆ Orthopnea
◆ Prominent jugular vein a waves
◆ Peripheral edema
◆ Diminished carotid pulses with delayed upstroke
◆ Apex of the heart may be displaced inferiorly and laterally
◆ Suprasternal thrill
◆ Split second heart sound (S_2) that develops as stenosis becomes more severe
◆ Prominent fourth heart sound (S_4)
◆ Harsh, rasping, mid- to late-peaking systolic murmur that's best heard at the base and commonly radiates to carotids and apex (see *Identifying the murmur of aortic stenosis*)

DIAGNOSTIC TEST RESULTS
◆ *Chest X-ray:* valvular calcification, left ventricular enlargement, pulmonary vein congestion, and in later stages, left atrial, pulmonary artery, right atrial, and right ventricular enlargement
◆ *Echocardiography:* decreased valve area, increased gradient, and increased left ventricular wall thickness
◆ *Cardiac catheterization:* increased pressure gradient across the aortic valve, increased left ventricular pressures, and presence of coronary artery disease
◆ *Electrocardiography:* left ventricular hypertrophy, atrial fibrillation, or other arrhythmia may show

Disorders

Treatment

♦ Periodic noninvasive evaluation of the severity of valve narrowing
♦ Lifelong treatment and management
♦ Low-sodium, low-fat, low-cholesterol diet
♦ Planned rest periods
♦ In adults, valve replacement after they become symptomatic with hemodynamic evidence of severe obstruction
♦ Percutaneous balloon aortic valvuloplasty
♦ In children without calcified valves, simple commissurotomy under direct visualization
♦ Ross procedure (for patients younger than age 5)

MEDICATIONS

♦ Cardiac glycosides
♦ Prophylactic antibiotics for infective endocarditis

Nursing interventions

♦ Place the patient in an upright position and administer oxygen as needed.
♦ Monitor vital signs, intake and output, and cardiac rhythm
♦ Give prescribed drugs.
♦ Provide a low-sodium, low-fat, low-cholesterol diet.
♦ Provide a bedside commode and alternate periods of activity and rest.
♦ Provide emotional support and encourage the patient to express his fears and concerns.
♦ Observe for signs and symptoms of heart failure and progressive aortic stenosis.
♦ Obtain daily weight.

After surgery

♦ Observe for signs and symptoms of thrombus formation.
♦ Monitor hemodynamics, arterial blood gas results, laboratory studies and chest X-ray results.

PATIENT TEACHING

♦ Explain the disorder, diagnostic testing, and treatment plan.
♦ Teach about the administration, dosage, and possible adverse effects of prescribed medications.
♦ Explain when to notify the practitioner of complications.
♦ Stress periodic rest in the patient's daily routine.
♦ Encourage leg elevation whenever the patient sits in a chair.
♦ Review dietary and fluid restrictions.
♦ Describe signs and symptoms of heart failure.
♦ Stress the importance of consistent follow-up care.
♦ Explain infective endocarditis prophylaxis.
♦ Teach the patient how to monitor pulse rate and rhythm.
♦ Refer the patient to a weight-reduction program if indicated.
♦ Refer the patient to a smoking-cessation program if indicated.

Identifying the murmur of aortic stenosis

A low-pitched, harsh crescendo-decrescendo murmur that radiates from the aortic valve area to the carotid artery characterizes aortic stenosis.

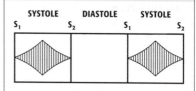

Appendicitis

Overview

Appendicitis, the most common major abdominal surgical disease, is the inflammation of the vermiform appendix. If left untreated, gangrene and perforation can develop within 36 hours, and it can be fatal. Appendicitis can occur at any age, but most cases occur between ages 11 and 20.

CAUSES
- Barium ingestion
- Fecal mass
- Foreign body
- Mucosal ulceration
- Neoplasm
- Stricture
- Viral infection

RISK FACTORS
- Adolescent male

PATHOPHYSIOLOGY
- Mucosal ulceration triggers inflammation, which temporarily obstructs the appendix.
- Obstruction causes mucus outflow, increasing pressure in the distended appendix; the appendix then contracts.
- Bacteria multiply and inflammation and pressure increase, restricting blood flow and causing thrombus and abdominal pain.

COMPLICATIONS
- Wound infection
- Intra-abdominal infection
- Fecal fistula
- Intestinal obstruction
- Incisional hernia
- Peritonitis (most common)
- Death

Assessment

HISTORY
- Abdominal pain that's initially generalized, then localizes in the right lower abdomen (McBurney's point)
- Anorexia
- Nausea, vomiting

PHYSICAL FINDINGS
- Low-grade fever, tachycardia
- Adjusting posture to decrease pain
- Guarding
- Normoactive bowel sounds, with possible constipation or diarrhea
- Rebound tenderness and spasm of the abdominal muscles
- Rovsing sign (pain in right lower quadrant that occurs with palpation of left lower quadrant)
- Psoas sign (abdominal pain that occurs when the patient flexes his hip when pressure applied to his knee)
- Obturator sign (abdominal pain that occurs when the hip is rotated)
- Absent abdominal tenderness or flank tenderness in patient with a retrocele or pelvic appendix

DIAGNOSTIC TEST RESULTS
- *White blood cell count:* moderately elevated with increased numbers of immature cells
- *Abdominal or transvaginal ultrasound:* appendiceal inflammation
- *Barium enema:* nonfilling appendix
- *Abdominal computed tomography scan:* suspected perforation or abscess

Treatment

◆ Nothing by mouth until after surgery, then gradual return to regular diet
◆ Appendectomy
◆ In suspected abcess, antibiotic therapy that's initiated before surgery
◆ Early postoperative ambulation
◆ Incentive spirometry

MEDICATIONS
◆ I.V. fluids
◆ Analgesics
◆ Antibiotics preoperatively and if peritonitis develops

Nursing interventions

◆ Maintain nothing-by-mouth status until surgery is performed.
◆ Administer I.V. fluids.

 Nursing alert
Avoid administering analgesics until the diagnosis is confirmed. Avoid administering cathartics or enemas that may rupture the appendix.

◆ Administer prescribed preoperative drugs.

After surgery
◆ Monitor vital signs and intake and output.
◆ Assess the patient's pain level, administer analgesics, and evaluate their effects.
◆ Provide wound care.

PATIENT TEACHING
◆ Explain the disorder, diagnostic testing, and treatment plan.
◆ Teach about the administration, dosage, and possible adverse effects of prescribed medications.

◆ Provide information about the surgical procedure and the expected postoperative care.
◆ Describe signs and symptoms of complications.
◆ Teach appropriate wound care.
◆ Review postoperative activity limitations.
◆ Refer the patient to a follow-up appointment with the surgeon or practitioner.

Arterial occlusive disease

Overview

Arterial occlusive disease, which has a higher incidence in patients with diabetes, is the obstruction or narrowing of the lumen of the aorta and its major branches. It may affect arteries, including the carotid, vertebral, innominate, subclavian, femoral, iliac, renal, mesenteric, and celiac. Prognosis depends on location of the occlusion and development of collateral circulation that counteracts reduced blood flow. Arteries in the legs are more commonly affected than other arteries.

CAUSES
◆ Atheromatous debris (plaques)
◆ Atherosclerosis
◆ Direct blunt or penetrating trauma
◆ Embolism
◆ Fibromuscular disease
◆ Immune arteritis
◆ Indwelling arterial catheter
◆ Raynaud's disease
◆ Thromboangiitis obliterans
◆ Thrombosis

RISK FACTORS
◆ Smoking
◆ Hypertension
◆ Dyslipidemia
◆ Diabetes mellitus
◆ Advanced age

PATHOPHYSIOLOGY
◆ Narrowing of vessel leads to interrupted blood flow, usually to the legs and feet.
◆ During times of increased activity or exercise, blood flow to surrounding muscles can't meet the metabolic demand, causing pain in affected areas.

COMPLICATIONS
◆ Severe ischemia
◆ Skin ulceration
◆ Gangrene
◆ Limb loss

Assessment

HISTORY
◆ One or more risk factors
◆ Family history of vascular disease
◆ Intermittent claudication
◆ Pain at rest
◆ Poor healing of wounds or ulcers
◆ Impotence
◆ Dizziness or near syncope
◆ Transient ischemic attack symptoms

PHYSICAL FINDINGS
◆ Trophic changes of involved arm or leg
◆ Diminished or absent pulses in arm or leg
◆ Presence of ischemic ulcers
◆ Pallor with elevation of arm or leg
◆ Dependent rubor
◆ Arterial bruit
◆ Hypertension
◆ Pain
◆ Pallor
◆ Pulselessness distal to the occlusion
◆ Paralysis and paresthesia occurring in the affected arm or leg
◆ Poikilothermy

DIAGNOSTIC TEST RESULTS
◆ *Arteriography:* type, location, degree of obstruction, establishment of collateral circulation
◆ *Ultrasonography and plethysmography:* decreased blood flow distal to the occlusion
◆ *Doppler ultrasonography:* relatively low-pitched sound and a monophasic waveform
◆ *EEG and computed tomography scan:* brain lesion
◆ *Segmental limb pressures and pulse volume measurements:* location and extent of the occlusion
◆ *Ophthalmodynamometry:* degree of obstruction in the internal carotid artery
◆ *Electrocardiogram:* cardiovascular disease

Treatment

- Smoking cessation
- Hypertension, diabetes, and dyslipidemia control
- Foot and leg care
- Weight control
- Low-fat, low-cholesterol, high-fiber diet
- Regular walking program
- Embolectomy
- Endarterectomy
- Atherectomy
- Laser angioplasty
- Endovascular stent placement
- Percutaneous transluminal angioplasty
- Laser surgery
- Patch grafting
- Bypass graft
- Lumbar sympathectomy
- Amputation
- Bowel resection

MEDICATIONS

- Antiplatelets
- Lipid-lowering agents
- Hypoglycemic agents
- Antihypertensives
- Thrombolytics
- Anticoagulation
- Niacin or vitamin B complex

Nursing interventions

For chronic arterial occlusive disease

- Provide measures to protect skin integrity, such as minimal pressure mattresses, heel protectors, a foot cradle, or a footboard.
- Avoid using restrictive clothing such as antiembolism stockings.
- Give prescribed drugs.
- Observe for complications.
- Allow the patient to express his fears and concerns.

For preoperative care during an acute episode

- Assess the patient's circulatory status.
- Give prescribed analgesics.

- Give prescribed heparin or thrombolytics.
- Avoid elevating or applying heat to the affected leg.

For postoperative care

- Evaluate circulatory status and observe for signs of hemorrhage.
- Monitor vital signs, intake and output, and neurologic status.
- Assess the patient's pain level, administer analgesics, and evaluate their effects.
- Assist with early ambulation, but don't allow the patient to sit for an extended period.
- Provide wound care.

PATIENT TEACHING

- Explain the disorder, diagnostic testing, and treatment plan.
- Teach about the administration, dosage, and possible adverse effects of prescribed medications.
- Provide information on surgical procedure and the expected postoperative care.
- Describe signs and symptoms of complications.
- Teach appropriate wound care.
- Review postoperative activity limitations.
- Refer the patient to a follow-up appointment with the surgeon or practitioner.
- Provide information on dietary restrictions and regular exercise program.
- Describe signs and symptoms of graft occlusion and arterial insufficiency and occlusion.
- Teach avoidance of wearing constrictive clothing, crossing legs, or wearing garters.
- Encourage risk factor modification.
- Stress importance of follow-up care.
- Refer the patient to a physical and occupational therapist as indicated.
- Refer the patient to a smoking-cessation program as indicated.

Asthma

Overview

A chronic reactive airway disorder, asthma involves episodic, reversible airway obstruction resulting from bronchospasms, increased mucus secretions, and mucosal edema. Signs and symptoms range from mild wheezing and dyspnea to life-threatening respiratory failure.

CAUSES
◆ Sensitivity to specific external allergens (extrinsic) or related to internal, nonallergenic factors (intrinsic)

Extrinsic
◆ Animal dander
◆ Food additives containing sulfites or other sensitizing substances
◆ House dust or mold
◆ Kapok or feather pillows
◆ Pollen

Intrinsic
◆ Emotional stress
◆ Genetic factors

Bronchoconstriction
◆ Cold air
◆ Drugs, such as aspirin, beta-adrenergic blockers, and nonsteroidal anti-inflammatory drugs
◆ Exercise
◆ Hereditary predisposition
◆ Psychological stress
◆ Sensitivity to allergens or irritants such as pollutants
◆ Tartrazine
◆ Viral infections

PATHOPHYSIOLOGY
◆ When tracheal and bronchial linings overreact to various stimuli, episodic smooth-muscle spasms occur that severely constrict the airways.
◆ Mucosal edema and thickened secretions further block the airways.
◆ Immunoglobulin (Ig) E antibodies, attached to histamine-containing mast cells and receptors on cell membranes, initiate intrinsic asthma attacks.
◆ When exposed to an antigen such as pollen, the IgE antibody combines with the antigen. On subsequent exposure to the antigen, mast cells degranulate and release mediators.
◆ The mediators cause the bronchoconstriction and edema of an asthma attack.
◆ During an asthma attack, expiratory airflow decreases, trapping gas in the airways and causing alveolar hyperinflation.
◆ Atelectasis may develop in some lung regions.
◆ The increased airway resistance causes labored breathing.

COMPLICATIONS
◆ Status asthmaticus
◆ Respiratory failure
◆ Death

Assessment

HISTORY
◆ Severe respiratory tract infections, especially in adults (intrinsic asthma)
◆ Irritants, emotional stress, fatigue, endocrine changes, temperature and humidity variations, and exposure to noxious fumes (may aggravate intrinsic asthma attacks)
◆ Dramatic, simultaneous onset of severe, multiple symptoms, or insidious, gradual increased respiratory distress
◆ Particular allergen exposure followed by a sudden onset of dyspnea and wheezing and tightness in the chest accompanied by a cough that produces thick, clear, or yellow sputum

PHYSICAL FINDINGS
◆ Visible dyspnea
◆ Ability to speak only a few words before pausing for breath
◆ Use of accessory respiratory muscles

- Diaphoresis
- Increased anteroposterior thoracic diameter
- Hyperresonance
- Tachycardia, tachypnea, mild systolic hypertension
- Inspiratory and expiratory wheezes
- Prolonged expiratory phase of respiration
- Diminished breath sounds
- Cyanosis, confusion, and lethargy (indicator of life-threatening status asthmaticus and respiratory failure)

DIAGNOSTIC TEST RESULTS

- *Arterial blood gas analysis:* hypoxemia
- *Serum IgE levels:* increased
- *Blood eosinophil count:* increased
- *Chest X-rays:* hyperinflation of the lungs with areas of focal atelectasis
- *Pulmonary function studies:* decreased peak flows and forced expiratory volume in 1 second, low-normal or decreased vital capacity, and increased total lung and residual capacities
- *Skin testing:* positive for specific allergens
- *Bronchial challenge testing:* clinical significance of identified allergens on the lungs
- *Pulse oximetry:* decreased oxygen saturation

Treatment

- Identification and avoidance of precipitating factors
- Desensitization to specific antigens
- Establishment and maintenance of patent airway
- Fluid replacement
- Activity as tolerated

MEDICATIONS

- Low-flow oxygen
- Bronchodilators
- Corticosteroids
- Histamine antagonists
- Immunomodulators
- Mast cell stabilizers
- Leukotriene antagonists
- Anticholinergic bronchodilators
- Antibiotics

Nursing interventions

- Give prescribed drugs.
- Place the patient in high Fowler's position and administer prescribed humidified oxygen.
- Encourage pursed-lip and diaphragmatic breathing.
- Assist with intubation and mechanical ventilation, if appropriate.
- Perform postural drainage and chest percussion, if tolerated.
- Suction an intubated patient as needed.
- Monitor vital signs, intake and output, and pulse oximetry.
- Evaluate breath sounds and response to treatment.
- Monitor for complications of corticosteroid treatment.

PATIENT TEACHING

- Explain the disorder, diagnostic testing, and treatment plan.
- Teach about the administration, dosage, and possible adverse effects of prescribed medications.
- Teach the signs and symptoms of an asthma attack and when to notify the practitioner.
- Assist with identification and avoidance of known allergens and irritants.
- Teach proper use of metered-dose inhaler or dry powder inhaler.
- Demonstrate pursed-lip and diaphragmatic breathing.
- Teach use of a peak flow meter and effective coughing techniques.
- Stress improtance of follow-up care.
- Refer the patient to a local asthma support group.

Atelectasis

Overview

Atelectasis is the incomplete expansion of alveolar clusters or lung segments, leading to partial or complete lung collapse. It may be chronic or acute and is common in patients after upper abdominal or thoracic surgery. Patients who have prompt removal of any airway obstruction, relief of hypoxia, and reexpansion of the collapsed lung have a good prognosis.

CAUSES
- Bronchial occlusion
- Bronchiectasis
- Bronchogenic carcinoma
- Cystic fibrosis
- External compression
- General anesthesia
- Idiopathic respiratory distress syndrome of the neonate
- Immobility
- Inflammatory lung disease
- Oxygen toxicity
- Pleural effusion
- Pulmonary edema
- Pulmonary embolism
- Sarcoidosis

PATHOPHYSIOLOGY
- Incomplete expansion causes certain regions of the lung to be removed from gas exchange process.
- Unoxygenated blood passes unchanged through these regions and produces hypoxia.
- Alveolar surfactant causes increased surface tension, permitting complete alveolar deflation.

COMPLICATIONS
- Hypoxemia
- Acute respiratory failure
- Pneumonia

Assessment

HISTORY
- Recent abdominal surgery
- Prolonged immobility
- Mechanical ventilation
- Central nervous system depression
- Smoking
- Chronic obstructive pulmonary disease
- Rib fractures, tight chest dressings

PHYSICAL FINDINGS
- Decreased chest wall movement
- Cyanosis
- Diaphoresis
- Substernal or intercostal retractions
- Anxiety
- Decreased fremitus
- Mediastinal shift to the affected side
- Dullness or flatness over lung fields
- End-inspiration crackles
- Decreased (or absent) breath sounds
- Tachycardia

DIAGNOSTIC TEST RESULTS
- *Arterial blood gas (ABG) analysis:* hypoxia
- *Chest X-rays:* characteristic horizontal lines in the lower lung zones and characteristic dense shadows
- *Bronchoscopy:* evidence of obstructing neoplasm, foreign body, or pneumonia
- *Pulse oximetry:* decreased oxygen saturation

Treatment

- Incentive spirometry
- Chest percussion and postural drainage
- Frequent coughing and deep-breathing exercises
- Bronchoscopy, if above measures fail
- Humidity

◆ Intermittent positive-pressure breathing therapy
◆ Radiation for obstructing neoplasm (may be needed)
◆ Increased fluids
◆ Activity as tolerated; bed rest discouraged
◆ Surgery, if obstructing neoplasm present

MEDICATIONS
◆ Bronchodilators
◆ Analgesics after surgery

Nursing interventions

◆ Give prescribed drugs.
◆ Encourage coughing and deep breathing.
◆ Reposition the patient often.
◆ Encourage and assist with ambulation as soon as possible.
◆ Encourage use of an incentive spirometer.
◆ Humidify inspired air.
◆ Encourage adequate fluid intake.
◆ Perform postural drainage and chest percussion and provide suctioning as needed.
◆ Offer the patient reassurance and emotional support.
◆ Monitor vital signs, intake and output, and pulse oximetry.
◆ Evaluate respiratory status (breath sounds, ABG results) per unit policy and clinical status.

PATIENT TEACHING
◆ Explain the disorder, diagnostic testing, and treatment plan.
◆ Teach about the administration, dosage, and possible adverse effects of prescribed medications.
◆ Demonstrate postural drainage and percussion, and coughing and deep-breathing exercises.

◆ Review importance of splinting incisions.
◆ Explain energy conservation techniques and stress-reduction strategies.
◆ Stress the importance of mobilization.
◆ Refer the patient to a smoking-cessation program if indicated.
◆ Refer the patient to a weight-reduction program if indicated.

Benign prostatic hyperplasia

Overview

Benign prostatic hyperplasia is the enlargement of the prostate gland, which causes compression of the urethra and overt urinary obstruction. This condition may be treated surgically or symptomatically, depending on the size of prostate, age and health of patient, and extent of obstruction.

CAUSES
◆ Exact cause unknown
◆ Possible link to hormonal activity

RISK FACTORS
◆ Age
◆ Intact testes

PATHOPHYSIOLOGY
◆ Changes occur in periurethral glandular tissue.
◆ The prostate enlarges and may extend into the bladder.
◆ The compression or distortion of the prostatic urethra obstructs urine outflow.
◆ Diverticulum may develop, causing urine retention.

COMPLICATIONS
◆ Acute or chronic renal failure
◆ Acute postobstructive diuresis
◆ Bladder diverticula and saccules
◆ Bladder wall trabeculation
◆ Detrusor muscle hypertrophy
◆ Hydronephrosis
◆ Paradoxical (overflow) incontinence
◆ Urethral stenosis
◆ Urinary stasis, urinary tract infection (UTI), or renal calculi

Assessment

HISTORY
◆ Decreased urine stream caliber and force
◆ Interrupted urinary stream
◆ Urinary hesitancy and frequency
◆ Difficulty initiating urination
◆ Nocturia, hematuria
◆ Dribbling, incontinence
◆ Urine retention

PHYSICAL FINDINGS
◆ Visible midline mass above the symphysis pubis
◆ Distended bladder
◆ Enlarged prostate on digital rectal examination

DIAGNOSTIC TEST RESULTS
◆ *Blood urea nitrogen and serum creatinine levels:* elevated, indicating possible impaired renal function
◆ *Bacterial count:* above 100,000/mm^3, indicating possible hematuria, pyuria, and UTI
◆ *Excretory urography:* presence of urinary tract obstruction, hydronephrosis, calculi or tumors, and bladder filling and emptying defects
◆ *Cystourethroscopy:* prostate enlargement, bladder wall changes, calculi, and raised bladder
◆ *International Prostate Symptom Score:* determines disorder's severity

Treatment

◆ Prostatic massage
◆ Short-term fluid restriction (prevents bladder distention)
◆ Transurethral resection of prostate
◆ Suprapubic (transvesical), retropubic (extravesical), or perineal prostatectomy
◆ Avoidance of lifting, performing strenuous exercises, and taking long automobile rides for at least 1 month after surgery
◆ Minimally invasive therapy such as heat therapy (laser, microwave energy), transurethral incision of the prostate, transurethral needle ablation of the prostate, or high-intensity ultrasound energy

MEDICATIONS

- Antibiotics, if infection present
- Alpha$_1$-adrenergic blockers
- Nonselective alpha blockers
- 5-alpha-reductase inhibitors
- Phytotherapeutic agents

Nursing interventions

- Give prescribed drugs.

 Nursing alert

Avoid giving sedatives, alcohol, antidepressants, or anticholinergics (which can worsen the obstruction).

- Provide I.V. therapy as ordered.
- Monitor vital signs, intake and output, and daily weight.
- Watch for signs of postobstructive diuresis, characterized by polyuria exceeding 2 L in 8 hours and excessive electrolyte losses.

After prostatic surgery

- Assess the patient's pain level, administer analgesics, and evaluate their effects.
- Monitor catheter function and drainage.
- Observe for signs of infection.

PATIENT TEACHING

- Explain the disorder, diagnostic testing, and treatment plan.
- Teach about the administration, dosage, and possible adverse effects of prescribed medications.
- Describe signs of UTI that should be reported.
- Stress follow-up care and when to seek medical care (for example, for fever, inability to void, or passing bloody urine).

Blood transfusion reaction

Overview

A blood transfusion reaction is a hemolytic response to the transfusion of mismatched blood or blood components. It's mediated by immune or nonimmune factors and the reaction can range from mild to severe.

CAUSES
◆ Transfusion with incompatible blood product

PATHOPHYSIOLOGY
◆ Recipient's antibodies, immunoglobulin (Ig) G or IgM, attach to donor red blood cells (RBCs), leading to widespread clumping and destruction of recipient's RBCs.
◆ Transfusion with Rh-incompatible blood triggers a less serious reaction, known as Rh isoimmunization, within several days to 2 weeks. (See *Understanding the Rh system.*)
◆ A febrile nonhemolytic reaction—the most common type of reaction—develops when cytotoxic or agglutinating antibodies in the recipient's plasma attack antigens on transfused lymphocytes, granulocytes, or plasma cells.

COMPLICATIONS
◆ Acute tubular necrosis leading to acute renal failure
◆ Anaphylactic shock
◆ Bronchospasm
◆ Disseminated intravascular coagulation
◆ Vascular collapse

Assessment

HISTORY
◆ Transfusion of blood product
◆ Chills, nausea, vomiting, chest tightness, or chest and back pain

PHYSICAL FINDINGS
◆ Rash
◆ Fever, tachycardia, hypotension
◆ Dyspnea, apprehension
◆ Dizziness
◆ Urticaria, angioedema
◆ Wheezing
◆ Blood oozing from mucous membranes or the incision site (in a surgical patient)
◆ Fever, an unexpected decrease in serum hemoglobin (Hb) level, frank blood in urine, and jaundice (in a hemolytic reaction)

DIAGNOSTIC TEST RESULTS
◆ *Serum Hb levels:* decreased
◆ *Serum bilirubin levels and indirect bilirubin levels:* increased
◆ *Urinalysis:* hemoglobinuria
◆ *Indirect Coombs' test or serum antibody screen:* positive for serum anti-A or anti-B antibodies
◆ *Prothrombin time:* increased
◆ *Fibrinogen level:* decreased
◆ *Blood urea nitrogen and serum creatinine levels:* increased

Treatment

◆ Immediate discontinuance of the transfusion
◆ Possible dialysis (if acute tubular necrosis occurs)
◆ Diet as tolerated
◆ Bed rest

MEDICATIONS
◆ I.V. normal saline solution
◆ Epinephrine
◆ Diphenhydramine (Benadryl)
◆ Corticosteroids
◆ Antipyretics
◆ Osmotic or loop diuretics
◆ Vasopressors

Nursing interventions

◆ Stop the blood transfusion and follow your facility's blood transfusion reaction policy and procedure.
◆ Administer supplemental oxygen as needed.
◆ Maintain a patent I.V. line with normal saline solution.
◆ Monitor vital signs, intake and output, and laboratory results.
◆ Administer medications as ordered by the physician.
◆ Assess for signs of shock.
◆ Report early signs of complications.
◆ Document the transfusion reaction on the patient's chart, noting the duration of the transfusion and the amount of blood absorbed.

PATIENT TEACHING
◆ Explain the disorder, diagnostic testing, and treatment plan.
◆ Teach about the administration, dosage, and possible adverse effects of prescribed medications.

Understanding the Rh system

The Rh system contains more than 45 antibodies and antigens. Of the world's population, about 85% are Rh positive, which means that their red blood cells carry the D or Rh antigen. The rest of the population are Rh negative and don't have this antigen.

Effects of sensitization
When an Rh-negative person receives Rh-positive blood for the first time, he becomes sensitized to the D antigen but shows no immediate reaction to it. If he receives Rh-positive blood a second time, he experiences a massive hemolytic reaction.

For example, an Rh-negative mother who gives birth to an Rh-positive baby is sensitized by the baby's Rh-positive blood. During her next Rh-positive pregnancy, her sensitized blood will cause a hemolytic reaction in the fetal circulation.

Preventing sensitization
To prevent the formation of antibodies against Rh-positive blood, an Rh-negative mother should receive $Rh_0(D)$ immune globulin (human) (RhoGAM) I.M. at 28 weeks' gestation and again within 72 hours after giving birth to an Rh-positive baby.

Botulism

Overview

Botulism is a life-threatening paralytic illness that results from an exotoxin produced by the gram-positive, anaerobic bacillus *Clostridium botulinum*. It occurs as botulism food poisoning, wound botulism, and infant botulism. (See *Infant botulism.*) It carries a 25% mortality rate, with death most commonly caused by respiratory failure during the first week of illness. If the onset of disease occurs within 24 hours of ingesting food, a critical and potentially fatal illness exists.

CAUSES
◆ *C. botulinum*

RISK FACTORS
◆ Eating improperly preserved foods
◆ Using injectable street drugs

PATHOPHYSIOLOGY
◆ Endotoxin acts at the neuromuscular junction of skeletal muscle, preventing acetylcholine release and blocking neural transmission, eventually resulting in paralysis.

COMPLICATIONS
◆ Respiratory failure
◆ Paralytic ileus
◆ Death

Assessment

HISTORY
◆ Consumption of home-canned food 18 to 30 hours before onset of symptoms
◆ Vertigo
◆ Sore throat
◆ Weakness
◆ Nausea and vomiting
◆ Constipation or diarrhea
◆ Diplopia
◆ Blurred vision
◆ Dysarthria
◆ Dysphagia
◆ Dyspnea
◆ Heroin use

PHYSICAL FINDINGS
◆ Ptosis
◆ Dilated, nonreactive pupils
◆ Appearance of dry, red, and crusted oral mucous membranes
◆ Abdominal distention with absent bowel sounds
◆ Descending weakness or paralysis of muscles in the extremities or trunk
◆ Deep tendon reflexes may be intact, diminished, or absent
◆ Unexplained postural hypotension
◆ Urinary retention
◆ Photophobia
◆ Slurred speech

DIAGNOSTIC TEST RESULTS
◆ *Mouse bioassay:* presence of toxin in the patient's serum, stool, or gastric contents
◆ *Electromyography:* diminished muscle action potential after a single supramaximal nerve stimulus

Treatment

- Supportive measures
- Early tracheotomy and ventilatory assistance in respiratory failure
- Nasogastric (NG) suctioning
- Total parenteral nutrition
- Bed rest
- Debridement of wounds to remove source of toxin-producing bacteria

MEDICATIONS

- I.V. or I.M. botulinum antitoxin (for adults)
- Botulism immunoglobulin (for infants)

Nursing interventions

- Obtain history of food intake for the past several days.
- Obtain family history of similar symptoms and food intake.
- Monitor neurologic status, and cardiac and respiratory function.
- Monitor vital signs, intake and output, and arterial blood gas levels.
- Administer I.V. fluids as ordered.
- Administer oxygen as needed.
- Perform NG suctioning as needed.
- Immediately report all cases of botulism to the local board of health.
- Assess cough and gag reflexes.

PATIENT TEACHING

- Explain the disorder, diagnostic testing, and treatment plan.
- Teach about the administration, dosage, and possible adverse effects of prescribed medications.

- Describe proper techniques in processing and preserving foods.
- Stress never tasting food from a bulging can or one with a peculiar odor and to be cautious about eating food from dented cans.
- Teach the patient to avoid feeding honey to infants (can be fatal if contaminated).

Infant botulism

Infant botulism, which usually afflicts neonates and infants between the ages of 6 weeks and 6 months, commonly results from the ingestion of spores of botulinum bacteria, which then grow in the intestines and release toxin. Honey or corn syrup is a common source of the toxin.

This disorder can produce floppy infant syndrome, characterized by constipation, a feeble cry, a depressed gag reflex, and an inability to suck. The infant also exhibits a flaccid facial expression, ptosis, and ophthalmoplegia–the result of cranial nerve deficits. As the disease progresses, the infant develops generalized weakness, hypotonia, areflexia, and sometimes a striking loss of head control. Almost 50% of affected infants develop respiratory arrest.

Intensive supportive care allows most infants to recover completely. Antitoxin therapy isn't recommended because of the risk of anaphylaxis.

Breast cancer

Overview

Breast cancer is the malignant proliferation of epithelial cells lining the ducts or lobules of the breast. Early detection and treatment signficantly impact the prognosis. With adjunctive therapy, 10-year (or longer) survival is 70% to 75% in patients with negative nodes, compared with 20% to 25% in those with positive nodes. Breast cancer is the second-leading cause of cancer death in women (after lung cancer) and the most common cancer in women.

CAUSES
◆ Unknown

RISK FACTORS
◆ Family history of breast cancer, particularly first-degree relatives, including mother, sister, maternal grandmother, and maternal aunt
◆ Positive test results for genetic mutations (BRCA 1 and BRCA 2)
◆ Being a premenopausal woman older than age 45

 Age considerations
A woman's risk for breast cancer increases by 17% at age 40 and by as much as 78% at age 50 and older.

◆ Long menstrual cycles
◆ Early onset of menses, late menopause
◆ Nulliparous or first pregnancy after age 30
◆ High-fat diet
◆ Endometrial or ovarian cancer
◆ History of unilateral breast cancer
◆ Radiation exposure
◆ Estrogen therapy
◆ Antihypertensive therapy
◆ Alcohol use and exposure to tobacco
◆ Obesity
◆ Preexisting fibrocystic disease

PATHOPHYSIOLOGY
◆ The lymphatic system and the bloodstream carry the disease through the right side of the heart to the lungs and to the other breast, chest wall, liver, bone, and the brain.
◆ Its classification varies, depending on the origin:
  • adenocarcinoma (ductal) (arising from the epithelium)
  • intraductal (developing within the ducts [includes Paget's disease of the breast])
  • infiltrating (occurring in the breast's parenchymal tissue)
  • inflammatory (rare) (growing rapidly and causing overlying skin to become edematous, inflamed, and indurated)
  • lobular carcinoma in situ (involving the lobes of glandular tissue)
  • medullary or circumscribed (enlarging tumor with rapid growth rate).

COMPLICATIONS
◆ Central nervous system effects
◆ Distant metastasis
◆ Infection
◆ Respiratory effects

Assessment

HISTORY
◆ Detection of a painless lump or mass in the breast
◆ Change in breast tissue
◆ History of risk factors
◆ Abnormal mammography

PHYSICAL FINDINGS
◆ Clear, milky, or bloody nipple discharge, nipple retraction, scaly skin around the nipple, and skin changes, such as dimpling or inflammation
◆ Arm edema
◆ Hard lump, mass, or thickening of breast tissue
◆ Lymphadenopathy
◆ Rash

DIAGNOSTIC TEST RESULTS

◆ *Alkaline phosphatase levels and liver function and scans of bone, brain, liver or other organs:* distant metastasis

◆ *Hormonal receptor assay:* presence of an estrogen-dependent or a progesterone-dependent tumor

◆ *In vitro diagnostic multivariate index:* likelihood of breast cancer returning within 5 to 10 years

◆ *Mammography:* irregular mass or calcification

◆ *Ultrasonography:* fluid-filled cyst or solid mass

◆ *Chest X-ray:* chest metastasis location

◆ *Fine-needle aspiration and excisional biopsy:* presence of malignant cells upon histologic examination

◆ *Magnetic resonance imaging:* presence of abnormal cells

Treatment

◆ Varies by stage and type of disease, patient's age and menopausal status, and any disfiguring effects of surgery

◆ Possible combination of surgery, radiation, chemotherapy, hormone therapy, and biological therapy

◆ Primary radiation therapy

◆ Preoperative breast irradiation

◆ Arm-stretching exercises after surgery

◆ Lumpectomy

◆ Partial, total, or modified radical mastectomy

MEDICATIONS

◆ Chemotherapy, such as a combination of drugs, including cyclophosphamide (Cytoxan), fluorouracil (5-FU), methotrexate (Rheumatrex), doxorubicin (Adriamycin), vincristine (Oncovin), paclitaxel (Onxol), and prednisone (Deltasone)

◆ Regimen of cyclophosphamide, methotrexate, and fluorouracil (in premenopausal and postmenopausal women)

◆ Antiestrogen therapy such as tamoxifen (Nolvadex)

◆ Hormonal therapy, including estrogen (Premarin), progesterone (Prometrium), androgen, or antiandrogen aminoglutethimide (Cytaden) therapy

Nursing interventions

◆ Give prescribed drugs.

◆ Provide emotional support to the patient and family.

◆ Provide postoperative wound care.

◆ Assess for postoperative complications.

◆ Monitor vital signs.

◆ Assess the patient's pain level, administer analgesics, and evaluate their effects.

PATIENT TEACHING

◆ Explain the disorder, diagnostic testing, and treatment plan.

◆ Teach about the administration, dosage, and possible adverse effects of prescribed medications.

◆ Provide activities or exercises that promote healing.

◆ Demonstrate breast self-examination and stress the importance of obtaining a clinical breast examination by a healthcare professional as recommended by the American Cancer Society.

 Nursing alert

The American Cancer Society recommends that women ages 20 to 30 receive a clinical breast examination every 3 years and that women older than age 40 receive one every year.

◆ Describe risks and signs and symptoms of recurrence.

◆ Stress avoidance of venipuncture or blood pressure monitoring on the affected arm.

◆ Explain how to avoid the development of lymphedema in the affected arm.

◆ Refer the patient to local and national support groups.

Bronchitis, chronic

Overview

Chronic bronchitis, a form of chronic obstructive pulmonary disease, is the inflammation of the bronchial tube linings and is characterized by excessive production of tracheobronchial mucus with a cough for at least 3 months each year for 2 consecutive years. Its severity is linked to the amount of cigarette smoke or other pollutants inhaled and inhalation duration. Development of significant airway obstruction is seen in few patients with chronic bronchitis. It can occur alone or with emphysema.

CAUSES
◆ Cigarette smoking
◆ Environmental pollution
◆ Organic or inorganic dusts and noxious gas exposure
◆ Possible genetic predisposition
◆ Allergies
◆ Viral or bacterial infection

PATHOPHYSIOLOGY
◆ Hypertrophy and hyperplasia of the bronchial mucous glands, increased goblet cells, ciliary damage, squamous metaplasia of the columnar epithelium, and chronic leukocytic and lymphocytic infiltration of bronchial walls occur.
◆ Additionally, there's widespread inflammation, airway narrowing, and mucus within the airways, all producing resistance in the small airways and, consequently, a severe ventilation-perfusion imbalance.

COMPLICATIONS
◆ Cor pulmonale
◆ Pulmonary hypertension
◆ Right ventricular hypertrophy
◆ Acute respiratory failure

Assessment

HISTORY
◆ Long-time smoker
◆ Frequent upper respiratory tract infections
◆ Productive cough
◆ Fatigue
◆ Headaches
◆ Exertional dyspnea
◆ Cough, initially prevalent in winter, but gradually becoming year-round
◆ Worsening coughing episodes
◆ Worsening dyspnea

PHYSICAL FINDINGS
◆ Cough producing copious gray, white, or yellow sputum
◆ Cyanosis
◆ Accessory respiratory muscle use
◆ Tachypnea
◆ Substantial weight gain
◆ Pedal edema
◆ Jugular vein distention
◆ Wheezing
◆ Prolonged expiratory time
◆ Rhonchi

DIAGNOSTIC TEST RESULTS
◆ *Arterial blood gas (ABG) analysis:* decreased partial pressure of oxygen, normal or increased partial pressure of carbon dioxide
◆ *Sputum culture:* numbers of microorganisms and neutrophils
◆ *Chest X-ray or computed tomography of the chest:* hyperinflation and increased bronchovascular markings
◆ *Pulmonary function tests:* increased residual volume, decreased vital capacity, forced expiratory flow, normal static compliance and diffusing capacity
◆ *Electrocardiography:* atrial arrhythmias; peaked P waves in leads II, III, and aV_F; and right ventricular hypertrophy

Treatment

- Smoking cessation
- Avoidance of air pollutants
- Chest physiotherapy and breathing exercises
- Ultrasonic or mechanical nebulizer treatments
- Adequate fluid intake
- High-calorie, protein-rich diet
- Activity as tolerated with frequent rest periods
- Tracheostomy with advanced disease

MEDICATIONS
- Oxygen therapy
- Antibiotics
- Bronchodilators
- Corticosteroids
- Diuretics

Nursing interventions

- Administer oxygen therapy as needed and monitor ABG results.
- Give prescribed drugs.
- Monitor vital signs, intake and output, pulse oximetry, and daily weight.
- Assess sputum production and respiratory status.
- Perform chest physiotherapy.
- Ensure adequate oral fluid intake.
- Provide a high-calorie, protein-rich diet.
- Offer small, frequent meals.
- Encourage energy-conservation techniques.
- Encourage daily activity.
- Provide frequent rest periods.
- Evaluate the patient's response to treatment.
- Encourage the patient to express his fears and concerns.

PATIENT TEACHING
- Explain the disorder, diagnostic testing, and treatment plan.
- Teach about the administration, dosage, and possible adverse effects of prescribed medications.
- Explain infection-control practices.
- Stress the importance of influenza and pneumococcus immunizations.
- Arrange for home oxygen therapy, if required.
- Teach postural drainage and chest percussion, and coughing and deep-breathing exercises.
- Teach proper inhaler use.
- Review dietary recommendations and the importance of adequate hydration.
- Explain how to avoid inhaled irritants and prevent bronchospasm.
- Refer the patient to a smoking-cessation program, if indicated.
- Refer the patient to the American Lung Association for information and support.

Burns

Overview

A burn is tissue injury that may affect muscles, bone, nerves, and blood vessels. Burns are classified by method and degree. Methods include thermal, chemical, electrical, light, cold, and radiation. Degrees of burns are based on the extent of tissue damage and include superficial partial-thickness, deep partial-thickness, and full-thickness. They're also termed mild, moderate, or severe based on the method of the burn, degree of burn, areas affected, age of the patient, and whether the patient has any preexisting physical or mental conditions.

CAUSES
◆ Thermal: flame, heat from fire, steam, hot liquid or objects
◆ Chemical: acids, bases, and caustics
◆ Electrical: electrical current, lightning
◆ Light: light sources, ultraviolet light
◆ Cold: frostbite, dry ice, helium, liquid nitrogen
◆ Radiation: nuclear source, ultraviolet light

PATHOPHYSIOLOGY
Superficial partial-thickness burns (first-degree)
◆ Burn is limited to the epidermis; it isn't life-threatening.

Deep partial-thickness burns (second-degree)
◆ The epidermis is destroyed along with some dermis.
◆ Blisters are thin-walled and fluid-filled.
◆ When blisters break, nerve endings are exposed to the air, causing pain.
◆ The barrier function of the skin is lost.

Full-thickness burns (third- and fourth-degree)
◆ Every body system and organ is affected.
◆ Damage extends into the subcutaneous tissue layer.
◆ Muscle, bone, and interstitial tissues are damaged.
◆ Interstitial fluids cause edema.
◆ An immediate immunologic response occurs.
◆ Threat of wound sepsis occurs.

COMPLICATIONS
◆ Infection
◆ Anemia
◆ Hypovolemic shock
◆ Malnutrition
◆ Multiple organ dysfunction syndrome
◆ Respiratory collapse
◆ Sepsis

Assessment

HISTORY
◆ Cause of the burn

PHYSICAL FINDINGS
◆ Based on extent and cause of burn
◆ Superficial, partial, or full-thickness tissue injury
◆ Respiratory distress and cyanosis
◆ Edema
◆ Alteration in pulse rate, strength, and regularity
◆ Stridor, wheezing, crackles, and rhonchi
◆ Third or fourth heart sound
◆ Hypotension

DIAGNOSTIC TEST RESULTS
◆ *Arterial blood gas levels:* evidence of smoke inhalation, decreased alveolar function, and hypoxia
◆ *Electrolyte levels:* abnormal from fluid losses and shifts
◆ *Blood urea nitrogen level:* increased from fluid losses
◆ *Glucose level:* decreased in children as a result of limited glycogen storage
◆ *Urinalysis:* myoglobinuria and hemoglobinuria
◆ *Carboxyhemoglobin level:* increased

- *Electrocardiography:* myocardial ischemia, injury, or arrhythmias, especially in electrical burns
- *Fiber-optic bronchoscopy:* edema of the airways

Treatment

- Removal of burn source (while maintaining personal safety)
- Airway, breathing, and circulation assessed and secured
- I.V. fluids
- Wound care
- Nothing by mouth until severity of burn established; then high-protein, high-calorie diet
- Increased hydration with high-calorie, high-protein drinks (not free water)
- Total parenteral nutrition (if patient is unable to take food by mouth)
- Activity with limitations based on extent and location of burn
- Physical therapy
- Loose tissue and blister debridement
- Escharotomy
- Skin grafting

MEDICATIONS
- Oxygen therapy
- Tetanus toxoid booster
- Analgesics
- Antibiotics
- Antianxiolytics
- Osmotic diuretics

Nursing interventions

- Maintain a patent airway.
- Monitor vital signs, cardiac rhythm, intake and output, and pulse oximetry.
- Assess respiratory and cardiovascular status.
- Assess the patient's pain level, administer analgesics, and evaluate their effects.
- Perform appropriate wound care.
- Administer I.V. fluids.

- Obtain daily weight.
- Observe for signs and symptoms of complications.
- Encourage the client to verbalize his feelings and provide support.

PATIENT TEACHING
- Explain the injury, diagnostic testing, and treatment plan.
- Teach about the administration, dosage, and possible adverse effects of prescribed medications.
- Explain infection control practices.
- Demonstrate appropriate wound care.
- Review signs and symptoms of complications.
- Refer the patient to rehabilitation, if appropriate.
- Review safety measures for prevention, if indicated.
- Refer the patient to psychological counseling, if needed.
- Refer the patient to resources and support services.

Candidiasis

Overview

Candidiasis is a mild, superficial fungal infection, but it can lead to severe disseminated infections and fungemia in the immunocompromised patient, transplant recipient, burn patient, low-birth-weight neonate, or a patient on hyperalimentation.

CAUSES
◆ In most cases, infection with *Candida albicans* or *C. tropicalis*

RISK FACTORS
◆ Maternal vaginitis present during vaginal birth
◆ Preexisting diabetes mellitus, cancer, or immunosuppressant illness
◆ Immunosuppressant drug use
◆ Radiation
◆ Aging
◆ Irritation from dentures
◆ I.V. or urinary catheterization
◆ Drug abuse
◆ Total parenteral nutrition
◆ Surgery
◆ Use of antibiotic agents

PATHOPHYSIOLOGY
◆ A change in the patient's resistance to infection, his immunocompromised state, and antibiotic use permits the sudden proliferation of *C. albicans* or *C. tropicalis.*

COMPLICATIONS
◆ Dissemination
◆ Failure of the kidneys, brain, GI tract, eyes, lungs, and heart
◆ Septic shock

Assessment

HISTORY
◆ Underlying illness
◆ Recent course of antibiotic or antineoplastic therapy
◆ Drug abuse
◆ Hyperalimentation
◆ Dysphagia
◆ Painful intercourse
◆ Indigestion or heartburn
◆ Unusual menstrual cramping

PHYSICAL FINDINGS
◆ Scaly, erythematous, papular rash, possibly covered with exudate and erupting in breast folds, between fingers, and at the axillae, groin, and umbilicus
◆ Red, swollen, darkened nail beds; occasionally, purulent discharge; possibly nail separation from the nail bed
◆ Scales in the mouth and throat
◆ Cracked tongue, bleeding gums
◆ White or yellow vaginal discharge, with local excoriation; white or gray raised patches on vaginal walls, with local inflammation
◆ Cream-colored or bluish white lacelike patches of exudate on the tongue, mouth, or pharynx that reveal bloody engorgement when scraped
◆ Hemoptysis, cough; coarse breath sounds in the infected lung fields
◆ Flank pain, dysuria, hematuria, cloudy urine with casts
◆ Headache, nuchal rigidity, seizures, focal neurologic deficits
◆ Blurred vision, orbital or periorbital pain, eye exudate, floating scotomata, and lesions with a white, cotton-ball appearance seen during ophthalmoscopy
◆ Chest pain and arrhythmias

DIAGNOSTIC TEST RESULTS
◆ *Fungal serological panel:* candidal organism
◆ *Urine culture:* candidal organism
◆ *Ultrasound or computed tomography scan:* identifies abscesses or lesions

Treatment

- ◆ Treatment of predisposing condition
- ◆ With oral infection, spicy food only as tolerated
- ◆ Activity as tolerated
- ◆ Surgical or percutaneous abscess drainage

MEDICATIONS
- ◆ Antifungals (oral, topical, or I.V.)
- ◆ Amphotericin B (Fungizone)
- ◆ Topical anesthetics

Nursing interventions

- ◆ Follow standard precautions.
- ◆ Give prescribed drugs.
- ◆ Provide a nonirritating mouthwash to loosen tenacious secretions and a soft toothbrush to avoid irritation.
- ◆ Observe high-risk patients daily for patchy areas, irritation, sore throat, oral and gingival bleeding, and other signs of superinfection.
- ◆ Assess the patient for underlying systemic causes.
- ◆ Monitor vital signs and laboratory values.

PATIENT TEACHING
- ◆ Explain the disorder, diagnostic testing, and treatment plan.
- ◆ Teach about the administration, dosage, and possible adverse effects of prescribed medications.
- ◆ Teach good oral hygiene practices.
- ◆ Explain to a woman in her third trimester of pregnancy the need for examination for vaginitis to protect her neonate from thrush infection at birth.

Cardiac tamponade

Overview

Cardiac tamponade is the increase of intrapericardial pressure caused by fluid accumulation in the pericardial sac which can result in impaired diastolic filling of the heart.

CAUSES

◆ Acute myocardial infarction
◆ Cardiac catheterization
◆ Cardiac surgery
◆ Chronic renal failure
◆ Connective tissue disorders
◆ Drug reaction
◆ Effusion in cancer, bacterial infections, tuberculosis and, rarely, acute rheumatic fever
◆ Hemorrhage from nontraumatic cause
◆ Hypothyroidism
◆ May be idiopathic
◆ Pericarditis
◆ Radiation therapy to the chest
◆ Trauma
◆ Viral, postirradiation, or idiopathic pericarditis

PATHOPHYSIOLOGY

◆ Progressive accumulation of fluid in the pericardial sac causes compression of the heart chambers.
◆ Compression of the heart chambers obstructs blood flow into the ventricles and reduces the amount of blood pumped out with each contraction.
◆ With each contraction more fluid accumulates, decreasing cardiac output.

COMPLICATIONS

◆ Cardiogenic shock
◆ Death

Assessment

HISTORY

◆ Presence of one or more causes
◆ Dyspnea
◆ Shortness of breath
◆ Chest pain
◆ Palpitations
◆ Light-headedness

PHYSICAL FINDINGS

◆ Vary with volume of fluid and speed of fluid accumulation
◆ Diaphoresis
◆ Anxiety and restlessness
◆ Pallor or cyanosis
◆ Jugular vein distention
◆ Chest discomfort relieved by sitting in a forward-leaning position
◆ Edema
◆ Rapid, weak pulses
◆ Hepatomegaly
◆ Decreased arterial blood pressure
◆ Increased central venous pressure
◆ Pulsus paradoxus
◆ Narrow pulse pressure
◆ Muffled heart sounds

DIAGNOSTIC TEST RESULTS

◆ *Chest X-rays:* slightly widened mediastinum and enlargement of the cardiac silhouette
◆ *Electrocardiography:* low-voltage complexes in the precordial leads
◆ *Echocardiography:* echo-free space, indicating fluid in the pericardial sac
◆ *Hemodynamic monitoring:* equalization of mean right atrial, right ventricular diastolic, pulmonary artery wedge, and left ventricular diastolic pressures

Treatment

- Pericardiocentesis
- Pericardial window
- Subxiphoid or complete pericardiotomy
- Thoracotomy
- Diet as tolerated
- Bed rest during acute episode

MEDICATIONS
- Oxygen
- Intravascular volume expander
- Inotropic agents
- Analgesics

Nursing interventions

- Administer oxygen therapy as needed.
- Assist with pericardiocentesis if necessary.
- Monitor vital signs, cardiac rhythm, pulse oximetry, and intake and output.
- Assess respiratory and cardiovascular status.
- Give prescribed drugs and evaluate the patient's response.
- Infuse I.V. solutions as ordered.
- Maintain the chest drainage system if used.
- Provide emotional support.
- Observe for signs and symptoms of complications.
- Assess the patient's pain level, administer analgesics as indicated, and evaluate their effects.

PATIENT TEACHING
- Explain the disorder, diagnostic testing, and treatment plan.
- Teach about the administration, dosage, and possible adverse effects of prescribed medications.

- Describe signs and symptoms of recurring tamponade and when to notify the practitioner.
- Review preoperative and postoperative care.

Cardiomyopathy, dilated

Overview

Dilated cardiomyopathy, also called *congestive cardiomyopathy*, is a disease of the heart muscle fibers that affects heart function.

CAUSES
◆ Cardiotoxic effects of drugs or alcohol
◆ Chemotherapy
◆ Drug hypersensitivity
◆ Hypertension
◆ Idiopathic
◆ Ischemic heart disease
◆ Peripartum syndrome related to preeclampsia and eclampsia
◆ Valvular disease
◆ Viral or bacterial infections
◆ Diabetes mellitus
◆ Severe coronary artery disease

PATHOPHYSIOLOGY
◆ Extensively damaged myocardial muscle fibers reduce contractility of the left ventricle.
◆ As systolic function declines, cardiac output falls.
◆ The sympathetic nervous system is stimulated to increase heart rate and contractility.
◆ When compensatory mechanisms can no longer maintain cardiac output, the heart begins to fail. (See *Recognizing dilated cardiomyopathy.*)

COMPLICATIONS
◆ Intractable heart failure
◆ Arrhythmias
◆ Emboli

Assessment

HISTORY
◆ Possible history of a disorder that can cause cardiomyopathy
◆ Gradual onset of shortness of breath, orthopnea, dyspnea on exertion, paroxysmal nocturnal dyspnea, fatigue, dry cough at night, palpitations, and vague chest pain
◆ Weight gain

PHYSICAL FINDINGS
◆ Peripheral edema
◆ Jugular vein distention
◆ Ascites
◆ Peripheral cyanosis
◆ Tachycardia even at rest and pulsus alternans in late stages
◆ Hepatomegaly and splenomegaly
◆ Narrow pulse pressure
◆ Irregular rhythms, diffuse apical impulses, pansystolic murmur
◆ Third and fourth heart sound gallop rhythms
◆ Pulmonary crackles

DIAGNOSTIC TEST RESULTS
◆ *Angiography:* rules out ischemic heart disease
◆ *Chest X-rays:* moderate to marked cardiomegaly and possible pulmonary edema
◆ *Echocardiography:* ventricular thrombi, global hypokinesis, and the degrees of left ventricular dilation and systolic dysfunction
◆ *Gallium scans:* dilated cardiomyopathy and myocarditis
◆ *Cardiac catheterization:* left ventricular dilation and dysfunction, elevated left ventricular and, commonly, right ventricular filling pressures, and diminished cardiac output
◆ *Transvenous endomyocardial biopsy:* identifies underlying disorder
◆ *Electrocardiography:* ischemic heart disease, arrhythmias, and intraventricular conduction defects

Disorders

Treatment

- Low-sodium diet, supplemented by vitamin therapy
- No ingestion of alcohol if cardiomyopathy caused by alcoholism
- Rest periods
- Heart transplantation
- Possible cardiomyoplasty
- Biventricular pacemaker insertion

MEDICATIONS
- Oxygen
- Cardiac glycoside
- Diuretics
- Angiotensin-converting enzyme inhibitors
- Anticoagulants
- Vasodilators
- Antiarrhythmics
- Beta-adrenergic blockers

Nursing interventions

- Administer oxygen as needed and monitor pulse oximetry.
- Monitor vital signs, cardiac rhythm, intake and output, and laboratory values.
- Provide periods of rest with required activities of daily living.
- Assist with active range-of-motion (ROM) exercises or provide passive ROM exercises.
- Provide a low-sodium diet.
- Obtain daily weight.
- Administer medications and evaluate the patient's response to treatment.
- Assess respiratory and cardiovascular status.
- Offer emotional support.
- Allow the patient and his family to express their fears and concerns and help them identify effective coping strategies.

PATIENT TEACHING
- Explain the disorder, diagnostic testing, and treatment plan.
- Teach about the administration, dosage, and possible adverse effects of prescribed medications.
- Review sodium and fluid restrictions.
- Describe signs and symptoms of worsening heart failure and provide instruction on when to notify the practitioner.
- Provide information on available support services.

Recognizing dilated cardiomyopathy

Characteristics of dilated cardiomyopathy include:
- greatly increased chamber size
- thinning of left ventricular muscle
- increased atrial chamber size
- increased myocardial mass
- normal ventricular inflow resistance
- decreased contractility.

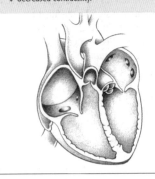

Cardiomyopathy, hypertrophic

Overview

Hypertrophic cardiomyopathy, also known as *hypertrophic obstructive cardiomyopathy* and *muscular aortic stenosis*, is a disease of cardiac muscle characterized by left ventricular hypertrophy.

CAUSES
◆ Associated with hypertension
◆ Transmission by autosomal dominant trait (about one-half of all cases)

PATHOPHYSIOLOGY
◆ The hypertrophied ventricle becomes stiff, noncompliant, and unable to relax during ventricular filling.
◆ Stiff walls resist filling and ventricular filling time is slowed.
◆ Compensation for decreased filling leads to hyperdynamic systolic dysfunction.
◆ Reduced ventricular filling leads to low cardiac output. (See *Recognizing hypertrophic cardiomyopathy.*)

COMPLICATIONS
◆ Pulmonary hypertension
◆ Heart failure
◆ Ventricular arrhythmias

Age considerations
Hypertrophic cardiomyopathy may trigger severe arrhythmias during the performance of heavy exercise, making it a major cause of death in young athletes.

Assessment

HISTORY
◆ Generally, no visible clinical features until disease is well advanced
◆ Blood flow to left ventricle abruptly reduced by atrial dilation and, sometimes, atrial fibrillation
◆ Possible family history of hypertrophic cardiomyopathy
◆ Orthopnea
◆ Dyspnea on exertion
◆ Anginal pain
◆ Fatigue
◆ Syncope, even at rest
◆ Palpitations

PHYSICAL FINDINGS
◆ Rapidly rising carotid arterial pulse possible
◆ Pulsus bisferiens
◆ Double or triple apical impulse, possibly displaced laterally
◆ Bibasilar crackles if heart failure is present
◆ Harsh systolic murmur heard after first heart sound at the apex near the left sternal border
◆ Possible fourth heart sound

DIAGNOSTIC TEST RESULTS
◆ *Chest X-rays:* mild to moderate increase in heart size
◆ *Thallium scan:* myocardial perfusion defects
◆ *Angiography:* dilated, diffusely hypokinetic left ventricle
◆ *Echocardiography:* left ventricular hypertrophy and a thick, asymmetrical intraventricular septum
◆ *Cardiac catheterization:* elevated left ventricular end-diastolic pressure and, possibly, mitral insufficiency
◆ *Electrocardiography:* left ventricular hypertrophy, ST-segment and T-wave abnormalities, Q waves in leads II, III, aV_F, and in V_4 to V_6 (because of hypertrophy, not infarction), left anterior hemiblock, left axis deviation, and ventricular and atrial arrhythmias

Treatment

- Cardioversion for atrial fibrillation
- Low-fat, low-sodium diet
- Fluid restrictions
- Avoidance of alcohol
- Individualized activity limitations
- Bed rest if necessary
- Ventricular myotomy alone or combined with mitral valve replacement
- Heart transplantation
- Implantable cardioverter-defibrillator insertion

MEDICATIONS

- Beta-adrenergic blockers
- Calcium channel blockers
- Amiodarone (Cordarone), unless atrioventricular block exists
- Antibiotic prophylaxis

Nursing interventions

- Monitor vital signs, cardiac rhythm, intake and output, and laboratory values.
- Assess respiratory and cardiovascular status.
- Provide periods of rest with required activities of daily living.
- Assist with active range-of-motion (ROM) exercises or provide passive ROM exercises.
- Provide a low-fat, low-sodium diet.
- Obtain daily weight.
- Administer medications and evaluate the patient's response to treatment.
- Offer emotional support.
- Allow the patient and his family to express their fears and concerns and help them identify effective coping strategies.

PATIENT TEACHING

- Explain the disorder, diagnostic testing, and treatment plan.
- Teach about the administration, dosage, and possible adverse effects of prescribed medications.
- Review sodium and fluid restrictions.
- Describe signs and symptoms of worsening heart failure and provide instruction on when to notify the practitioner.
- Provide information on available support services.
- Stress the need for antibiotic prophylaxis before dental work or surgery to prevent infective endocarditis.

Recognizing hypertrophic cardiomyopathy

Characteristics of hypertrophic cardiomyopathy include:

- normal right and decreased left chamber size
- left ventricular hypertrophy
- thickened interventricular septum (hypertrophic obstructive cardiomyopathy)
- atrial chamber size increased on left
- increased myocardial mass
- increased ventricular inflow resistance
- increased or decreased contractility.

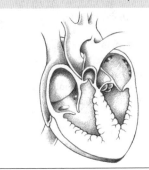

Cardiomyopathy, restrictive

Overview

The least common type of cardiomyopathy, restrictive cardiomyopathy is a disease of the heart muscle fibers that results in restrictive filling and reduced diastolic volume of either one or both ventricles. It's irreversible if severe.

CAUSES
◆ Carcinoid heart disease
◆ Heart transplant
◆ Idiopathic or associated with other disease (for example, amyloidosis or endomyocardial fibrosis)
◆ Mediastinal radiation

PATHOPHYSIOLOGY
◆ Stiffness of the ventricle is caused by left ventricular hypertrophy and endocardial fibrosis and thickening, thus reducing the ventricle's ability to relax and fill during diastole.
◆ Failure of the rigid myocardium to contract completely during systole causes decreased cardiac output. (See *Recognizing restrictive cardiomyopathy.*)

COMPLICATIONS
◆ Heart failure
◆ Arrhythmias
◆ Systemic or pulmonary embolization
◆ Sudden death

Assessment

HISTORY
◆ Fatigue
◆ Viral infection
◆ Dyspnea
◆ Orthopnea
◆ Chest pain

PHYSICAL FINDINGS
◆ Peripheral edema
◆ Liver engorgement and tenderness
◆ Ascites
◆ Peripheral cyanosis
◆ Pallor
◆ Third and fourth heart sound gallop rhythms (caused by heart failure)
◆ Systolic murmurs

DIAGNOSTIC TEST RESULTS
◆ *Complete blood count:* eosinophilia
◆ *Chest X-ray:* cardiomegaly
◆ *Radionuclide imaging:* increased diffuse uptake in cardiac amyloidosis
◆ *Echocardiography:* left ventricular muscle mass, normal or reduced left ventricular cavity size, and decreased systolic function
◆ *Electrocardiography:* low-voltage hypertrophy, atrioventricular conduction defects, and arrhythmias
◆ *Cardiac catheterization:* reduced systolic function and myocardial infiltration and increased left ventricular end-diastolic pressures

Treatment

◆ Treatment of underlying cause
◆ Low-sodium diet
◆ Initially, bed rest, then activity as tolerated
◆ Permanent pacemaker
◆ Heart transplantation

MEDICATIONS
◆ Digoxin (Lanoxin)
◆ Diuretics
◆ Vasodilators
◆ Angiotensin-converting enzyme inhibitors
◆ Anticoagulants
◆ Corticosteroids

Nursing interventions

◆ Give prescribed drugs.
◆ Monitor vital signs, cardiac rhythm, intake and output, and hemodynamic parameters.
◆ Provide emotional support.
◆ Provide appropriate diversions for the patient restricted to prolonged bed rest.
◆ Obtain daily weight.

PATIENT TEACHING
◆ Explain the disorder, diagnostic testing, and treatment plan.
◆ Teach about the administration, dosage, and possible adverse effects of prescribed medications.
◆ Review sodium and fluid restrictions.
◆ Describe signs and symptoms of worsening heart failure and when to notify the practitioner.
◆ Provide information on available support services.
◆ Stress the importance of recording daily weight and reporting weight gain of 2 lb (0.9 kg) or more.

Recognizing restrictive cardiomyopathy

Characteristics of restrictive cardiomyopathy include:
◆ decreased ventricular chamber size
◆ left ventricular hypertrophy
◆ increased atrial chamber size
◆ normal myocardial mass
◆ increased ventricular inflow resistance
◆ decreased contractility.

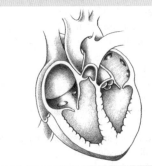

Carpal tunnel syndrome

Overview

Carpal tunnel syndrome is the compression of the median nerve in the wrist and results in numbness, tingling, and pain in the hand and wrist. It's the most common nerve entrapment syndrome. Carpal tunnel syndrome may pose a serious occupational health problem, requiring a change in occupation.

Causes
◆ Exact cause unknown
◆ Acute sprain that may damage the median nerve
◆ Arthritis
◆ Amyloidosis
◆ Dislocation
◆ Edema-producing conditions
◆ Gout
◆ Repetitive wrist motions involving excessive flexion or extension
◆ Tumors

Risk factors
◆ Obesity
◆ Diabetes
◆ Pregnancy
◆ Alcoholism
◆ Hypothyroidism
◆ Renal failure

Pathophysiology
◆ A space-occupying lesion or direct pressure within the carpal canal increases pressure on the median nerve, resulting in compression.
◆ Compression of the median nerve interrupts normal function. (See *The carpal tunnel.*)

Complications
◆ Tendon inflammation
◆ Compression
◆ Neural ischemia
◆ Permanent nerve damage with loss of movement and sensation

Assessment

History
◆ Occupation or hobby requiring strenuous or repetitive use of the hands
◆ Condition that causes swelling in carpal tunnel structures
◆ Weakness, pain, burning, numbness, or tingling that occurs in one or both hands
◆ Paresthesia that worsens at night and in the morning
◆ Pain that spreads to the forearm and, in severe cases, as far as the shoulder
◆ Pain that can be relieved by shaking hands vigorously or dangling the arms at sides

Physical findings
◆ Inability to make a fist
◆ Fingernails may be atrophied, with surrounding dry, shiny skin

Diagnostic test results
◆ *Magnetic resonance imaging:* identifies causitive lesions
◆ *Electromyography:* median nerve motor conduction delay of more than 5 msec
◆ *Digital electrical stimulation:* median nerve compression
◆ *Phalen test:* positive
◆ *Tinel test:* positive

Treatment

◆ Initially, conservative: wrist splinting, possible occupation change, correction of underlying disorder
◆ Activity as tolerated, restrictions or therapy as prescribed
◆ Surgical nerve decompression
◆ Neurolysis

Medications
◆ Nonsteroidal anti-inflammatory drugs
◆ Corticosteroids
◆ Vitamin B complex

Nursing interventions

- Promote self-care.
- Assess the patient's pain level, administer analgesics as ordered, and evaluate their effects.
- Assist with prescribed exercises.
- Evaluate color, sensation, and motion of the affected hand.
- Apply a splint to the affected wrist, as ordered.
- If surgery is performed, assess the incision and provide wound care.

PATIENT TEACHING

- Explain the disorder, diagnostic testing, and treatment plan.
- Teach about the administration, dosage, and possible adverse effects of prescribed medications.
- Demonstrate splint application.
- Review exercises recommended by physical therapy.
- Refer the patient for occupational counseling if a job change is necessary.

The carpal tunnel

The carpal tunnel is clearly visible in this palmar view and cross section of a right hand. Note the median nerve, flexor tendons of fingers, and blood vessels passing through the tunnel on their way from the forearm to the hand.

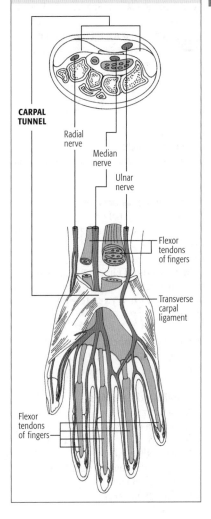

CARPAL TUNNEL

Radial nerve

Median nerve

Ulnar nerve

Flexor tendons of fingers

Transverse carpal ligament

Flexor tendons of fingers

Cataract

Overview

A cataract is opacity of the eye's lens or lens capsule that causes gradual vision loss. Cataracts commonly affect both eyes, although a traumatic cataract is usually unilateral. Cataracts can be classified as senile, congenital, traumatic, complicated, or toxic.

 Age considerations

Cataracts are most prevalent in people older than age 70. More than one-half of all people older than age 80 in the United States have a cataract or have had surgery to remove a cataract.

CAUSES

Senile cataracts
◆ Chemical changes in lens proteins in elderly patients

Congenital cataracts
◆ Congenital anomaly
◆ Genetic causes (usually autosomal dominant)
◆ Inborn errors of metabolism
◆ Maternal rubella infection during the first trimester
◆ Sex-linked cause (with recessive cataracts)

Traumatic cataracts
◆ Foreign bodies, causing aqueous or vitreous humor to enter lens capsule

Complicated cataracts
◆ Atopic dermatitis
◆ Diabetes mellitus
◆ Glaucoma
◆ Hypoparathyroidism
◆ Ionizing radiation or infrared rays
◆ Retinal detachment
◆ Retinitis pigmentosa
◆ Uveitis

Toxic cataracts
◆ Drug or chemical toxicity from dinitrophenol, ergot, naphthalene, phenothiazines, or corticosteroids

PATHOPHYSIOLOGY
◆ Clouded lens blocks light shining through the cornea.
◆ Images cast onto the retina are blurred.
◆ A hazy image is interpreted by the brain.

COMPLICATIONS
◆ Complete vision loss

Postoperative
◆ Loss of vitreous humor
◆ Wound dehiscence
◆ Hyphema
◆ Pupillary block glaucoma
◆ Retinal detachment
◆ Infection

Assessment

HISTORY
◆ Painless, gradual vision loss
◆ Blinding glare from headlights with night driving
◆ Poor reading vision
◆ Annoying glare
◆ Poor vision in bright sunlight
◆ Better vision in dim light than in bright light (central opacity)
◆ Diplopia
◆ Fading of colors
◆ Frequent changes in eyeglass prescriptions

PHYSICAL FINDINGS
◆ Milky white pupil on inspection with a penlight
◆ Grayish white area behind the pupil (advanced cataract)
◆ Red reflex lost (mature cataract)

DIAGNOSTIC TEST RESULTS
◆ *Indirect ophthalmoscopy:* dark area in the normally homogeneous red reflex
◆ *Slit-lamp examination:* lens opacity
◆ *Visual acuity test:* degree of vision loss

Treatment

◆ Eyeglasses and contact lenses before surgery
◆ Sunglasses in bright light
◆ Lamps to provide reflected lighting rather than direct lighting, decreasing glare and aiding vision
◆ Restricted activity according to vision loss
◆ Lens extraction and implantation of intraocular lens
◆ Extracapsular or intracapsular cataract extraction
◆ Phacoemulsification (emulsifying and aspirating the cataract using an ultrasonic needle)

MEDICATIONS
For cataract removal
◆ Nonsteroidal anti-inflammatory drugs
◆ Short-acting local anesthetic

Nursing interventions

◆ Perform routine postoperative care.
◆ Assist with early ambulation.
◆ Administer eye drops as ordered.
◆ Apply an eye shield or eye patch postoperatively as ordered.
◆ Monitor vital signs and visual acuity.
◆ Observe for complications of surgery.

PATIENT TEACHING
◆ Explain the disorder, diagnostic testing, and treatment plan.
◆ Teach about the administration, dosage, and possible adverse effects of prescribed medications.

 Nursing alert

Stress the need to avoid activities that increase intraocular pressure, such as straining with coughing, bowel movements, or lifting.
◆ Demonstrate proper instillation of ophthalmic ointment or drops.
◆ Stress the importance of follow-up care.

Cellulitis

Overview

Cellulitis is an acute infection of the dermis and subcutaneous tissue that causes cell inflammation. It may follow damage to the skin, such as a bite or wound. With timely treatment, the prognosis is usually good.

CAUSES

◆ Bacterial infections, usually by *Staphylococcus aureus* and group A beta-hemolytic streptococci
◆ Extension of a skin wound or ulcer
◆ Fungal infections
◆ Furuncles or carbuncles

RISK FACTORS

◆ Venous and lymphatic compromise
◆ Edema
◆ Diabetes mellitus
◆ Underlying skin lesion
◆ Chronic steroid use
◆ Prior trauma
◆ Advanced age (associated with thrombophlebitis from lower extremity cellulitis)

PATHOPHYSIOLOGY

◆ A break in skin integrity almost always precedes the infection.
◆ As the offending organism invades the compromised area, it overwhelms the defensive cells, including the neutrophils, eosinophils, basophils, and mast cells that normally contain and localize the inflammation.
◆ As cellulitis progresses, the organism invades tissue around the initial wound site.

COMPLICATIONS

◆ Sepsis
◆ Deep vein thrombosis
◆ Progression of cellulitis
◆ Local abscesses
◆ Thrombophlebitis
◆ Lymphangitis
◆ Amputation

Assessment

HISTORY

◆ Presence of one or more risk factors
◆ Tenderness
◆ Pain at the site and possibly surrounding area
◆ Erythema and warmth
◆ Edema
◆ Possible fever, chills, malaise

PHYSICAL FINDINGS

◆ Erythema with indistinct margins
◆ Drainage or leakage of clear yellow fluid from the skin
◆ Large blisters
◆ Fever
◆ Warmth and tenderness of the skin
◆ Regional lymph node enlargement and tenderness
◆ Red streaking visible in skin proximal to area of cellulitis

DIAGNOSTIC TEST RESULTS

◆ *White blood cell count:* mild leukocytosis
◆ *Erythrocyte sedimentation rate:* elevated
◆ *Culture and Gram stain:* causative organism

Treatment

◆ Immobilization and elevation of the affected extremity
◆ Moist heat to affected area
◆ Well-balanced diet
◆ Bed rest (with severe infection)
◆ Possible tracheostomy (with severe cellulitis of head and neck)
◆ Possible abscess drainage
◆ Amputation (with gas-forming cellulitis [gangrene])

MEDICATIONS

◆ Antibiotics
◆ Topical antifungals
◆ Analgesics

Nursing interventions

◆ Give prescribed drugs.
◆ Elevate the affected extremity.
◆ Apply moist heat, as ordered.
◆ Encourage a well-balanced diet and adequate fluid intake.
◆ Encourage the patient to verbalize his feelings and concerns.
◆ Institute safety precautions.
◆ Monitor vital signs and laboratory results.
◆ Assess the patient's pain level, administer analgesics, and evaluate their effects.
◆ Observe for signs and symptoms of complications.

PATIENT TEACHING
◆ Explain the disorder, diagnostic testing, and treatment plan.
◆ Teach about the administration, dosage, and possible adverse effects of prescribed medications.
◆ Demonstrate how to use warm compresses.
◆ Explain the signs and symptoms of complications.
◆ Review ways to prevent injury and trauma.
◆ Refer the patient for management of diabetes mellitus, if indicated.

Cerebral contusion

Overview

A cerebral contusion is ecchymosis of brain tissue that results from injury to the head.

CAUSES
- Acceleration-deceleration or coup-contrecoup injuries
- Falls
- Gun-shot wounds
- Head trauma
- Motor vehicle collisions
- Stab wounds

RISK FACTORS
- Unsteady gait
- Participation in contact sports
- Receiving anticoagulant therapy

PATHOPHYSIOLOGY
- Trauma to the head causes tearing or twisting of the structures and blood vessels of the brain.
- Scattered hemorrhages form over the brain's surface.
- Functional disruption occurs and may be prolonged.

COMPLICATIONS
- Intracranial hemorrhage
- Hematoma
- Tentorial herniation
- Respiratory failure
- Seizures
- Neurologic deficits
- Brain hemorrhage
- Increased intracranial pressure

Assessment

HISTORY
- Head injury or motor vehicle accident
- Loss of consciousness
- Seizure

PHYSICAL FINDINGS
- Unconscious patient: pale and motionless, altered vital signs
- Conscious patient: drowsy or easily disturbed
- Abnromal pupil size or reaction
- Nausea, vomiting
- Memory loss or forgetfulness
- Scalp wound
- Possible involuntary evacuation of bowel and bladder
- Hemiparesis
- Personality changes

DIAGNOSTIC TEST RESULTS
- *Computed tomography, magnetic resonance imaging:* areas of damage
- *Electroencephalography, cerebral angiography:* areas of damage and interrupted blood flow

Treatment

- Establishing a patent airway
- I.V. fluid administration
- Minimizing environmental stimuli
- Nothing by mouth until fully conscious
- Activity based on neurologic status
- Initially, bed rest, with proper positioning with head of bed raised to promote drainage
- Craniotomy
- Suturing open wounds

MEDICATIONS
- Nonopioid analgesics
- Anticonvulsants
- Antibiotics
- Corticosteroids

Nursing interventions

◆ Maintain a patent airway.
◆ Monitor vital signs and neurologic status.
◆ Give prescribed drugs.

 Nursing alert
Avoid giving aspirin because it increases the chance of bleeding.

◆ Protect the client from injury.
◆ Check for cerebrospinal fluid leakage.

PATIENT TEACHING

◆ Explain the disorder, diagnostic testing, and treatment plan.
◆ Teach about the administration, dosage, and possible adverse effects of prescribed medications.
◆ Stress the need to avoid coughing, sneezing, or blowing the nose until after recovery.
◆ Describe how to detect and report mental status changes.
◆ Explain the need to avoid contact sports.
◆ Stress the importance of avoiding smoking and alcohol.
◆ Describe the signs and symptoms of complications.
◆ Refer the patient to a social worker for further support and counseling, as needed.

Cholelithiasis, cholecystitis, and related disorders

Overview

Cholelithiasis, the leading biliary tract disease, is the formation of calculi (gallstones) in the gallbladder. Cholecystitis, a related disorder, is the acute or chronic inflammation of the gallbladder. Choledocholithiasis is a partial or complete biliary obstruction. Cholangitis is an infected bile duct commonly linked to choledocholithiasis. Gallstone ileus is the obstruction of the small bowel related to gallstone formation.

CAUSES
◆ Cholelithiasis: precipitation of cholesterol and bile salts
◆ Cholecystitis: gallstone lodged in the cystic duct
◆ Acute cholecystitis: gallbladder's inability to fill or empty from trauma, reduced blood supply, prolonged immobility, chronic dieting, adhesions, prolonged anesthesia, and opioid abuse
◆ Choledocholithiasis: gallstones lodged in the common bile duct
◆ Gallstone ileus: gallstone lodged in the small bowel

RISK FACTORS
◆ High-calorie, high-cholesterol diet
◆ Obesity
◆ Elevated estrogen levels from hormonal contraceptive use, postmenopausal hormone replacement therapy, or pregnancy
◆ Diabetes mellitus, ileal disease, hemolytic disorders, hepatic disease (cirrhosis), or pancreatitis
◆ Rapid weight loss

PATHOPHYSIOLOGY
◆ Calculi formation in the biliary system causes obstruction.
◆ Obstruction of the hepatic duct leads to intrahepatic retention of bile and increased release of bilirubin into the bloodstream.
◆ Obstruction of the cystic duct leads to inflammation of the gallbladder and increased gallbladder contraction and peristalsis.
◆ Obstruction of bile causes impairment of digestion and absorption of lipids.

COMPLICATIONS
Cholelithiasis
◆ Cholangitis
◆ Cholecystitis
◆ Choledocholithiasis
◆ Gallstone ileus

Cholecystitis
◆ Gallbladder complications, such as empyema, hydrops or mucocele, and gangrene
◆ Chronic cholecystitis and cholangitis

Choledocholithiasis
◆ Cholangitis
◆ Obstructive jaundice
◆ Pancreatitis
◆ Secondary biliary cirrhosis

Cholangitis
◆ Septic shock
◆ Death

Gallstone ileus
◆ Bowel obstruction

Assessment

HISTORY
◆ May be asymptomatic (even when X-rays reveal gallstones)

Gallbladder attack
◆ Sudden onset of severe steady or aching pain in the midepigastric region or the right upper abdominal quadrant
◆ Pain radiating to the back, between the shoulder blades or over the right shoulder blade, or just to the shoulder area
◆ Attack occurring after eating a fatty meal or a large meal after fasting for an extended time
◆ Nausea, vomiting, and chills

◆ Low-grade fever
◆ History of indigestion, vague abdominal discomfort, belching, and flatulence after eating high-fat meals or snacks

PHYSICAL FINDINGS

◆ Severe pain
◆ Pallor
◆ Diaphoresis
◆ Low-grade fever (high fever in cholangitis)
◆ Exhaustion
◆ Jaundice (chronic)
◆ Dark-colored urine and clay-colored stools
◆ Tachycardia
◆ Murphy's sign
◆ Palpable, painless, sausagelike mass (calculus-filled gallbladder without ductal obstruction)
◆ Hypoactive bowel sounds

DIAGNOSTIC TEST RESULTS

◆ *Serum alkaline phosphatase, lactate dehydrogenase, aspartate aminotransferase, icteric index, and total bilirubin studies:* elevated (during attack)
◆ *White blood cell count:* slightly elevated (during attack)
◆ *Abdominal X-rays:* radiopaque gallstones containing calcium; porcelain gallbladder, limy bile, and gallstone ileus
◆ *Gallbladder ultrasonography:* cholelithiasis in most patients, distinction between obstructive and nonobstructive jaundice; calculi as small as 2 mm
◆ *Endoscopic retrograde cholangiopancreatography:* gallstones, narrowing of the bile ducts
◆ *Oral cholecystography (gradually being replaced by ultrasonography):* gallstones
◆ *Technetium-labeled iminodiacetic acid gallbladder scan:* cystic duct obstruction and acute or chronic cholecystitis
◆ *Percutaneous transhepatic cholangiography imaging performed under fluoroscopic guidance:* obstructive jaundice, visualization of calculi in the ducts

Treatment

◆ Endoscopic retrograde cholangiopancreatography to visualize and remove calculi
◆ Lithotripsy
◆ Low-fat diet
◆ Nothing by mouth (if surgery is required)
◆ Cholecystectomy (laparoscopic or abdominal), cholecystectomy with operative cholangiography, choledochostomy, or exploration of the common bile duct

MEDICATIONS

◆ Gallstone dissolution therapy, such as with ursodiol (Actigall)
◆ Bile salts
◆ Analgesics
◆ Antispasmodics
◆ Anticholinergics
◆ Antiemetics
◆ Antibiotics

Nursing interventions

◆ Give prescribed drugs.
◆ Assess the patient's pain level, administer analgesics, and evaluate their effects.

After surgery

◆ Observe for signs and symptoms of complications.
◆ Assess the wound site and provide wound care.
◆ Check T-tube patency and drainage.

PATIENT TEACHING

◆ Explain the disorder, diagnostic testing, and treatment plan.
◆ Teach about the administration, dosage, and possible adverse effects of prescribed medications.
◆ Demonstrate how to breathe deeply, cough, expectorate, and perform leg exercises that are necessary after surgery.
◆ Review dietary modifications.
◆ Teach appropriate wound care.

Cirrhosis

Overview

Cirrhosis is a chronic disease that causes hepatic dysfunction. Types of cirrhosis include Laënnec's, postnecrotic, biliary, and idiopathic.

CAUSES

Laënnec's or micronodular cirrhosis
◆ Chronic alcoholism
◆ Malnutrition

Postnecrotic or macronodular cirrhosis
◆ Viral hepatitis
◆ Exposure to such liver toxins as arsenic, carbon tetrachloride, and phosphorus

Biliary cirrhosis
◆ Prolonged biliary tract obstruction or inflammation

Idiopathic cirrhosis (cryptogenic)
◆ Chronic inflammatory bowel disease
◆ Sarcoidosis

RISK FACTORS
◆ Alcoholism
◆ Toxins
◆ Biliary obstruction
◆ Hepatitis
◆ Metabolic disorders

PATHOPHYSIOLOGY
◆ Diffuse destruction and fibrotic regeneration of hepatic cells occurs.
◆ Necrotic tissue yields to fibrosis.
◆ Liver structure and normal vasculature are altered.
◆ Blood and lymph flow are impaired.
◆ Hepatic insufficiency occurs.

COMPLICATIONS
◆ Portal hypertension
◆ Bleeding esophageal varices
◆ Hepatic encephalopathy
◆ Hepatorenal syndrome
◆ Death

Assessment

HISTORY
◆ Chronic alcoholism
◆ Malnutrition
◆ Viral hepatitis
◆ Exposure to liver toxins, such as arsenic and certain medications
◆ Prolonged biliary tract obstruction or inflammation

Early stage
◆ Vague signs and symptoms
◆ Abdominal pain
◆ Diarrhea, constipation
◆ Fatigue
◆ Loss of appetite
◆ Nausea, vomiting
◆ Muscle cramps

Later stage
◆ Chronic dyspepsia
◆ Constipation
◆ Jaundice
◆ Pruritus
◆ Weight loss
◆ Bleeding tendency, such as frequent nosebleeds, easy bruising, and bleeding gums
◆ Hepatic encephalopathy

PHYSICAL FINDINGS
◆ Telangiectasis on the cheeks
◆ Spider angiomas on the face, neck, arms, and trunk
◆ Gynecomastia
◆ Umbilical hernia
◆ Distended abdominal blood vessels
◆ Ascites
◆ Testicular atrophy
◆ Palmar erythema
◆ Clubbed fingers
◆ Thigh and leg edema
◆ Ecchymosis
◆ Jaundice
◆ Palpable, large, firm liver with a sharp edge (early finding)
◆ Enlarged spleen

◆ Asterixis
◆ Slurred speech, paranoia, hallucinations

DIAGNOSTIC TEST RESULTS

◆ *Liver enzymes, such as alanine aminotransferase, aspartate aminotransferase, total serum bilirubin:* elevated
◆ *Indirect bilirubin:* elevated
◆ *Total serum albumin and protein levels:* decreased
◆ *Prothrombin time:* prolonged
◆ *Hemoglobin, hematocrit, and serum electrolyte levels:* decreased
◆ *Vitamins A, C, and K:* deficient
◆ *Urine levels of bilirubin and urobilinogen:* increased
◆ *Fecal urobilinogen levels:* decreased
◆ *Ammonia levels:* elevated
◆ *Abdominal X-rays:* increased liver and spleen size, and cysts or gas in the biliary tract or liver; liver calcification; massive ascites
◆ *Computed tomography and liver scans:* increased liver size, liver masses, possible obstructed hepatic blood flow
◆ *Radioisotope liver scans:* increased liver size, decreased blood flow, or obstruction
◆ *Liver biopsy:* hepatic tissue destruction and fibrosis
◆ *Esophagogastroduodenoscopy:* bleeding esophageal varices, stomach irritation or ulceration, and duodenal bleeding and irritation

Treatment

◆ Removal or alleviation of underlying cause
◆ Paracentesis for ascites
◆ Esophageal balloon tamponade for bleeding
◆ Sclerotherapy
◆ I.V. fluids
◆ Transfusion of blood products
◆ Restricted sodium consumption and high-calorie diet
◆ Restricted fluid intake
◆ Cessation of alcohol consumption

◆ Frequent rest periods, as needed
◆ Peritoneovenous shunt
◆ Portal-systemic shunts
◆ Transplantation

MEDICATIONS

◆ Vitamin and nutritional supplements
◆ Antacids
◆ Potassium-sparing diuretics
◆ Beta-adrenergic blockers and vasopressin
◆ Ammonia detoxicant
◆ Antiemetics

Nursing interventions

◆ Give prescribed I.V. fluids, blood products, and drugs.
◆ Encourage the client to verbalize his feelings and provide support.
◆ Provide appropriate skin care.
◆ Monitor vital signs and laboratory values.
◆ Assess hydration and nutritional status.
◆ Measure abdominal girth and take weight daily.
◆ Observe for signs of bleeding.
◆ Assess and maintain skin integrity.
◆ Monitor for changes in mentation and behavior.

PATIENT TEACHING

◆ Explain the disorder, diagnostic testing, and treatment plan.
◆ Teach about the administration, dosage, and possible adverse effects of prescribed medications.
◆ Review dietary modifications.
◆ Stress the need to abstain from alcohol and avoid sedatives and acetaminophen (hepatotoxic).
◆ Encourage follow-up care.
◆ Refer the patient to Alcoholics Anonymous if appropriate.
◆ Refer the patient for psychological counseling if needed.

Clostridium difficile infection

Overview

Clostridium difficile is a gram-positive anaerobic bacterium that typically causes antibiotic-related diarrhea. Symptoms range from asymptomatic carrier states to severe pseudomembranous colitis caused by exotoxins (toxin A is an enterotoxin and toxin B is a cytotoxin).

CAUSES
- Antibiotics that disrupt the bowel flora
- Enemas and intestinal stimulants
- Some antifungal and antiviral agents
- Transmission from infected person

RISK FACTORS
- Contaminated equipment and surfaces
- Antibiotics
- Abdominal surgery
- Antineoplastic agents that have an antibiotic activity
- Immunocompromised state

PATHOPHYSIOLOGY
- Antibiotics may trigger toxin production.
- Toxin A mediates alteration in fluid secretion, enhances inflammation, and causes leakage of albumin from the postcapillary venules.
- Toxin B causes damage and exfoliation to the superficial epithelial cells and inhibits adenosine diphosphate ribosylation of Rho proteins.
- Both toxins cause electrophysiologic alterations of colonic tissue.

COMPLICATIONS
- Electrolyte abnormalities
- Hypovolemic shock
- Toxic megacolon
- Colonic perforation
- Peritonitis
- Sepsis
- Hemorrhage
- Pseudomembranous colitis

Assessment

HISTORY
- Recent antibiotic therapy
- Abdominal pain
- Cramping

PHYSICAL FINDINGS
- Soft, unformed, or watery diarrhea (more than three stools in a 24-hour period) that may be foul smelling or grossly bloody
- Abdominal tenderness
- Fever

DIAGNOSTIC TEST RESULTS
- *Cell cytotoxin test:* presence of toxins A and B
- *Stool culture:* presence of *C. difficile*

Treatment

- Withdrawal of causative antibiotic
- Avoidance of antimotility agents
- Good skin care
- Well-balanced diet
- Increased fluid intake if appropriate
- Rest periods if fatigued

MEDICATIONS
- Metronidazole (Flagyl)
- Vancomycin (Vancocin)
- Low-dose vancomycin (if relapse and previous treatment was metronidazole)
- Combination of vancomycin and rifampin (Rifadin)
- *Saccharomyces boulardii* (a yeast) with metronidazole or vancomycin and biologic vaccines to restore the normal GI flora (experimental)
- Lactobacillus
- Cholestyramine (Questran)

Nursing interventions

♦ Give prescribed drugs.
♦ Institute enteric precautions for those with active diarrhea.
♦ Enforce proper hand washing for all visitors.
♦ Make sure reusable equipment is disinfected before it's used on another patient.
♦ Monitor vital signs, intake and output, and laboratory results.
♦ Observe for signs and symptoms of complications.
♦ Assess the patient's response to treatment.
♦ Note amount and characteristics of stools.
♦ Assess and maintain skin integrity.

PATIENT TEACHING
♦ Explain the disorder, diagnostic testing, and treatment plan.
♦ Teach about the administration, dosage, and possible adverse effects of prescribed medications.
♦ Demonstrate proper hand-washing technique.
♦ Stress proper disinfection of contaminated clothing or household items.
♦ Review dietary and fluid needs.
♦ Describe signs and symptoms of dehydration.

Complex regional pain syndrome

Disorders

Overview

Complex regional pain syndrome (CRPS), also known as *reflex sympathetic dystrophy* or *causalgia*, is a chronic pain condition that results from abnormal healing after minor or major injury to a bone, muscle, or nerve. It generally affects one of the arms, legs, hands, or feet; however, it can spread.

CAUSES
◆ Exact cause unknown

 Age consideration
CRPS most commonly occurs in adults between the ages of 40 and 60.

RISK FACTORS
◆ Trauma
◆ Neurologic disorder
◆ Herpes zoster infection
◆ Myocardial infarction
◆ Musculoskeletal disorder (shoulder rotator cuff injury)
◆ Malignancy

PATHOPHYSIOLOGY
◆ Abnormal functioning of the sympathetic nervous system causes symptoms commonly disproportionate to the injury's severity.
◆ Interference with normal signals for sensations, temperature, and blood flow may be caused by impaired communication between the damaged nerves of the sympathetic nervous system and the brain.

COMPLICATIONS
◆ Impaired mobility
◆ Depression

Assessment

HISTORY
◆ Injury
◆ Intense burning or aching pain
◆ Severe pain that worsens after activity
◆ Muscle spasms

PHYSICAL FINDINGS
◆ Altered blood flow, feeling either warm or cool to the touch, with discoloration, sweating, or swelling to the affected extremity
◆ Skin, hair, and nail changes
◆ Skin sensitivity
◆ Impaired mobility and weakness

Stages of complex regional pain syndrome

Complex regional pain syndrome is divided into three stages. The stages aren't always distinct and not all of the signs may be present.

Stage	Duration	Pain, swelling, and immobility
I (acute)	◆ May begin within hours, days, or weeks of the injury; lasts several weeks	◆ Gradual or abrupt onset of severe aching, throbbing, and burning pain at site of injury ◆ May be accompanied by sensitivity to touch, swelling, muscle spasm, stiffness, and limited mobility
II (subacute or dystrophic)	◆ Lasts 3 to 6 months	◆ Continuous burning, aching, or throbbing pain that's more severe than stage I ◆ Spreading of swelling that changes from soft to brawny and firm ◆ Loss of range of motion, muscle wasting
III (chronic or atrophic)	◆ Lasts more than 6 months	◆ Proximal spreading of pain; may be intractable, but sometimes lessens and stabilizes ◆ More distinct dystrophic changes and irreversible tissue damage ◆ Muscle atrophy and contractures

♦ Muscle wasting (see *Stages of complex regional pain syndrome*)

DIAGNOSTIC TEST RESULTS
♦ *Bone X-rays:* diffuse inceased activity with increased uptake and scintigraphic abnormalities
♦ *Quantitative sensory testing:* determines heat and pain threshholds

Treatment
♦ Physical, cold, or heat therapy
♦ Occupational and recreational therapy
♦ Activity as tolerated
♦ Surgical sympathectomy
♦ Transcutaneous electrical nerve stimulator (TENS)
♦ Biofeedback
♦ Spinal cord stimulation
♦ Intrathecal pump

MEDICATIONS
♦ Anti-inflammatories
♦ Antidepressants
♦ Vasodilators
♦ Analgesics
♦ Nerve blocks
♦ Morphine pump

Nursing interventions
♦ Assess the patient's pain level, administer analgesics, and evaluate their effects.
♦ Offer alternate methods of pain control, such as massage.
♦ Provide emotional support.
♦ Apply antiembolism stockings.
♦ Apply heat or cold therapy.
♦ Monitor pain control.
♦ Monitor effects of medications.
♦ Monitor blood glucose level.

PATIENT TEACHING
♦ Explain the disorder, diagnostic testing, and treatment plan.
♦ Teach about the administration, dosage, and possible adverse effects of prescribed medications.
♦ Teach relaxation techniques.
♦ Provide information about the TENS unit and implantable pump, as indicated.
♦ Refer the patient for home therapy or for physical or occupational therapy.
♦ Refer the patient to a pain care specialist.
♦ Refer the patient for psychological counseling and support groups, as indicated.

Skin	Hair and nails	Osteoporosis
♦ Warm, red, dry skin at onset; changes to bluish and becomes cold and sweaty	♦ Accelerated hair and nail growth	♦ Early osteoporosis symptoms
♦ Cool, pale, bluish, sweaty	♦ Altered hair growth; cracked, grooved, or ridged nails	♦ More apparent osteoporosis
♦ Thin, shiny	♦ Increasingly brittle and ridged nails	♦ Marked diffuse osteoporosis

Coronary artery disease

Overview

Coronary artery disease (CAD) is heart disease that results from atherosclerosis, which causes narrowing of coronary arteries over time. Its primary effect is the loss of oxygen and nutrients to myocardial tissue because of diminished coronary blood flow.

CAUSES
◆ Atherosclerosis
◆ Dissecting aneurysm
◆ Infectious vasculitis
◆ Syphilis
◆ Congenital defects
◆ Coronary artery spasm

RISK FACTORS
◆ Family history
◆ High cholesterol level
◆ Smoking
◆ Diabetes
◆ Hormonal contraceptives
◆ Obesity
◆ Sedentary lifestyle
◆ Stress
◆ Increased homocystine levels

PATHOPHYSIOLOGY
◆ Increased blood levels of low-density lipoprotein (LDL) irritate or damage the inner layer of coronary vessels.
◆ LDL enters the vessel after damaging the protective barrier, accumulates, and forms a fatty streak.
◆ Smooth muscle cells move to the inner layer to engulf the fatty substance, produce fibrous tissue, and stimulate calcium deposition.
◆ Cycle continues, resulting in transformation of the fatty streak into fibrous plaque and, eventually, a CAD lesion evolves.
◆ Oxygen deprivation forces the myocardium to shift from aerobic to anaerobic metabolism, leading to accumulation of lactic acid and reduction of cellular pH.

◆ The combination of hypoxia, reduced energy availability, and acidosis rapidly impairs left ventricular function.
◆ The strength of contractions in the affected myocardial region is reduced as the fibers shorten inadequately, resulting in less force and velocity.
◆ Wall motion is abnormal in the ischemic area, resulting in less blood being ejected from the heart with each contraction.

COMPLICATIONS
◆ Arrhythmias
◆ Myocardial infarction (MI)
◆ Heart failure

Assessment

HISTORY
◆ Angina that may radiate to the left arm, neck, jaw, or shoulder blade
◆ Commonly occurs after physical exertion but may also follow emotional excitement, exposure to cold, or a large meal
◆ Symptoms that cause the patient to awaken from sleep
◆ Nausea
◆ Vomiting
◆ Fainting
◆ Sweating
◆ Stable angina (predictable and relieved by rest or nitrates)
◆ Unstable angina (increases in frequency and duration and is more easily induced and generally indicates extensive or worsening disease and, if untreated, may progress to MI)
◆ Crescendo angina (an effort-induced pain that occurs with increasing frequency and with decreasing provocation)
◆ Prinzmetal's or variant angina pectoris (severe pain that occurs at rest without provocation or effort)

PHYSICAL FINDINGS
◆ Cool extremities
◆ Xanthoma
◆ Arteriovenous nicking of the eye

- Obesity
- Hypertension
- Positive Levine sign (holding fist to chest)
- Decreased or absent peripheral pulses

DIAGNOSTIC TEST RESULTS
- *Myocardial perfusion imaging with thallium 201 during treadmill exercise:* "cold spots," indicating ischemic areas
- *Pharmacologic myocardial perfusion imaging:* decreased blood flow in arteries with stenosis proportional to the percentage of occlusion
- *Multiple-gated acquisition scanning:* cardiac tissue injury
- *Coronary angiography:* location and degree of coronary artery stenosis or obstruction, collateral circulation, and the condition of the artery beyond the narrowing
- *Echocardiography:* abnormal wall motion
- *Electrocardiography:* ischemic changes during angina
- *Stress testing:* ST-segment changes during exercise or medication administration, indicating ischemia

Treatment

...ction techniques essential, es-
...wn stressors precipitate pain
...ifications, such as smoking
...intaining ideal body

...m, low-cholesterol

...graft
...nvasive surgery

...right ...t

...ary ar-
...ment
...easure-
...s, wall

- Beta-adrenergic blockers
- Calcium channel blockers
- Antiplatelets
- Antilipemics
- Antihypertensives
- Estrogen replacement therapy

Nursing interventions

- Assess the patient's pain level, administer analgesics, and evaluate their effects.
- Administer medications as ordered.
- Observe for signs and symptoms that may signify worsening of the patient's condition.
- Assess cardiovascular status.
- Monitor vital signs and cardiac rhythm.

PATIENT TEACHING
- Explain the disorder, diagnostic testing, and treatment plan.
- Teach about the administration, dosage, and possible adverse effects of prescribed medications.
- Review risk factors for CAD and encourage lifestyle modifications as indicated.
- Identify activities that precipitate episodes of pain.
- Teach effective coping mechanisms to deal with stress.
- Stress the importance of follow-up care.
- Review dietary modifications.
- Explain the importance of regular, moderate exercise.
- Refer the patient to a weight-loss program if needed.
- Refer the patient to a smoking-cessation program if needed.
- Refer the patient to a cardiac rehabilitation program if indicated.

Cr

Cor pulmonale

Overview

Cor pulmonale, also called *right-sided heart failure*, is hypertrophy and dilation of the right ventricle secondary to disease affecting the structure or function of the lungs or their vasculature. It can occur at the end stage of various chronic disorders of the lungs, pulmonary vessels, chest wall, or respiratory control center.

CAUSES

◆ Bronchial asthma
◆ Chronic obstructive pulmonary disease
◆ Cystic fibrosis
◆ Disorders affecting the pulmonary parenchyma
◆ External vascular obstruction resulting from a tumor or aneurysm
◆ High altitude
◆ Interstitial lung disease
◆ Kyphoscoliosis
◆ Muscular dystrophy
◆ Obesity
◆ Obstructive sleep apnea
◆ Pectus excavatum (funnel chest)
◆ Poliomyelitis
◆ Primary pulmonary hypertension
◆ Pulmonary emboli
◆ Vasculitis

PATHOPHYSIOLOGY

◆ An occluded vessel impairs the heart's ability to generate enough pressure.
◆ Increased blood flow creates pulmonary hypertension.
◆ Pulmonary hypertension increases the heart's workload.
◆ To compensate, the right ventricle hypertrophies to force blood through the lungs.
◆ In response to hypoxia, the bone marrow produces more red blood cells, causing polycythemia.
◆ The blood's viscosity increases, further ___ating pulmonary hypertension. This ___ increases the right ventricle's ___ausing heart failure.

COMPLICATIONS

◆ Left-sided heart failure
◆ Hepatomegaly
◆ Shock
◆ Death
◆ Pulmonary hypertension
◆ Pleural effusions
◆ Thromboembolism caused by polycythemia

Assessment

HISTORY

◆ Dyspnea
◆ Chronic productive cough
◆ Fatigue
◆ Weakness
◆ Exercise intolerance

PHYSICAL FINDINGS

◆ Cyanosis
◆ Wheezing respirations
◆ Tachypnea
◆ Dependent edema
◆ Distended jugular veins
◆ Enlarged, tender liver
◆ Hepatojugular reflex
◆ Tachycardia
◆ Pansystolic murmur at the lower left sternal border

DIAGNOSTIC TEST RESULTS

◆ *Arterial blood gas analysis:* decreased partial pressure of arterial oxygen (usually less than 70 mm Hg and rarely more tha___ 90 mm Hg)
◆ *Brain natriuretic peptide level:* eleva___
◆ *Hematocrit:* typically over 50%
◆ *Serum hepatic tests, aspartate amin___ transferase levels:* elevated
◆ *Echocardiography and angiograph___* ventricular enlargement
◆ *Chest X-rays:* large central pulm___ teries and right ventricular enlarg___
◆ *Magnetic resonance imaging:* ___ ment of the right ventricular m___ thickness, and ejection fracti___

◆ *Cardiac catheterization:* pulmonary vascular pressures
◆ *Electrocardiography:* arrhythmias, such as premature atrial and ventricular contractions and atrial fibrillation during severe hypoxia; right bundle-branch block; right axis deviation; prominent P waves; and an inverted T wave in right precordial leads
◆ *Pulmonary function studies:* underlying pulmonary disease
◆ *Pulmonary artery catheterization:* increased right ventricular and pulmonary artery pressures
◆ *Hemodynamic profile:* increased pulmonary vascular resistance

PATIENT TEACHING
◆ Explain the disorder, diagnostic testing, and treatment plan.
◆ Teach about the administration, dosage, and possible adverse effects of prescribed medications.
◆ Review dietary restrictions.
◆ Describe signs and symptoms of complications.
◆ Refer the patient for home services as indicated.
◆ Stress the importance of follow-up care.

Treatment

◆ Treatment of underlying disorder
◆ Phlebotomy if necessary
◆ Low-sodium diet
◆ Fluid restrictions
◆ Limited activity or bed rest

MEDICATIONS
◆ Oxygen
◆ Diuretics
◆ Calcium channel blockers
◆ Cardiac glycosides
◆ Antibiotics
◆ Vasodilators
◆ Anticoagulant therapy
◆ Methylxanthines
◆ Endothelin receptor antagonists

Nursing interventions

◆ Administer oxygen therapy as needed and monitor pulse oximetry.
◆ Give prescribed drugs.
◆ Monitor vital signs, intake and output, and laboratory results.
◆ Assess respiratory status.
◆ Monitor for signs and symptoms of complications.

Crohn's disease

Overview

Crohn's disease is an inflammatory bowel disease that may affect any part of the GI tract but commonly involves the terminal ileum. Fifty percent of cases involve the colon and small bowel; 33%, terminal ileum; 10% to 20%, only the colon. This disorder extends through all layers of the intestinal wall and may involve regional lymph nodes and mesentery.

CAUSES
◆ Exact cause unknown
◆ Lymphatic obstruction and infection among contributing factors

RISK FACTORS
◆ History of allergies
◆ Immune disorders
◆ Genetic predisposition (one or more affected relatives in 10% to 20% of patients; sometimes occurs in monozygotic twins)

PATHOPHYSIOLOGY
◆ Crohn's disease involves slow, progressive inflammation of the bowel.
◆ Lymphatic obstruction is caused by enlarged lymph nodes.
◆ Edema, mucosal ulceration, fissures, and abscesses occur.
◆ Elevated patches of closely packed lymph follicles (Peyer's patches) develop in the small intestinal lining.
◆ Fibrosis occurs, thickening the bowel wall and causing stenosis.
◆ Inflamed bowel loops adhere to other diseased or normal loops.
◆ The diseased bowel becomes thicker, shorter, and narrower.

COMPLICATIONS
◆ Anal fistula
◆ Perineal abscess
◆ Fistulas of the bladder or vagina or to skin in an old scar area
◆ ▬stinal obstruction
◆ Bowel perforation
◆ Nutritional deficiencies caused by malabsorption and maldigestion

Assessment

HISTORY
◆ Gradual onset of signs and symptoms, marked by periods of remission and exacerbation
◆ Fatigue and weakness
◆ Fever, flatulence, nausea
◆ Steady, colicky, or cramping abdominal pain that usually occurs in the right lower abdominal quadrant
◆ Diarrhea that may worsen after emotional upset or ingestion of poorly tolerated foods, such as milk, fatty foods, and spices
◆ Weight loss

PHYSICAL FINDINGS
◆ Possible soft or semiliquid stool usually without gross blood
◆ Right lower abdominal quadrant tenderness or distention
◆ Possible abdominal mass indicating adherent loops of bowel
◆ Hyperactive bowel sounds
◆ Bloody diarrhea
◆ Perianal and rectal abscesses

DIAGNOSTIC TEST RESULTS
◆ *Fecal occult blood testing:* positive
◆ *Hemoglobin (Hb) and hematocrit levels:* decreased
◆ *White blood cell count and erythrocyte sedimentation rate:* increased
◆ *Serum potassium, calcium, magnesium, and Hb levels:* decreased
◆ *Vitamin B_{12} and folate:* deficiency
◆ *Small bowel X-rays:* irregular mucosa, ulceration, and stiffening
◆ *Barium enema:* string sign (segments of stricture separated by normal bowel), fissures and narrowing of the lumen
◆ *Sigmoidoscopy and colonoscopy:* patchy areas of inflammation, coarse irregularity

(cobblestone appearance) of the mucosal surface

◆ *Biopsy:* granulomas in up to 50% of all specimens

Treatment

◆ Stress reduction
◆ Avoidance of foods that worsen diarrhea
◆ Avoidance of raw fruits and vegetables if blockage occurs
◆ Adequate caloric, protein, and vitamin intake
◆ Parenteral nutrition if necessary
◆ Reduced activity
◆ Surgery for acute intestinal obstruction
◆ Colectomy with ileostomy

MEDICATIONS
◆ Corticosteroids
◆ Immunosuppressants
◆ Sulfonamides
◆ Anti-inflammatories
◆ Antibacterials and antiprotozoals
◆ Antidiarrheals
◆ Opioids
◆ Vitamin supplements
◆ Antispasmodics

Nursing interventions

◆ Assess GI status and monitor the amount and consistency of stools.
◆ Provide meticulous skin care after each bowel movement.
◆ Schedule patient care to include rest periods throughout the day.
◆ Assist with dietary modification.
◆ Give prescribed iron supplements and blood transfusions.
◆ Give prescribed analgesics.
◆ Provide emotional support to the patient and his family.
◆ Monitor vital signs, intake and output, and laboratory results.
◆ Obtain daily weight.
◆ Observe for signs of infection or obstruction.

PATIENT TEACHING
◆ Explain the disorder, diagnostic testing, and treatment plan.
◆ Teach about the administration, dosage, and possible adverse effects of prescribed medications.
◆ Review dietary restrictions.
◆ Describe signs and symptoms of complications.
◆ Refer the patient for home services as indicated.
◆ Stress the importance of adequate rest.
◆ Teach how the patient can reduce sources of stress.
◆ Refer the patient to a smoking-cessation program if appropriate.
◆ Refer the patient to an enterostomal therapist if indicated.
◆ Stress the importance of follow-up care.

Deep vein thrombosis

Disorders

Overview

Deep vein thrombosis (DVT), an acute condition characterized by inflammation and thrombus formation, mainly affects the veins of the lower leg, but can also affect upper body veins. The development of a thrombus may cause vessel occlusion or embolization, resulting in pulmonary embolism, stroke, myocardial infarction (MI), and possibly death. (See *Major venous pathways of the leg.*)

CAUSES
◆ Thrombus formation in a deep vein
◆ Possibly idiopathic

RISK FACTORS
◆ Age older than 60
◆ Hypercoagulable condition
◆ Fracture of the spine, pelvis, femur, or tibia
◆ Hormonal contraceptives
◆ Neoplasms
◆ Pregnancy and childbirth
◆ Prolonged bed rest
◆ Surgery
◆ Trauma
◆ Obesity
◆ Sepsis
◆ Venulitis
◆ MI
◆ Inflammatory bowel disease
◆ Heart failure
◆ Peripherally inserted central catheter

PATHOPHYSIOLOGY
◆ Alterations in the epithelial lining cause platelet aggregation and fibrin entrapment of red blood cells, white blood cells, and additional platelets.
◆ The thrombus initiates a chemical inflammatory process in the vessel epithelium that leads to fibrosis, which may occlude the vessel lumen or embolize.

COMPLICATIONS
◆ Pulmonary embolism
◆ Chronic venous insufficiency
◆ Stroke
◆ MI

Assessment

HISTORY
◆ Asymptomatic in up to 50% of patients with DVT
◆ Possible tenderness, aching, or severe pain in the affected leg or arm; fever, chills, and malaise

PHYSICAL FINDINGS
◆ Redness, swelling, and tenderness of the affected leg or arm
◆ Possible positive Homans' sign
◆ Positive cuff sign
◆ Possible warm feeling in affected leg or arm
◆ Lymphadenitis in cases of extensive vein involvement

DIAGNOSTIC TEST RESULTS
◆ *D-dimer:* elevated
◆ *Doppler ultrasonography:* reduced blood flow to a specific area and any obstruction to the venous flow, particularly in iliofemoral DVT
◆ *Venography:* thrombi in the affected extremity
◆ *Plethysmography (more sensitive than ultrasonography in detecting DVT):* decreased circulation distal to the affected area
◆ *Phlebography:* filling defects, diverted blood flow, confirmation of diagnosis

Treatment

◆ Application of warm, moist compresses to the affected area
◆ Bed rest with elevation of the affected extremity
◆ Simple ligation to vein, plication, or clipping
◆ Embolectomy
◆ Caval interruption with transvenous placement of a vena cava filter

◆ Antiembolism stockings, sequential compression devices, ambulation or lower extremity exercises (preventive measures)

MEDICATIONS
◆ Anticoagulants
◆ Thrombolytics
◆ Analgesics

Nursing interventions

◆ Enforce bed rest and elevate the patient's affected arm or leg, but avoid compressing the popliteal space.
◆ Apply warm compresses or a covered aquathermia pad.
◆ Give prescribed analgesics.
◆ Mark, measure, and record the circumference of the affected arm or leg daily, and compare this measurement with that of the other arm or leg.
◆ Give prescribed anticoagulants and monitor coagulation studies.
◆ Perform or encourage range-of-motion exercises.
◆ Encourage ambulation.
◆ Observe for signs and symptoms of bleeding while on anticoagulants.
◆ Monitor vital signs and pulse oximetry.
◆ Observe for complication signs and symptoms.

PATIENT TEACHING
◆ Explain the disorder, diagnostic testing, and treatment plan.
◆ Teach about the administration, dosage, and possible adverse effects of prescribed medications.
◆ Stress the importance of follow-up blood studies to monitor anticoagulant therapy.
◆ Instruct the patient to avoid prolonged sitting or standing.
◆ Demonstrate proper application and use of antiembolism stockings.
◆ Explain the importance of adequate hydration.

Major venous pathways of the leg

Thrombophlebitis can occur in any leg vein. It most commonly occurs at valve sites.

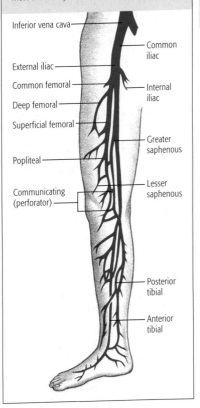

Inferior vena cava
Common iliac
External iliac
Common femoral
Internal iliac
Deep femoral
Superficial femoral
Greater saphenous
Popliteal
Lesser saphenous
Communicating (perforator)
Posterior tibial
Anterior tibial

Diabetes insipidus

Overview

A disorder of water balance regulation, diabetes insipidus (DI) is characterized by decreased antidiuretic hormone secretion, resulting in excessive fluid intake and hypotonic polyuria. DI may be primary or secondary. An impaired or absent thirst mechanism increases the risk of complications.

CAUSES
- Certain medications such as lithium
- Congenital malformation of the central nervous system
- Damage to hypothalamus or pituitary gland
- Failure of the kidneys to respond to vasopressin (nephrogenic DI)
- Failure of vasopressin secretion in response to normal physiologic stimuli
- Familial
- Granulomatous disease
- Idiopathic
- Infection
- Neurosurgery, skull fracture, or head trauma
- Pregnancy (gestational DI)
- Psychogenic
- Trauma
- Tumors
- Vascular lesions

PATHOPHYSIOLOGY
- Vasopressin (antidiuretic hormone) is synthesized in the hypothalamus and stored by the posterior pituitary gland.
- Once released into the general circulation, vasopressin acts on the distal and collecting tubules of the kidneys.
- Vasopressin increases the water permeability of the tubules and causes water reabsorption.
- The absence of vasopressin allows filtered water to be excreted in the urine instead of being reabsorbed.

COMPLICATIONS
- Hypovolemia
- Hyperosmolality
- Circulatory collapse
- Hydronephrosis

Assessment

HISTORY
- Abrupt onset of extreme polyuria
- Extreme thirst
- Extraordinarily large oral fluid intake
- Weight loss
- Dizziness, weakness, fatigue
- Constipation
- Nocturia

PHYSICAL FINDINGS
- Signs of dehydration
- Fever
- Dyspnea
- Pale, voluminous urine
- Poor skin turgor
- Tachycardia
- Decreased muscle strength
- Hypotension

DIAGNOSTIC TEST RESULTS
- *Urinalysis:* colorless urine with low osmolality and specific gravity
- *Serum sodium level:* increased
- *Serum osmolality:* increased
- *Serum vasopressin level:* decreased
- *24-hour urine test:* specific gravity decreased, volume increased
- *Blood urea nitrogen and creatinine levels:* elevated
- *Dehydration test or water deprivation test:* increased urine osmolality after vasopressin administration (exceeding 9%)

Treatment

◆ Identification and treatment of underlying cause
◆ Control of fluid balance
◆ Dehydration prevention
◆ Free access to oral fluids
◆ Low-sodium diet (nephrogenic DI)

MEDICATIONS
◆ Vasopressin (Pitressin)
◆ Synthetic vasopressin analogue
◆ Vasopressin stimulant
◆ Thiazide diuretics (nephrogenic DI)
◆ I.V. fluids: 5% dextrose in water (serum sodium level greater than 1,500 mEq/L), normal saline solution (serum sodium level less than 150 mEq/L)

Nursing interventions

◆ Administer medications and I.V. fluids as ordered.
◆ Monitor vital signs, cardiac rhythm, intake and output, urine specific gravity, and serum electrolytes.
◆ Provide meticulous skin and mouth care.
◆ Obtain daily weight.
◆ Observe for signs and symptoms of hypovolemic shock.
◆ Assess for changes in mental or neurologic status.

PATIENT TEACHING
◆ Explain the disorder, diagnostic testing, and treatment plan.
◆ Teach about the administration, dosage, and possible adverse effects of prescribed medications.
◆ Review signs and symptoms of dehydration and when to notify the practitioner.
◆ Stress the importance of maintaining fluid balance.
◆ Explain the need for medical identification jewelry.
◆ Stress the importance of follow-up care.

Diabetes mellitus

Overview

Diabtese mellitus (DM), a chronic disease of absolute or relative insulin deficiency or resistance, is characterized by disturbances in carbohydrate, protein, and fat metabolism. There are two primary forms: type 1, characterized by absolute insulin insufficiency, and type 2, characterized by insulin resistance with varying degrees of insulin secretory defects. About one-third of patients with DM are undiagnosed.

CAUSES
- Autoimmune disease (type 1)
- Genetic factors

RISK FACTORS
- Viral infections (type 1)
- Obesity (type 2)
- Physiologic or emotional stress
- Sedentary lifestyle (type 2)
- Pregnancy
- Medication, such as thiazide diuretics, adrenal corticosteroids, and hormonal contraceptives

PATHOPHYSIOLOGY
- The effects of DM result from insulin deficiency or resistance to endogenous insulin.
- Insulin allows glucose transport into the cells for use as energy or storage as glycogen.
- Insulin also stimulates protein synthesis and free fatty acid storage in the adipose tissues.
- Insulin deficiency compromises the body tissues' access to essential nutrients for fuel and storage.

COMPLICATIONS
- Ketoacidosis
- Hyperosmolar hyperglycemic nonketotic syndrome
- Cardiovascular disease
- Peripheral vascular disease
- Retinopathy, blindness
- Nephropathy
- Diabetic dermopathy
- Impaired resistance to infection
- Cognitive depression

Assessment

HISTORY
- Polyuria, nocturia
- Dehydration
- Polydipsia
- Dry mucous membranes
- Poor skin turgor
- Weight loss, hunger
- Weakness, fatigue
- Vision changes
- Frequent skin and urinary tract infections
- Dry, itchy skin
- Sexual problems
- Numbness or pain in the hands or feet
- Postprandial feeling of nausea or fullness
- Nocturnal diarrhea

Type 1
- Rapidly developing symptoms

Type 2
- Vague, long-standing symptoms that develop gradually
- Family history of DM
- Pregnancy
- Severe viral infection
- Other endocrine diseases
- Recent stress or trauma
- Use of drugs that increase blood glucose levels

PHYSICAL FINDINGS
- Retinopathy or cataract formation
- Skin changes, especially on the legs and feet, poor skin turgor
- Muscle wasting and loss of subcutaneous fat (type 1)
- Obesity, particularly in the abdominal area (type 2)

- Dry mucous membranes
- Decreased peripheral pulses
- Cool skin temperature
- Diminished deep tendon reflexes
- Orthostatic hypotension
- Characteristic "fruity" breath odor in ketoacidosis
- Possible signs of hypovolemia and shock in ketoacidosis and hyperosmolar hyperglycemic state

DIAGNOSTIC TEST RESULTS

- *Fasting plasma glucose level:* greater than or equal to 126 mg/dl on at least two occasions
- *Random blood glucose level:* greater than or equal to 200 mg/dl
- *2-hour postprandial blood glucose level:* greater than or equal to 200 mg/dl
- *Glycosylated hemoglobin (HbA$_{1C}$):* increased
- *Urinalysis:* acetone or glucose
- *Ophthalmologic examination:* diabetic retinopathy

Treatment

- American Diabetes Association recommendations to reach target glucose, HbA$_{1C}$ lipid, and blood pressure levels
- Exercise and diet control
- Tight glycemic control to prevent complications
- Modest caloric restriction for weight loss or maintenance
- Regular aerobic exercise
- Pancreas transplantation

MEDICATIONS

- Exogenous insulin (type 1 or possibly type 2)
- Oral antihyperglycemic drugs (type 2)
- Electrolyte replacement

Nursing interventions

- Give prescribed drugs and monitor the patient's response.
- Monitor vital signs, daily weight, capillary glucose levels, and laboratory values.
- Provide an appropriate diet.
- Provide meticulous skin care, especially to the feet and legs.
- Encourage adequate fluid intake.
- Encourage the patient to verbalize his feelings and offer emotional support.
- Assess renal status.
- Observe for signs of complications.
- Give rapidly absorbed carbohydrates for hypoglycemia or, if the patient is unconscious, glucagon or I.V. dextrose as ordered.
- Administer I.V. fluids and insulin replacement for hyperglycemic crisis as ordered.

PATIENT TEACHING

- Explain the disorder, diagnostic testing, and treatment plan.
- Teach about the administration, dosage, and possible adverse effects of prescribed medications.
- Explain the signs and symptoms of complications and when to notify the practitioner.
- Review dietary recommendations and prescribed exercise program.
- Demonstrate self-monitoring of blood glucose.
- Stress the importance of foot care and monitoring for wounds.
- Explain the importance of follow-up care.
- Explain the need for annual regular ophthalmologic examinations.
- Refer the patient to a dietitian.
- Refer adult patients who are planning families to preconception counseling.
- Refer the patient to the American Diabetes Association to obtain additional information and support.

Disseminated intravascular coagulation

Overview

A syndrome of activated coagulation, disseminated intravascular coagulation (DIC) is characterized by bleeding or thrombosis. It complicates diseases and conditions that accelerate clotting, causing occlusion of small blood vessels, organ necrosis, depletion of circulating clotting factors and platelets, and activation of the fibrinolytic system.

CAUSES
♦ Disorders that produce necrosis, such as extensive burns and trauma
♦ Infection, sepsis
♦ Neoplastic disease
♦ Obstetric complications
♦ Other disorders, such as heatstroke, shock, incompatible blood transfusion, drug reactions, cardiac arrest, surgery necessitating cardiopulmonary bypass, acute respiratory distress syndrome, diabetic ketoacidosis, pulmonary embolism, and sickle cell anemia

PATHOPHYSIOLOGY
♦ Typical accelerated clotting results in generalized activation of prothrombin and a consequent excess of thrombin.
♦ Excess thrombin converts fibrinogen to fibrin, producing fibrin clots in the microcirculation.
♦ This process consumes exorbitant amounts of coagulation factors (especially platelets, factor V, prothrombin, fibrinogen, and factor VIII), causing thrombocytopenia, deficiencies in factors V and VIII, hypoprothrombinemia, and hypofibrinogenemia.
♦ Circulating thrombin activates the fibrinolytic system, which lyses fibrin clots into fibrinogen degradation products (FDPs).
♦ The hemorrhage that occurs may be due largely to the anticoagulant activity of FDPs and depletion of plasma coagulation factors.

COMPLICATIONS
♦ Renal failure
♦ Hepatic damage
♦ Stroke
♦ Ischemic bowel
♦ Respiratory failure
♦ Death (mortality is greater than 50%)

Assessment

HISTORY
♦ Abnormal bleeding without a history of a serious hemorrhagic disorder; bleeding may occur at all bodily orifices
♦ Possible presence of one of the causes of DIC
♦ Possible signs of bleeding into the skin, such as cutaneous oozing, petechiae, ecchymoses, and hematomas
♦ Possible bleeding from surgical or invasive procedure sites, such as incisions or venipuncture sites
♦ Possible nausea and vomiting; severe muscle, back, and abdominal pain; chest pain; hemoptysis; epistaxis; seizures; and oliguria
♦ Possible GI bleeding, hematuria

PHYSICAL FINDINGS
♦ Petechiae
♦ Acrocyanosis
♦ Dyspnea, tachypnea
♦ Mental status changes, including confusion

DIAGNOSTIC TEST RESULTS
♦ *Serum platelet count:* decreased (less than 150,000/ml)
♦ *Serum fibrinogen level:* decreased (less than 170 mg/dl)
♦ *Prothrombin time:* prolonged (more than 19 seconds)

◆ *Partial thromboplastin time:* prolonged (more than 40 seconds)
◆ *FDPs:* increased (commonly greater than 45 mcg/ml, or positive at less than 1:100 dilution)
◆ *D-dimer test (specific fibrinogen test for DIC):* positive result at less than 1:8 dilution
◆ *Thrombin time:* prolonged
◆ *Blood clotting factors V and VIII:* diminished
◆ *Complete blood count:* hemoglobin levels less than 10 g/dl

Treatment

◆ Treatment of the underlying condition
◆ Possible supportive care alone if the patient isn't actively bleeding
◆ Activity as tolerated

MEDICATIONS
If the patient is actively bleeding
◆ Administration of blood, fresh frozen plasma, platelets, or packed red blood cells
◆ Cryoprecipitate
◆ Antithrombin III
◆ Fluid replacement

Nursing interventions

◆ Observe for signs of bleeding.
◆ Give prescribed oxygen therapy.
◆ Monitor vital signs, cardiac rhythm, pulse oximetry, intake and output, and laboratory studies.
◆ Assess respiratory, cardiovascular, and renal status.
◆ Provide adequate rest periods.
◆ Assess the patient's pain level, administer analgesics, and evaluate their effects.
◆ Reposition the patient every 2 hours and provide meticulous skin care.
◆ Protect the patient from injury.
◆ Obtain daily weight.
◆ Observe for signs and symptoms of complications.

PATIENT TEACHING
◆ Explain the disorder, diagnostic testing, and treatment plan.
◆ Teach about the administration, dosage, and possible adverse effects of prescribed medications.
◆ Review signs and symptoms of complications.

Diverticular disease

Overview

Diverticular disease involves bulging pouches (diverticula) in the GI wall that push the mucosal lining through surrounding muscle. The most common affected site is the sigmoid colon, but diverticula may develop anywhere from the proximal end of the pharynx to the anus. Diverticular disease of the ileum (Meckel's diverticulum) is the most common congenital anomaly of the GI tract. Types of diverticular disease are *diverticulosis*—when diverticula are present but don't cause symptoms—and *diverticulitis*—when diverticula become inflamed, possibly causing complications.

CAUSES
◆ Defects in colon wall strength
◆ Diminished colonic motility and increased intraluminal pressure

RISK FACTORS
◆ Age
◆ Low-fiber diet

PATHOPHYSIOLOGY
◆ Pressure in the intestinal lumen is exerted on weak areas, such as points where blood vessels enter the intestine, causing a break in the muscular continuity of the GI wall, creating a diverticulum.
◆ Diverticulitis occurs when retained undigested food mixed with bacteria accumulates in the diverticulum, forming a hard mass (fecalith). This substance cuts off the blood supply to the diverticulum's thin walls, increasing its susceptibility to attack by colonic bacteria.
◆ Inflammation follows bacterial infection, causing abdominal pain.

COMPLICATIONS
◆ Ruptured diverticula that cause abdominal abscesses or peritonitis
◆ Intestinal obstruction
◆ Rectal hemorrhage
◆ Portal pyemia
◆ Fistula

Assessment

HISTORY
Diverticulosis
◆ May be symptom-free
◆ Occasional intermittent pain in the left lower abdominal quadrant, which may be relieved by defecation or the passage of flatus
◆ Alternating bouts of constipation and diarrhea

Diverticulitis
◆ History of diverticulosis
◆ Low fiber consumption
◆ Recent consumption of foods containing seeds or kernels or indigestible roughage, such as celery and corn
◆ Complaints of moderate dull or steady pain in the left lower abdominal quadrant, aggravated by straining, lifting, or coughing
◆ Mild nausea, gas, diarrhea, or intermittent bouts of constipation, sometimes accompanied by rectal bleeding

PHYSICAL FINDINGS
Diverticulitis
◆ Distressed appearance
◆ Left lower quadrant abdominal tenderness
◆ Low-grade fever
◆ Palpable mass

Acute diverticulitis
◆ Muscle spasms
◆ Signs of peritoneal irritation
◆ Guarding and rebound tenderness

DIAGNOSTIC TEST RESULTS
◆ *Complete blood count:* leukocytosis
◆ *Erythrocyte sedimentation rate:* diverticulitis
◆ *Stool test for occult blood:* positive for diverticulitis (in 25% of patients)

◆ *Barium studies:* barium filled diverticula or outlines (not when diverticula blocked by impacted stools; not performed for acute diverticulitis because of potential rupture)
◆ *Radiography:* colonic spasm if irritable bowel syndrome accompanies diverticular disease
◆ *Abdominal X-rays:* rules out perforation
◆ *Computed tomography scan of the abdomen:* abscess presence
◆ *Colonoscopy or flexible sigmoidoscopy:* diverticula or inflamed mucosa (tests usually not done in acute phase)
◆ *Biopsy:* rules out cancer

Treatment

For diverticulosis
◆ No treatment required for asymptomatic diverticulosis
◆ Liquid or low-residue diet (if experiencing pain)
◆ Increased water consumption if appropriate
◆ High-residue diet (if not in pain)

For severe diverticulitis
◆ Nasogastric (NG) decompression
◆ Nothing by mouth
◆ Bed rest
◆ Colon resection
◆ Possible temporary colostomy to drain abscesses, to rest the colon for 6 to 8 weeks, to correct rupture, or to treat cases refractory to medical treatment

MEDICATIONS
For diverticulosis
◆ Stool softeners
◆ Bulk medication

For diverticulitis
◆ Antibiotics
◆ Analgesics
◆ Antispasmodics
◆ I.V. therapy for severe diverticulitis

Nursing interventions

◆ Assess the patient's pain level, administer analgesics, and evaluate their effects.
◆ Monitor vital signs and intake and output.
◆ Enforce bed rest for acute diverticulitis.
◆ Provide the prescribed diet.
◆ Monitor stools for color, consistency, and frequency.
◆ Provide preoperative care as indicated.

After colon resection
◆ Perform wound care.
◆ Encourage coughing and deep breathing and use of incentive spirometer.
◆ Administer I.V. fluids and prescribed drugs.
◆ Provide colostomy care if appropriate.
◆ Perform NG drainage if appropriate.
◆ Look for signs and symptoms of complications.
◆ Observe for signs of infection and postoperative bleeding.

PATIENT TEACHING
◆ Explain the disorder, diagnostic testing, and treatment plan.
◆ Teach about the administration, dosage, and possible adverse effects of prescribed medications.
◆ Review signs and symptoms of complications.
◆ Review dietary recommendations.
◆ Provide instruction on colostomy care, if appropriate.
◆ Refer the patient to an enterostomal therapist if appropriate.

Emphysema

Overview

Emphysema, the most common cause of death from respiratory disease in the United States, is a chronic lung disease characterized by permanent enlargement of air spaces distal to the terminal bronchioles and by exertional dyspnea. It's one of several diseases usually labeled collectively as chronic obstructive pulmonary disease or chronic obstructive lung disease.

CAUSES
- Cigarette smoking
- Genetic deficiency of alpha$_1$-antitrypsin

PATHOPHYSIOLOGY
- Recurrent inflammation associated with the release of proteolytic enzymes from lung cells causes abnormal, irreversible enlargement of the air spaces distal to the terminal bronchioles.
- This enlargement leads to the destruction of alveolar walls, which results in a breakdown of elasticity.

COMPLICATIONS
- Recurrent respiratory tract infections
- Cor pulmonale
- Respiratory failure
- Peptic ulcer disease
- Spontaneous pneumothorax
- Pneumomediastinum

Assessment

HISTORY
- Smoking
- Shortness of breath
- Chronic cough
- Anorexia and weight loss
- Malaise

PHYSICAL FINDINGS
- Barrel chest
- Pursed-lip breathing
- Use of accessory muscles
- Cyanosis
- Clubbed fingers and toes
- Tachypnea
- Decreased tactile fremitus
- Decreased chest expansion
- Hyperresonance
- Decreased breath sounds
- Crackles
- Inspiratory wheeze
- Prolonged expiratory phase with grunting respirations
- Distant heart sounds

DIAGNOSTIC TEST RESULTS
- *Arterial blood gas analysis:* decreased partial pressure of oxygen, normal partial pressure of carbon dioxide until late in the disease.
- *Red blood cell count:* increased hemoglobin level late in the disease
- *Chest X-ray:* flattened diaphragm, reduced vascular markings at the lung periphery, overaeration of the lungs, a vertical heart, enlarged anteroposterior chest diameter, large retrosternal air space
- *Pulmonary function tests:* increased residual volume and total lung capacity, reduced diffusing capacity, increased inspiratory flow
- *Electrocardiography:* tall, symmetrical P waves in leads II, III, and aV$_F$; a vertical QRS axis; signs of right ventricular hypertrophy late in the disease

Treatment

- Chest physiotherapy
- Possible transtracheal catheterization and home oxygen therapy
- Mechanical ventilation (in acute exacerbations)
- Adequate hydration
- High-protein, high-calorie diet
- Activity as tolerated
- Chest tube insertion for pneumothorax

MEDICATIONS
- Oxygen
- Bronchodilators

- Anticholinergics
- Mucolytics
- Corticosteroids
- Antibiotics

Nursing interventions

- Give prescribed drugs.
- Perform chest physiotherapy.
- Provide a high-calorie, protein-rich diet.
- Monitor vital signs, intake and output, and pulse oximetry.
- Obtain daily weight.
- Observe for signs and symptoms of complications.
- Assess respiratory status per unit policy.
- Note the patient's activity tolerance and provide frequent rest periods.
- Provide supportive care.
- Help the patient adjust to lifestyle changes necessitated by a chronic illness.

PATIENT TEACHING

- Explain the disorder, diagnostic testing, and treatment plan.
- Teach about the administration, dosage, and possible adverse effects of prescribed medications.
- Review signs and symptoms of complications.
- Teach techniques for conserving energy.
- Stress the importance of smoking cessation and avoiding areas where smoking occurs.
- Explain the importance of receiving an annual influenza vaccine.
- Teach about home oxygen therapy if indicated.
- Demonstrate coughing and deep breathing exercises.
- Demonstrate the proper use of handheld inhalers.
- Explain the need for a high-calorie, protein-rich diet and adequate oral fluid intake.
- Identify respiratory irritants and ways to avoid them.
- Stress the importance of follow-up care.

- Refer the family of patients with familial emphysema for alpha$_1$-antitrypsin deficiency screening.

Endocarditis

Overview

Endocarditis is an infection of the endocardium, heart valves (most commonly the mitral), or cardiac prosthesis. There are three types: native valve (acute and subacute) endocarditis, prosthetic valve (early and late) endocarditis, and endocarditis related to I.V. drug abuse (usually involving the tricuspid valves). Rheumatic valvular disease occurs in about 25% of all cases.

CAUSES

Native valve endocarditis
◆ Alpha-hemolytic *Streptococcus* or enterococci (subacute form)
◆ Group B hemolytic *Streptococcus*
◆ *Staphylococcus aureus*

Prosthetic valve
◆ Alpha-hemolytic *Streptococcus,* enterococci, and *Staphylococcus* (late, 60 days or more after implant)
◆ *Staphylococcus,* gram-negative bacilli, and *Candida* (early, within 60 days after implant)

Related to I.V. drug abuse
◆ *S. aureus*

PATHOPHYSIOLOGY
◆ Fibrin and platelets cluster on valve tissue and engulf circulating bacteria or fungi. (See *Degenerative changes in endocarditis.*)
◆ This produces vegetation, which in turn may cover the valve surfaces, causing deformities and destruction of valvular tissue and may extend to the chordae tendineae, causing them to rupture, leading to valvular insufficiency.
◆ Vegetative growth on the heart valves, endocardial lining of a heart chamber, or the endothelium of a blood vessel may embolize to the spleen, kidneys, central nervous system, and lungs.

COMPLICATIONS
◆ Peripheral vascular occlusion
◆ Left-sided heart failure
◆ Valve stenosis or insufficiency
◆ Myocardial erosion
◆ Embolic debris lodged in the small vasculature of the visceral tissue
◆ Splenic, renal, cerebal, or pulmonary infarction

Assessment

HISTORY
◆ Predisposing condition, such as heart failure or I.V. drug use
◆ Nonspecific symptoms, such as weakness, fatigue, weight loss, anorexia, arthralgia, night sweats, and intermittent fever that may recur for weeks
◆ Dyspnea and chest pain

PHYSICAL FINDINGS
◆ Petechiae on the skin (especially common on the upper anterior trunk) and on the buccal, pharyngeal, or conjunctival mucosa
◆ Splinter hemorrhages under the nails
◆ Clubbing of the fingers in patients with long-standing disease
◆ Heart murmur in all patients except those with early acute endocarditis and I.V. drug users with tricuspid valve infection
◆ Osler's nodes
◆ Roth's spots
◆ Janeway lesions
◆ A murmur that changes suddenly or a new murmur that develops in the presence of fever (classic physical sign)
◆ Splenomegaly in long-standing disease
◆ Dyspnea, tachycardia, and bibasilar crackles possible with left-sided heart failure

DIAGNOSTIC TEST RESULTS
◆ *Blood cultures (three or more during a 24- to 48-hour period):* causative organism (in up to 90% of patients)

◆ *White blood cell count and differential:* normal or elevated

◆ *Complete blood count and anemia panel:* normocytic, normochromic anemia (in subacute native valve endocarditis)

◆ *Erythrocyte sedimentation rate and serum creatinine levels:* elevated

◆ *Serum rheumatoid factor:* positive in about 50% of all patients with endocarditis lasting longer than 6 weeks

◆ *Urinalysis:* proteinuria and microscopic hematuria

◆ *Echocardiography:* valvular damage in up to 80% of patients with native valve disease

◆ *Electrocardiography:* atrial fibrillation and other arrhythmias that accompany valvular disease

Treatment

◆ Selection of anti-infective drug based on type of infecting organism and sensitivity studies

◆ If blood cultures are negative (10% to 20% of subacute cases), possible I.V. antibiotic therapy (usually for 4 to 6 weeks) against probable infecting organism

◆ Sufficient fluid intake

◆ Bed rest

◆ With severe valvular damage, especially aortic insufficiency or infection of a cardiac prosthesis, possible corrective surgery if refractory heart failure develops or if an infected prosthetic valve must be replaced

MEDICATIONS

◆ Aspirin

◆ Antibiotics

Nursing interventions

◆ Administer oxygen therapy and monitor pulse oximetry.

◆ Assess cardiovascular and respiratory status.

◆ Monitor vital signs and cardiac rhythm.

◆ Stress the importance of bed rest.

◆ Administer medications as ordered.

◆ Observe for signs and symptoms of complications.

PATIENT TEACHING

◆ Explain the disorder, diagnostic testing, and treatment plan.

◆ Teach about the administration, dosage, and possible adverse effects of prescribed medications.

◆ Review signs and symptoms of complications.

◆ Explain the need for prophylactic antibiotics before dental work and some surgical procedures.

◆ Recommend proper dental hygiene and avoiding flossing the teeth.

◆ Describe the signs and symptoms of endocarditis and when to notify the practitioner.

◆ Encourage follow-up care with cardiologist.

Degenerative changes in endocarditis

This illustration shows typical vegetations on the endocardium produced by fibrin and platelet deposits on infection sites.

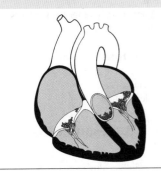

Fibromyalgia syndrome

Overview

Fibramyalgia syndrome (FMS) is a diffuse pain syndrome formerly known as *fibrositis*. It's observed in up to 15% of patients seen in general rheumatology practice and 5% of general medicine clinic patients.

CAUSES
- Unknown
- May be multifactorial and influenced by stress, physical conditioning, abnormal-quality sleep, and neuroendocrine, psychiatric, or hormonal factors
- May be a primary disorder or associated with underlying disease such as infection

PATHOPHYSIOLOGY
- Blood flow to the muscle is decreased (because of poor muscle aerobic conditioning, rather than other physiologic abnormalities).
- Blood flow in the thalamus and caudate nucleus is decreased, leading to a lowered pain threshold.
- Endocrine dysfunction—such as abnormal pituitary-adrenal axis responses or abnormal levels of the neurotransmitter serotonin in brain centers—affects pain and sleep.
- The functioning of other pain-processing pathways is abnormal.

COMPLICATIONS
- Pain
- Depression
- Sleep deprivation

Assessment

HISTORY
- Diffuse, dull, aching pain across neck and shoulders and in lower back and proximal limbs
- Pain typically worse in the morning, sometimes with stiffness; can be exacerbated by stress, lack of sleep, weather changes, and inactivity
- Sleep disturbances with frequent arousal and fragmented sleep or frequent waking throughout the night (patient unaware of arousals)
- Possible report of irritable bowel syndrome, tension headaches, puffy hands, and paresthesia

PHYSICAL FINDINGS
- Tender points from moderate amount of pressure to a specific location (see *Tender points of fibromyalgia*)

DIAGNOSTIC TEST RESULTS
- *Diagnostic testing in FMS not associated with an underlying disease:* generally negative for significant abnormalities

Treatment

- Massage therapy
- Ultrasound treatments
- Regular, low-impact aerobic exercise program such as water aerobics
- Preexercise and postexercise stretching to minimize injury
- Low-fat, high-complex carbohydrate diet

MEDICATIONS
- Amitriptyline, nortriptyline, or cyclobenzaprine
- Tricyclic antidepressants and serotonin reuptake inhibitors
- Nonsteroidal anti-inflammatory drugs
- Magnesium supplements
- Steroid or lidocaine injections
- Pramipexole (Mirapex), a dopamine agonist (helpful in some patients)

Nursing interventions

◆ Assess the patient's pain level, administer analgesics, and evaluate their effects.
◆ Suggest alternate methods to relieve pain, such as relaxation techniques and massage.
◆ Provide emotional support.
◆ Encourage the patient to perform regular stretching exercises safely and effectively.
◆ Monitor sensory disturbances.
◆ Evaluate the patient's level of fatigue and watch for signs of depression.

PATIENT TEACHING

◆ Explain the disorder, diagnostic testing, and treatment plan.
◆ Teach about the administration, dosage, and possible adverse effects of prescribed medications.
◆ Stress the importance of exercise in maintaining muscle conditioning, improving energy and, possibly, improving sleep quality.
◆ Teach alternate methods of pain relief, such as relaxation techniques.
◆ Review dietary recommendations.
◆ Refer the patient to appropriate counseling as needed.

Tender points of fibromyalgia

The patient with fibromyalgia syndrome may complain of specific areas of tenderness, which are shown in the illustrations below.

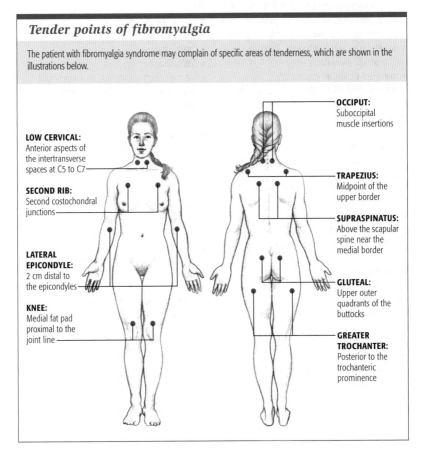

LOW CERVICAL:
Anterior aspects of the intertransverse spaces at C5 to C7

SECOND RIB:
Second costochondral junctions

LATERAL EPICONDYLE:
2 cm distal to the epicondyles

KNEE:
Medial fat pad proximal to the joint line

OCCIPUT:
Suboccipital muscle insertions

TRAPEZIUS:
Midpoint of the upper border

SUPRASPINATUS:
Above the scapular spine near the medial border

GLUTEAL:
Upper outer quadrants of the buttocks

GREATER TROCHANTER:
Posterior to the trochanteric prominence

Gastritis

Overview

Gastritis is the acute or chronic inflammation of the gastric mucosa. The acute form is the most common stomach disorder. Gastritis may occur with other serious conditions, such as atrophy of the stomach.

CAUSES
Acute gastritis
◆ Chronic ingestion of irritating foods and alcohol
◆ Complication of acute illness
◆ Drugs such as aspirin and other nonsteroidal anti-inflammatory agents (in large doses), cytotoxic agents, caffeine, corticosteroids, antimetabolites, and indomethacin
◆ Endotoxins released from infecting bacteria, such as staphylococci, *Escherichia coli*, and salmonella
◆ Ingested poisons, especially dichlorodiphenyltrichloroethane, ammonia, mercury, carbon tetrachloride, or corrosive substances

Chronic gastritis
◆ *Helicobacter pylori* infection (common in nonerosive gastritis)
◆ Pernicious anemia, renal disease, or diabetes mellitus
◆ Recurring exposure to irritating substances, such as drugs, alcohol, cigarette smoke, and environmental agents

RISK FACTORS
◆ Age older than 60
◆ Exposure to toxic substances
◆ Hemodynamic disorder

PATHOPHYSIOLOGY
Acute gastritis
◆ The protective mucosal layer is altered.
◆ Acid secretion produces mucosal reddening, edema, and superficial surface erosion.

Chronic gastritis
◆ The gastric mucosa progressively thins and degenerates.

COMPLICATIONS
◆ Hemorrhage
◆ Bowel obstruction
◆ Peritonitis
◆ Gastric cancer

Assessment

HISTORY
◆ One or more causative agents
◆ Rapid onset of symptoms (acute gastritis)
◆ Epigastric discomfort
◆ Indigestion
◆ Cramping
◆ Anorexia
◆ Nausea, hematemesis, and vomiting
◆ Coffee-ground emesis or melena (if GI bleeding is present)

PHYSICAL FINDINGS
◆ Possible normal appearance
◆ Grimacing
◆ Restlessness
◆ Pallor
◆ Tachycardia
◆ Hypotension
◆ Abdominal distention, tenderness, and guarding
◆ Normoactive to hyperactive bowel sounds

DIAGNOSTIC TEST RESULTS
◆ *Guaiac test:* positive for occult blood in vomitus or stools or both, indicating gastric bleeding
◆ *Hemoglobin (Hb) level and hematocrit:* decreased
◆ *Urea breath test:* H. pylori
◆ *Upper GI endoscopy within 24 hours of bleeding:* inflammation of gastric mucosa
◆ *Biopsy:* inflammatory process

Treatment

- Elimination of cause
- For massive bleeding: blood transfusion, iced saline gastric lavage, or angiography with vasopressin
- Nothing by mouth (if bleeding occurs)
- Elimination of irritating foods
- Encouraging activity and mobilization as tolerated
- Vagotomy, pyloroplasty (when conservative treatment fails)
- Partial or total gastrectomy (rarely)

MEDICATIONS
- Histamine antagonists
- Antacids
- Proton pump inhibitors
- Prostaglandins
- Vitamin B_{12}
- Dual therapy: antibiotic and proton pump inhibitor
- Triple therapy: two antibiotics and bismuth subsalicylate (Pepto-Bismol)

Nursing interventions

- Give prescribed drugs and I.V. fluids.
- Assist the patient with diet modification.
- Consult a dietitian as necessary.
- Provide physical and emotional support.

With acute bleeding
- Monitor vital signs, intake and output, and laboratory values.
- Administer blood products as ordered.
- Prepare for endoscopy or surgery, as appropriate.
- Assess cardiovascular status.
- Observe for signs and symptoms of complications.

PATIENT TEACHING
- Explain the disorder, diagnostic testing, and treatment plan.
- Teach about the administration, dosage, and possible adverse effects of prescribed medications.
- Identify lifestyle and diet modifications needed.
- Provide preoperative teaching if surgery is necessary.
- Explain stress reduction techniques.
- Refer the patient to a smoking-cessation program if indicated.

Gastroesophageal reflux disease

Overview

Gastroesophageal reflux disease (GERD), commonly called *heartburn*, is the backflow of gastric or duodenal contents, or both, into the esophagus and past the lower esophageal sphincter (LES) without associated belching or vomiting. This reflux of gastric acid causes acute epigastric pain, usually after a meal.

CAUSES
- Any condition or position that increases intra-abdominal pressure
- Hiatal hernia with incompetent sphincter
- Pyloric surgery (alteration or removal of the pylorus), which allows reflux of bile or pancreatic juice

RISK FACTORS
- Any agent that lowers LES pressure: acidic and fatty food, alcohol, cigarettes, anticholinergics (atropine [Sal-Tropine], belladonna, propantheline [Pro-Banthine]) or other drugs (morphine, diazepam [Valium], calcium channel blockers, meperidine [Demerol])
- Nasogastric intubation for more than 4 days

PATHOPHYSIOLOGY
- Reflux occurs when LES pressure is deficient or pressure in the stomach exceeds LES pressure. The LES relaxes, and gastric contents regurgitate into the esophagus.
- The degree of mucosal injury is based on the amount and concentration of refluxed gastric acid, proteolytic enzymes, and bile acids.

COMPLICATIONS
- Reflux esophagitis
- Esophageal stricture
- Esophageal ulcer
- Barrett's esophagus (metaplasia and possible increased risk of neoplasm)
- Anemia from esophageal bleeding
- Reflux aspiration leading to chronic pulmonary disease

Assessment

HISTORY
- Minimal or no symptoms in one-third of patients
- Heartburn typically occurring $1\frac{1}{2}$ to 2 hours after eating
- Heartburn worsening with vigorous exercise, bending, lying down, wearing tight clothing, coughing, constipation, and obesity
- Reported relief by using antacids or sitting upright
- Regurgitation without nausea or belching
- Feeling of fluid accumulation in the throat without a sour or bitter taste
- Chronic pain radiating to the neck, jaws, and arms that may mimic angina pectoris
- Nocturnal hypersalivation and wheezing
- Chronic cough

PHYSICAL FINDINGS
- Odynophagia (sharp substernal pain on swallowing), possibly followed by a dull substernal ache
- Bright red or dark brown blood in vomitus
- Laryngitis and morning hoarseness
- Chronic cough

DIAGNOSTIC TEST RESULTS
- *Barium swallow with fluoroscopy:* evidence of recurrent reflux
- *Esophageal acidity test:* degree of gastroesophageal reflux
- *Gastroesophageal scintillation testing:* reflux
- *Esophageal manometry:* abnormal LES pressure and sphincter incompetence
- *Acid perfusion (Bernstein) test:* esophagitis
- *Esophagoscopy and biopsy:* pathologic changes in the mucosa

Treatment

◆ Lifestyle modifications
◆ Positional therapy
◆ Treatment of underlying cause
◆ Weight reduction, if appropriate
◆ Avoidance of acidic or fatty foods
◆ Avoidance of eating 2 hours before sleep
◆ Lifting restrictions after surgical treatment
◆ Hiatal hernia repair
◆ Vagotomy or pyloroplasty
◆ Esophagectomy

MEDICATIONS
◆ Antacids
◆ Cholinergics
◆ Histamine-2 receptor antagonists
◆ Proton pump inhibitors

Nursing interventions

◆ Assist with identifying areas requiring lifestyle and dietary modification.
◆ Offer emotional and psychological support.

AFTER SURGERY
◆ Assess the patient's respiratory status.
◆ Assess the patient's pain level, administer analgesics, and evaluate their effects.
◆ Monitor vital signs, intake and output, and pulse oximetry.
◆ Observe type and amount of chest tube drainage if indicated.
◆ Assess bowel function and resume the patient's diet as ordered.

PATIENT TEACHING
◆ Explain the disorder, diagnostic testing, and treatment plan.
◆ Teach about the administration, dosage, and possible adverse effects of prescribed medications.
◆ Identify appropriate lifestyle and diet modifications.
◆ Describe recommended positional therapy (keeping head elevated after eating).

◆ Assist with identification of situations or activities that increase intra-abdominal pressure.
◆ Explain the signs and symptoms of complications and when to notify the practitioner.

Glaucoma

Overview

Glaucoma is an eye disorder characterized by high intraocular pressure (IOP) and optic nerve damage. There are two forms: open-angle glaucoma (also known as *chronic, simple,* or *wide-angle glaucoma*), which begins insidiously and progresses slowly, and angle-closure glaucoma (also known as *acute* or *narrow-angle glaucoma*), which occurs suddenly and can cause permanent vision loss in 48 to 72 hours. Glaucoma is a leading cause of blindness, accounting for about 12% of newly diagnosed blindness in the United States.

CAUSES
Open-angle glaucoma
◆ Degenerative changes

Angle-closure glaucoma
◆ Anatomically narrow angle between the iris and the cornea
◆ Trauma, pupillary dilation, stress, or ocular changes that push the iris forward

RISK FACTORS
Open-angle glaucoma
◆ Family history
◆ Myopia
◆ Ethnic origin

Angle-closure glaucoma
◆ Family history
◆ Cataracts
◆ Hyperopia

PATHOPHYSIOLOGY
Open-angle glaucoma
◆ Degenerative changes in the trabecular meshwork block the flow of aqueous humor from the eye, increasing IOP and resulting in optic nerve damage.

Angle-closure glaucoma
◆ Obstruction to the outflow of aqueous humor is caused by an anatomically narrow angle between the iris and the cornea.
◆ IOP increases suddenly.

COMPLICATIONS
◆ Varying degrees of vision loss
◆ Total blindness

Assessment

HISTORY
Open-angle glaucoma
◆ Possibly no symptoms
◆ Dull, morning headache
◆ Mild aching in the eyes
◆ Loss of peripheral vision
◆ Halos around lights
◆ Reduced visual acuity (especially at night) not corrected by glasses

Angle-closure glaucoma
◆ Pain and pressure over the eye
◆ Blurred vision
◆ Decreased visual acuity
◆ Halos around lights
◆ Nausea and vomiting (from increased IOP)

PHYSICAL FINDINGS
◆ Unilateral eye inflammation
◆ Cloudy cornea
◆ Moderately dilated pupil, nonreactive to light
◆ With gentle fingertip pressure to the closed eyelids, one eye feels harder than the other (in angle-closure glaucoma)

DIAGNOSTIC TEST RESULTS
◆ *Tonometry measurement:* increased IOP
◆ *Slit-lamp examination:* effects of glaucoma on the anterior eye structures
◆ *Gonioscopy:* angle of the eye's anterior chamber

◆ *Ophthalmoscopy:* cupping of the optic disk (see *Optic disk changes*)
◆ *Perimetry or visual field tests:* extent of peripheral vision loss
◆ *Fundus photography:* optic disk changes

Treatment

◆ Reduction of IOP by decreasing aqueous humor production with medications
◆ Bed rest (with acute angle-closure glaucoma)

For glaucoma nonrefractive to drug therapy
◆ Argon laser trabeculoplasty
◆ Trabeculectomy

For angle-closure glaucoma
◆ Laser iridectomy
◆ Surgical peripheral iridectomy
◆ In end-stage glaucoma, tube shunt or valve

MEDICATIONS
◆ Topical adrenergic agonists
◆ Cholinergic agonists
◆ Beta-adrenergic blockers
◆ Topical or oral carbonic anhydrase inhibitors

Nursing interventions

◆ Give prescribed drugs.
◆ Prepare for surgery if indicated.
◆ After surgery, protect the affected eye.
◆ Encourage ambulation immediately after surgery.
◆ Encourage the patient to express his concerns related to the chronic condition.
◆ Monitor vital signs.
◆ Assess the patient's response to treatment and visual acuity.

PATIENT TEACHING
◆ Explain the disorder, diagnostic testing, and treatment plan.
◆ Teach about the administration, dosage, and possible adverse effects of prescribed medications.
◆ Stress the need for meticulous compliance with prescribed drug therapy.
◆ Explain the need for modification of the patient's environment for safety.
◆ Describe the signs and symptoms that require immediate medical attention such as sudden vision change or eye pain.
◆ Stress the importance of glaucoma screening for early detection and prevention.

Optic disk changes

Ophthalmoscopy and slit-lamp examination show cupping of the optic disk, as shown, which is characteristic of glaucoma.

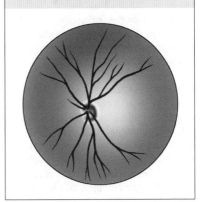

Glomerulonephritis

Overview

Glomerulonephritis, also called *acute post-streptococcal glomerulonephritis,* is inflammation of the glomeruli in the kidney, usually after a streptococcal infection. It can affect adequate kidney function and may result in renal failure.

CAUSES
◆ Immunoglobulin A nephropathy (Berger's disease)
◆ Impetigo
◆ Lipoid nephrosis
◆ *Streptococcal* infection of the respiratory tract

Chronic glomerulonephritis
◆ Focal glomerulosclerosis
◆ Goodpasture's syndrome
◆ Hemolytic uremic syndrome
◆ Membranoproliferative glomerulonephritis
◆ Membranous glomerulopathy
◆ Poststreptococcal glomerulonephritis
◆ Rapidly progressive glomerulonephritis
◆ Systemic lupus erythematosus

PATHOPHYSIOLOGY
◆ The epithelial or podocyte layer of the glomerular membrane is disturbed.
◆ Acute poststreptococcal glomerulonephritis results from antigen-antibody complexes becoming trapped and collecting in glomerular capillary membranes after infection with group A beta-hemolytic streptococci.
◆ Antigens stimulate the formation of antibodies.
◆ Circulating antigen-antibody complexes become lodged in the glomerular capillaries.
◆ Complement activation is initiated and immunologic substances are released that lyse cells and increase membrane permeability.
◆ Antibody damage to basement membranes causes crescent formation.

◆ Antibody or antigen-antibody complexes in the glomerular capillary wall activate biochemical mediators of inflammation—complement, leukocytes, and fibrin.
◆ Lysosomal enzymes are released that damage the glomerular cell walls and cause a proliferation of the extracellular matrix, affecting glomerular blood flow.
◆ Membrane permeability increases and protein filtration is enhanced.
◆ Membrane damage leads to platelet aggregation, and platelet degranulation releases substances that increase glomerular permeability.

COMPLICATIONS
◆ Pulmonary edema
◆ Heart failure
◆ Sepsis
◆ Renal failure
◆ Severe hypertension
◆ Cardiac hypertrophy

Assessment

HISTORY
◆ Sudden onset of proteinuria
◆ Sudden onset of red blood cells (RBCs) and casts in urine
◆ Decreased urination
◆ Recent streptococcal infection of the respiratory tract

PHYSICAL FINDINGS
◆ Smoky or coffee-colored urine
◆ Dyspnea
◆ Periorbital edema
◆ Increased blood pressure

DIAGNOSTIC TEST RESULTS
◆ *Throat culture:* beta-hemolytic streptococci
◆ *Electrolyte, blood urea nitrogen, and creatinine levels:* increased
◆ *Serum protein level:* decreased
◆ *Hemoglobin level:* decreased (chronic glomerulonephritis)
◆ *Antistreptolysin-O titers:* elevated

◆ *Streptozyme and anti-DNase B levels:* elevated
◆ *Serum complement levels:* abnormally low
◆ *Urinalysis:* RBCs, white blood cells, mixed cell casts, fibrin-degradation products, protein, and C3 protein
◆ *Kidney-ureter-bladder X-ray:* bilateral kidney enlargement (acute glomerulonephritis)
◆ *X-ray:* symmetrical contraction with normal pelves and calyces (chronic glomerulonephritis)
◆ *Renal biopsy:* confirmation of diagnosis

Treatment

◆ Treatment of the primary disease
◆ Correction of electrolyte imbalance
◆ Dialysis
◆ Plasmapheresis
◆ Fluid restriction
◆ Sodium restriction
◆ Bed rest
◆ Kidney transplant

MEDICATIONS
◆ Antibiotics
◆ Anticoagulants
◆ Diuretics
◆ Vasodilators
◆ Corticosteroids

Nursing interventions

◆ Monitor vital signs, intake and output, and laboratory values.
◆ Assess renal status.
◆ Provide appropriate skin care and oral hygiene.
◆ Encourage the patient to express his feelings about the disorder.
◆ Give prescribed drugs.
◆ Obtain daily weight.
◆ Observe for signs and symptoms of complications.

PATIENT TEACHING
◆ Explain the disorder, diagnostic testing, and treatment plan.
◆ Teach about the administration, dosage, and possible adverse effects of prescribed medications.
◆ Describe signs and symptoms of complications.
◆ Teach the patient to obtain and record daily weight and to report increases of 2 lb (0.9 kg) in 1 day or 5 lb (2.3 kg) in 1 week.
◆ Stress the importance of follow-up care.

Guillain-Barré syndrome

Overview

A form of polyneuritis, Guillain-Barré syndrome is an acute, rapidly progressive, and potentially fatal condition. It has three phases: acute, beginning from the first symptom and ending in 1 to 3 weeks; plateau, lasting several days to 2 weeks; and recovery, coinciding with remyelination and axonal process regrowth and extending over 4 to 6 months and possibly up to 2 to 3 years. Recovery may not be complete.

CAUSES
◆ Unknown

RISK FACTORS
◆ Surgery
◆ Rabies or swine influenza vaccination
◆ Viral illness
◆ Hodgkin's disease or other malignant disease
◆ Lupus erythematosus

PATHOPHYSIOLOGY
◆ Segmented demyelination of peripheral nerves occurs, preventing normal transmission of electrical impulses.
◆ Sensorimotor nerve roots are affected; autonomic nerve transmission may also be affected.

COMPLICATIONS
◆ Thrombophlebitis
◆ Pressure ulcers
◆ Contractures
◆ Muscle wasting
◆ Aspiration
◆ Respiratory tract infections
◆ Life-threatening respiratory and cardiac compromise

Assessment

HISTORY
◆ Minor febrile illness 1 to 4 weeks before current symptoms
◆ Tingling and numbness (paresthesia) in the legs
◆ Progression of symptoms to arms, trunk and, finally, the face
◆ Stiffness and pain in the calves

PHYSICAL FINDINGS
◆ Muscle weakness (the major neurologic sign)
◆ Sensory loss, usually in the legs (spreads to arms)
◆ Difficulty talking, chewing, and swallowing
◆ Paralysis of the ocular, facial, and oropharyngeal muscles
◆ Loss of position sense
◆ Diminished or absent deep tendon reflexes

DIAGNOSTIC TEST RESULTS
◆ *Cerebrospinal fluid (CSF) analysis:* normal white blood cell count, elevated protein count and, in severe disease, increased CSF pressure
◆ *Electromyography:* repeated firing of the same motor unit instead of widespread sectional stimulation
◆ *Nerve conduction studies:* marked slowing of nerve conduction velocities

Treatment

◆ Supportive measures
◆ Emotional support
◆ Maintenance of skin integrity
◆ Possible endotracheal (ET) intubation or tracheotomy

- Fluid volume replacement
- Plasmapheresis
- Possible tube feedings with ET intubation
- Adequate caloric intake
- Exercise program to prevent contractures
- Possible tracheostomy
- Possible gastrostomy or jejunotomy feeding tube insertion

MEDICATIONS
- I.V. beta-adrenergic blockers
- Parasympatholytics
- I.V. immune globulin

Nursing interventions

- Assess musculoskeletal status to determine progression of muscle weakness.
- Assess respiratory status.
- Monitor vital signs and pulse oximetry.
- Give prescribed drugs.
- Establish a means of communication before intubation is required, if possible.
- Reposition the patient every 2 hours and assess skin integrity.
- Provide skin care.
- Encourage coughing and deep breathing and use of incentive spirometer.
- Provide passive range-of-motion exercises.
- Apply sequential compression stockings when the patient is in bed.
- Provide emotional support.
- Observe for signs and sympoms of complications.

PATIENT TEACHING
- Explain the disorder, diagnostic testing, and treatment plan.
- Teach about the administration, dosage, and possible adverse effects of prescribed medications.

- Describe signs and symptoms of complications.
- Refer the patient to physical rehabilitation sources as indicated.
- Refer the patient to occupational and speech rehabilitation resources as indicated.
- Refer the patient and his family to the Guillain-Barré Syndrome Foundation for additional information and support.

Headache

Overview

A headache is head pain that usually occurs as a symptom of an underlying disorder. Tension headache is the most common type of head pain. A migraine headache is more severe and involves photophobia, sleep disruption, and depression.

CAUSES
Headache
- Allergy
- Caffeine withdrawal
- Disorder of the scalp, teeth, extracranial arteries, or external or middle ear
- Emotional stress
- Environmental stimuli
- Fatigue
- Glaucoma
- Head trauma or tumors
- Hypertension
- Hypoxia
- Inflammation of the eyes or mucosa of the nasal or paranasal sinuses
- Intracranial bleeding, abscess, or aneurysm
- Menstruation
- Muscle spasms of the face, neck, or shoulders
- Overuse of over-the-counter headache medications (rebound headache)
- Psychological disorders
- Systemic disorder
- Tension (muscle contraction)
- Underlying intracranial disorder
- Vasodilators

Migraine
- Constriction and dilation of intracranial and extracranial arteries
- Associated with depression, epilepsy, hereditary hemorrhagic telangiectasia, ischemic stroke, and Tourette syndrome

PATHOPHYSIOLOGY
Headache
- Sustained muscle contractions directly deform pain receptors.

- Inflammation or direct pressure affects the cranial nerves.
- Pain-sensitive structures respond, including the skin; scalp; muscles; arteries; veins; cranial nerves V, VII, IX, and X; and cervical nerves 1, 2, and 3.

Migraine
- Biochemical abnormalities occur, including the release of neurokinin A and calcitonin, a gene-related peptide that dilates vessels and triggers inflammation, stimulating the trigeminocervical complex.
- The thalamus and cortex then register pain and trigger autonomic symptoms.

COMPLICATIONS
- Worsening of existing hypertension
- Loss of work or the ability to perform activities of daily living
- Stroke
- Substance dependency

Assessment

HISTORY
Headache
- Onset (acute, recurrent, or chronic)
- Location (frontal, temporal, occipital, or cervical), characteristics (frequency and intensity), and duration (continuous or intermittent)
- Precipitating factors: tension, menstruation, loud noises, caffeine, alcohol consumption, stress, allergies, medications, and lights.
- Aggravating factors: coughing, sneezing, and sunlight
- Associated symptoms: nausea or vomiting, weakness, facial pain, scotomas, gait disturbance, fever, and tingling in the face, lips, or hands
- Efforts to relieve: analgesics, ice packs, and a darkened room
- Familial history of headaches
- Impact on activities of daily living

Migraine
- Unilateral, throbbing pain that gradually becomes more generalized

◆ Scintillating scotoma, hemianopsia, unilateral paresthesias, or speech disorders preceding the migraine

◆ Associated irritability, anorexia, nausea or vomiting, photophobia, sensitivity to noise or visual disturbances

◆ Feeling of heaviness of the limbs or tingling in the lips, hands, or feet

PHYSICAL FINDINGS
Headache
◆ Findings based on cause
◆ If no underlying problem, normal physical findings
◆ Possible crepitus or tender spots of the head and neck

Migraine
◆ Possible extraocular muscle palsies
◆ Possible ptosis
◆ Possible hemiparesis, hemiplegia, staggering gait, or sensory disturbances

DIAGNOSTIC TEST RESULTS
◆ *Skull X-rays*: skull fracture (with trauma)
◆ *Sinus X-rays*: sinusitis
◆ *Computed tomography scan*: tumor, subarachnoid hemorrhage, other intracranial pathology, sinus pathology
◆ *Magnetic resonance imaging*: tumor
◆ *Lumbar puncture:* increased intracranial pressure suggesting tumor, edema, or hemorrhage
◆ *Electroencephalography*: alterations in the brain's electrical activity suggesting intracranial lesion, head injury, meningitis, or encephalitis

Treatment

◆ Identification and elimination of causative factors (including environmental)
◆ Yoga, meditation, or other relaxation therapy
◆ Psychotherapy if emotional stress involved
◆ For migraine patient, adequate oral fluid intake and avoidance of dietary triggers

◆ For migraine patient, bed rest in dark, quiet room

MEDICATIONS
Headache and migraine
◆ Nonsteroidal anti-inflammatory drugs (NSAIDs)
◆ Analgesics
◆ Sedatives
◆ Muscle relaxants

Migraine
◆ NSAIDs
◆ Combination analgesics
◆ Ergotamine preparations
◆ Beta-adrenergic blockers
◆ Tricyclic antidepressants
◆ Calcium channel blockers
◆ Selective serotonin receptor agonists
◆ Serotonin antagonists
◆ Antiemetics
◆ Anticonvulsants

Nursing interventions

◆ Monitor vital signs, especially blood pressure.
◆ Assess the patient's pain level, administer analgesics, and evaluate their effects.
◆ Encourage the use of relaxation techniques.
◆ Keep the patient's room dark and quiet.
◆ Place ice packs on the patient's forehead or a cold cloth over his eyes.

PATIENT TEACHING
◆ Explain the disorder, diagnostic testing, and treatment plan.
◆ Review the administration, dosage, and possible adverse effects of prescribed medications.
◆ Teach methods to prevent migraine occurrence.
◆ Review beneficial lifestyle changes.
◆ Teach nonpharmacologic strategies for treating migraines.
◆ Recommend monitoring headaches with a headache diary.
◆ Refer the patient to the National Headache Foundation.

Heart failure

Overview

Heart failure is insufficient cardiac output caused by fluid buildup in the heart. It may occur from a damaged myocardium or an impaired left or right ventricle. Compensatory mechanisms cause cardiac muscle fibers to stretch, resulting in ventricular hypertrophy in chronic conditions.

CAUSES
- Acute blood loss
- Anemia
- Arrhythmias
- Cardiomyopathy
- Constrictive pericarditis
- Coronary artery disease
- Hypertension
- Increased salt or water intake
- Infections (severe)
- Ischemic heart disease
- Mitral or aortic insufficiency
- Mitral stenosis secondary to rheumatic heart disease or constrictive pericarditis
- Myocarditis
- Pregnancy or childbirth
- Pulmonary embolism
- Severe physical or mental stress
- Thyrotoxicosis
- Valvular disease

PATHOPHYSIOLOGY
Left-sided heart failure
- Pumping ability of the left ventricle fails and cardiac output falls.
- Blood backs up into the left atrium and lungs, causing pulmonary congestion.

Right-sided heart failure
- Ineffective contractile function of the right ventricle leads to blood backing up into the right atrium and the peripheral circulation, which results in peripheral edema and engorgement of the liver and other organs.

COMPLICATIONS
- Pulmonary edema
- Thomboembolism
- Organ failure, especially the brain and kidneys
- Myocardial infarction
- Cardiac arrhythmias
- Activity intolerance

Assessment

HISTORY
- A disorder or condition that can precipitate heart failure
- Dyspnea or paroxysmal nocturnal dyspnea
- Peripheral edema
- Fatigue
- Weakness
- Exercise intolerance
- Insomnia
- Anorexia
- Nausea
- Sense of abdominal fullness (particularly in right-sided heart failure)
- Substance abuse

PHYSICAL FINDINGS
Left-sided heart failure
- Dyspnea on exertion
- Moist, bibasilar crackles, rhonchi, and expiratory wheezing
- Tachycardia
- Restlessness, confusion
- Cough producing pink, frothy sputum
- Pale, cool, clammy skin
- Diaphoresis
- Lateral displacement of PMI
- Pulsus alternans
- Third and fourth heart sounds
- Decreased urinary output

Right-sided heart failure
- Jugular vein distention
- Hepatojugular reflex
- Hepatomegaly
- Right upper quadrant pain
- Weight gain
- Peripheral edema
- Ascites
- Cyanosis
- Decreased pulse pressure

- Decreased pulse oximetry
- Decreased urinary output

DIAGNOSTIC TEST RESULTS

- *B-type natriuretic peptide immunoassay*: elevated
- *Chest X-rays*: increased pulmonary vascular markings, interstitial edema, or pleural effusion and cardiomegaly
- *Pulse oximetry*: decreased
- *Arterial blood gas analysis*: hypoxia
- *Electrocardiography*: ischemia, atrial or ventricular enlargement, or arrhythmias
- *Pulmonary artery pressure monitoring*: elevated pulmonary artery and pulmonary artery wedge pressures, left ventricular end diastolic pressure in left-sided heart failure, and elevated right atrial or central venous pressure in right-sided heart failure
- *Echocardiography:* left ventricular hypertrophy and dilation and decreased ejection fraction

Treatment

- Semi-Fowler's position
- Elevation of lower extremities
- Sodium and fluid restriction
- Calorie restriction, if indicated
- Low-fat diet, if indicated
- Bed rest while acute, then activity as tolerated (walking encouraged)
- Surgical replacement (for valvular dysfunction with recurrent acute heart failure)
- Heart transplantation
- Ventricular assist device
- Biventricular pacemeaker
- Implantable cardioverter-defibrillator insertion
- Stent placement
- Antiembolism stockings

MEDICATIONS

- Oxygen therapy
- Diuretics
- Human B-type natriuretic peptide: nesiritide (Natrecor)
- Angiotensin receptor blockers
- Angiotensin-converting enzyme inhibitors
- Inotropic drugs
- Vasodilators
- Morphine sulfate
- Phosphodiesterase enzyme inhibitors
- Potassium supplements
- Selective aldosterone-blocking agent: eplerenone (Inspra)
- Beta-adrenergic blockers

Nursing interventions

- Place the patient in semi-Fowler's position, and give supplemental oxygen.
- Provide continuous cardiac monitoring in acute and advanced stages.
- Assess for peripheral edema and other signs and symptoms of fluid overload.
- Monitor vital signs, cardiac rhythm, intake and output, and laboratory values.
- Auscultate for abnormal heart and breath sounds and report changes immediately.
- Assist the patient with range-of-motion exercises.
- Apply antiembolism stockings, and check for calf pain and tenderness.
- Obtain daily weight.

PATIENT TEACHING

- Explain the disorder, diagnostic testing, and treatment plan.
- Teach about the administration, dosage, and possible adverse effects of prescribed medications.
- Describe signs and symptoms of worsening heart failure and explain when to notify the practitioner.
- Review dietary and fluid restrictions.
- Explain the need to obtain a weight every morning at the same time (before eating, after urinating) and to keep a record of weight. Instruct the patient to report weekly weight gain of 5 lb (2.5 kg) or more.
- Stress the importance of follow-up care.
- Refer the patient to a smoking-cessation program if appropriate.

Heat syndrome

Overview

Heat syndrome is the increase of body temperature caused by the body's inability to compensate for increased heat production or decreased heat loss. The three categories of heat syndrome are: heat cramps (normal to high temperature with muscle cramping), heat exhaustion (acute heat injury with hyperthermia caused by dehydration), and heatstroke (extreme hyperthermia with thermoregulatory failure).

CAUSES
◆ Behavior such as excessive exercise, not opening windows or using air conditioning in extreme heat, or wearing inappropriate clothing for the temperature
◆ Dehydration
◆ Drugs, such as phenothiazines, anticholinergics, and amphetamines
◆ Endocrine disorders
◆ Heart disease
◆ Hot environment without ventilation
◆ Illness
◆ Inadequate fluid intake
◆ Infection (fever)
◆ Lack of acclimatization
◆ Neurologic disorder
◆ Sudden discontinuation of Parkinson's disease medications

RISK FACTORS
◆ Obesity
◆ Salt and water depletion
◆ Alcohol use
◆ Poor physical condition
◆ Age

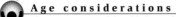

Age considerations

The very young and the elderly are the most susceptible to heat syndrome. Symptoms may develop quickly.

◆ Socioeconomic status
◆ Athletes
◆ History of chronic diseases

PATHOPHYSIOLOGY
◆ Normal regulation of temperature is by evaporation (30% of body's heat loss) or vasodilation. When heat is generated or gained by the body faster than it can be dissipated, the thermoregulatory mechanism is stressed and eventually fails.
◆ Failure of the thermoregulatory mechanism causes hyperthermia to accelerate.
◆ Cerebral edema and cerebrovascular congestion occur.
◆ Cerebral perfusion pressure increases and cerebral perfusion decreases.
◆ Tissue damage occurs when temperature exceeds 107.6° F (42° C), resulting in tissue necrosis, organ dysfunction, and failure.

COMPLICATIONS
◆ Hypovolemic shock
◆ Cardiogenic shock
◆ Cardiac arrhythmias
◆ Renal failure
◆ Disseminated intravascular coagulation
◆ Hepatic failure
◆ Cerebral edema

Assessment

HISTORY
Heat cramps
◆ Strenuous activity

Heat exhaustion
◆ Prolonged activity in a very warm or hot environment
◆ Muscle cramps
◆ Nausea and vomiting
◆ Thirst
◆ Weakness
◆ Headache
◆ Fatigue
◆ Sweating
◆ Tachycardia

Heatstroke
◆ Exposure to high temperature
◆ Signs and symptoms of heat exhaustion
◆ Blurred vision
◆ Confusion
◆ Hallucinations
◆ Decreased muscle coordination
◆ Syncope

PHYSICAL FINDINGS

Heat cramps

- Muscle twitching and spasms
- Weakness
- Severe muscle cramps
- Nausea

Heat exhaustion

- Rectal temperature 100.4° F (38° C) to 104° F (40° C)
- Pale skin
- Thready, rapid pulse
- Cool, moist skin
- Decreased blood pressure
- Irritability
- Syncope
- Impaired judgment
- Hyperventilation

Heatstroke

- Rectal temperature of at least 105° F (40.5° C)
- Red, diaphoretic, hot skin in early stages
- Gray, dry, hot skin in later stages
- Tachycardia
- Slightly elevated blood pressure in early stages; decreased blood pressure in later stages
- Tachypnea
- Decreased level of consciousness
- Altered mental status
- Cheyne-Stokes respirations
- Anhidrosis (late sign)

DIAGNOSTIC TEST RESULTS

- *Serum electrolytes*: elevated, which may show hyponatremia and hypokalemia
- *Arterial blood gas levels:* respiratory alkalosis
- *Complete blood count*: leukocytosis and thrombocytopenia
- *Coagulation studies*: increased bleeding and clotting times
- *Urinalysis*: concentrated urine and proteinuria with tubular casts and myoglobinuria
- *Blood urea nitrogen*: elevated
- *Serum calcium level*: decreased
- *Serum phosphorus level*: decreased
- *Myoglobinuria*: rhabdomyolysis

Treatment

Heat cramps and heat exhaustion

- Cool environment
- Oral or I.V. fluid administration
- Adequate ventilation

Heatstroke

- Lowering the body temperature as rapidly as possible
- Evaporation, hypothermia blankets, and ice packs to the groin, axillae, and neck
- Supportive respiratory and cardiovascular measures
- Increased hydration, cool liquids only
- Avoidance of caffeine and alcohol
- Rest periods as needed

Nursing interventions

- Perform rapid cooling procedures.
- Provide supportive measures.
- Provide adequate fluid intake.
- Give prescribed drugs.
- Monitor vital signs, cardiac rhythm, intake and output, and pulse oximetry readings.
- Observe for signs and symptoms of complications.

PATIENT TEACHING

- Explain the disorder, diagnostic testing, and treatment plan.
- Teach about the administration, dosage, and possible adverse effects of prescribed medications.
- Describe how to avoid reexposure to high temperatures.
- Stress the need to maintain adequate fluid intake and adequate ventilation.
- Recommend wearing loose clothing while exercising and activity limitation in hot weather.
- Refer the patient to social services if appropriate.

Hemophilia

Overview

An incurable hereditary bleeding disorder resulting from a deficiency of specific clotting factors, hemophilia is characterized by greatly prolonged coagulation time. Hemophilia is the most common X-linked genetic disease. Hemophilia A (classic hemophilia), the most common type, results from factor VIII deficiency. Hemophilia B (Christmas disease) results from factor IX deficiency.

CAUSES
◆ Acquired immunologic process
◆ Hemophilia A and B inherited as X-linked recessive traits
◆ Spontaneous mutation

PATHOPHYSIOLOGY
◆ A low level or absence of the blood protein necessary for clotting causes a disruption of the normal intrinsic coagulation cascade.
◆ Abnormal bleeding, which may be mild, moderate, or severe, depending on the degree of protein factor deficiency, is produced.
◆ After a platelet plug at a bleeding site, the lack of clotting factors impairs formation of a stable fibrin clot.
◆ Immediate hemorrhage isn't prevalent and delayed bleeding is common; the severity depends upon the degree of deficiency.

COMPLICATIONS
◆ Pain, swelling, extreme tenderness, and permanent joint and muscle deformity
◆ Peripheral neuropathies, pain, paresthesia, and muscle atrophy
◆ Ischemia and gangrene
◆ Hypovolemic shock and death

Assessment

HISTORY
◆ Familial history of bleeding disorders
◆ Prolonged bleeding with circumcision or a large cephalo-hematoma at birth
◆ Concomitant illness
◆ Pain and swelling in a weight-bearing joint, such as the hip, knee, or ankle
◆ With mild hemophilia or after minor trauma, lack of spontaneous bleeding, but prolonged bleeding with major trauma or surgery
◆ Moderate hemophilia producing only occasional spontaneous bleeding episodes
◆ Severe hemophilia causing spontaneous bleeding
◆ Prolonged bleeding after surgery or trauma or joint pain caused by spontaneous bleeding into muscles or joints
◆ Signs of internal bleeding, such as abdominal, chest, or flank pain; episodes of hematuria or hematemesis; and tarry stools
◆ Activity or movement limitations and need for assistive devices, such as splints, canes, or crutches

PHYSICAL FINDINGS
◆ Hematomas on extremities, torso, or both
◆ Joint swelling in episodes of bleeding into joints
◆ Limited and painful joint range of motion in episodes of bleeding into joints

DIAGNOSTIC TEST RESULTS
Hemophilia A
◆ *Factor VIII assay:* 30% of normal or less
◆ *Coagulation studies:* abnormal

Hemophilia B
◆ *Factor IX assay:* deficient
◆ *Coagulation studies:* abnormal

Hemophilia A or B
◆ *Degree of factor severity:* mild (factor levels 5% to 30% of normal), moderate (fac-

tor levels 1% to 5% of normal), or severe (factor levels less than 1% of normal)

Treatment

◆ Measures to stop bleeding, such as pressure to the bleeding site
◆ Foods high in vitamin K
◆ Activity as guided by the degree of factor deficiency

MEDICATIONS
◆ Aminocaproic acid (Amicar)

Hemophilia A
◆ Cryoprecipitated antihemophilic factor (AHF), lyophilized AHF, or both
◆ Desmopressin (Stimate)

Hemophilia B
◆ Factor IX concentrate

Nursing interventions

During bleeding episodes
◆ Apply pressure to bleeding sites.
◆ Give the deficient clotting factor or plasma, as ordered, until bleeding stops.
◆ Observe for signs and symptoms of decreased tissue perfusion.
◆ Apply cold compresses or ice bags, and elevate the injured part.
◆ To prevent recurrence of bleeding, restrict activity for 48 hours after bleeding is under control.
◆ Assess the patient's pain level, administer analgesics, and evaluate their effects.
◆ Avoid administering I.M. injections, aspirin, and aspirin-containing drugs.
◆ Monitor vital signs and laboratory values.

During bleeding into a joint
◆ Immediately elevate the joint.
◆ Perform range-of-motion exercises at least 48 hours after the bleeding is controlled.

◆ Restrict weight bearing until bleeding stops and swelling subsides.
◆ Apply ice packs and elastic bandages to alleviate pain.
◆ Monitor vital signs.

PATIENT TEACHING
◆ Explain the disorder, diagnostic testing, and treatment plan.
◆ Teach about the administration, dosage, and possible adverse effects of prescribed medications.
◆ Explain the benefits of regular isometric exercises.
◆ Teach safety measures, such as wearing protective devices during activities and avoiding contact sports.
◆ Teach measures to decrease bleeding.
◆ Describe signs and symptoms of complications.

 Nursing alert
Stress the importance of avoiding aspirin, combination medications that contain aspirin, and over-the-counter non-steroidal anti-inflammatory drugs. Instruct the patient to use acetaminophen instead.

◆ Explain the importance of good dental care and the need to check with the practitioner before dental extractions or surgery.
◆ Teach the need to wear medical identification at all times.
◆ Refer new patients to a hemophilia treatment center for evaluation.

Hepatic encephalopathy

Overview

A central nervous system dysfunction, hepatic encephalopathy develops as a complication of aggressive fulminant hepatitis or chronic hepatic disease. It's most common in patients with cirrhosis. The acute form occurs with acute fulminant hepatic failure and may be fatal; the chronic form occurs with chronic liver disease and is usually reversible. The prognosis in advanced stages is extremely poor, even with vigorous treatment.

CAUSES
◆ Exact cause unknown
◆ Ammonia intoxication of the brain

RISK FACTORS
◆ Excessive protein intake
◆ Sepsis
◆ Excessive accumulation of nitrogenous body wastes (from constipation or GI hemorrhage)
◆ Bacterial action on protein and urea to form ammonia
◆ Hepatitis
◆ Diuretic therapy
◆ Alcoholism
◆ Fluid and electrolyte imbalance (especially metabolic alkalosis)
◆ Hypoxia
◆ Azotemia
◆ Impaired glucose metabolism
◆ Infection
◆ Use of sedatives, general anesthetics, diuretics, tranquilizers, and analgesics

PATHOPHYSIOLOGY
◆ Ammonia produced by protein breakdown in the bowel normally is metabolized to urea in the liver. When portal blood shunts past the liver, ammonia directly enters the systemic circulation and is carried to the brain.
◆ Shunting may result from the collateral venous circulation that develops in portal hypertension or from surgically created portal systemic shunts.
◆ Cirrhosis further compounds this problem because impaired hepatocellular function prevents conversion of ammonia that reaches the liver.

COMPLICATIONS
◆ Irreversible coma
◆ Death

Assessment

HISTORY
Prodromal stage
◆ Slight personality changes, such as agitation, belligerence, disorientation, and forgetfulness
◆ Trouble concentrating or thinking clearly
◆ Fatigue
◆ Mental changes, such as confusion and disorientation
◆ Sleep-wake reversal

Impending stage
◆ Mental changes, such as confusion and disorientation

Stuporous stage
◆ Marked mental confusion

Comatose stage
◆ Unable to arouse

PHYSICAL FINDINGS
Prodromal stage
◆ Slurred or slowed speech
◆ Slight tremor
◆ Unkempt appearance

Impending stage
◆ Tremors that have progressed to asterixis
◆ Lethargy
◆ Aberrant behavior
◆ Apraxia
◆ Possible incontinence
◆ Hyperactive deep tendon reflexes (DTRs)

Stuporous stage
◆ Drowsy and stuporous
◆ Noisy and abusive when aroused
◆ Hyperventilation
◆ Muscle twitching
◆ Asterixis

Comatose stage
◆ Absence of DTRs
◆ Obtunded
◆ Seizures
◆ Hyperactive reflexes
◆ Positive Babinski's sign
◆ Fetor hepaticus (musty, sweet breath odor)

DIAGNOSTIC TEST RESULTS
◆ *Serum ammonia levels:* elevated
◆ *Serum bilirubin level:* elevated
◆ *Prothrombin time:* prolonged
◆ *Electroencephalography:* slowing waves, increased amplitude of waves, and triphasic waves as the disease progresses

Treatment

◆ Elimination of the underlying cause
◆ I.V. fluid administration
◆ Control of GI bleeding
◆ Life-support measures (if appropriate)
◆ Bowel cleansing
◆ Limited protein intake (1.0 to 1.5 grams/kg)
◆ Avoidance of alcohol
◆ Nothing by mouth (with decreased responsiveness)
◆ Parenteral or enteric feedings if appropriate
◆ Bed rest until condition improves
◆ Possible liver transplant

MEDICATIONS
◆ Lactulose (Cholac)
◆ Neomycin (Neo-fradin)
◆ Potassium supplements
◆ Salt-poor albumin
◆ Benzodiazepine antagonists

Nursing interventions

◆ Assess the patient's level of consciousness.
◆ Monitor vital signs, intake and output, and laboratory values.
◆ Promote rest, comfort, and a quiet atmosphere.
◆ Give prescribed drugs.
◆ Obtain daily weight and abdominal girth measurements.
◆ Provide safety measures.
◆ Reposition the patient every 2 hours, assess skin integrity, and provide skin care.
◆ Perform passive range-of-motion exercises.
◆ Provide emotional support.
◆ Observe for signs and symptoms of complications.

PATIENT TEACHING
◆ Explain the disorder, diagnostic testing, and treatment plan.
◆ Teach about the administration, dosage, and possible adverse effects of prescribed medications.
◆ Describe signs of complications or worsening symptoms.
◆ Review dietary modifications.
◆ Refer the patient to social services as indicated.

Hepatitis, viral

Overview

Viral hepatitis is an infection and inflammation of the liver caused by a virus. There are six recognized types—A, B, C, D, E, and G. The most common types are hepatitis A, B, and C.

CAUSES
◆ Infection with the causative virus

Type A
◆ Transmission by the fecal-oral route
◆ Ingestion of contaminated food, milk, or water

Type B
◆ Transmission by contact with contaminated human blood, secretions, and stool
◆ Perinatal transmission

Type C
◆ Transmission primarily through needles shared by I.V. drug users or used in tattooing, through blood transfusions, or through shared paraphernalia used for sniffing cocaine

Type D
◆ Found only in patients with an acute or a chronic episode of hepatitis B

Type E
◆ Transmission by fecal-oral route via contaminated water

Type G
◆ Thought to be blood-borne, with transmission similar to that of hepatitis B and C

PATHOPHYSIOLOGY
◆ Hepatic inflammation caused by the virus leads to diffuse injury and edema of the interstitium and necrosis of hepatocytes.
◆ Hypertrophy and hyperplasia of Kupffer cells and cells of the sinusoidal lining occurs.
◆ Bile obstruction may occur.

COMPLICATIONS
◆ Life-threatening fulminant hepatitis
◆ Chronic active hepatitis (hepatitis B and C)
◆ Syndrome resembling serum sickness, characterized by arthralgia or arthritis, rash, and angioedema
◆ Primary liver cancer (hepatitis B and C)
◆ In hepatitis D, mild or asymptomatic form of hepatitis B flares into severe, progressive chronic active hepatitis and cirrhosis

Assessment

HISTORY
◆ No signs or symptoms in 50% to 60% of people with hepatitis B
◆ No signs or symptoms in 80% of people with hepatitis C
◆ Revelation of a transmission source

Prodromal stage
◆ Patient easily fatigued, with generalized malaise
◆ Anorexia, mild weight loss
◆ Depression
◆ Headache, photophobia
◆ Weakness
◆ Arthralgia, myalgia (hepatitis B)
◆ Nausea or vomiting
◆ Changes in the senses of taste and smell

Clinical jaundice stage
◆ Pruritus
◆ Abdominal pain or tenderness
◆ Indigestion
◆ Anorexia
◆ Possible jaundice of sclerae, mucous membranes, and skin

Posticteric stage
◆ Most symptoms decreasing or subsided

PHYSICAL FINDINGS
Prodromal stage
◆ Fever (100° to 102° F [37.8° to 38.9° C])
◆ Dark urine
◆ Clay-colored stools

Clinical jaundice stage
◆ Rashes, erythematous patches, or hives
◆ Abdominal tenderness in the right upper quadrant
◆ Enlarged and tender liver
◆ Splenomegaly
◆ Cervical adenopathy

Posticteric stage
◆ Decrease in liver enlargement

DIAGNOSTIC TEST RESULTS
◆ *Hepatitis profile*: antibodies specific to the causative virus, establishing type
  ● *Hepatitis A antibody:* confirms diagnosis
  ● *Hepatitis B surface antigens and hepatitis B antibodies*: confirms diagnosis
  ● *Serologic testing:* positive for hepatitis A, B, and C (performed 1 month or more after diagnosis because test is initially negative in types A, B, and C)
  ● *Intrahepatic delta antigens or immunoglobulin (Ig) M antidelta antigens:* acute type D hepatitis
  ● *IgM and IgG antidelta antigens:* chronic type D hepatitis
  ● *Hepatitis E antigens:* positive for hepatitis E
  ● *Hepatitis G ribonucleic acid*: positive for hepatitis G (serologic assays in development)
◆ *Serum aspartate aminotransferase and serum alanine aminotransferase levels*: increased in prodromal stage of acute viral hepatitis
◆ *Serum alkaline phosphatase levels*: slightly increased
◆ *Serum bilirubin level*: elevated in clinical jaundice stage
◆ *Prothrombin time:* prolonged
◆ *White blood cell count*: transient neutropenia and lymphopenia, followed by lymphocytosis
◆ *Liver biopsy*: chronic hepatitis

Treatment
◆ Stopping or slowing hepatic damage and relieving symptoms
◆ Parenteral feeding if appropriate
◆ Small, frequent, high-calorie, high-protein meals (reduced protein intake if signs develop of precoma—lethargy, confusion, mental changes)
◆ Avoidance of alcohol
◆ Frequent rest periods as needed
◆ Avoidance of contact sports and strenuous activity
◆ Possible liver transplant (hepatitis C)

MEDICATIONS
◆ Standard Ig
◆ Vaccine
◆ Interferon alfa-2b (hepatitis B and C)
◆ Antiemetics
◆ Cholestyramine (Questran)
◆ Lamivudine (Epivir) (hepatitis B)
◆ Ribavirin (Virazole) (hepatitis C)

Nursing interventions
◆ Give prescribed drugs.
◆ Encourage oral fluid intake.
◆ Provide rest periods during the day.
◆ Monitor and assess the patient's hydration and nutritional status.
◆ Obtain daily weight.
◆ Monitor stools for color, consistency, amount, and frequency.
◆ Observe for signs and symptoms of complications.

PATIENT TEACHING
◆ Explain the disorder, diagnostic testing, and treatment plan.
◆ Teach about the administration, dosage, and possible adverse effects of prescribed medications.
◆ Explain measures to prevent to spread of disease
◆ Stress the importance of abstaining from alcohol.
◆ Explain the need for follow-up care.
◆ Refer the patient to Alcoholics Anonymous if indicated.

Herniated intervertebral disk

Overview

A herniated intervertebral disk is caused by the rupture of fibrocartilaginous material that surrounds the disk, resulting in the protrusion of the nucleus pulposus. The protrusion puts pressure on spinal nerve roots or the spinal cord and causes back pain and other symptoms of nerve root irritation. Disk space L4 to L5 is the most common site of herniation but it also occurs at L5 to S1, L2 to L3, L3 to L4, C6 to C7, and C5 to C6.

CAUSES
◆ Degenerative disk disease
◆ Direct injury
◆ Improper lifting or twisting
◆ Obesity

RISK FACTORS
◆ Advanced age
◆ Congenitally small lumbar spinal canal
◆ Osteophytes along the vertebrae
◆ Work environment

PATHOPHYSIOLOGY
◆ Ligament and posterior capsule of the disk are usually torn, allowing the nucleus pulposus to extrude, compressing the nerve root.
◆ Occasionally, the injury tears the entire disk loose, causing protrusion onto the nerve root or compression of the spinal cord.
◆ Large amounts of extruded nucleus pulposus or complete disk herniation of the capsule and nucleus pulposus may compress the spinal cord.

COMPLICATIONS
◆ Neurologic deficits
◆ Bowel and bladder dysfunction
◆ Sexual dysfunction

Assessment

HISTORY
◆ Previous traumatic injury or back strain
◆ Unilateral, lower back pain
◆ Pain that may radiate to the buttocks, legs, and feet
◆ Pain that may begin suddenly, subside in a few days, and then recur at shorter intervals with progressive intensity
◆ Sciatic pain beginning as a dull ache in the buttocks, worsening with Valsalva's maneuver, coughing, sneezing, or bending
◆ Pain that may subside with rest
◆ Muscle spasms
◆ Chronic repetitive injury
◆ Constipation or incontinence
◆ Urgency difficulties or incontinence

PHYSICAL FINDINGS
◆ Limited ability to bend forward
◆ Posture favoring the affected side
◆ Gait difficulty
◆ Muscle atrophy in later stages
◆ Tenderness over the affected region
◆ Radicular pain with straight leg raising in lumbar herniation
◆ Increased pain with neck movement in cervical herniation
◆ Referred upper trunk pain with cervical neck compression
◆ Weakness in affected area

DIAGNOSTIC TEST RESULTS
◆ *X-rays of the spine*: degenerative changes
◆ *Myelography*: herniation level
◆ *Computed tomography scan*: bone and soft-tissue abnormalities, spinal canal compression
◆ *Magnetic resonance imaging*: soft-tissue abnormalities at the site of herniation
◆ *Electromyography*: muscle response to nerve stimulation
◆ *Nerve conduction studies*: sensory and motor loss

Treatment

◆ Initially conservative and symptomatic, unless neurologic impairment progresses rapidly
◆ Possible pelvic or cervical traction
◆ Supportive devices such as a brace
◆ Heat or ice applications
◆ Transcutaneous electrical nerve stimulation
◆ Chemonucleolysis

 Nursing alert
Confirm that the patient isn't allergic to meat tenderizers before beginning therapy.

◆ Avoidance of repetitive activity
◆ Bed rest, initially
◆ Prescribed exercise program
◆ Physical therapy
◆ Laminectomy or hemilaminectomy
◆ Spinal fusion
◆ Microdiskectomy

MEDICATIONS

◆ Nonsteroidal anti-inflammatory drugs
◆ Steroids
◆ Muscle relaxants
◆ Analgesics

Nursing interventions

◆ Assess the patient's pain level, administer analgesics, and evaluate their effects.
◆ Monitor neurologic and musculoskeletal status.
◆ Offer supportive care.
◆ Encourage self-care.
◆ Help the patient to identify activities that promote rest and relaxation.
◆ Apply sequential compression stockings when the patient is in bed.
◆ Assist with leg and back-strengthening exercises.
◆ Encourage adequate oral fluid intake.
◆ Encourage coughing and deep-breathing exercises.
◆ Provide meticulous skin care.

After surgery

◆ Enforce bed rest as ordered.
◆ Use the logrolling technique to turn the patient.
◆ Assist the patient with ambulation.
◆ Provide wound care.

 Nursing alert
Immediately report colorless moisture on the dressing or excessive drainage .

PATIENT TEACHING

◆ Explain the disorder, diagnostic testing, and treatment plan.
◆ Review the administration, dosage, and possible adverse effects of prescribed medications.
◆ Review activity restrictions and use of brace, if prescribed.
◆ Review preoperative and postoperative care if indicated.
◆ Teach relaxation techniques and proper body mechanics.
◆ Describe signs and symptoms of complications.
◆ Refer the patient to physical therapy if indicated.
◆ Refer the patient to occupational therapy if indicated.
◆ Refer the patient to a weight-reduction program if appropriate.

Herpes zoster

Overview

Herpes zoster, also called *shingles,* is the acute unilateral and segmental inflammation of dorsal root ganglia due to the reactivation of the varicella virus. It's most common in people ages 50 to 70; people who had chickenpox at a young age may have a higher risk. Patients who have received a bone marrow transplant are especially at risk.

CAUSES
◆ Dormant varicella zoster virus (the herpesvirus that also causes chickenpox) that reactivates

PATHOPHYSIOLOGY
◆ Herpes zoster erupts when the varicella virus reactivates after dormancy in the cerebral ganglia (extramedullary ganglia of the cranial nerves) or the ganglia of posterior nerve roots.
◆ The virus may multiply as it reactivates, and antibodies remaining from the initial infection may neutralize it.
◆ Without opposition from effective antibodies, the virus continues to multiply in the ganglia, destroys neurons, and spreads down the sensory nerves to the skin, causing localized vascular eruptions along dermatome pathways.

COMPLICATIONS
◆ Deafness
◆ Bell's palsy
◆ Secondary skin infection
◆ Postherpetic neuralgia
◆ Meningoencephalitis
◆ Cutaneous dissemination
◆ Ocular involvement with facial zoster
◆ Hepatitis
◆ Pneumonitis
◆ Peripheral motor weakness
◆ Guillain-Barré syndrome
◆ Cranial nerve syndrome

Assessment

HISTORY
◆ Typically no history of exposure to others with the varicella zoster virus
◆ Fever
◆ Malaise
◆ Pain within the affected dermatome
◆ Pleurisy
◆ Musculoskeletal pain
◆ Severe, deep pain
◆ Pruritus
◆ Paresthesia or hyperesthesia (usually affecting the trunk and occasionally the arms and legs)

PHYSICAL FINDINGS
◆ Small, red, vesicular skin lesions spread unilaterally around the thorax or vertically over the arms or legs
◆ Vesicles possibly filled with clear fluid or pus
◆ Vesicles drying, forming scabs, or even becoming gangrenous (see *A look at herpes zoster*)
◆ Enlarged regional lymph nodes

Geniculate involvement
◆ Vesicle formation in the external auditory canal with ipsilateral facial palsy
◆ Hearing loss, dizziness, and loss of taste

Trigeminal involvement
◆ Eye pain
◆ Corneal and scleral damage and impaired vision
◆ Conjunctivitis, extraocular weakness, ptosis, and paralytic mydriasis
◆ Secondary glaucoma

DIAGNOSTIC TEST RESULTS
◆ *Vesicular fluid and infected tissue analyses:* eosinophilic intranuclear inclusions and varicella virus
◆ *Antibody staining and identification under fluorescent light:* differentiation of herpes zoster from herpes simplex virus

- *Varicella antibodies globulin measurement:* elevated
- *Cerebrospinal fluid analysis:* increased protein levels, possibly pleocytosis
- *Lumbar puncture:* increased pressure

Treatment

- Transcutaneous peripheral nerve stimulation (for postherpetic neuralgia)
- Soothing baths
- Cold compresses

 Age considerations
Patients age 60 or older should receive a single-dose herpes zoster vaccine.

MEDICATIONS
- Antivirals
- Antipruritics
- Analgesics
- Tricyclic antidepressants
- Demulcent and skin protectant
- Systemic antibiotic (for secondary bacterial infections)
- Corticosteroids
- Sedatives
- Patient-controlled analgesia

Nursing interventions

- Give prescribed drugs, as ordered, and evaluate the patient's response to treatment.
- Assess pain level; administer analgesics as indicated and evaluate their effectiveness.
- Maintain meticulous hygiene to prevent spreading the infection to other parts of the patient's body.
- With open lesions, follow contact isolation precautions to prevent the spread of infection.
- Monitor lesions and assess for signs and symptoms of infection.

PATIENT TEACHING
- Explain the disorder, diagnostic testing, and treatment plan.
- Teach about the administration, dosage, and possible adverse effects of prescribed medications.
- Explain the use of a soft toothbrush, use of a saline- or bicarbonate-based mouthwash and oral anesthetics to decrease discomfort from oral lesions.
- Advise the patient to eat soft foods.
- Explain the need for meticulous hygiene.
- Instruct the patient to avoid scratching the lesions to prevent spreading the infection to other body parts.
- Tell the patient to apply a cold compress if vesicles rupture.
- Refer the patient to an ophthalmologist for ocular involvement.
- Refer the patient to a pain management specialist for postherpetic neuralgia.

A look at herpes zoster

Unilateral vesicular lesions that appear in a dermatomal pattern are characteristic of herpes zoster. The lesions are fluid-filled vesicles that dry and form scabs after about 10 days.

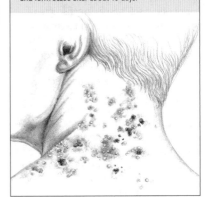

Hip fracture

Overview

A hip fracture is the break in the head or neck of the femur (usually the head). It's the most common fall-related injury resulting in hospitalization and the leading cause of disability among older adults. Hip fractures affect more than 200,000 people annually and may permanently change a person's level of functioning and independence. They can be fatal in almost 25% of patients within 1 year of the fracture. White women are more likely to fracture hips than non-white women and men.

 Age considerations
One in five women fractures a hip by age 80.

CAUSES
◆ Cancer metastasis
◆ Falls
◆ Osteoporosis
◆ Skeletal disease
◆ Trauma

PATHOPHYSIOLOGY
◆ With bone fracture, the periosteum and blood vessels in the marrow, cortex, and surrounding soft tissues are disrupted.
◆ This disruption results in bleeding from the damaged ends of the bone and from the neighboring soft tissue.
◆ Clot formation occurs within the medullary canal, between the fractured bone ends, and beneath the periosteum.
◆ Bone tissue immediately adjacent to the fracture dies, and the necrotic tissue causes an intense inflammatory response.
◆ Vascular tissue invades the fracture area from surrounding soft tissue and marrow cavity within 48 hours, increasing blood flow to the entire bone.
◆ Bone-forming cells in the periosteum, endosteum, and marrow are activated to produce subperiosteal procallus along the outer surface of the shaft and over the broken ends of the bone.

◆ Collagen and matrix, which become mineralized to form callus, are synthesized by osteoblasts within the procallus.
◆ During the repair process, remodeling occurs; unnecessary callus is resorbed, and trabeculae are formed along stress lines.
◆ New bone, not scar tissue, is formed over the healed fracture.

COMPLICATIONS
◆ Pneumonia
◆ Infection
◆ Venous thrombosis
◆ Pressure ulcers
◆ Social isolation
◆ Depression
◆ Bladder and bowel dysfunction
◆ Deep vein thrombosis
◆ Pulmonary embolus
◆ Hip dislocation or nonunion
◆ Death

Assessment

HISTORY
◆ Falls or trauma to the bones
◆ Pain in the affected hip and leg
◆ Pain worsened by movement

PHYSICAL FINDINGS
◆ Outward rotation of affected extremity
◆ Affected extremity possibly appearing shorter
◆ Limited or abnormal range of motion (ROM)
◆ Pain with movement
◆ Edema and discoloration of the surrounding tissue
◆ In an open fracture, bone protruding through the skin

DIAGNOSTIC TEST RESULTS
◆ *X-rays*: fracture location
◆ *Computed tomography scan*: abnormalities in complicated fractures

Treatment

- Depends on age, comorbidities, cognitive functioning, support systems, and functional ability
- Possible skin traction
- Non-weight-bearing transfers
- Well-balanced diet
- Foods rich in vitamins C and A, calcium, and protein
- Adequate vitamin D
- Bed rest, initially
- Ambulation as soon as possible after surgery
- Physical therapy
- Total hip arthroplasty
- Hemiarthroplasty
- Percutaneous pinning
- Internal fixation using a compression screw and plate

MEDICATIONS
- Analgesics
- Heparin (given prophylactically for deep vein thrombosis)

Nursing interventions

- Give prescribed drugs.
- Give prescribed prophylactic anticoagulation after surgery.
- Maintain traction.
- Maintain proper body alignment and posturing.
- Use logrolling techniques to turn the patient in bed.
- Maintain non-weight-bearing status.
- Increase the patient's activity level as prescribed.
- Consult physical therapy as early as possible.
- Assist with active ROM exercises to unaffected limbs.
- Encourage coughing and deep-breathing exercises.
- Provide skin care, keeping the patient's skin clean and dry.
- Encourage good nutrition; offer high-protein, high-calorie snacks.
- Perform daily wound care.
- Monitor vital signs, intake and output, pain, and mobility and ROM.
- Monitor for complications, signs of bleeding, and signs and symptoms of infection.
- Assess the incision and dressings and skin integrity.
- Monitor coagulation study results
- Monitor the neurovascular status of the affected extremity.

PATIENT TEACHING
- Explain the disorder, diagnostic testing, and treatment plan.
- Teach about the administration, dosage, and possible adverse effects of prescribed medications.
- Demonstrate ROM exercises.
- Teach about meticulous skin care and wound care.
- Teach proper body alignment and use of assistive devices.
- Describe signs of infection.
- Reinforce need for coughing and deep-breathing exercises and incentive spirometry.
- Explain activity restrictions, necessary lifestyle changes, and safe ambulation practices.
- Provide guidance on nutritious diet and adequate fluid intake.
- Refer the patient to physical and occupational therapy programs as indicated.
- Refer the patient to home health or intermediate care.

Hodgkin's disease

Overview

Hodgkin's disease, also known as *Hodgkin's lymphoma*, is a neoplastic disorder characterized by painless, progressive enlargement of the lymph nodes, spleen, and other lymphoid tissue. It's most common in people ages 15 to 38, except in Japan, where it occurs exclusively in people older than age 50.

CAUSES
◆ Unknown

RISK FACTORS
◆ Genetic factors
◆ Viral factors
◆ Environmental factors

PATHOPHYSIOLOGY
◆ Enlarged lymphoid tissue results from proliferation of lymphocytes, histiocytes, eosinophils, and Reed-Sternberg cells (see *Recognizing Reed-Sternberg cells*).
◆ Untreated Hodgkin's disease follows a variable but progressive and ultimately fatal course.

COMPLICATIONS
◆ Multiple organ failure
◆ Toxic effects of treatment, such as myocardial damage, sterility, and opportunistic infections

Assessment

HISTORY
◆ Painless swelling of a cervical, axillary, or inguinal lymph node
◆ Persistent fever and night sweats
◆ Weight loss despite an adequate diet, resulting in fatigue and malaise
◆ Increasing susceptibility to infection

PHYSICAL FINDINGS
◆ Edema of the face and neck and jaundice
◆ Enlarged, rubbery lymph nodes in the neck that enlarge during periods of fever and then revert to normal size

DIAGNOSTIC TEST RESULTS
◆ *Hematologic tests:* mild to severe normocytic, normochromic anemia in 50% of patients; elevated, normal, or reduced white blood cell count and differential; any combination of neutrophilia, lymphocytopenia, monocytosis, and eosinophilia
◆ *Serum alkaline phosphatase levels:* elevated, indicating liver or bone involvement
◆ *Lymph node biopsy:* presence of Reed-Sternberg cells, abnormal histiocyte proliferation, and nodular fibrosis and necrosis; level of lymph node and organ involvement
◆ *Staging laparotomy:* direct pathologic staging to evaluate spread of disease

Treatment

◆ Radiation therapy and short-term chemotherapy for patients with stage I or II disease
◆ Radiation therapy and chemotherapy for patients with stage III disease
◆ High-dose chemotherapy or stem cell transplant and possible radiation for patients with relapsed Hodgkin's disease
◆ Autologous bone marrow transplantation or autologous peripheral blood sternal transfusions and immunotherapy
◆ Well-balanced, high-calorie, high-protein diet
◆ Frequent rest periods

MEDICATIONS
◆ Chemotherapy
◆ Rituximab (Rituxan)
◆ Antiemetics
◆ Sedatives
◆ Antidiarrheals

Nursing interventions

◆ Provide a well-balanced, high-calorie, high-protein diet.
◆ Provide frequent rest periods.
◆ Give prescribed drugs.
◆ Provide emotional support.
◆ Evaluate the patient's response to treatment and observe for complications.
◆ Assess the patient's pain level, administer analgesics, and evaluate their effects.
◆ Monitor vital signs, temperature, daily weight, and lymph node status.
◆ Observe for signs and symptoms of infection or dehydration.

PATIENT TEACHING
◆ Explain the disorder, diagnostic testing, and treatment plan.
◆ Teach about the administration, dosage, and possible adverse effects of prescribed medications.
◆ Review signs and symptoms of infection.
◆ Stress the importance of maintaining good nutrition and pacing activities to counteract therapy-induced fatigue.
◆ Explain the need to avoid crowds and people with known infections.
◆ Refer the patient to appropriate resources and support services.

Recognizing Reed-Sternberg cells

The illustration below shows Reed-Sternberg cells. Note the large, distinct nucleoli.

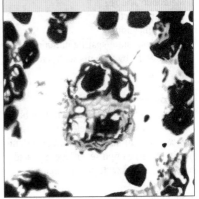

Hyperkalemia

Overview

Hyperkalemia, which is commonly induced by treatments for other disorders, is an excessive serum level of the potassium anion. (The normal range for serum potassium is 3.5 to 5 mEq/L.) Hyperkalemia occurs in up to 8% of hospitalized patients in the United States.

CAUSES
◆ Adrenal gland insufficiency
◆ Burns
◆ Certain drugs
◆ Crushing injuries
◆ Decreased urinary excretion of potassium
◆ Dehydration
◆ Diabetic acidosis
◆ Increased intake of potassium
◆ Multiple blood transfusions
◆ Metabolic acidosis
◆ Renal dysfunction or failure
◆ Severe infection
◆ Use of potassium-sparing diuretics such as triamterene by patients with renal disease

PATHOPHYSIOLOGY
◆ Potassium facilitates contraction of both skeletal and smooth muscles, including myocardial contraction, and figures prominently in nerve impulse conduction, acid-base balance, enzyme action, and cell membrane function.
◆ Slight deviation in serum levels can produce profound clinical consequences.
◆ Potassium imbalance can lead to muscle weakness and flaccid paralysis because of an ionic imbalance in neuromuscular tissue excitability.

COMPLICATIONS
◆ Cardiac arrhythmia
◆ Metabolic acidosis
◆ Cardiac arrest
◆ Paralytic ileus

Assessment

HISTORY
◆ Irritability
◆ Paresthesia
◆ Muscle weakness
◆ Nausea
◆ Abdominal cramps
◆ Diarrhea

PHYSICAL FINDINGS
◆ Hypotension
◆ Irregular heart rate
◆ Irregular heart rhythm (see *Clinical effects of hyperkalemia*)

DIAGNOSTIC TEST RESULTS
◆ *Serum potassium level:* greater than 5 mEq/L
◆ *Arterial pH:* decreased
◆ *Electrocardiography:* tall, tented T wave; widened QRS complex, prolonged PR interval, flattened or absent P waves, depressed ST segment

Treatment

◆ Treatment of the underlying cause
◆ Hemodialysis or peritoneal dialysis
◆ Low potassium diet (for chronic hyperkalemia)

MEDICATIONS
◆ Rapid infusion of 10% calcium gluconate (to decrease myocardial irritability)
◆ Insulin and 10% to 50% glucose I.V.
◆ Sodium polystyrene sulfonate (Kayexalate) with 70% sorbitol
◆ Sodium bicarbonate

Nursing interventions

◆ Check the serum sample for hemolysis.
◆ Give prescribed drugs.
◆ Implement safety measures.
◆ Be alert for signs of hypokalemia after treatment.
◆ Monitor serum electrolytes levels, cardiac rhythm, and intake and output.

PATIENT TEACHING

◆ Explain the disorder, diagnostic testing and treatment plan.
◆ Teach about the administration, dosage, and possible adverse effects of prescribed medications.
◆ Teach how to monitor intake and output.
◆ Explain measures for preventing hyperkalemia.
◆ Describe a potassium-restricted diet.

Clinical effects of hyperkalemia

Here's how hyperkalemia affects various body systems.

Body system	Effects
Cardiovascular	◆ Tachycardia and later bradycardia, electrocardiogram changes (tented and elevated T waves, widened QRS complex, prolonged PR interval, flattened or absent P waves, depressed ST segment), cardiac arrest (with levels greater than 7 mEq/L)
Gastrointestinal	◆ Nausea, diarrhea, abdominal cramps
Genitourinary	◆ Oliguria, anuria
Musculoskeletal	◆ Muscle weakness, flaccid paralysis
Neurologic	◆ Hyperreflexia progressing to weakness, numbness, tingling, flaccid paralysis
Other	◆ Metabolic acidosis

Hypertension

Overview

Hypertension, the intermittent or sustained elevation of diastolic or systolic blood pressure, usually is benign at first before slowly progressing to an accelerated or malignant state. The two major types are essential (also called *primary* or *idiopathic*) hypertension and secondary hypertension, which results from renal disease or another identifiable cause. Essential hypertension accounts for 90% to 95% of cases.

The stages of hypertension are classified according to systolic and diastolic pressure readings. Prehypertension is characterized by a systolic blood pressure between 120 and 139 mm Hg and a diastolic blood pressure between 80 and 89 mm Hg. Stage I hypertension involves a systolic range of 140 to 159 and a diastolic range of 90 to 99 mm Hg. A systolic blood pressure greater than 160 mm Hg and a diastolic pressure greater than 100 mm Hg characterizes stage II hypertension.

 Nursing alert

Malignant hypertension, a severe, fulminant form that arises from either type of hypertension, is considered a medical emergency.

CAUSES
◆ Sleep apnea
◆ Chronic kidney disease
◆ Primary aldosteronism
◆ Cushing's syndrome
◆ Pheochromocytoma
◆ Thyroid or parathyroid disease

RISK FACTORS
◆ Family history
◆ Being black
◆ Stress
◆ Obesity
◆ High-sodium, high-saturated fat diet
◆ Tobacco use
◆ Hormonal contraceptive use
◆ Excessive alcohol intake
◆ Sedentary lifestyle
◆ Aging
◆ Metabolic syndrome

PATHOPHYSIOLOGY
◆ Changes in the arteriolar bed cause increased peripheral vascular resistance.
◆ Abnormally increased tone in the sympathetic nervous system originates in the vasomotor system centers, causing increased peripheral vascular resistance.
◆ Increased blood volume results from renal or hormonal dysfunction.
◆ Increased arteriolar thickening is caused by genetic factors, leading to increased peripheral vascular resistance.
◆ Abnormal renin release results in the formation of angiotensin II, which constricts the arterioles and increases blood volume.

COMPLICATIONS
◆ Cardiac disease
◆ Left ventricular hypertrophy
◆ Renal failure
◆ Blindness
◆ Stroke

Assessment

HISTORY
◆ In many cases, no symptoms; disorder is revealed incidentally during evaluation for another disorder or during a routine blood pressure screening program
◆ Symptoms that reflect the effect of hypertension on the organ systems, such as renal insufficiency and atherosclerosis
◆ Awakening with a headache in the occipital region, which subsides spontaneously after a few hours
◆ Dizziness, fatigue, and confusion
◆ Palpitations, chest pain, dyspnea
◆ Epistaxis
◆ Hematuria
◆ Blurred vision

PHYSICAL FINDINGS
◆ Bounding pulse
◆ Fourth heart sound
◆ Peripheral edema in late stages
◆ Hemorrhages, exudates, and papilledema of the eye in late stages if hypertensive retinopathy is present

• Pulsating abdominal mass, suggesting an abdominal aneurysm
• Elevated blood pressure on at least two consecutive occasions after initial screenings (prehypertension range: 120 to 139/80 to 89 mm Hg; stage I hypertension
• Bruits over the abdominal aorta and femoral arteries or the carotids

DIAGNOSTIC TEST RESULTS

• *Urinalysis:* presence of protein, red blood cells, or white blood cells, suggesting renal disease; presence of glucose, suggesting diabetes mellitus
• *Serum potassium levels:* less than 3.5 mEq/L, indicating adrenal dysfunction (primary hyperaldosteronism)
• *Blood urea nitrogen levels:* normal or elevated to more than 20 mg/dl, suggesting renal disease
• *Serum creatinine levels:* normal or elevated to more than 1.5 mg/dl, suggesting renal disease
• *Excretory urography:* renal atrophy, indicating chronic renal disease; one kidney more than 5/8″ (1.6 cm) shorter than the other suggests unilateral renal disease
• *Chest X-rays:* cardiomegaly
• *Renal arteriography:* renal artery stenosis
• *Electrocardiography:* left ventricular hypertrophy or ischemia
• *Oral captopril challenge:* renovascular hypertension
• *Ophthalmoscopy:* arteriovenous nicking and, in hypertensive encephalopathy, edema

Treatment

• Based on stage of hypertension and its cause
• Weight control, limiting alcohol, regular exercise, and smoking cessation
• Correction of the underlying cause (for secondary hypertension)
• Low-saturated fat, low-sodium diet
• Adequate intake of fruits and vegetables

MEDICATIONS

• Diuretics
• Alpha-adrenergic blockers
• Beta-adrenergic blockers
• Calcium channel blockers
• Angiotensin-converting enzyme inhibitors
• Alpha-receptor antagonists
• Vasodilators
• Angiotensin-receptor blockers
• Aldosterone-receptor blockers

Nursing interventions

• Monitor vital signs, especially blood pressure.
• Give prescribed drugs, as ordered, and evaluate the patient's response to treatment.
• Encourage dietary changes as appropriate.
• Help the patient identify risk factors and modify his lifestyle as appropriate.
• Assess for signs and symptoms of target end-organ damage.

PATIENT TEACHING

• Explain the disorder, diagnostic testing, and treatment plan.
• Review the administration, dosage, and possible adverse effects of prescribed medications.
• Demonstrate how to use a self-monitoring blood pressure cuff and record the reading in a journal for review by the practitioner.
• Stress the importance of compliance with antihypertensive therapy and establishing a daily routine for taking prescribed drugs.
• Tell the patient to report adverse effects of drugs.
• Review needed lifestyle modifications and the need for a routine exercise program, particularly aerobic walking.
• Explain dietary restrictions.
• Stress the importance of follow-up care.
• Refer the patient to stress-reduction therapies or support groups as needed.
• Refer the patient to weight-reduction or smoking-cessation groups as needed.

Hyperthyroidism

Overview

Hyperthyroidism, also known as *thyrotoxicosis,* is an alteration in thyroid function in which thyroid hormones (TH) exert greater than normal responses. Thyrotoxicoses not associated with hyperthyroidism include subacute thyroiditis, ectopic thyroid tissue, and ingestion of excessive TH. Graves' disease, also known as *toxic diffuse goiter,* is an autoimmune disease and the most common cause of hyperthyroidism. Treatment depends on the underlying cause.

CAUSES
- Genetic and immunologic factors
- Graves' disease
- Increased thyroid-stimulating hormone (TSH) secretion
- Thyroid cancer
- Toxic multinodular goiter
- Diabetic ketoacidosis
- Excessive iodine intake
- Infection
- Stress
- Surgery
- Toxemia of pregnancy

PATHOPHYSIOLOGY
- In Graves' disease, thyroid-stimulating antibodies bind to and stimulate the TSH receptors of the thyroid gland; the trigger for this disease is unclear.
- Hyperthyroidism associated with the production of autoantibodies is possibly caused by a defect in the function of suppressor T-lymphocytes that allows the formation of these autoantibodies.

COMPLICATIONS
- Arrhythmias
- Left ventricular hypertrophy
- Heart failure
- Muscle weakness and atrophy
- Paralysis
- Osteoporosis
- Vitiligo
- Skin hyperpigmentation
- Corneal ulcers
- Myasthenia gravis
- Impaired fertility
- Decreased libido
- Gynecomastia
- Thyrotoxic crisis or thyroid storm
- Hepatic or renal failure

Assessment

HISTORY
- Nervousness, tremor
- Heat intolerance
- Weight loss despite increased appetite
- Sweating
- Frequent bowel movements
- Palpitations
- Poor concentration
- Shaky handwriting
- Clumsiness
- Emotional instability and mood swings
- Thin, brittle nails
- Hair loss
- Nausea and vomiting
- Weakness and fatigue
- Oligomenorrhea or amenorrhea
- Fertility problems
- Diminished libido
- Diplopia

PHYSICAL FINDINGS
- Enlarged thyroid (goiter)
- Exophthalmos
- Tremor
- Smooth, warm, flushed skin
- Fine, soft hair
- Premature graying and increased hair loss
- Friable nails and onycholysis
- Pretibial myxedema
- Thickened skin
- Accentuated hair follicles
- Tachycardia at rest
- Full, bounding pulses
- Arrhythmias, especially atrial fibrillation

- Wide pulse pressure
- Possible systolic murmur
- Dyspnea
- Hepatomegaly
- Hyperactive bowel sounds
- Weakness, especially in proximal muscles, and atrophy
- Possible generalized or localized paralysis
- Gynecomastia in males
- Increased tearing

DIAGNOSTIC TEST RESULTS
- *Radioimmunoassay:* increased serum triiodothyronine and thyroxine concentrations
- *Serum protein-bound iodine level:* increased
- *Serum cholesterol and total lipid levels:* decreased
- *TSH level:* decreased
- *Thyroid scan:* increased uptake of iodine 131 (^{131}I)
- *Ultrasonography:* subclinical ophthalmopathy

Treatment

- Subtotal (partial) thyroidectomy
- Surgical decompression
- Adequate caloric intake
- Activity as tolerated

MEDICATIONS
- Treatment with a single oral dose of ^{131}I for women past reproductive age or men and women not planning to have children
- Thyroid hormone antagonists
- Beta-adrenergic antagonists
- Calcium channel blockers
- Corticosteroids
- Sedatives

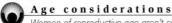 **Age considerations**

Women of reproductive age aren't candidates for ^{131}I treatment because of the risk of destroying a developing fetus's thyroid.

Nursing interventions

- Monitor vital signs, daily weight, intake and output, and serum electrolyte levels.
- Minimize physical and emotional stress.
- Balance rest and activity periods.
- Consult a dietitian to ensure the patient has a nutritious diet with adequate calories and fluids.
- Offer small, frequent meals.
- Provide meticulous skin care.
- Encourage the patient to verbalize his feelings and provide emotional support.
- Help the patient identify and develop coping strategies.
- Give prescribed drugs.
- Avoid excessive palpation of the thyroid.

After thyroidectomy
- Monitor for signs and symptoms of hypocalcemia
- Change dressings and perform wound care as ordered.
- Keep the patient in semi-Fowler's position.
- Support the patient's head and neck with sandbags.

PATIENT TEACHING
- Explain the disorder, diagnostic testing, and treatment plan.
- Teach about the administration, dosage, and possible adverse effects of prescribed medications.
- Explain the need for regular medical follow-up visits.
- Instruct the patient to notify the practitioner if signs and symptoms of hypothyroidism occur.
- Stress the importance of wearing medical identification jewelry.
- Explain precautions required for ^{131}I therapy.
- Describe signs and symptoms of hypothyroidism.

Hypocalcemia

Overview

Hypocalcemia involves deficient serum levels of calcium (a serum calcium level less than 8.5 mg/dL or ionized calcium level less than 1 mmol/L). Insufficient calcium in the cells affects cell function, blood coagulation, neural transmission, and bone health.

CAUSES
◆ Hypoalbuminemia
◆ Hypomagnesemia
◆ Hyperphosphetemia
◆ Hypoparathyroidism
◆ Inadequate dietary intake of calcium and vitamin D
◆ Malabsorption or loss of calcium from the GI tract
◆ Osteomalacia
◆ Overcorrection of acidosis
◆ Pancreatic insufficiency
◆ Hepatic or renal insufficiency
◆ Severe infections or burns
◆ Toxic shock syndrome
◆ Certain medications

PATHOPHYSIOLOGY
◆ Together with phosphorous, calcium is responsible for the formation and structure of bones and teeth.
◆ Calcium helps maintain cell structure and function.
◆ It plays a role in cell membrane permeability and impulse transmission.
◆ It affects the contraction of cardiac muscle, smooth muscle, and skeletal muscle.
◆ It also participates in the blood-clotting process.

COMPLICATIONS
◆ Laryngeal spasm
◆ Seizures
◆ Cardiac arrhythmia
◆ Respiratory arrest

Assessment

HISTORY
◆ Evidence of underlying cause
◆ Anxiety
◆ Irritability
◆ Seizures
◆ Muscle cramps
◆ Diarrhea
◆ Shortness of breath
◆ Numbness and tingling of distal extremities

PHYSICAL FINDINGS
◆ Twitching (see *Clinical effects of hypocalcemia*)
◆ Carpopedal spasm
◆ Dry skin
◆ Tetany
◆ Hypotension
◆ Confusion
◆ Positive Chvostek's and Trousseau's signs

DIAGNOSTIC TEST RESULTS
◆ *Serum calcium level:* less than 8.5 mg/dl
◆ *Ionized calcium level:* less than 1.0 mmol/L
◆ *Electrocardiography:* lengthened QT interval, prolonged ST segment, and arrhythmias

Treatment

◆ Treatment of the underlying cause
◆ Supportive treatment for life-threatening symptoms
◆ Smoking cessation
◆ Avoidance of caffeine and alcohol, which inhibit calcium absorption

MEDICATIONS
◆ Oral calcium and vitamin D supplements
◆ Calcium gluconate or calcium chloride I.V.

Nursing interventions

♦ Provide safety measures and institute seizure precautions if appropriate.
♦ Give prescribed calcium replacement.
♦ Assess I.V. sites if administering calcium I.V. (infiltration causes sloughing).
♦ Monitor vital signs, cardiac rhythm, and calcium levels.

PATIENT TEACHING
♦ Explain the disorder, diagnostic testing, and treatment plan.

♦ Teach about the administration, dosage, and possible adverse effects of prescribed medications.
♦ Explain proper administration of calcium supplements.
♦ Tell the patient to avoid overuse of laxatives, which contain phosphorous.
♦ Stress the importance of following a high-calcium diet.
♦ Refer the patient to a dietitian and social services if indicated.

Clinical effects of hypocalcemia

Here's how hypocalcemia affects various body systems.

Body system	Effects
Cardiovascular	♦ Arrhythmias, hypotension, lengthened QT interval, prolonged ST segment
Gastrointestinal	♦ Increased GI motility, diarrhea
Musculoskeletal	♦ Paresthesia, tetany or painful tonic muscle spasms, facial spasms, abdominal cramps, muscle cramps, spasmodic contractions
Neurologic	♦ Anxiety, irritability, twitching around mouth, laryngospasm, seizures, Chvostek's sign, Trousseau's sign
Other	♦ Blood-clotting abnormalities

Hypokalemia

Overview

Hypokalemia, which occurs in about 80% of patients who receive diuretics, is a deficient serum level of the potassium anion. Hypokalemia affects up to 20% of hospitalized patients, but it's significant in about 4% to 5%. The normal serum potassium level range is narrow (3.5 to 5 mEq/L), and a slight decrease can be life-threatening.

CAUSES
◆ Acid-base imbalances
◆ Bartter's syndrome
◆ Certain drugs, especially potassium-wasting diuretics, steroids, and certain sodium-containing antibiotics (carbenicillin)
◆ Chronic alcoholism
◆ Chronic renal disease, with tubular potassium wasting
◆ Cushing's syndrome
◆ Cystic fibrosis
◆ Excessive GI or urinary losses, such as vomiting, gastric suction, diarrhea, dehydration, anorexia, or chronic laxative abuse
◆ Excessive ingestion of licorice
◆ Hyperglycemia
◆ Low-potassium diet
◆ Primary hyperaldosteronism
◆ Prolonged potassium-free I.V. therapy
◆ Severe serum magnesium deficiency
◆ Trauma (injury, burns, or surgery)

PATHOPHYSIOLOGY
◆ Potassium facilitates contraction of skeletal and smooth muscles, including myocardial contraction.
◆ Potassium figures prominently in nerve impulse conduction, acid-base balance, enzyme action, and cell membrane function.
◆ Potassium imbalance can lead to muscle weakness and flaccid paralysis because of an ionic imbalance in neuromuscular tissue excitability.

COMPLICATIONS
◆ Cardiac arrhythmia
◆ Cardiac arrest
◆ Rhabdomyolysis

Assessment

HISTORY
◆ Muscle weakness
◆ Paresthesia
◆ Abdominal cramps
◆ Anorexia
◆ Nausea, vomiting
◆ Constipation
◆ Polyuria

PHYSICAL FINDINGS
◆ Hyporeflexia (see *Clinical effects of hypokalemia*)
◆ Weak, irregular pulse
◆ Orthostatic hypotension
◆ Decreased bowel sounds

DIAGNOSTIC TEST RESULTS
◆ *Serum potassium level:* less than 3.5 mEq/L
◆ *Bicarbonate and pH levels:* elevated
◆ *Serum glucose level:* slightly elevated
◆ *Electrocardiogram:* flattened T wave, depressed ST segment and U wave, premature ventricular contractions

Treatment

◆ Treatment of the underlying cause
◆ Supportive measures for life-threatening symptoms
◆ High-potassium diet

MEDICATIONS
◆ Potassium chloride supplement (I.V. or oral)

Nursing interventions

◆ Give prescribed drugs.
◆ Be alert for signs of hyperkalemia after treatment.
◆ Administer I.V. fluids.
◆ Monitor the patient's vital signs, cardiac rhythm, intake and output, and serum potassium levels.
◆ Assess respiratory status.

PATIENT TEACHING
◆ Explain the disorder, diagnostic testing, and treatment plan.
◆ Teach about the administration, dosage, and possible adverse effects of prescribed medications.
◆ Stress the need for a high-potassium diet.
◆ Describe warning signs and symptoms to report to the practitioner.

Clinical effects of hypokalemia

Here's how hypokalemia affects various body systems.

Body system	Effects
Cardiovascular	◆ Dizziness, hypotension, arrhythmias, electrocardiogram changes (flattened T waves, depressed ST segment and U waves, prolonged QT interval, premature ventricular contractions), cardiac arrest (with levels less than 2.5 mEq/L)
Gastrointestinal	◆ Nausea, vomiting, anorexia, diarrhea, abdominal distention, paralytic ileus, or decreased peristalsis
Genitourinary	◆ Polyuria
Musculoskeletal	◆ Muscle weakness and fatigue, leg cramps
Neurologic	◆ Malaise, irritability, confusion, mental depression, speech changes, decreased reflexes, respiratory paralysis
Other	◆ Metabolic alkalosis

Hypomagnesemia

Overview

Hypomagnesemia, a relatively common imbalance, is a deficient serum level of the magnesium cation (less than 1.7 mg/dl). It occurs in 10% to 20% of hospitalized patients, including 50% to 60% of patients in the intensive care unit, and 25% of alcoholics.

CAUSES
- Administration of parenteral fluids without magnesium salts
- Certain drugs
- Chronic alcoholism
- Chronic diarrhea
- Diabetic acidosis
- Excessive release of adrenocortical hormones
- Hyperaldosteronism
- Hypercalcemia
- Hyperparathyroidism or hypoparathyroidism
- Hypothermia
- Inflammatory bowel disease
- Malabsorption syndrome
- Nasogastric suctioning
- Postoperative complications after bowel resection
- Prolonged diuretic therapy
- Severe dehydration
- Starvation or malnutrition
- Syndrome of inappropriate antidiuretic hormone

RISK FACTORS
- Sepsis
- Serious burns
- Wounds requiring debridement

PATHOPHYSIOLOGY
- Magnesium enhances neuromuscular integration and stimulates parathyroid hormone secretion, regulating intracellular fluid calcium levels.
- Magnesium may also regulate skeletal muscles through its influence on calcium utilization by depressing acetylcholine release at synaptic junctions.
- It activates many enzymes for proper carbohydrate and protein metabolism, aids in cell metabolism and the transport of sodium and potassium across cell membranes, and influences sodium, potassium, calcium, and protein levels.
- About one-third of magnesium taken into the body is absorbed through the small intestine and is eventually excreted in the urine; the remaining, unabsorbed magnesium is excreted in the stool.

COMPLICATIONS
- Laryngeal stridor
- Seizures
- Respiratory depression
- Cardiac arrhythmia
- Cardiac arrest

Assessment

HISTORY
- Dysphagia
- Mood changes
- Nausea
- Vomiting
- Drowsiness
- Confusion
- Leg and foot cramps
- Seizure

PHYSICAL FINDINGS
- Tachycardia
- Hypertension (see *Clinical effects of hypomagnesemia*)
- Muscle weakness, tremors, twitching
- Hyperactive deep tendon reflexes
- Chvostek's and Trousseau's signs
- Cardiac arrhythmia

DIAGNOSTIC TEST RESULTS
- Serum magnesium level: less than 1.5 mEq/L
- *Serum potassium and calcium levels:* below normal
- *Electrocardiography:* abnormalities, such as prolonged QT interval and atrioventricular block

Treatment

◆ Treatment of the underlying cause
◆ Supportive treatment of life-threatening symptoms
◆ Magnesium-rich diet
◆ Cessation of alcohol consumption

MEDICATIONS
◆ Magnesium salts
◆ Magnesium sulfate
◆ Potassium and calcium replacement as indicated

Nursing interventions

◆ Institute seizure precautions.
◆ Give prescribed drugs.
◆ Report abnormal serum electrolyte levels immediately.
◆ Ensure patient safety.
◆ Monitor the patient's vital signs, cardiac rhythm, intake and output, and serum magnesium and electrolyte levels.
◆ Assess respiratory status.

PATIENT TEACHING
◆ Explain the disorder, diagnostic testing, and treatment plan.
◆ Teach about the administration, dosage, and possible adverse effects of prescribed medications.
◆ Instruct the patient to avoid drugs that deplete magnesium, such as diuretics and laxatives.
◆ Explain the need to adhere to a high-magnesium diet.
◆ Describe dangerous signs and symptoms and when to report them to the practitioner.
◆ Refer the patient to Alcoholics Anonymous if appropriate.

Disorders

Clinical effects of hypomagnesemia

Here's how hypomagnesemia affects various body systems.

Body system	Effects
Cardiovascular	◆ Arrhythmias, vasomotor changes (vasodilation and hypotension) and, occasionally, hypertension
Neurologic	◆ Confusion, delusions, hallucinations, seizures
Neuromuscular	◆ Hyperirritability, tetany, leg and foot cramps, Chvostek's sign (facial muscle spasms induced by tapping the branches of the facial nerve)

Hypothyroidism

Overview

Hypothryoidism, a clinical condition characterized by decreased circulating levels of thyroid hormones (TH) or a resistance to them, is classified as primary or secondary. Severe hypothyroidism is also known as *myxedema*.

CAUSES
- Hashimoto's thyroiditis (most common cause)
- Amyloidosis
- Antithyroid drugs
- Congenital defects
- Drugs, such as iodides and lithium
- Endemic iodine deficiency
- External radiation to the neck
- Hypothalamic failure to produce thyrotropin-releasing hormone
- Inflammatory conditions
- Pituitary failure to produce thyroid-stimulating hormone (TSH)
- Pituitary tumor
- Postpartum pituitary necrosis
- Radioactive iodine therapy
- Sarcoidosis
- Thyroid gland surgery
- Idiopathic

PATHOPHYSIOLOGY
- In primary hypothyroidism, loss of thyroid tissue leads to a decrease in TH production.
- This decrease results in increased TSH secretion, which leads to a goiter.
- In secondary hypothyroidism, the pituitary typically fails to synthesize or secrete adequate amounts of TSH or target tissues fail to respond to normal blood levels of TH.
- Either type may progress to myxedema, which is clinically more severe and considered a medical emergency.

COMPLICATIONS
Cardiovascular
- Hypercholesterolemia
- Arteriosclerosis
- Ischemic heart disease
- Peripheral vascular disease
- Hypertension
- Cardiomegaly
- Heart failure
- Pleural and pericardial effusion

GI
- Achlorhydria
- Anemia
- Dynamic colon
- Megacolon
- Intestinal obstruction
- Bleeding tendencies

Other
- Conductive or sensorineural deafness
- Psychiatric disturbances
- Carpal tunnel syndrome
- Benign intracranial hypertension
- Impaired fertility
- Myxedema coma

Assessment

HISTORY
- Vague and varied symptoms that developed slowly over time
- Energy loss, fatigue
- Forgetfulness
- Sensitivity to cold
- Unexplained weight gain
- Constipation
- Anorexia
- Decreased libido
- Menorrhagia
- Paresthesia
- Joint stiffness
- Muscle cramping or pain

PHYSICAL FINDINGS
- Slight mental slowing to severe obtundation
- Thick, dry tongue
- Hoarseness; slow, slurred speech
- Dry, flaky, inelastic skin
- Puffy face, hands, and feet
- Periorbital edema; drooping upper eyelids

- Dry, sparse hair with patchy hair loss
- Loss of outer third of eyebrow
- Thick, brittle nails with transverse and longitudinal grooves
- Ataxia, intention tremor, nystagmus
- Doughy skin that feels cool
- Weak pulse and bradycardia
- Muscle weakness
- Sacral or peripheral edema
- Delayed reflex relaxation time
- Possible goiter
- Absent or decreased bowel sounds
- Hypotension
- A gallop or distant heart sounds
- Adventitious breath sounds
- Abdominal distention or ascites

DIAGNOSTIC TEST RESULTS

- *Radioimmunoassay:* decreased serum levels of triiodothyronine and thyroxine
- *Serum TSH level:* increased with thyroid insufficiency, decreased with hypothalamic or pituitary insufficiency
- *Serum cholesterol, alkaline phosphatase, and triglycerides levels:* elevated
- *Serum electrolyte levels:* low in myxedema coma
- *Arterial blood gas analysis:* decreased pH and increased partial pressure of carbon dioxide in myxedema coma
- *Skull X-rays, computed tomography scan, and magnetic resonance imaging:* pituitary or hypothalamic lesions

Treatment

- Supportive measures for life-threatening symptoms (myxedema coma)
- Low-fat, low-cholesterol, high-fiber, low-sodium diet
- Possibly fluid restriction
- Surgery for underlying cause, such as pituitary tumor

MEDICATIONS

- Synthetic hormones: levothyroxine (Synthroid), liothyronine (Cytomel)

Nursing interventions

- Give prescribed drugs.
- Provide adequate rest periods.
- Provide a high-bulk, low-calorie diet with fluid restrictions, as ordered.
- Keep the patient warm as needed.
- Help the patient develop effective coping strategies.
- Monitor vital signs, intake and output, and daily weight.
- Assess cardiovascular and respiratory status.
- Observe for and document bowel sounds, abdominal distention, and frequency of bowel movements.
- Observe for signs and symptoms of hyperthyroidism.

PATIENT TEACHING

- Explain the disorder, diagnostic testing, and treatment plan.
- Teach about the administration, dosage, and possible adverse effects of prescribed medications.
- Describe dangerous signs and symptoms and when to notify the practitioner.
- Stress the need for lifelong hormone replacement therapy.
- Explain the need to wear a medical identification bracelet and the importance of keeping accurate records of daily weight.
- Explain the need to follow a well-balanced, high-fiber, low-sodium diet.
- Refer the patient and family members to a mental health professional for additional counseling if needed.

Intestinal obstruction

Overview

Commonly a medical emergency, an intestinal obstruction is the partial or complete blockage of the small or large bowel lumen. Without treatment, complete obstruction in any part of bowel can cause death within hours from shock and vascular collapse.

CAUSES
Mechanical obstruction
◆ Adhesions
◆ Carcinomas
◆ Compression of the bowel wall from stenosis, intussusception, volvulus of the sigmoid or cecum, tumors, and atresia
◆ Foreign bodies
◆ Strangulated hernias

Nonmechanical obstruction
◆ Electrolyte imbalances
◆ Neurogenic abnormalities
◆ Paralytic ileus
◆ Thrombosis or embolism of mesenteric vessels
◆ Toxicity, such as that associated with uremia or generalized infection

RISK FACTORS
◆ Abdominal surgery
◆ Radiation therapy
◆ Gallstones
◆ Inflammatory bowel disease

PATHOPHYSIOLOGY
◆ Mechanical or nonmechanical (neurogenic) blockage of the lumen occurs.
◆ Fluid, air, or gas collects near the site.
◆ Peristalsis increases temporarily in an attempt to break through the blockage.
◆ Intestinal mucosa is injured, and distention at and above the site of obstruction occurs.
◆ Venous blood flow is impaired, and normal absorptive processes stop.
◆ Water, sodium, and potassium are secreted by the bowel into the fluid pooled in the lumen.

◆ With small-bowel obstruction, loss of gastric acid, dehydration, and metabolic alkalosis occur.
◆ With large-bowel obstruction, loss of alkaline intestinal fluids lead to metabolic acidosis.

COMPLICATIONS
◆ Bowel perforation
◆ Peritonitis
◆ Septicemia
◆ Secondary infection
◆ Metabolic alkalosis or acidosis
◆ Death

Assessment

HISTORY
◆ Recent change in bowel habits
◆ Hiccups
◆ Malaise
◆ Thirst

Mechanical obstruction
◆ Colicky pain
◆ Nausea, vomiting
◆ Constipation

Nonmechanical obstruction
◆ Diffuse abdominal discomfort
◆ Fecal vomitus
◆ Severe abdominal pain (if obstruction results from vascular insufficiency or infarction)

PHYSICAL FINDINGS
Mechanical obstruction
◆ Distended abdomen
◆ Borborygmi and rushes (occasionally loud enough to be heard without a stethoscope)
◆ Abdominal tenderness
◆ Rebound tenderness

Nonmechanical obstruction
◆ Abdominal distention
◆ Decreased bowel sounds (early), then absent bowel sounds

Diagnostic test results

◆ *Serum sodium, chloride, and potassium levels:* decreased
◆ *White blood cell count:* elevated
◆ *Serum amylase level:* increased (if pancreas is irritated by a bowel loop)
◆ *Blood urea nitrogen:* increased (with dehydration)
◆ *Abdominal X-rays:* presence and location of intestinal gas or fluid; in small bowel obstruction, presence of characterisic "stepladder" pattern
◆ *Barium enema:* distended, air-filled colon or a closed loop of sigmoid with extreme distention (in sigmoid volvulus)

Treatment

◆ Surgery (type dependent on blockage cause); for paralytic ileus, nonoperative therapy usually attempted first
◆ Surgical resection with anastomosis, colostomy, or ileostomy
◆ Bowel decompression to relieve vomiting and distention
◆ Supportive measures for life-threatening signs and symptoms
◆ Nothing by mouth (if surgery is planned)
◆ High-fiber diet after obstruction is relieved
◆ Bed rest during acute phase
◆ Postoperatively, avoidance of lifting and contact sports

Medications

◆ Broad-spectrum antibiotics
◆ Analgesics
◆ Electrolyte supplements as indicated
◆ Parenteral nutrition until bowel is functioning

Nursing interventions

◆ Insert a nasogastric (NG) tube and monitor its function and drainage.
◆ Maintain the patient in semi-Fowler's position.
◆ Provide mouth and nose care.
◆ Begin and maintain I.V. therapy as ordered.
◆ Give prescribed drugs.
◆ Monitor vital signs and laboratory studies.
◆ Assess bowel sounds and monitor for signs of returning peristalsis.
◆ Assess the patient's pain level, administer analgesics, and evaluate their effects.
◆ Assess the patient's hydration and nutritional status.
◆ Provide postoperative wound care.

Patient teaching

◆ Explain the disorder, diagnostic testing, and treatment plan.
◆ Teach about the administration, dosage, and possible adverse effects of prescribed medications.
◆ Demonstrate techniques for coughing and deep breathing and use of incentive spirometry.
◆ Teach incision care and review signs and symptoms of complications.
◆ Teach colostomy or ileostomy care if appropriate.
◆ Explain postoperative activity limitations.
◆ Stress the importance of following a structured bowel regimen, particularly if the patient had a mechanical obstruction from fecal impaction.
◆ Refer the patient to an enterostomal therapist if indicated.
◆ Teach about a high-fiber diet

Disorders

Irritable bowel syndrome

Overview

Irritable bowel syndrome (IBS), also known as *spastic colon, spastic colitis,* and *mucous colitis,* is a common GI condition marked by chronic or periodic diarrhea alternating with constipation and excessive flatus. It's accompanied by straining and abdominal cramps that are relieved after defecation. Initial episodes usually occur in the late teens to 20s.

CAUSES
♦ Anxiety and stress
♦ Dietary factors, such as fiber, raw fruits, coffee, alcohol, and foods that are cold, highly seasoned, or laxative in nature

POSSIBLE TRIGGERS
♦ Allergy to certain foods or drugs
♦ Hormones
♦ Lactose intolerance
♦ Laxative abuse

PATHOPHYSIOLOGY
♦ The precise etiology is unclear.
♦ A change occurs in bowel motility, reflecting an abnormality in the neuromuscular control of intestinal smooth muscle.
♦ The disorder may reflect a hypersensitivity to gastrin or cholecystokinin.

COMPLICATIONS
♦ Diverticulitis and colon cancer
♦ Chronic inflammatory bowel disease

Assessment

HISTORY
♦ Chronic constipation, diarrhea, or both
♦ Lower abdominal pain (typically in the left lower quadrant), usually relieved by defecation or passage of gas
♦ Small stools with visible mucus or pasty, pencil-like stools instead of diarrhea
♦ Dyspepsia
♦ Abdominal bloating
♦ Heartburn
♦ Faintness and weakness
♦ Contributing psychological factors, such as a recent stressful life change, that may have triggered or aggravated symptoms
♦ Anxiety and fatigue

PHYSICAL FINDINGS
♦ Normal bowel sounds
♦ Tympany over a gas-filled bowel
♦ Abdominal distention

DIAGNOSTIC TEST RESULTS
♦ *Barium enema:* colonic spasm and a tubular appearance of the descending colon; rules out certain other disorders, such as diverticula, tumors, and polyps
♦ *Sigmoidoscopy:* spastic contractions

Treatment

♦ Stress management
♦ Lifestyle modifications
♦ Initially, elimination diet
♦ Avoidance of sorbitol, nonabsorbable carbohydrates, and foods that contain lactose
♦ Increased bulk and fluids in diet
♦ Regular exercise program

MEDICATIONS
♦ Anticholinergic, antispasmodic drugs
♦ Antidiarrheals
♦ Laxatives, bulking agents
♦ Antiemetics
♦ Simethicone (Mylicon)
♦ Mild sedatives
♦ Tricyclic antidepressants

Nursing interventions

◆ Because the patient with IBS isn't hospitalized, nursing interventions almost always focus on patient teaching.
◆ Monitor the patient's weight, diet, and bowel activity.

PATIENT TEACHING
◆ Explain the disorder, diagnostic testing, and treatment plan.
◆ Teach about the administration, dosage, and possible adverse effects of prescribed medications.
◆ Review dietary plans.
◆ Stress the importance of drinking 8 to 10 glasses of water or other compatible fluids daily.
◆ Review appropriate lifestyle changes that reduce stress.
◆ Recommend smoking cessation.
◆ Stress the importance of regular physical examinations.

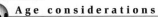 **Age considerations**

For patients older than age 40, emphasize the need for colorectal cancer screening, including annual proctosigmoidoscopy and rectal examinations.

◆ Refer the patient for counseling if appropriate.

Latex allergy

Overview

A latex allergy is an immunoglobulin (Ig) E-mediated immediate hypersensitivity to natural latex-containing products. Reactions, which range from local dermatitis to life-threatening anaphylactic events, affect 10% to 30% of health care workers and 20% to 68% of patients with spina bifida and urogenital abnormalities.

CAUSES
◆ Frequent contact with latex-containing products (see *Products that contain latex*)

RISK FACTORS
◆ Being a medical or dental professional
◆ Working in a latex manufacturing or supply company
◆ Having spina bifida or other conditions that require multiple surgeries involving latex material
◆ History of asthma or other allergies, especially to bananas, avocados, tropical fruits, or chestnuts
◆ History of multiple intra-abdominal or genitourinary surgeries
◆ History of frequent intermittent urinary catheterization

PATHOPHYSIOLOGY
◆ Mast cells release histamine and other secretory products in response to contact with latex-containing products.
◆ Vascular permeability increases, and vasodilation and bronchoconstriction occur.
◆ Chemical sensitivity dermatitis, a type IV delayed hypersensitivity reaction to the chemicals used to produce latex, occurs.
◆ Sensitized T lymphocytes are triggered in a cell-mediated allergic reaction, stimulating the proliferation of other lymphocytes and mononuclear cells, resulting in tissue inflammation and contact dermatitis.

COMPLICATIONS
◆ Respiratory obstruction
◆ Systemic vascular collapse
◆ Death

Assessment

HISTORY
◆ Exposure to latex

PHYSICAL FINDINGS
◆ Contact dermatitis
◆ Signs of anaphylaxis (throat edema, respiratory distress)
◆ Rash
◆ Angioedema
◆ Conjunctivitis
◆ Wheezing, stridor

DIAGNOSTIC TEST RESULTS
◆ *Radioallergosorbent test:* specific IgE antibodies to latex (safest for use in patients with a history of type I hypersensitivity)
◆ *History and physical assessment:* latex allergy diagnosis
◆ *Patch test reaction:* positive, as indicated by hives with itching or redness

Disorders

Treatment

◆ Use of latex-free products to prevent exposure and to decrease hypersensitivity exacerbation
◆ Supportive measures for life-threatening signs and symptoms

MEDICATIONS
◆ Corticosteroids
◆ Antihistamines
◆ Histamine-2 receptor blockers

Acute treatment
◆ Epinephrine (1:1,000)
◆ Oxygen therapy
◆ Volume expanders
◆ I.V. vasopressors
◆ Aminophylline and albuterol

Nursing interventions

◆ Maintain the patient's airway, breathing, and circulation as indicated.
◆ Give prescribed drugs.
◆ Monitor the patient for sensitivity to tropical nuts or bananas.
◆ Keep the patient's environment latex-free.
◆ Monitor the patient's vital signs and respiratory status.

PATIENT TEACHING
◆ Explain the disorder, diagnostic testing, and treatment plan.
◆ Teach about the administration, dosage, and possible adverse effects of prescribed medications.
◆ Stress the potential for a life-threatening reaction.
◆ Explain the importance of wearing medical identification jewelry that identifies the patient's latex allergy.
◆ Demonstrate how to use an epinephrine autoinjector.
◆ Review common products that contain latex.

Products that contain latex

Keep in mind that these products contain latex.

Medical products
◆ Adhesive bandages
◆ Airways, Levin tube
◆ Handheld resuscitation bags
◆ Blood pressure cuff, tubing, and bladder
◆ Catheters
◆ Catheter leg straps
◆ Dental dams
◆ Elastic bandages
◆ Electrode pads
◆ Fluid-circulating hypothermia blankets
◆ Hemodialysis equipment
◆ I.V. catheters
◆ Latex or rubber gloves
◆ Medication vials
◆ Pads for crutches
◆ Protective sheets
◆ Reservoir breathing bags
◆ Rubber airways and endotracheal tubes
◆ Tape
◆ Tourniquets

Nonmedical products
◆ Adhesive tape
◆ Balloons (excluding Mylar)
◆ Cervical diaphragms
◆ Condoms
◆ Disposable diapers
◆ Elastic stockings
◆ Glue
◆ Latex paint
◆ Nipples and pacifiers
◆ Rubber bands
◆ Tires

Legionnaires' disease

Overview

Legionnaires' disease, an acute bronchopneumonia produced by a gram-negative bacteria, ranges from mild illness, with or without pneumonitis, to serious multilobed pneumonia. Mortality may be as high as 15%. Epidemic outbreaks may occur, usually in late summer and early fall; however, outbreaks may be limited to a few cases.

CAUSES
◆ *Legionella pneumophila*, an aerobic, gram-negative bacillus that's most likely transmitted by air
◆ Water distribution systems (such as whirlpool spas and decorative fountains) and air-conditioning vents, which are reservoirs for the organism

RISK FACTORS
◆ Older age
◆ Being immunocompromised
◆ Chronic underlying disease
◆ Alcoholism
◆ Smoking

PATHOPHYSIOLOGY
◆ Legionella organisms enter the lungs after aspiration or inhalation.
◆ Although alveolar macrophages phagocytize *Legionella*, the organisms aren't killed and proliferate intracellularly.
◆ The cells rupture, releasing *Legionella*, and the cycle starts again.
◆ Lesions develop a nodular appearance and alveoli become filled with fibrin, neutrophils, and alveolar macrophages.

COMPLICATIONS
◆ Hypoxia and acute respiratory failure
◆ Renal failure
◆ Septic shock

Assessment

HISTORY
◆ Presence at a suspected infection source
◆ Prodromal symptoms, including anorexia, malaise, myalgia, and headache

PHYSICAL FINDINGS
◆ Cough
◆ Shortness of breath
◆ Rapidly rising fever with chills
◆ Grayish or rust-colored, nonpurulent, occasionally blood-streaked sputum
◆ Chest pain
◆ Tachypnea
◆ Bradycardia (in about 50% of patients)
◆ Altered level of consciousness
◆ Dullness over areas of secretions and consolidation or pleural effusions
◆ Fine crackles that develop into coarse crackles as the disease progresses

DIAGNOSTIC TEST RESULTS
◆ *Gram staining:* numerous neutrophils but no organism
◆ *Bronchial washings or thoracentesis:* definitive diagnosis through organism isolation from respiratory secretions
◆ *Direct immunofluorescence or indirect fluorescent serum antibody testing:* definitive identification of *L. pneumophila*
◆ *Complete blood count:* leukocytosis
◆ *Erythrocyte sedimentation rate:* increased
◆ *Arterial blood gas (ABG) analysis:* decreased partial pressure of arterial oxygen, initially decreased partial pressure of arterial carbon dioxide
◆ *Serum sodium level:* less than 131 mg/L
◆ *Chest X-ray:* patchy, localized infiltration that progresses to multilobed consolidation (usually involving the lower lobes) and pleural effusion; opacification of the entire lung in fulminant disease

Treatment

◆ Oxygen administration with mechanical ventilation as needed
◆ Fluid replacement

MEDICATIONS
◆ Antibiotics
◆ Antipyretics
◆ Vasopressors (with shock)

Nursing interventions

◆ Give tepid sponge baths or use hypothermia blankets to lower fever.
◆ Replace fluids and electrolytes as needed.
◆ Institute seizure precautions.
◆ Give prescribed drugs.
◆ Monitor vital signs, pulse oximetry, and ABG values.
◆ Assess respiratory and neurologic status.

PATIENT TEACHING
◆ Explain the disorder, diagnostic testing, and treatment plan.
◆ Teach about the administration, dosage, and possible adverse effects of prescribed medications.
◆ Explain how to prevent infection and the importance of disinfecting the water supply.
◆ Review the purpose of postural drainage and how to perform coughing and deep-breathing exercises.
◆ Demonstrate proper hand washing and disposal of soiled tissues to prevent disease transmission.
◆ Explain the importance of smoking cessation.
◆ Refer the patient to a pulmonologist if necessary.

Overview

The most common form of cancer among children, acute leukemia is the malignant proliferation of white blood cell (WBC) precursors, or blasts, in bone marrow or lymph tissue. Common forms include acute lymphoblastic (lymphocytic) leukemia (ALL) and acute myeloblastic (myelogenous) leukemia (AML). ALL treatment induces remissions in 90% of children (average survival: 5 years) and in 65% of adults (average survival: 1 to 2 years). With AML, average survival is 1 year after diagnosis, even with aggressive treatment.

 Age considerations

ALL treatment induces remission in children 90% of the time with an average survival of 5 years. In adults, there's a 65% remission rate with 1 year average survival.

CAUSES
◆ Unknown

RISK FACTORS
◆ Radiation (especially prolonged exposure)
◆ Certain chemicals and drugs
◆ Viruses
◆ Genetic abnormalities
◆ Chronic exposure to benzene

In children
◆ Down syndrome
◆ Ataxia
◆ Telangiectasia
◆ Congenital disorders, such as albinism and congenital immunodeficiency syndrome

PATHOPHYSIOLOGY
◆ Immature, nonfunctioning WBCs appear to accumulate first in the tissue where they originate (lymphocytes in lymphatic tissue and granulocytes in bone marrow).
◆ The immature, nonfunctioning WBCs spill into the bloodstream and overwhelm red blood cells (RBCs) and platelets, and then they infiltrate other tissues.

COMPLICATIONS
◆ Infection
◆ Organ malfunction through encroachment or hemorrhage

Assessment

HISTORY
◆ Sudden onset of high fever
◆ Abnormal bleeding
◆ Fatigue and night sweats
◆ Weakness, lassitude, recurrent infections, and chills
◆ Abdominal or bone pain

PHYSICAL FINDINGS
◆ Tachycardia, palpitations, and a systolic ejection murmur
◆ Decreased ventilation
◆ Pallor
◆ Lymph node enlargement
◆ Liver or spleen enlargement

DIAGNOSTIC TEST RESULTS
◆ *Blood counts:* anemia, thrombocytopenia, and neutropenia
◆ *WBC differential:* affected cell type
◆ *Computed tomography:* affected organs
◆ *Cerebrospinal fluid analysis:* abnormal WBC invasion of the central nervous system
◆ *Bone marrow aspiration and biopsy:* proliferation of immature WBCs (confirm acute leukemia and the type of cells involved)
◆ *Lumbar puncture:* meningeal involvement

Treatment

◆ Blood product transfusions
◆ Bone marrow transplantation (in some patients)
◆ Radiation treatment for brain or testicular infiltration
◆ Chemotherapy and radiation treatment, depending on diagnosis
◆ Well-balanced diet
◆ Frequent rest periods

MEDICATIONS

◆ Combination therapy antineoplastics
◆ Corticosteroids
◆ Anti-infective agents, such as antibiotics, antifungals, and antiviral drugs
◆ Granulocyte colony-stimulating factor injections (in acute monoblastic leukemia)

Nursing interventions

◆ Encourage the patient to verbalize his feelings, and provide comfort.
◆ Provide adequate hydration.
◆ Administer blood products as necessary.
◆ Give prescribed drugs.
◆ Provide frequent mouth care and saline rinses.
◆ Observe for signs and symptoms of treatment complications.
◆ Assess the patient's hydration and nutritional status.
◆ Monitor the patient's vital signs.
◆ Observe for signs and symptoms of bleeding.
◆ Provide frequent rest periods.

PATIENT TEACHING

◆ Explain the disorder, diagnostic testing, and treatment plan.
◆ Teach about the administration, dosage, and possible adverse effects of prescribed medications.

◆ Explain the need to use a soft toothbrush and to avoid hot, spicy foods and commercial mouthwashes.
◆ Review signs and symptoms of complications.
◆ Stress the importance of planned rest periods during the day.
◆ Refer the patient to available resources and support services.

Liver failure

Overview

Liver failure is the inability of the liver to function properly, usually as the end result of liver disease. It causes a complex syndrome involving the impairment of various organs and body functions. (See *Understanding liver functions.*) Two conditions occurring in liver failure are hepatic encephalopathy and hepatorenal syndrome. Liver transplantation is the only cure.

CAUSES
- Acetaminophen toxicity
- Cirrhosis
- Liver cancer
- Nonviral hepatitis
- Viral hepatitis

PATHOPHYSIOLOGY
- Manifestations of liver failure include hepatic encephalopathy and hepatorenal syndrome.

Hepatic encephalopathy
- The liver can no longer detoxify the blood.
- Liver dysfunction and collateral vessels that shunt blood around the liver to the systemic circulation permit toxins absorbed from the GI tract to circulate freely to the brain.
- The liver can't convert ammonia to urea, which the kidneys normally excrete.
- Ammonia blood levels rise, and the ammonia is delivered to the brain.
- Short-chain fatty acids, serotonin, tryptophan, and false neurotransmitters may also accumulate in the blood.

Hepatorenal syndrome
- The kidneys appear to be normal but abruptly stop functioning.
- Blood volume expands, hydrogen ions accumulate, and electrolyte disturbances occur.

- Vasoactive substances accumulate, causing inappropriate renal arteriole constriction, leading to decreased glomerular filtration and oliguria.
- Vasoconstriction may also be a compensatory response to portal hypertension and the pooling of blood in the splenic circulation.

COMPLICATIONS
- Variceal bleeding
- GI hemorrhage
- Coma
- Death

Assessment

HISTORY
- Liver disorder
- Fatigue
- Weight loss
- Nausea
- Anorexia
- Pruritus

PHYSICAL FINDINGS
- Jaundice
- Abdominal tenderness
- Splenomegaly
- Ascites
- Peripheral edema
- Decreased level of consciousness

DIAGNOSTIC TEST RESULTS
- *Liver function test:* elevated levels of aspartate aminotransferase, alanine aminotransferase, alkaline phosphatase, and bilirubin
- *Blood studies:* anemia, impaired red blood cell production, prolonged bleeding and clotting times, low blood glucose levels, and increased serum ammonia levels
- *Urine osmolarity:* increased

Treatment

- Paracentesis to remove ascitic fluid
- Balloon tamponade or sclerosis to control bleeding varices
- Low-protein, high-carbohydrate diet
- Activity as tolerated
- Shunt placement
- Liver transplantation

MEDICATIONS

- Lactulose (Cephulac)
- Potassium-sparing diuretics (for ascites)
- Potassium supplements
- Vasoconstrictors (for variceal bleeding)
- Vitamin K

Nursing interventions

- Monitor the patient's level of consciousness, vital signs, intake and output, and laboratory values.
- Administer I.V fluids and prescribed drugs.
- Observe for signs and symptoms of bleeding.
- Reorient the patient as needed.
- Provide a safe environment.
- Provide emotional support.
- Obtain daily weight and abdominal girth measurements.

PATIENT TEACHING

- Explain the disorder, diagnostic testing, and treatment plan.
- Teach about the administration, dosage, and possible adverse effects of prescribed medications.
- Review the signs and symptoms of complications and when to notify the practitioner.
- Stress the importance of following a low-protein diet and of avoiding alcohol.
- Refer the patient to available support services as appropriate.

Understanding liver functions

To understand how liver disease affects the body, you need to understand its main functions. The liver:
- detoxifies poisonous chemicals, including alcohol and drugs (prescribed and over-the-counter as well as illegal substances)
- makes bile to help digest food
- stores energy by stockpiling sugar (carbohydrates, glucose, and fat) until needed
- stores iron reserves as well as vitamins and minerals
- manufactures new proteins
- produces important plasma proteins necessary for blood coagulation, including prothrombin and fibrinogen
- serves as a site for hematopoiesis during fetal development.

Lung cancer

Overview

The most frequent cause of death from cancer for men and women ages 50 to 75, lung cancer is a malignant tumor arising from the respiratory epithelium. The most common types are epidermoid (squamous cell), adenocarcinoma, small-cell (oat cell), and large-cell (anaplastic). Usually, occurrence is on the wall or epithelium of the bronchial tree.

CAUSES
◆ Exact cause unknown

RISK FACTORS
◆ Smoking
◆ Exposure to carcinogenic and industrial air pollutants, such as asbestos, arsenic, chromium, coal dust, iron oxides, nickel, radioactive dust, and uranium
◆ Genetic predisposition

PATHOPHYSIOLOGY
◆ Individuals with lung cancer demonstrate bronchial epithelial changes progressing from squamous cell alteration or metaplasia to carcinoma in situ.
◆ Tumors originating in the bronchi are thought to be more mucus producing.
◆ Partial or complete obstruction of the airway occurs with tumor growth, resulting in lobar collapse distal to the tumor.
◆ Early metastasis to other thoracic structures, such as hilar lymph nodes or the mediastinum, occurs.
◆ Distant metastasis to the brain, liver, bone, and adrenal glands occurs.

COMPLICATIONS
◆ Metastasis
◆ Tracheal obstruction
◆ Esophageal compression with dysphagia
◆ Phrenic nerve paralysis with hemidiaphragm elevation and dyspnea
◆ Sympathetic nerve paralysis with Horner's syndrome
◆ Spinal cord compression

◆ Lymphatic obstruction with pleural effusion
◆ Hypoxemia
◆ Neoplastic and paraneoplastic syndromes, including Pancoast's syndrome and syndrome of inappropriate secretion of antidiuretic hormone

Assessment

HISTORY
◆ Possibly no symptoms
◆ Exposure to carcinogens
◆ Coughing
◆ Hemoptysis
◆ Shortness of breath
◆ Hoarseness
◆ Fatigue

PHYSICAL FINDINGS
◆ Dyspnea on exertion
◆ Digital clubbing
◆ Edema of the face, neck, and upper torso
◆ Dilated chest and abdominal veins (superior vena cava syndrome)
◆ Weight loss
◆ Enlarged lymph nodes
◆ Enlarged liver
◆ Decreased breath sounds
◆ Wheezing
◆ Pleural friction rub

DIAGNOSTIC TEST RESULTS
◆ *Cytologic sputum analysis:* evidence of pulmonary malignancy
◆ *Liver function test:* abnormal, especially with metastasis
◆ *Chest X-rays:* advanced lesions (may be visible up to 2 years before signs and symptoms appear), tumor size and location
◆ *Chest computed tomography (CT) and bronchography contrast studies:* size, location and spread of lesion, malignant pleural effusion
◆ *Positron emission tomography:* primary and metastatic sites
◆ *Magnetic resonance imaging:* tumor invasion

- *Bronchoscopy:* cytologic and histologic study of tumor from bronchoscopic washings
- *Needle biopsy of the lungs:* confirms diagnosis in 80% of patients
- *Tissue biopsy of metastatic sites (including supraclavicular and mediastinal lymph nodes and pleura):* disease extent
- *Thoracentesis:* presence of malignant cells upon pleural fluid chemical and cytologic examination
- *Exploratory thoracotomy:* retrieval of a biopsy specimen

Treatment

- Various combinations of surgery, radiation therapy, and chemotherapy to improve prognosis
- Palliative (most treatments)
- Preoperative and postoperative radiation therapy
- Laser therapy (experimental)
- Well-balanced diet
- Activity as tolerated, according to breathing capacity
- Partial removal of lung (wedge resection, segmental resection, lobectomy, or radical lobectomy)
- Total removal of lung (pneumonectomy or radical pneumonectomy)

MEDICATIONS
- Combination antineoplastic therapy
- Erlotinib (Tarceva)
- Bevacizumab (Avastin)
- Oxygen therapy

Nursing interventions

- Assess the patient's pain level, administer analgesics, and evaluate their effects.
- Provide supportive care and encourage the patient to verbalize his feelings.
- Give prescribed drugs.
- Monitor chest tube function and drainage.
- Observe for postoperative complications.
- Provide wound care.
- Monitor vital signs, pulse oximetry, and sputum production.
- Assess hydration and nutritional status.

PATIENT TEACHING
- Explain the disorder, diagnostic testing, and treatment plan.
- Teach about the administration, dosage, and possible adverse effects of prescribed medications.
- Describe procedures and equipment.
- Demonstrate chest physiotherapy and exercises to prevent shoulder stiffness.
- Refer smokers to local branches of the American Cancer Society or Smokenders.
- Provide information about group therapy, individual counseling, and hypnosis.
- Refer the patient to available resources and support services.

Lymphoma, non-Hodgkin's

Overview

Non-Hodgkin's lymphoma, also called *malignant lymphoma* and *lymphosarcoma*, is a heterogeneous group of malignant diseases that originate in lymph glands and other lymphoid tissue. It's usually classified according to histologic, anatomic, and immunomorphic characteristics developed by the National Cancer Institute. Non-Hodgkin's lymphoma is three times more common than Hodgkin's disease.

CAUSES
◆ Exact cause unknown

RISK FACTORS
◆ History of autoimmune disease

PATHOPHYSIOLOGY
◆ Non-Hodgkin's lymphoma seems to be similar to Hodgkin's disease, but Reed-Sternberg cells aren't present, and the lymph node destruction is different.
◆ Lymphoid tissue is characterized by a pattern of either diffuse or nodular infiltration. Nodular lymphomas yield a better prognosis than the diffuse form, but in both forms the prognosis is less hopeful than in Hodgkin's disease.

COMPLICATIONS
◆ Hypercalcemia
◆ Hyperuricemia
◆ Lymphomatosis
◆ Meningitis
◆ Anemia
◆ Liver, kidney, and lung problems (with tumor growth)
◆ Increased intracranial pressure (with central nervous system involvement)

Assessment

HISTORY
◆ Symptoms mimic those of Hodgkin's disease
◆ Painless, swollen lymph glands that may have appeared and disappeared over several months
◆ Complaints of fatigue, malaise, weight loss, fever, and night sweats
◆ Trouble breathing, cough (usually children)

PHYSICAL FINDINGS
◆ Enlarged tonsils and adenoids
◆ Rubbery nodes in the cervical and supraclavicular areas

DIAGNOSTIC TEST RESULTS
◆ *Complete blood count:* anemia
◆ *Uric acid levels:* normal or elevated
◆ *Calcium levels:* elevated, from bone lesions
◆ *Chest X-rays; lymphangiography; liver, bone, and spleen scans; computed tomography of the abdomen; and excretory urography:* disease progression
◆ *Biopsies of lymph nodes, tonsils, bone marrow, liver, bowel, skin, or from exploratory laparotomy:* differentiation of non-Hodgkin's lymphoma from Hodgkin's disease

Treatment

◆ Radiation therapy mainly during the localized stage of the disease
◆ Total nodal irradiation (usually effective in nodular and diffuse lymphomas)
◆ Well-balanced, high-calorie, high-protein diet
◆ Increased fluid intake
◆ Limited activity with frequent rest periods

◆ Debulking procedure (subtotal or, in some cases, total gastrectomy) before chemotherapy for perforation (common in patients with gastric lymphomas)
◆ Stem cell transplantation

MEDICATIONS
◆ Combination chemotherapy regimens
◆ Radioimmunotherapy: ibritumomab tiuxetant (Zevalin), tositumomab and iodine 131 tositumomab (Bexxar)
◆ Rituximab (Rituxan)

Nursing interventions

◆ Assess the patient's pain level, administer analgesics, and evaluate their effects.
◆ Give prescribed drugs.
◆ Provide frequent rest periods.
◆ Encourage the patient to verbalize his feelings, and provide support.
◆ Observe for adverse effects of treatment, such as nausea, vomiting, stomatitis, and pain.
◆ Monitor vital signs.
◆ Assess hydration and nutritional status.

PATIENT TEACHING
◆ Explain the disorder, diagnostic testing, and treatment plan.
◆ Teach about the administration, dosage, and possible adverse effects of prescribed medications.
◆ Explain preoperative and postoperative procedures.
◆ Review the dietary plan.
◆ Advise the patient to perform mouth care using a soft-bristled toothbrush and avoid commercial mouthwashes.
◆ Describe symptoms that require immediate attention.
◆ Refer the patient to available resources and support services.

Meningitis

Overview

Meningitis, an inflammation of brain and spinal cord meninges, develops rapidly and causes serious illness within 24 hours, usually after the onset of respiratory symptoms. It may affect all three meningeal membranes—the dura mater, the arachnoid membrane, and the pia mater.

CAUSES

◆ Bacterial infection, usually with *Neisseria meningitidis* and *Streptococcus pneumoniae*
◆ Fungal infection
◆ Protozoal infection
◆ Secondary to another bacterial infection such as pneumonia
◆ Skull fracture, penetrating head wound, lumbar puncture, or ventricular shunting procedures
◆ Viral infection

PATHOPHYSIOLOGY

◆ Inflammation of pia-arachnoid and subarachnoid space progresses to congestion of adjacent tissues.
◆ Nerve cells are destroyed.
◆ Intracranial pressure (ICP) increases because of exudates.
◆ Effects of increased ICP can include engorged blood vessels, disrupted blood supply, edema of the brain tissue, thrombosis, rupture, and acute hydrocephalus.

COMPLICATIONS

◆ Visual impairment, optic neuritis
◆ Cranial nerve palsies
◆ Deafness
◆ Paresis or paralysis
◆ Endocarditis
◆ Coma
◆ Vasculitis
◆ Cerebral infarction
◆ Seizures

Assessment

HISTORY

◆ Headache
◆ Fever
◆ Nausea, vomiting
◆ Weakness
◆ Myalgia
◆ Photophobia
◆ Confusion, delirium
◆ Seizures

PHYSICAL FINDINGS

◆ Meningismus
◆ Rigors
◆ Profuse sweating
◆ Kernig's and Brudzinski's signs (elicited in only 50% of adults)
◆ Declining level of consciousness
◆ Cranial nerve palsies
◆ Rash (with meningococcemia)
◆ Focal neurologic deficits such as visual field defects
◆ Signs of increased ICP in later stages

DIAGNOSTIC TEST RESULTS

◆ *White blood cell count:* leukocytosis
◆ *Blood cultures:* positive, depending on the pathogen (in bacterial meningitis)
◆ *Coagglutination test:* causative agent
◆ *Xpert EV test:* positive for Enterovirus (in viral meningitis)
◆ *Chest X-rays:* coexisting pneumonia
◆ *Computed tomography and magnetic resonance imaging*: evidence of complications and a parameningeal source of infection
◆ *Lumbar puncture and cerebrospinal fluid (CSF) analysis:* increased opening pressure (due to inflammation), neutrophilic pleocytosis, elevated protein level, hypoglycorrhachia, positive Gram stain, positive culture, decreased glucose level (milky or cloudy CSF)

Treatment

- Fever reduction
- Fluid therapy
- Bed rest (in acute phase)

MEDICATIONS

- Oxygen therapy
- Antipyretics
- Antibiotics
- Antiarrhythmics
- Osmotic diuretics
- Anticonvulsants

Nursing interventions

- Maintain respiratory isolation for the first 24 hours (with meningococcal meningitis).
- Assess the patient's pain level, administer analgesics, and evaluate their effects.
- Give prescribed oxygen.
- Encourage active range-of-motion (ROM) exercises when appropriate.
- Provide passive ROM exercises when appropriate.
- Maintain adequate nutrition and hydration.
- Provide meticulous skin and mouth care.
- Give prescribed drugs.
- Assess neurologic status.
- Monitor the patient's vital signs, pulse oximetry, and intake and output.
- Observe for signs and symptoms of cranial nerve involvement and increased ICP.
- Monitor respiratory status.

PATIENT TEACHING

- Explain the disorder, diagnostic testing, and treatment plan.
- Teach about the administration, dosage, and possible adverse effects of prescribed medications.
- Explain the contagion risks for close contacts.
- Demonstrate exercises to promote muscle strength and mobility.
- Teach about polysaccharide meningococcal vaccine and pneumococcal vaccine.
- Refer the patient to community resources as indicated.

Metabolic acidosis and alkalosis

Disorders

Overview

These acid-base disorders are characterized by abnormal levels of acid and bicarbonate (HCO_3^-) in the blood. Both may cause metabolic, respiratory, and renal responses that produce characteristic symptoms, most notably, hypoventilation. Metabolic acidosis is characterized by a gain in acids or a loss of bases from the plasma. Metabolic alkalosis is characterized by a loss of acid or a gain of bases.

 Nursing alert
Severe or untreated metabolic acid-base disorders can be fatal.

CAUSES
Metabolic acidosis
- Dieting
- Lactic acidosis
- Renal insufficiency and failure
- Diarrhea, intestinal malabsorption, or loss of sodium bicarbonate from the intestines
- Salicylate intoxication, exogenous poisoning
- Hypoaldosteronism
- Potassium-sparing diuretics use

Metabolic alkalosis
- Gastric fluid loss
- Diuretic use
- Congenital chloride diarrhea
- Cystic fibrosis
- Primary aldosteronism
- Bartter syndrome
- Excessive licorice ingestion

PATHOPHYSIOLOGY
Metabolic acidosis
- Underlying mechanisms are a loss of HCO_3^- from extracellular fluid, an accumulation of metabolic acids, or a combination of the two.
- Acidosis is a result of an accumulation of metabolic acids (unmeasured anions) if the anion gap is greater than 14 mEq/L. If the anion gap is normal (8 to 14 mEq/L), loss of HCO_3^- may be the cause.

- An overproduction of ketone bodies may be related when glucose supplies have been used and the body draws on fat stores for energy.

Metabolic alkalosis
- Underlying mechanisms include a loss of hydrogen ions (acid), a gain in HCO_3^-, or both.
- A partial pressure of arterial carbon dioxide ($Paco_2$) level more than 45 mm Hg (possibly as high as 60 mm Hg) indicates that the lungs are compensating for the alkalosis. The kidneys are more effective at compensating; however, they're far slower than the lungs.

COMPLICATIONS
- Respiratory failure
- Cardiac arrhythmia
- Seizure

Assessment

HISTORY
- Underlying condition that affects acid-base balance
- Change in level of consciousness
- Generalized weakness
- History of vomiting or GI fluid loss
- Diuretic use
- Change in mental status or personality
- Paresthesia

PHYSICAL FINDINGS
- Confusion
- Hypotension
- Loss of reflexes
- Muscle twitching
- Nausea and vomiting
- Paresthesia
- Polyuria
- Weakness
- Cardiac arrhythmias
- Decreased rate and depth of respirations

Metabolic acidosis

◆ Hyperkalemic signs and symptoms, including abdominal cramping, diarrhea, muscle weakness, and electrocardiogram changes
◆ Kussmaul's respirations
◆ Fruity breath odor
◆ Signs of dehydration, such as poor skin turgor, thirst, decreased blood pressure

Metabolic alkalosis

◆ Anorexia
◆ Positive Trousseau's and Chvostek's signs
◆ Tetany, if serum calcium levels are borderline or low

DIAGNOSTIC TEST RESULTS

◆ *Arterial blood gas (ABG) studies (metabolic acidosis):* pH less than 7.35, $Paco_2$ less than 34 mm Hg as respiratory compensatory mechanisms take hold, HCO_3^- level 22 mEq/L or greater
◆ *ABG studies (metabolic alkalosis):* pH greater than 7.45, HCO_3^- greater than 26 mEq/L, $Paco_2$ greater than 45 mm Hg (indicates attempts at respiratory compensation)
◆ *Potassium level:* abnormal
◆ *Urine pH:* less than 4.5 with metabolic acidosis, about 7 with metabolic alkalosis
◆ *Serum ketone bodies:* present with metabolic acidosis
◆ *Lactic acid level:* elevated with lactic acidosis
◆ *Anion gap:* greater than 14 mEq/L in metabolic acidosis, lactic acidosis, ketoacidosis, aspirin overdose, alcohol poisoning, renal failure, or other conditions characterized by accumulation of organic acids, sulfates, or phosphates; 12 mEq/L or less in normal anion gap metabolic acidosis from HCO_3^- loss, GI or renal loss, increased acid load (hyperalimentation fluids), rapid I.V. saline solution administration, or other conditions characterized by loss of bicarbonate
◆ *Electrocardiography:* abnormalities

Treatment

◆ Treatment of underlying cause
◆ Supportive measures for life-threatening signs and symptoms
◆ Dialysis

MEDICATION

◆ Electrolyte supplements
◆ I.V. fluids
◆ Antidiarrheal agents
◆ Antiemetics
◆ Vasopressors
◆ I.V. sodium bicarbonate (metabolic acidosis)
◆ Hydrochloric acid (metabolic alkalosis)
◆ Carbonic anhydrase inhibitors (metabolic alkalosis)

Nursing interventions

◆ Monitor vital signs, pulse oximetry, intake and output, laboratory values, and ABG values.
◆ Assess neurologic, cardiovascular, and respiratory systems.
◆ Monitor electrocardiograms for arrhythmias.
◆ Administer supplemental oxygen if indicated.
◆ Provide seizure precautions and safety measures for the patient with altered thought processes.
◆ Reposition the patient every 2 hours, and provide skin care.

PATIENT TEACHING

◆ Explain the disorder, diagnostic testing, and treatment plan.
◆ Teach about the administration, dosage, and possible adverse effects of prescribed medications.
◆ Explain the underlying cause of the disorder and how to prevent reoccurence.
◆ Refer the patient to appropriate agencies for supportive care and further teaching.

Metabolic syndrome

Overview

Metabolic syndrome is a cluster of symptoms triggered by insulin resistance from abdominal fat, obesity, high blood pressure, and high levels of blood glucose, triglycerides, and cholesterol. It's associated with increased risk of diabetes, heart disease, and stroke. Metabolic syndrome is also known as *syndrome X, insulin resistance syndrome, dysmetabolic syndrome,* and *multiple metabolic syndrome.*

CAUSES
◆ Genetic predisposition

RISK FACTORS
◆ Obesity
◆ High fat, high-carbohydrate diet
◆ Insufficient physical activity
◆ Aging
◆ Hyperinsulinemia and impaired glucose tolerance
◆ Prior heart attack

PATHOPHYSIOLOGY
◆ Glucose doesn't respond to insulin's attempt to guide it into storage cells. The result is insulin resistance.
◆ To overcome this resistance, the pancreas produces excess insulin, which causes damage to arterial lining.
◆ Excessive insulin secretion also promotes fat storage deposits and prevents fat breakdown.
◆ This series of events can lead to diabetes, blood clots, and coronary events.

COMPLICATIONS
◆ Coronary artery disease
◆ Diabetes
◆ Hyperlipidemia
◆ Premature death

Assessment

HISTORY
◆ Familial history
◆ Hypertension
◆ High low-density lipoprotein (LDL) and triglyceride levels
◆ Low high-density lipoprotein (HDL) levels
◆ Abdominal obesity
◆ Sedentary lifestyle
◆ Poor diet

PHYSICAL FINDINGS
◆ Abdominal obesity

DIAGNOSTIC TEST RESULTS
◆ *Glucose level:* elevated
◆ *LDL and triglyceride levels:* increased
◆ *HDL level:* decreased
◆ *Blood glucose tests:* equal to or greater than 100 mg/dl
◆ *Serum uric acid level:* elevated
◆ *Blood pressure:* greater than 130/85 mm Hg

Treatment

◆ Weight-reduction program
◆ Low alcohol intake
◆ Diet high in complex carbohydrates and low in refined carbohydrates and cholesterol
◆ At least 20 minutes daily of physical activity
◆ Smoking cesstion

MEDICATIONS
◆ Oral antidiabetic agents
◆ Antihypertensives
◆ Statins

Nursing interventions

◆ Promote lifestyle changes and give appropriate support.
◆ Monitor the patient's blood pressure and laboratory values.

PATIENT TEACHING

◆ Explain the disorder, diagnostic testing, and treatment plan.
◆ Teach about the administration, dosage, and possible adverse effects of prescribed medications.
◆ Teach the principles of a healthy diet and the relationship of diet, inactivity, and obesity to metabolic syndrome (see *Why abdominal obesity is dangerous*).
◆ Refer the patient to appropriate support services for lifestyle changes.

Why abdominal obesity is dangerous

People with excess weight around the waist have a greater risk of developing metabolic syndrome than people with excess weight around the hips. That's because intra-abdominal fat tends to be more resistant to insulin than fat in other areas of the body. Insulin resistance increases the release of free fatty acid into the portal system, leading to increased apolipoprotein B, increased low-density lipoprotein, decreased high-density lipoprotein, and increased triglyceride levels. As a result, the risk of cardiovascular disease increases.

Methicillin-resistant *Staphylococcus aureus*

Disorders

Overview

Methicillin-resistant *Staphylococcus aureus* (MRSA) is treatment-resistant mutation of the common bacterium *S. aureus*. It's easily spread by direct person-to-person contact and is endemic in nursing homes, long-term care facilities, and community facilities.

CAUSES
◆ MRSA that enters a health care facility through an infected or colonized patient (symptom-free carrier of the bacteria) or colonized health care worker
◆ Transmission of bacteria mainly by health care workers' hands

RISK FACTORS
◆ Immunosuppression
◆ Prolonged facility stays
◆ Extended therapy with multiple or broad-spectrum antibiotics
◆ Proximity to others colonized or infected with MRSA

PATHOPHYSIOLOGY
◆ 90% of *S. aureus* isolates or strains are penicillin-resistant, and about 27% of all *S. aureus* isolates are resistant to methicillin, a penicillin derivative. These strains may also resist cephalosporins, aminoglycosides, erythromycin, tetracycline, and clindamycin.
◆ When natural defense systems break down (after invasive procedures, trauma, or chemotherapy), the usually benign bacteria can invade tissue, proliferate, and cause infection.

◆ The most frequent colonization site is the anterior nares (40% of adults and most children become transient nasal carriers). The groin, armpits, and intestines are less common colonization sites.

COMPLICATIONS
◆ Sepsis
◆ Death

Assessment

HISTORY
◆ Possible MRSA risk factors

PHYSICAL FINDINGS
◆ Signs and symptoms related to the primary diagnosis (respiratory, cardiac, or other major system symptoms) in symptomatic patients

DIAGNOSTIC TEST RESULTS
◆ *Cultures from suspicious wounds, skin, urine, or blood:* positive for MRSA

Treatment

◆ Contact isolation for wound, skin, and urine infection; respiratory isolation for sputum infection
◆ No treatment for patients with colonization only
◆ High-protein diet
◆ Rest periods as needed

MEDICATIONS
◆ Linezolid (Zyvox)

Nursing interventions

♦ Follow proper hand-washing technique.
♦ Maintain contact precautions and standard precautions.
♦ Provide emotional support to the patient and family members.
♦ Consider grouping infected patients together and having the same nursing staff care for them.
♦ Monitor the patient's vital signs and culture results.
♦ Observe for signs and symptoms of complications.

PATIENT TEACHING

♦ Explain the disorder, diagnostic testing, and treatment plan.
♦ Teach about the administration, dosage, and possible adverse effects of prescribed medications.
♦ Teach the difference between MRSA infection and colonization.
♦ Demonstrate proper hand-washing technique.
♦ Explain contact precautions to visitors.
♦ Refer the patient to an infectious disease specialist if indicated.

Mitral stenosis

Overview

Mitral stenosis is the narrowing of the mitral valve orifice. A normal orifice measurement is 3 to 6 cm; with mild mitral stenosis, the measurement is 2 cm; with moderate mitral stenosis, 1 to 2 cm; and with severe mitral stenosis, 1 cm. Two-thirds of all patients with mitral stenosis are female, and the condition occurs in about 40% of patients with rheumatic heart disease.

CAUSES
◆ Atrial myxoma
◆ Congenital anomalies
◆ Endocarditis
◆ Use of fenfluramine and phentermine combination (Fen-phen)
◆ Rheumatic fever

PATHOPHYSIOLOGY
◆ Valve leaflets become diffusely thickened by fibrosis and calcification.
◆ The mitral commissures and the chordae tendineae fuse and shorten, the valvular cusps become rigid, and the valve's apex becomes narrowed.
◆ This narrowing obstructs blood flow from the left atrium to the left ventricle, resulting in incomplete emptying.
◆ Left atrial volume and pressure increase, and the atrial chamber dilates.
◆ Increased resistance to blood flow causes pulmonary hypertension, right ventricular hypertrophy, and eventually, right-sided heart failure and reduced cardiac output.

COMPLICATIONS
◆ Cardiac arrhythmias, especially atrial fibrillation
◆ Thromboembolism

Assessment

HISTORY
Mild mitral stenosis
◆ Asymptomatic

Moderate to severe mitral stenosis
◆ Gradual decline in exercise tolerance
◆ Dyspnea on exertion, shortness of breath
◆ Paroxysmal nocturnal dyspnea
◆ Orthopnea
◆ Weakness
◆ Fatigue
◆ Palpitations
◆ Cough

PHYSICAL FINDINGS
◆ Hemoptysis
◆ Peripheral and facial cyanosis
◆ Malar rash
◆ Jugular vein distention
◆ Ascites
◆ Peripheral edema
◆ Hepatomegaly
◆ A loud first heart sound or opening snap
◆ A diastolic murmur at the apex (see *Identifying the murmur of mitral stenosis*)
◆ Crackles
◆ Resting tachycardia, irregularly irregular heart rhythm

DIAGNOSTIC TEST RESULTS
◆ *Chest X-rays:* left atrial and ventricular enlargement (in severe mitral stenosis), straightening of the left border of the cardiac silhouette, enlarged pulmonary arteries, dilation of the upper lobe pulmonary veins, and mitral valve calcification
◆ *Echocardiography:* thickened mitral valve leaflets and left atrial enlargement
◆ *Cardiac catheterization:* a diastolic pressure gradient across the valve, elevated pulmonary artery wedge pressure (greater than 15 mm Hg), and pulmonary artery pressure in the left atrium with severe pulmonary hypertension
◆ *Electrocardiography:* right axis deviation, and in 40% to 50% of cases, atrial fibrillation

Treatment

- Synchronized electrical cardioversion to correct uncontrolled atrial fibrillation
- Sodium-restricted diet
- Activity as tolerated
- Commissurotomy or valve replacement
- Percutaneous balloon valvuloplasty

MEDICATIONS

- Digoxin (Lanoxin)
- Diuretics
- Oxygen therapy
- Beta-adrenergic blockers
- Calcium channel blockers
- Anticoagulants
- Antiarrhythmics
- Infective endocarditis antibiotic prophylaxis
- Nitrates

Nursing interventions

- Provide oxygen therapy and monitor pulse oximetry.
- Stress the importance of rest periods if needed.
- Place the patient in an upright position to relieve dyspnea, if needed.
- Provide a low-sodium diet.
- Monitor the patient's vital signs, cardiac rhythm, and intake and output.
- Assess the patient's respiratory status.
- Observe for signs and symptoms of complications.
- Apply sequential compression stockings while in bed.

PATIENT TEACHING

- Explain the disorder, diagnostic testing, and treatment plan, including preoperative and postoperative procedures.
- Teach about the administration, dosage, and possible adverse effects of prescribed medications.
- Explain the need to plan for periodic rest in daily routine.
- Review dietary restrictions.
- Describe signs and symptoms to report to the practitioner.
- Stress the importance of consistent follow-up care.
- Stress the need to use prophylactic antibiotics for invasive procedures such as dental work.

Identifying the murmur of mitral stenosis

A low, rumbling crescendo-decrescendo murmur in the mitral valve area characterizes mitral stenosis.

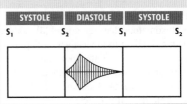

Mitral valve prolapse

Overview

Mitral valve prolapse (MVP) is a condition involving the prolapse of a portion of the mitral valve (MV) into the left atrium during ventricular contraction (systole). This condition is more prevalent in women than in men, and it's usually detected in young adulthood.

CAUSES
◆ Heart disease
◆ Congenital heart disease
◆ Connective tissue disorders

PATHOPHYSIOLOGY
◆ Myxomatous degeneration of MV leaflets with redundant tissue leads to prolapse of the MV into the left atrium during systole.
◆ In some patients, this degeneration results in leakage of blood into the left atrium from the left ventricle.

COMPLICATIONS
◆ Arrhythmias
◆ Infective endocarditis
◆ Mitral insufficiency from chordal rupture

Assessment

HISTORY
◆ Usually asymptomatic
◆ Possible fatigue, syncope, palpitations, chest pain, or dyspnea on exertion

PHYSICAL FINDINGS
◆ Orthostatic hypotension
◆ Mid-to-late systolic click and late systolic murmur

DIAGNOSTIC TEST RESULTS
◆ *Echocardiography:* MVP with or without mitral insufficiency
◆ *Electrocardiography:* usually normal but possible atrial or ventricular arrhythmia
◆ *Signal-averaged electrocardiography:* ventricular and supraventricular arrhythmias
◆ *Holter monitor (worn 24 hours):* arrhythmia

Treatment

◆ Regular monitoring
◆ Decreased caffeine intake
◆ Fluid intake to maintain hydration
◆ Regular exercise program

MEDICATIONS
◆ Antibiotic prophylaxis
◆ Beta-adrenergic blockers
◆ Anticoagulants
◆ Antiarrhythmics

Nursing interventions

◆ Provide reassurance and comfort if the patient experiences anxiety.
◆ Provide rest periods as needed.
◆ Monitor the patient's vital signs and cardiac rhythm.
◆ Assess cardiovascular status and observe for signs and symtpoms of mitral valve insufficiency.

Patient teaching

◆ Explain the disorder, diagnostic testing, and treatment plan, including preoperative and postoperative procedures.
◆ Teach about the administration, dosage, and possible adverse effects of prescribed medications.
◆ Explain the importance of hydration and the need to decrease caffeine intake.
◆ Stress the need for antibiotic prophylaxis before dental or surgical procedures, as indicated. (Not all patients with MVP require antibiotic prophylaxis.)
◆ Teach about a Holter monitor as needed.

Multiple sclerosis

Overview

Multiple sclerosis (MS), a neurodegenerative disorder caused by progressive demyelination of white matter of brain and spinal cord, is characterized by exacerbations and remissions of symptoms. Prognosis varies, with 70% of MS patients leading active lives with prolonged remissions.

CAUSES
◆ Exact cause unknown
◆ Allergic response
◆ Autoimmune response of the nervous system
◆ Possible genetic factors
◆ Slow-acting viral infection

RISK FACTORS
◆ Trauma
◆ Anoxia
◆ Toxins
◆ Nutritional deficiencies
◆ Vascular lesions
◆ Anorexia nervosa

TRIGGERING EVENTS
◆ Emotional stress
◆ Fatigue
◆ Pregnancy
◆ Acute respiratory tract infections

PATHOPHYSIOLOGY
◆ Sporadic patches of demyelination occur in the central nervous system, resulting in widespread and varied neurologic dysfunction. (See *Describing multiple sclerosis.*)

COMPLICATIONS
◆ Injuries from falls
◆ Urinary tract infection
◆ Contractures
◆ Pressure ulcers
◆ Pneumonia
◆ Depression

Assessment

HISTORY
◆ Symptoms related to the extent and site of myelin destruction, extent of remyelination, and adequacy of subsequently restored synaptic transmission
◆ Symptoms that are transient or lasting for hours or weeks
◆ Blurred vision or diplopia and sensory impairment (the first signs)
◆ Urinary problems
◆ Emotional lability
◆ Dysphagia
◆ Bowel disturbances (involuntary evacuation or constipation)
◆ Fatigue and weakness (typically the most disabling symptom)

PHYSICAL FINDINGS
◆ Muscle weakness of the involved area
◆ Spasticity, hyperreflexia
◆ Intention tremor
◆ Gait ataxia
◆ Paralysis, ranging from monoplegia to quadriplegia
◆ Nystagmus, scotoma
◆ Optic neuritis
◆ Ophthalmoplegia

DIAGNOSTIC TEST RESULTS
◆ *Cerebrospinal fluid analysis:* mononuclear cell pleocytosis, elevated total immunoglobulin (Ig) G levels, presence of oligoclonal IgG
◆ *Magnetic resonance imaging:* focal lesions (most sensitive test)
◆ *Electroencephalography:* abnormalities (in one-third of patients)
◆ *Evoked potential study:* slowed conduction of nerve impulses

Treatment

◆ Symptomatic treatment for acute exacerbations and related signs and symptoms
◆ High-fluid and high-fiber diet (for constipation)
◆ Frequent rest periods

MEDICATIONS

◆ I.V. steroids followed by oral steroids
◆ Immunosuppressants
◆ Antimetabolites
◆ Alkylating agents
◆ Biological response modifiers
◆ Antidepressants
◆ Glatiramer acetate (Copaxone)

Nursing interventions

◆ Provide emotional and psychological support.
◆ Assist with the physical therapy program.
◆ Provide adequate rest periods.
◆ Provide bowel and bladder training if indicated.
◆ Give prescribed drugs and evaluate the patient's response.
◆ Assess sensory and muscle response.
◆ Observe for signs and symptoms of complications.

PATIENT TEACHING

◆ Explain the disorder, diagnostic testing, and treatment plan.
◆ Teach about the administration, dosage, and possible adverse effects of prescribed medications.
◆ Explain the need to avoid stress, infections, and fatigue.
◆ Stress the importance of maintaining independence.

◆ Teach how to avoid exposure to bacterial and viral infections.
◆ Review nutritional needs and the importance of adequate fluid intake and regular urination.
◆ Refer the patient to the National Multiple Sclerosis Society and to physical and occupational rehabilitation programs, as indicated.

Describing multiple sclerosis

The various types (or stages) of multiple sclerosis (MS) include:

◆ *relapsing-remitting*—clear relapses (or acute attacks or exacerbations) with full recovery and lasting disability; disease doesn't worsen between attacks

◆ *primary progressive*—steadily progressing or worsening with minor recovery or plateaus (uncommon; may involve different brain and spinal cord damage from other forms)

◆ *secondary progressive*—beginning as a pattern of clear-cut relapses and recovery but becoming steadily progressive and worsening between acute attacks

◆ *progressive-relapsing*—steadily progressing from the onset but also involving clear, acute attacks (rare).

Differential diagnosis must rule out spinal cord compression, foramen magnum tumor (which may mimic the exacerbations and remissions of MS), multiple small strokes, syphilis or another infection, thyroid disease, and chronic fatigue syndrome.

Myocardial infarction

Overview

Myocardial infarction (MI) results from reduced blood flow through one or more coronary arteries having myocardial ischemia and necrosis. The infarction site depends on the vessels involved. Men and postmenopausal women are more susceptible to MI than premenopausal women. Sudden death may be the first and only indication of MI.

CAUSES
◆ Atherosclerosis
◆ Coronary artery stenosis or spasm
◆ Platelet aggregation
◆ Thrombosis

RISK FACTORS
◆ Increased age (40 to 70)
◆ Being postmenopausal
◆ Diabetes mellitus
◆ Elevated serum triglyceride, low-density lipoprotein, and cholesterol levels, and decreased serum high-density lipoprotein levels
◆ Excessive intake of saturated fats, carbohydrates, or salt
◆ Hypertension
◆ Obesity
◆ Family history of coronary artery disease (CAD)
◆ Sedentary lifestyle
◆ Smoking
◆ Stress or type A personality
◆ Use of drugs, such as amphetamines or cocaine

PATHOPHYSIOLOGY
◆ One or more coronary arteries become occluded.
◆ If coronary occlusion causes ischemia lasting longer than 30 to 45 minutes, irreversible myocardial cell damage and muscle death occur.
◆ Every MI has a central area of necrosis surrounded by an area of hypoxic injury. This injured tissue is potentially viable and may be salvaged if circulation is restored, or it may progress to necrosis.

COMPLICATIONS
◆ Arrhythmias
◆ Cardiogenic shock
◆ Heart failure causing pulmonary edema
◆ Pericarditis
◆ Rupture of the atrial or ventricular septum or of the ventricular wall
◆ Ventricular aneurysm
◆ Cerebral or pulmonary emboli
◆ Extension of the original infarction
◆ Mitral insufficiency

Assessment

HISTORY
◆ Possible CAD with increasing anginal frequency, severity, or duration
◆ Persistent, crushing substernal pain or pressure possibly radiating to the left arm, jaw, neck, and shoulder blades, and possibly persisting for 12 or more hours (cardinal symptom of MI); pain possibly absent in women, elderly patients or those with diabetes; pain possibly mild and with confusion and indigestion in others
◆ A feeling of impending doom, fatigue, nausea, vomiting, and shortness of breath
◆ Unusual fatigue, shortness of breath, weakness and dizziness, especially in women

PHYSICAL FINDINGS
◆ Extreme anxiety and restlessness
◆ Dyspnea
◆ Diaphoresis
◆ Tachycardia
◆ Hypertension
◆ Bradycardia and hypotension in inferior MI
◆ Third and fourth heart sounds and paradoxical splitting of the second heart sound (in ventricular dysfunction)
◆ Systolic murmur of mitral insufficiency
◆ Pericardial friction rub (in transmural MI) or pericarditis

- Dizziness
- Weakness

DIAGNOSTIC TEST RESULTS
- *Serum creatine kinase (CK) and CK-MB isoenzyme levels*: elevated
- *Serum lactate dehydrogenase levels:* elevated
- *Myoglobin:* detected within 1 to 4 hours after MI
- *Troponin I levels:* elevated
- *Nuclear medicine scans:* acutely damaged muscle
- *Myocardial perfusion imaging:* "cold spot" during the first few hours after a transmural MI
- *Echocardiography:* ventricular wall dyskinesia (ejection fraction) in transmural MI
- *Serial 12-lead electrocardiography:* ST-segment depression in subendocardial MI, ST-segment elevation and Q waves in transmural MI
- *Cardiac catheterization:* vessel occlusion

Treatment

- Pacemaker implantation or electrical cardioversion for arrhythmias
- Intra-aortic balloon pump for cardiogenic shock
- Low-fat, low-cholesterol diet
- Initially, bed rest with bedside commode, then activity as tolerated
- Coronary artery bypass graft
- Percutaneous transluminal coronary angioplasty (PTCA) and stenting

MEDICATIONS
- Oxygen therapy
- I.V. thrombolytic therapy started within 3 hours of onset of symptoms
- Aspirin
- Nitrates
- Analgesic: I.V. morphine
- Antiarrhythmics
- Calcium channel blockers
- I.V. heparin
- Inotropic agents
- Beta-adrenergic blockers
- Angiotensin-converting enzyme inhibitors
- Platelet aggregation inhibitor: abciximab (ReoPro)
- Stool softeners
- Antianxiety agents if indicated

Nursing interventions

- Assess the patient's pain level, administer analgesics, and evaluate their effects.
- Monitor the patient's vital signs, cardiac rhythm, pulse oximetry, and laboratory values.
- Assess the patient's cardiovascular status.
- Obtain an electrocardiogram during episodes of chest pain.
- Provide frequent rest periods.
- Provide a low-cholesterol, low-sodium diet with caffeine-free beverages.
- Apply sequential compression stockings while the patient is in bed.
- Provide emotional support and help to reduce stress and anxiety.
- Provide sheath care post PTCA or cardiac catheterization per facility policy.
- Observe for signs and symptoms of complications.

PATIENT TEACHING
- Explain the disorder, diagnostic testing, and treatment plan.
- Teach about the administration, dosage, and possible adverse effects of prescribed medications.
- Review dietary and activity restrictions.
- Describe types of chest pain to report to the practitioner.
- Refer the patient to a cardiac rehabilitation program and a smoking-cessation or weight-reduction program, if needed.

Necrotizing fasciitis

Overview

Necrotizing fasciitis, commonly called *flesh-eating disease,* is a progressive, rapidly spreading inflammatory infection of the deep fascia. It has a mortality rate of 70% to 80%.

Causes

◆ Group A beta-hemolytic streptococci and *Staphylococcus aureus,* alone or together (most common primary infecting bacteria)
◆ More than 80 types of the causative bacteria (*Streptococcus pyogenes*)

Risk factors

◆ Surgery
◆ Insect bite
◆ Older age
◆ Being immunocompromised
◆ History of chronic illness
◆ Steroid use

Pathophysiology

◆ Infecting bacteria enter the host through a local tissue injury or a breach in a mucous membrane barrier.
◆ Organisms proliferate in an environment of tissue hypoxia caused by trauma, recent surgery, or a medical condition that compromises the patient.
◆ Necrosis of the surrounding tissue results, accelerating the disease process by creating a favorable environment for organisms to proliferate.
◆ The fascia and fat tissues are destroyed, resulting in secondary necrosis of subcutaneous tissue.

Complications

◆ Renal failure
◆ Septic shock
◆ Myositis
◆ Myonecrosis
◆ Amputation

Assessment

History

◆ Associated risk factors
◆ Pain
◆ Tissue injury

Physical findings

◆ Rapidly progressing erythema at the site of insult
◆ Fluid-filled blisters and bullae (indicate rapid progression of the necrotizing process)
◆ Large areas of gangrenous skin by days 4 and 5
◆ Extensive necrosis of the subcutaneous tissue by days 7 to 10
◆ Fever
◆ Sepsis
◆ Hypovolemia
◆ Hypotension
◆ Respiratory insufficiency
◆ Deterioration in level of consciousness
◆ Signs of sepsis

Diagnostic test results

◆ *Tissue biopsy:* bacteria and polymorphonuclear cell infiltration of deep dermis, fascia, and muscular planes; necrosis of fatty and muscular tissue
◆ *Microorganism cultures:* causative organism
◆ *Gram stain and tissue biopsy:* causative organism
◆ *X-rays:* presence of subcutaneous gas
◆ *Computed tomography scan:* location of necrosis
◆ *Magnetic resonance imaging:* areas of necrosis, areas requiring surgical debridement

Treatment

◆ Wound care
◆ Hyperbaric oxygen therapy
◆ High-protein, high-calorie diet
◆ Increased fluid intake
◆ Bed rest until treatment is effective
◆ Immediate surgical debridement, fasciectomy, or amputation

MEDICATIONS
◆ Antimicrobials
◆ Analgesics

Nursing interventions

◆ Give prescribed drugs.
◆ Provide supportive care and supplemental oxygen as appropriate.
◆ Provide emotional support.
◆ Observe for signs and symptoms of complications.
◆ Monitor vital signs.
◆ Provide wound care and assess healing.
◆ Assess the patient's pain level, administer analgesics, and evaluate their effects.

PATIENT TEACHING
◆ Explain the disorder, diagnostic testing, and treatment plan.
◆ Teach about the administration, dosage, and possible adverse effects of prescribed medications.
◆ Stress the importance of strict sterile technique and proper hand-washing technique for wound care.
◆ Describe signs and symptoms of complications.
◆ Refer the patient for follow-up care with an infectious disease specialist and surgeon as indicated.

◆ Refer the patient for physical rehabilitation if indicated.
◆ Refer the patient to the National Necrotizing Fasciitis Foundation for information and support.

Obesity

Overview

Obesity, the second-leading cause of preventable deaths in the United States, is a 25% excess of body fat for men, more than 33% for women, or having a body mass index (BMI) of 30 or greater (see *BMI measurements*). Obesity affects one in five childen in the United States, and 30% to 50% of adults are overweight.

CAUSES
◆ Excessive caloric intake combined with inadequate energy expenditure
◆ Abnormal absorption of nutrients
◆ Environmental factors
◆ Genetic predisposition
◆ Hypothalamic dysfunction of hunger and satiety centers
◆ Impaired action of GI and growth hormones and of hormonal regulators such as insulin
◆ Psychological factors
◆ Socioeconomic status

PATHOPHYSIOLOGY
◆ Fat cells increase in size in response to dietary intake.
◆ When the cells can no longer expand, they increase in number.
◆ With weight loss, the size of the fat cells decreases, but the number of cells doesn't.

COMPLICATIONS
◆ Respiratory difficulties
◆ Hypertension
◆ Cardiovascular disease
◆ Diabetes mellitus
◆ Renal disease
◆ Gallbladder disease
◆ Psychosocial difficulties
◆ Premature death

Assessment

HISTORY
◆ Increasing weight
◆ Complications of obesity
◆ Dyspnea on exertion
◆ Snoring
◆ Joint pain

PHYSICAL FINDINGS
◆ Large abdomen
◆ Large neck circumference

DIAGNOSTIC TEST RESULTS
◆ *Standard height and weight table:* indicators of obesity
◆ *Caliper measurements:* increased total body fat
◆ *BMI calculation:* 30 or greater

Treatment

◆ Behavior modification techniques
◆ Psychological counseling
◆ Reduction in daily caloric intake
◆ Increase in daily activity level
◆ Vertical banded gastroplasty
◆ Gastric bypass surgery
◆ Management of comorbidities

Nursing interventions

◆ Treat complications of obesity as indicated.

◆ Obtain a diet history.

◆ Promote increased physical activity as appropriate.

◆ Assist with dietary choices.

◆ Monitor the patient's vital signs, intake, and output.

◆ Obtain weight and calculate BMI.

PATIENT TEACHING

◆ Explain the disorder, diagnostic testing, and treatment plan.

◆ Teach about the administration, dosage, and possible adverse effects of prescribed medications.

◆ Review dietary guidelines and safe weight-loss practices.

◆ Refer the patient to a weight-reduction program.

◆ Explain the need for long-term maintenance after the patient's desired weight is achieved.

BMI measurements

Use these steps to calculate body mass index (BMI):

◆ Multiply weight in pounds by 705.
◆ Divide this number by height in inches.
◆ Then divide this by height in inches again.
◆ Compare results to these standards:
  ● 18.5 to 24.9: normal
  ● 25 to 29.9: overweight
  ● 30 to 39.9: obese
  ● 40 or greater: morbidly obese.

Osteoarthritis

Overview

Osteoarthritis, the most common form of arthritis, is the chronic degeneration of joint cartilage. Disability ranges from minor limitation to near immobility. Osteoarthritis most commonly affects the hips and knees.

CAUSES
◆ Advancing age
◆ Congenital abnormality
◆ Endocrine disorders such as diabetes mellitus
◆ Hereditary (possibly)
◆ Metabolic disorders such as chondrocalcinosis
◆ Secondary osteoarthritis
◆ Traumatic injury

PATHOPHYSIOLOGY
◆ Joint cartilage deteriorates.
◆ Reactive new bone forms at the margins and subchondral areas.
◆ Breakdown of chondrocytes occurs.
◆ Cartilage flakes irritate synovial lining.
◆ The cartilage lining becomes fibrotic and joint movement is limited.
◆ Synovial fluid leaks into bone defects, causing cysts.

COMPLICATIONS
◆ Flexion contractures
◆ Subluxation
◆ Deformity
◆ Ankylosis
◆ Bony cysts
◆ Gross bony overgrowth
◆ Central cord syndrome
◆ Nerve root compression
◆ Cauda equina syndrome

Assessment

HISTORY
◆ Predisposing traumatic injury
◆ Deep, aching joint pain
◆ Pain after exercise or weight bearing
◆ Pain possibly relieved by rest
◆ Stiffness in morning and after exercise
◆ Joint aches during changes in weather
◆ "Grating" feeling when the joint moves
◆ Limited movement

PHYSICAL FINDINGS
◆ Contractures
◆ Joint swelling
◆ Muscle atrophy
◆ Deformity of the involved areas
◆ Gait abnormalities
◆ Hard nodes that may be red, swollen, and tender on the distal and proximal interphalangeal joints (see *Signs of osteoarthritis*)
◆ Loss of finger dexterity
◆ Muscle spasms, limited movement, and joint instability

DIAGNOSTIC TEST RESULTS
◆ *Synovial fluid analysis:* rules out inflammatory arthritis
◆ *Joint X-ray:* narrowing of the joint space or margin, cystlike bony deposits in the joint space and margins, sclerosis of the subchondral space, joint deformity or articular damage, bony growths at weight-bearing areas, possible joint fusion
◆ *Radionuclide bone scan:* rules out inflammatory arthritis
◆ *Magnetic resonance imaging:* affected joint, adjacent bones, disease progression
◆ *Arthroscopy:* articular cartilage degeneration, soft-tissue swelling

Treatment

- Activity as tolerated
- Physical therapy
- Assistive mobility devices
- Weight loss if indicated
- Arthroplasty (partial or total)
- Arthrodesis
- Osteoplasty
- Osteotomy

MEDICATIONS
- Analgesics
- Antispasmodics

Nursing interventions

- Allow adequate time for self-care, and assist as needed.
- Assess the patient's pain level, administer analgesics, and evaluate their effects.
- Apply hot soaks and paraffin dips to affected hand joints.
- Apply a cervical collar, if ordered, for affected cervical spinal joints.
- Assist with range-of-motion (ROM) exercises.
- Apply elastic supports or braces.

PATIENT TEACHING
- Explain the disorder, diagnostic testing, and treatment plan.
- Teach about the administration, dosage, and possible adverse effects of prescribed medications.
- Explain the need for adequate rest during the day, after exertion, and at night.
- Review ways to conserve energy.
- Teach about safety measures and devices at home.
- Demonstrate ROM exercises.
- Stress the need to acheive and maintain proper body weight.
- Review dietary recommendations if indicated.
- Demonstrate the use of crutches or other orthopedic devices.
- Refer the patient to occupational or physical therapist as indicated.

Signs of osteoarthritis

Heberden's nodes appear on the dorsolateral aspect of the distal interphalangeal joints. These bony and cartilaginous enlargements are usually hard and painless. They typically occur in middle-aged and elderly patients with osteoarthritis. Bouchard's nodes are similar to Heberden's nodes but are less common and appear on the proximal interphalangeal joints.

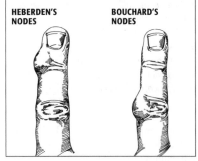

HEBERDEN'S NODES   BOUCHARD'S NODES

Osteomyelitis

Overview

Osteomyelitis, a chronic or acute pyogenic bone infection, originates elsewhere in the body and migrates to the bone, causing pain. With prompt treatment, the acute form has a good prognosis, but the chronic form has a poor prognosis.

CAUSES
◆ *Escherichia coli*
◆ Fungi or viruses
◆ Minor traumatic injury
◆ *Proteus vulgaris*
◆ *Pseudomonas aeruginosa*
◆ *Staphylococcus aureus*
◆ *Streptococcus pyogenes*

RISK FACTORS
◆ Older age
◆ Obesity
◆ Immunosuppression
◆ Diabetes
◆ Rheumatoid arthritis
◆ Long-term steroid therapy

PATHOPHYSIOLOGY
◆ Organisms settle in a hematoma or weakened area and spread directly to bone.
◆ Pus is produced and pressure builds within the rigid medullary cavity.
◆ Pus is forced through the haversian canals.
◆ A subperiosteal abscess forms.
◆ Bone is deprived of its blood supply.
◆ Necrosis results and new bone formation is stimulated.
◆ Dead bone detaches and exits through an abscess or the sinuses.
◆ Osteomyelitis becomes chronic.

COMPLICATIONS
◆ Chronic infection
◆ Skeletal deformities
◆ Joint deformities
◆ Disturbed bone growth in children
◆ Differing leg lengths
◆ Impaired mobility

Assessment

HISTORY
◆ Previous injury, surgery, or primary infection
◆ Sudden, severe pain in the affected bone
◆ Pain unrelieved by rest that worsens with motion
◆ Chills, nausea, malaise

PHYSICAL FINDINGS
◆ Tachycardia
◆ Elevated temperature
◆ Swelling over the infection site
◆ Restricted movement of affected area
◆ Tenderness and warmth over the infection site
◆ Pus drainage

DIAGNOSTIC TEST RESULTS
◆ *Computed tomography scan and magnetic resonance imaging:* extent of infection
◆ *White blood cell count:* leukocytosis
◆ *Erythrocyte sedimentation rate:* increased
◆ *Blood culture:* pathogen identification
◆ *X-rays:* bone involvement
◆ *Bone scans:* early infection

Treatment

◆ Hyperbaric oxygen therapy
◆ Free tissue transfers
◆ High-protein diet, rich in vitamin C
◆ Bed rest
◆ Immobilization of involved bone and joint with a cast or traction
◆ Surgical drainage of pus
◆ Local muscle flaps
◆ Sequestrectomy
◆ Amputation for chronic and unrelieved symptoms

MEDICATIONS
◆ I.V. fluids as needed
◆ I.V. antibiotics
◆ Analgesics
◆ Intracavitary instillation of antibiotics for open wounds

Nursing interventions

◆ Assess the patient's pain level, administer analgesics, and evaluate their effects.
◆ Protect the affected area from injury.
◆ Provide emotional support.
◆ Promote and allow adequate time for self-care.
◆ Allow frequent rest periods.
◆ Provide wound care using strict sterile technique.
◆ Reposition the patient every 2 hours and provide skin care.
◆ Monitor vital signs.

PATIENT TEACHING

◆ Explain the disorder, diagnostic testing, and treatment plan.
◆ Teach about the administration, dosage, and possible adverse effects of prescribed medications.
◆ Review techniques for promoting rest and relaxation.
◆ Demonstrate wound site care.
◆ Describe signs of recurring infection and stress the importance of follow-up examinations.
◆ Refer the patient for occupational therapy as appropriate.

Osteoporosis

Overview

Osteoporosis, the loss of calcium and phosphate from bones, increases a person's vulnerability to fractures. It may occur as a primary disorder or secondary to underlying disease. Primary osteoporosis has three types: postmenopausal (type I), senile (type II), and idiopathic. Postmenopausal osteoporosis is caused by a lack of estrogen. It typically affects women ages 51 to 75. Senile osteoporosis is related to an imbalance between the rate of bone breakdown and the rate of bone formation. It's most common in patients older than age 75. Idiopathic osteoporosis, which has no known cause, occurs in children and young adults.

CAUSES
- Exact cause unknown
- Alcoholism
- Bone immobilization
- Hyperthyroidism
- Lactose intolerance
- Liver disease
- Malabsorption
- Malnutrition
- Osteogenesis imperfecta
- Prolonged therapy with steroids or heparin
- Rheumatoid arthritis
- Scurvy
- Sudeck's atrophy (localized in hands and feet, with recurring attacks)

RISK FACTORS
- Mild, prolonged negative calcium balance
- Declining gonadal adrenal function
- Faulty protein metabolism (caused by estrogen deficiency)
- Sedentary lifestyle
- Menopause

PATHOPHYSIOLOGY
- The rate of bone resorption accelerates as the rate of bone formation decelerates.
- Decreased bone mass results and bones become porous and brittle.

COMPLICATIONS
- Bone fractures (vertebrae, femoral neck, distal radius)

Assessment

HISTORY
- Postmenopausal woman
- Preexisting condition
- Snapping sound or sudden pain in lower back when bending down to lift something
- Possible slow development of pain (over several years)
- With vertebral collapse, backache and pain radiating around the trunk
- Pain aggravated by movement or jarring

PHYSICAL FINDINGS
- Humped back
- Markedly aged appearance
- Loss of height
- Aching bone pain
- Muscle spasm
- Decreased spinal movement with flexion more limited than extension

DIAGNOSTIC TEST RESULTS
- *Dual- or single-photon absorptiometry:* bone mass measurement
- *Parathyroid hormone level:* elevated
- *X-rays:* characteristic degeneration in the lower thoracolumbar vertebrae
- *Computed tomography scan:* spinal bone loss
- *Bone scans:* injured or diseased areas
- *Bone biopsy:* thin, porous, otherwise normal bone

Treatment

- Fracture prevention
- Reduction and immobilization of fractures
- Supportive devices
- Diet rich in vitamin D, calcium, and protein
- Weight-bearing exercise and activity
- Open reduction and internal fixation for femur fractures

MEDICATIONS

- Hormone replacement therapy (in females)
- Bisphosphonates
- Androgens (males)
- Parathyroid hormone
- Selective estrogen-receptor modulators
- Calcium and vitamin D supplements
- Calcitonin (Miacalcin)

Nursing interventions

- Encourage careful positioning and ambulation.
- Promote weight-bearing exercises and participation in physical therapy program.
- Promote self-care and assist as needed.
- Maintain safety precautions.
- Assess the patient's pain level, administer analgesics, and evaluate their effects.
- Evaluate nutritional status.
- Assess joint mobility.

PATIENT TEACHING

- Explain the disorder, diagnostic testing, and treatment plan.
- Teach about the administration, dosage, and possible adverse effects of prescribed medications.
- Review exercise recommendations.
- Advise sleeping on a firm mattress and avoiding excessive bed rest.

- Demonstrate how to use a back brace if appropriate.
- Demonstrate proper body mechanics.
- Recommend home safety devices.
- Review dietary recommendations, including limiting alcohol intake.
- Stress smoking cessation.
- Teach cast care, if appropriate.
- Refer the patient for physical and occupational therapy as appropriate.

Pancreatitis

Overview

Pancreatitis, which occurs in acute and chronic forms, is the inflammation of the pancreas that causes autodigestion of the gland. The acute form has a 10% mortality rate; the chronic form can cause irreversible tissue damage, which tends to progress to significant pancreatic function loss.

Causes
- Idiopathic
- Alcoholism
- Biliary tract disease
- Metabolic or endocrine disorders
- Pancreatic cysts or tumors
- Penetrating peptic ulcers
- Penetrating trauma
- Viral or bacterial infection

Risk factors
- Use of glucocorticoids, sulfonamides, thiazides, and hormonal contraceptives
- Renal failure and kidney transplantation
- Endoscopic retrograde cholangiopancreatography (ERCP)
- Heredity
- Emotional or neurogenic factors
- Trauma to the abdomen or back

Pathophysiology
- Enzymes normally excreted into the duodenum by the pancreas are activated in the pancreas or its ducts and start to autodigest pancreatic tissue.
- Consequent inflammation causes intense pain, third-spacing of large fluid volumes, pancreatic fat necrosis with consumption of serum calcium, and, occasionally, hemorrhage.

Complications
- Diabetes mellitus
- Massive hemorrhage
- Shock and coma
- Acute respiratory distress syndrome
- Atelectasis and pleural effusion
- Pneumonia
- Paralytic ileus
- Pancreatic abscess and cancer
- Pseudocysts
- Renal failure
- Respiratory failure

Assessment

History
- Intense epigastric pain centered close to the umbilicus and radiating to the back, between the 10th thoracic and 6th lumbar vertebrae
- Abdominal pain aggravated by fatty foods, alcohol consumption, or recumbent position
- Weight loss with nausea and vomiting
- One or more risk factors
- Steatorrhea (with chronic pancreatitis)

Physical findings
- Hypotension
- Tachycardia
- Fever
- Dyspnea, orthopnea
- Generalized jaundice
- Cullen's sign (bluish periumbilical discoloration)
- Turner's sign (bluish flank discoloration)
- Abdominal tenderness, rigidity, and guarding

Diagnostic test results
- *Serum amylase and lipase levels:* elevated
- *White blood cell count:* elevated
- *Serum bilirubin level:* elevated
- *Urine amylase level:* increased
- *Serum glucose level:* transiently elevated
- *Lipid and trypsin levels:* elevated in stools
- *Computed tomography scans and ultrasonography:* increased pancreatic diameter, pancreatic cysts, and pseudocysts
- *ERCP:* ductal system abnormalities, findings that differentiate pancreatitis from other disorders
- *Ranson score:* severity of acute pancreatitis (see *Ranson score*)

Treatment

- Supportive measures for life-threatening signs and symptoms
- Blood transfusions for hemorrhage
- Nasogastric suctioning
- Nothing by mouth; once crisis starts to resolve, low-fat, low-protein feedings
- Alcohol and caffeine abstention
- Sphincterotomy (chronic pancreatitis)
- Pancreaticojejunostomy

MEDICATIONS

- I.V. fluids
- Analgesics
- Antacids
- Histamine antagonists
- Antibiotics
- Anticholinergics
- Total parenteral nutrition
- Pancreatic enzymes
- Insulin
- Albumin

Nursing interventions

- Monitor the patient's respiratory status and provide oxygen therapy.
- Assess the patient's pain level, administer analgesics, and evaluate their effects.
- Give prescribed drugs and I.V. therapy.
- Provide emotional support.
- Monitor the patient's vital signs, pulse oximetry, intake and output, and laboratory values.
- Maintain nasogastric tube function and monitor drainage.
- Obtain daily weight.
- Assess the patient's hydration and nutritional status.

PATIENT TEACHING

- Explain the disorder, diagnostic testing, and treatment plan.
- Teach about the administration, dosage, and possible adverse effects of prescribed medications.
- Promote identification and avoidance of acute pancreatitis triggers.
- Review dietary recommendations.
- Refer the patient to community resource and support services as needed.

Ranson score

The Ranson score evaluates 11 criteria to predict the severity of acute pancreatitis. This score should be determined within the first 48 hours of symptom onset. To determine the score, assign 1 point for each condition present.

Criteria present on admission

- Age older than 55
- White blood cell count greater than 16,000/ul
- Blood glucose level greater than 200 mg/dl
- Lactate dehydrogenase greater than 350 international units/L
- Aspartate aminotransferase greater than 250 international units/L

Criteria developing during the first 48 hours

- Hematocrit decrease of more than 10%
- Blood urea nitrogen greater than 8 mg/dl
- Serum calcium level less than 8 mg/dl
- Arterial oxygen saturation less than 60 mm Hg
- Base deficit greater than 4 mmol/L
- Estimated fluid sequestration greater than 600 ml

Total Ranson score

0 to 2: minimal mortality
3 to 5: 10% to 20% mortality
Greater than 5: greater than 50% mortality

Parkinson's disease

Disorders

Overview

Parkinson's disease, one of the most common crippling diseases in the United States, is a neurodegenerative disorder that affects motor function, causing progressive deterioration with muscle rigidity, akinesia, and involuntary tremors. Death commonly results from aspiration pneumonia.

CAUSES
- Usually unknown
- Drug-induced (haloperidol [Haldol], methyldopa [Aldomet], reserpine [Serpalan])
- Exposure to toxins, such as manganese dust and carbon monoxide
- Possible genetic or viral cause
- Type A encephalitis

RISK FACTORS
- Middle age or older

PATHOPHYSIOLOGY
- Dopaminergic neurons degenerate, causing loss of available dopamine.
- Dopamine deficiency prevents affected brain cells from performing their normal inhibitory function.
- Excess excitatory acetylcholine occurs at synapses.
- Nondopaminergic receptors are also involved.
- Motor neurons are depressed.

COMPLICATIONS
- Injury from falls
- Aspiration pneumonia
- Urinary tract infections
- Pressure ulcers
- Pneumonia
- Depression
- Dementia
- Sleep problems
- Sexual dysfunction

Assessment

HISTORY
- Muscle rigidity
- Akinesia
- Insidious (unilateral pill-roll) tremor, which increases during stress or anxiety and decreases with purposeful movement and sleep
- Dysphagia
- Fatigue with activities of daily living
- Muscle cramps of legs, neck, and trunk
- Increased perspiration
- Insomnia
- Mood changes

PHYSICAL FINDINGS
- High-pitched, monotonous voice
- Dysarthria
- Drooling
- Masklike facial expression
- Difficulty walking
- Lack of parallel motion in gait
- Loss of posture control with walking
- Oculogyric crises (eyes fixed upward with involuntary tonic movements)
- Muscle rigidity causing resistance to passive muscle stretching
- Loss of balance
- Tremors of hands and feet
- Oily skin

DIAGNOSTIC TEST RESULTS
- *Computed tomography scan or magnetic resonance imaging:* rules out other disorders such as intracranial tumors

Treatment

- Environmental safety measures
- Assistance with activities of daily living
- Small, frequent meals with high-bulk foods
- Physical therapy and occupational therapy
- Assistive devices for ambulation
- Surgery: stereotaxic neurosurgery, destruction of ventrolateral nucleus of thalamus, deep brain stimulation, or neural transplantation

MEDICATIONS

- Dopamine replacement drugs
- Catechol-O-methyltransferase inhibitors
- Anticholinergics
- Monoamine oxidase (MAO)-B inhibitors
- *N*-methyl-D-aspartic inhibitors
- Dopamine agonists
- Selective serotonin reuptake inhibitors

Nursing interventions

- Maintain swallowing precautions; assess for signs of aspiration.
- Initiate fall prevention measures.
- Provide frequent rest periods.
- Assess the patient's hydration and nutritional status.
- Provide emotional and psychological support.
- Assist with ambulation and range-of-motion (ROM) exercises, and encourage participation in physical therapy program.
- Monitor the patient's vital signs and intake and output.
- Observe for and document adverse reactions to medications.
- Assess the patient's neurologic status; postoperatively, observe for signs of hemorrhage and increased intracranial pressure.

PATIENT TEACHING

- Explain the disorder, diagnostic testing, and treatment plan.
- Teach about the administration, dosage, and possible adverse effects of prescribed medications.
- Teach measures to prevent pressure ulcers and contractures.
- Review household safety measures.
- Demonstrate ROM exercises.
- Teach the patient about aspiration precautions.
- Refer the patient for occupational and physical rehabilitation as indicated.

Peptic ulcer

Overview

Peptic ulcers, which are circumscribed lesions in the mucosal membrane of the lower esophagus, stomach, duodenum, or jejunum, occur in two major chronic forms: duodenal ulcers and gastric ulcers. About 80% of peptic ulcers are duodenal ulcers affecting the proximal part of the small intestine and follow a chronic course characterized by remissions and exacerbations. Gastric ulcers are most common in middle-aged and elderly men, especially those who are poor, undernourished, or chronic users of aspirin or alcohol.

CAUSES
◆ *Helicobacter pylori*
◆ Nonsteroidal anti-inflammatory drug (NSAID) or glucocorticoid use
◆ Pathologic hypersecretory states

RISK FACTORS
◆ Type A blood (for gastric ulcer)
◆ Type O blood (for duodenal ulcer)
◆ Exposure to irritants
◆ Cigarette smoking
◆ Trauma
◆ Psychogenic factors
◆ Normal aging

PATHOPHYSIOLOGY
◆ *H. pylori* releases a toxin that promotes mucosal inflammation and ulceration.
◆ In a peptic ulcer resulting from *H. pylori*, acid isn't the dominant cause of bacterial infection but contributes to the consequences.
◆ Ulceration stems from inhibition of prostaglandin synthesis, increased gastric acid and pepsin secretion, reduced gastric mucosal blood flow, or decreased cytoprotective mucus production.

COMPLICATIONS
◆ GI hemorrhage
◆ Abdominal or intestinal infarction
◆ Ulcer penetration into attached structures

Assessment

HISTORY
◆ Periods of symptom exacerbation and remission, with remissions lasting longer than exacerbations
◆ One or more risk factors
◆ Left epigastric pain described as heartburn or indigestion, accompanied by a feeling of fullness or distention

Gastric ulcer
◆ Recent weight or appetite loss
◆ Nausea or vomiting
◆ Pain triggered or worsened by eating

Duodenal ulcer
◆ Pain relieved by eating that may occur 2 to 3 hours after food intake
◆ Pain that awakens the patient from sleep
◆ Weight gain

PHYSICAL FINDINGS
◆ Pallor
◆ Epigastric tenderness
◆ Hyperactive bowel sounds

DIAGNOSTIC TEST RESULTS
◆ *Complete blood count:* anemia
◆ *Occult blood test:* positive in stools
◆ *Venous blood sample: H. pylori* antibodies
◆ *White blood cell count:* elevated
◆ *Urea breath test:* low levels of exhaled carbon-13
◆ *Barium swallow or upper GI and small-bowel series:* collection of barium, usually in the lesser curvature or posterior wall of the stomach, indicating ulcers of 3 mm to 5 mm
◆ *Upper GI tract X-rays:* mucosal abnormalities
◆ *Upper GI endoscopy or esophagogastroduodenoscopy:* evidence of an ulcer in the intestinal lining
◆ *Cytologic studies and biopsy:* rule out *H. pylori* or cancer
◆ *Gastric secretory studies:* hyperchlorhydria

Treatment

- Treatment of symptoms
- Iced saline GI lavage, possibly containing norepinephrine (for active bleeding)
- Blood transfusions
- Laser or cautery during endoscopy
- Stress reduction
- Smoking cessation
- Avoidance of dietary irritants
- Nothing by mouth (if GI bleeding is evident)
- Surgery (varies with ulcer location and extent; major operations include bilateral vagotomy, pyloroplasty, and gastrectomy)

MEDICATIONS

For *H. pylori*
- Amoxicillin (Amoxil), clarithromycin (Biaxin), and omeprazole (Prilosec)

For gastric or duodenal ulcer
- Proton pump inhibitors
- Antacids
- Histamine-receptor antagonists or gastric acid pump inhibitors
- Coating agents for duodenal ulcer
- Antisecretory agents if ulcer resulted from NSAID use and NSAIDs must be continued
- Sedatives (for gastric ulcer)
- Anticholinergics (for duodenal ulcers; usually contraindicated in gastric ulcers)
- Prostaglandin analogs

Nursing interventions

- Monitor the patient's vital signs and laboratory values.
- Observe for signs and symptoms of bleeding.
- Give prescribed drugs.
- Administer blood products as ordered.
- Maintain nasogastric tube function and monitor drainage.
- Assess the patient's pain level, administer analgesics, and evaluate their effects.
- Assess the patient's GI, hydration, and nutritional status.

- If the patient had surgery, provide wound care.
- Observe for signs and symptoms of complications.
- Provide six small meals or small hourly meals as ordered.
- Offer emotional support.

PATIENT TEACHING
- Explain the disorder, diagnostic testing, and treatment plan.
- Teach about the administration, dosage, and possible adverse effects of prescribed medications.
- Warn about using over-the-counter medications, especially aspirin, products containing aspirin, and NSAIDs, unless the practitioner approves.
- Advise against caffeine and alcohol intake during exacerbations.
- Assist with identifying appropriate lifestyle changes.
- Review dietary modifications.
- Refer the patient to a smoking-cessation program if indicated.

Pericarditis

Overview

Pericarditis, which occurs in acute and chronic forms, is the inflammation of the pericardium, the fibroserous sac that envelops, supports, and protects the heart. The acute form can be fibrinous or effusive and is characterized by serous, purulent, or hemorrhagic exudate. The chronic form, also known as *constrictive pericarditis,* is characterized by dense fibrous pericardial thickening.

CAUSES
◆ Aortic aneurysm with pericardial leakage
◆ Bacterial, fungal, or viral infection (in infectious pericarditis)
◆ Chest trauma
◆ Certain drugs, such as hydralazine (Apresoline) or procainamide (Pronestyl)
◆ High-dose chest radiation
◆ Hypersensitivity or autoimmune disease
◆ Idiopathic factors
◆ Myocardial infarction (MI)
◆ Myxedema with cholesterol deposits in the pericardium
◆ Neoplasms (primary or metastatic)
◆ Radiation
◆ Rheumatologic conditions
◆ Tuberculosis
◆ Uremia

PATHOPHYSIOLOGY
◆ Pericardial tissue is damaged by bacteria or another substance that releases chemical mediators of inflammation into surrounding tissue.
◆ Friction occurs as the inflamed layers rub against each other.
◆ Chemical mediators dilate blood vessels and increase vessel permeability.
◆ Vessel walls leak fluids and proteins, causing extracellular edema.

COMPLICATIONS
◆ Pericardial effusion
◆ Cardiac tamponade

Assessment

HISTORY
◆ One or more risk factors
◆ Sharp, sudden pain, usually starting over the sternum and radiating to the neck, shoulders, back, and arms
◆ Pleuritic pain, increasing with deep inspiration and decreasing when the patient sits up and leans forward
◆ Dyspnea
◆ Chest pain (may mimic MI pain)

PHYSICAL FINDINGS
◆ Pericardial friction rub
◆ Diminished apical impulse
◆ Fluid retention, ascites, hepatomegaly (resembling those of chronic right-sided heart failure)
◆ Tachycardia with pericardial effusion
◆ Pallor, clammy skin, hypotension, pulsus paradoxus, jugular vein distention, and dyspnea with cardiac tamponade

DIAGNOSTIC TEST RESULTS
◆ *White blood cell count:* elevated, especially in infectious pericarditis
◆ *Erythrocyte sedimentation rate:* elevated
◆ *Serum creatine kinase-MB levels:* slightly elevated with associated myocarditis
◆ *Pericardial fluid culture:* causative organism in bacterial or fungal pericarditis
◆ *Echocardiography:* echo-free space between the ventricular wall and the pericardium, indicating pericardial effusion
◆ *High-resolution computed tomography and magnetic resonance imaging:* pericardial thickness
◆ *Electrocardiography:* initial ST-segment elevation across the precordium

Treatment

- Management of the underlying disorder
- Bed rest as long as fever and pain persist
- Surgical drainage
- Pericardiocentesis
- Partial pericardectomy (for recurrent pericarditis) or total pericardectomy (for constrictive pericarditis)

MEDICATIONS
- Nonsteroidal anti-inflammatory drugs
- Corticosteroids
- Antibiotics

Nursing interventions

- Administer oxygen therapy.
- Monitor the patient's vital signs, pulse oximetry, cardiac rhythm, and hemodynamic values.
- Assess the patient's cardiovascular status.
- Administer prescribed drugs.
- Assess the patient's pain level, administer analgesics, and evaluate their effects.
- Place the patient upright to relieve dyspnea and chest pain.
- Provide appropriate postoperative care.

PATIENT TEACHING
- Explain the disorder, diagnostic testing, and treatment plan.
- Teach about the administration, dosage, and possible adverse effects of prescribed medications.
- Describe how to perform deep-breathing and coughing exercises.
- Explain the need to resume daily activities slowly.
- Explain the importance of follow-up care.

Peritonitis

Overview

Peritonitis, which can be acute or chronic, is an inflammation of the peritoneum that may extend throughout the peritoneum or localize as an abscess. It commonly decreases intestinal motility and causes intestinal distention with gas.

CAUSES
◆ Bacterial or chemical inflammation
◆ GI tract perforation from appendicitis, diverticulitis, peptic ulcer, or ulcerative colitis
◆ Ruptured ectopic pregnancy
◆ Peritoneal dialysis
◆ Ascites

PATHOPHYSIOLOGY
◆ Bacteria invade the peritoneum after inflammation and perforation of the GI tract.
◆ Fluid containing protein and electrolytes accumulates in the peritoneal cavity; normally transparent, the peritoneum becomes opaque, red, inflamed, and edematous.
◆ Infection may localize as an abscess rather than disseminate as a generalized infection.

COMPLICATIONS
◆ Abscess
◆ Septicemia
◆ Respiratory compromise
◆ Bowel obstruction
◆ Shock

Assessment

HISTORY
Early phase
◆ Vague, generalized abdominal pain
◆ If localized, pain over a specific area, usually the inflammation site
◆ If generalized, diffuse pain over the abdomen

With progression
◆ Increasingly severe and constant abdominal pain that increases with movement and respirations
◆ Possible referral of pain to shoulder or thoracic area
◆ Anorexia, nausea, and vomiting
◆ Inability to pass stools and flatus
◆ Hiccups

PHYSICAL FINDINGS
◆ Fever
◆ Tachycardia
◆ Hypotension
◆ Shallow breathing
◆ Signs of dehydration
◆ Positive bowel sounds (early), absent bowel sounds (later)
◆ Abdominal rigidity
◆ General abdominal tenderness
◆ Rebound tenderness
◆ Lying still with knees flexed

DIAGNOSTIC TEST RESULTS
◆ *Complete blood count:* leukocytosis
◆ *Abdominal X-rays:* edematous and gaseous distention of the small and large bowel, air in the abdominal cavity, with perforation of a visceral organ
◆ *Chest X-rays:* elevation of the diaphragm
◆ *Computed tomography scan:* fluid and inflammation
◆ *Paracentesis:* permits bacterial culture testing of exudate

Treatment

◆ I.V. fluids
◆ Nasogastric (NG) intubation
◆ Nothing by mouth until bowel function returns, then gradual increase in diet
◆ Bed rest until the patient's condition improves
◆ Surgery (varies according to the cause)

MEDICATIONS
◆ Antibiotics
◆ I.V. fluids
◆ Electrolyte replacement
◆ Analgesics
◆ Total parenteral nutrition if necessary

Nursing interventions

◆ Assess the patient's GI, hydration, and nutritional status.
◆ Assess the patient's pain level, administer analgesics, and evaluate their effects.
◆ Monitor the patient's vital signs, intake and output, and pulse oximetry.
◆ Give prescribed drugs.
◆ Encourage early postoperative ambulation.
◆ Provide emotional support.
◆ Maintain NG tube function and monitor drainage.
◆ Provide wound care.
◆ Observe for signs and symptoms of complications.

PATIENT TEACHING
◆ Explain the disorder, diagnostic testing, and treatment plan.
◆ Teach about the administration, dosage, and possible adverse effects of prescribed medications.
◆ Demonstrate coughing and deep-breathing techniques.
◆ Describe signs and symptoms of complications.
◆ Teach proper wound care.
◆ Review activity limitations.

Pheochromocytoma

Overview

A pheochromocytoma, which is the most common cause of adrenal medullary hypersecretion, is a catecholamine-producing tumor that's typically benign and usually derived from adrenal medullary cells. These tumors usually produce norepinephrine; large tumors secrete epinephrine and norepinephrine.

CAUSES
- Unknown
- Possibly an inherited autosomal dominant trait
- Drugs that cause hypertensive crisis, including opiates, anesthetic agents, dopamine antagonists, contrast dye, tricyclic antidepressants, and cocaine
- Hypertensive crisis caused by childbirth

PATHOPHYSIOLOGY
- An autonomous tumor produces excessive amounts of catecholamine.
- The tumor stems from a chromaffin cell tumor of the adrenal medulla or sympathetic ganglia (more commonly in the right adrenal gland than in the left).
- Extra-adrenal pheochromocytomas may occur in the abdomen, thorax, urinary bladder, and neck and in association with the 9th and 10th cranial nerves.

COMPLICATIONS
- Stroke
- Retinopathy
- Irreversible kidney damage
- Acute pulmonary edema
- Cholelithiasis
- Cardiac arrhythmias
- Heart failure

Assessment

HISTORY
- Unpredictable episodes of hypertensive crisis
- Paroxysmal symptoms suggesting a seizure disorder or anxiety attack
- Hypertension that responds poorly to conventional treatment
- Hypotension or shock after surgery or diagnostic procedures
- Childbirth

During paroxysms or crises
- Throbbing headache
- Palpitations
- Blurred vision
- Nausea and vomiting
- Severe diaphoresis
- Feelings of impending doom
- Precordial or abdominal pain
- Moderate weight loss
- Dizziness or light-headedness when moving to an upright position

PHYSICAL FINDINGS
During paroxysms or crises
- Hypertension
- Tachypnea
- Pallor or flushing
- Profuse sweating
- Tremor
- Seizures
- Tachycardia

DIAGNOSTIC TEST RESULTS
- *Vanillylmandelic acid and metanephrine levels:* increased in a 24-hour urine specimen
- *Total plasma catecholamine levels:* 10 to 50 times higher than normal on direct assay
- *Adrenal gland computed tomography (CT) scan or magnetic resonance imaging:* intra-adrenal lesions
- *CT scan, chest X-rays, or abdominal aortography:* extra-adrenal pheochromocytoma
- *Iodine-131–meta-iodobenzylguanidine scintiscan:* pheochromocytoma location or confirmation

Treatment

- Surgical removal of tumor
- High-protein diet with adequate calories
- Rest during acute attacks

MEDICATIONS

- Alpha-adrenergic receptor blockers
- Vasodilators
- Beta-adrenergic receptor blockers
- Tyrosine kinase inhibitors
- I.V. fluids

Nursing interventions

- Monitor the patient's vital signs and orthostatic blood pressures.
- Give prescribed drugs.
- Provide emotional support.
- Consult a dietitian as needed.
- Monitor the patient's serum glucose level.
- Obtain daily weight.
- Assess the patient's cardiovascular and neurologic status and renal function.
- Observe for signs and symptoms of complications.
- Provide wound care after surgery.
- Assess the patient's pain level, administer analgesics, and evaluate their effects.

PATIENT TEACHING

- Explain the disorder, diagnostic testing, and treatment plan.
- Teach about the administration, dosage, and possible adverse effects of prescribed medications.
- Describe ways to prevent paroxysmal attacks.
- Review signs and symptoms of adrenal insufficiency.
- Stress the importance of wearing medical identification jewelry.
- Teach the patient how to obtain and monitor blood pressure readings.
- Refer family members for genetic counseling if autosomal dominant transmission of pheochromocytoma is suspected.

Pleural effusion and empyema

Overview

A pleural effusion, which can be classified as exudative or transudative, is fluid accumulation in the pleural space. Empyema is the presence of pus in the pleural effusion.

CAUSES

Exudative pleural effusion
◆ Pleural infection
◆ Pleural inflammation
◆ Pleural malignancy

Transudative pleural effusion
◆ Cardiovascular disease
◆ Hepatic disease
◆ Hypoproteinemia
◆ Renal disease

Empyema
◆ Infected wound
◆ Intra-abdominal infection
◆ Lung abscess
◆ Pulmonary infection
◆ Thoracic surgery

PATHOPHYSIOLOGY
◆ Typically, fluid and other blood components migrate through the walls of intact capillaries bordering the pleura.
◆ In exudative effusion, inflammatory processes increase capillary permeability. Exudative effusion is less watery and contains high concentrations of white blood cells (WBCs) and plasma proteins.
◆ In transudative effusion, fluid is watery and diffuses out of the capillaries if hydrostatic pressure increases or capillary oncotic pressure decreases.
◆ Empyema occurs when pulmonary lymphatics become blocked, leading to outpouring of contaminated lymphatic fluid into the pleural space.

COMPLICATIONS
◆ Atelectasis
◆ Infection
◆ Hypoxemia
◆ Pneumothorax

Assessment

HISTORY
◆ Underlying pulmonary disease
◆ Shortness of breath
◆ Chest pain
◆ Malaise

PHYSICAL FINDINGS
◆ Fever
◆ Trachea deviated away from the affected side
◆ Dullness and decreased tactile fremitus over the effusion
◆ Diminished or absent breath sounds
◆ Pleural friction rub
◆ Bronchial breath sounds
◆ Foul-smelling sputum in empyema

DIAGNOSTIC TEST RESULTS
◆ *Pleural fluid analysis (transudative effusion):* specific gravity less than 1.015, less than 3 g/dl of protein present
◆ *Pleural fluid analysis (exudative effusion):* ratio of protein in pleural fluid to protein in serum 0.5 or higher, lactate dehydrogenase (LD) level of 200 international units or higher, ratio of LD in pleural fluid to LD in serum 0.6 or higher
◆ *Pleural fluid analysis (empyema):* microorganisms present, WBC count increased, glucose level decreased
◆ *Chest X-rays:* pleural effusions, loculated pleural effusions, or small pleural effusions
◆ *Thorax computed tomography scan:* pleural effusions
◆ *Tuberculin skin test:* tuberculosis
◆ *Pleural biopsy:* carcinoma

Treatment

◆ Thoracentesis
◆ Thoracoscopy
◆ Possible chest tube insertion
◆ Possible chemical pleurodesis (usually for recurrent pleural effusions)
◆ High-calorie diet
◆ Thoracotomy with decortication (removal of fibrous tissue over lung)

MEDICATIONS
◆ Antibiotics
◆ Oxygen therapy

Nursing interventions

◆ Administer prescribed drugs.
◆ Provide oxygen therapy.
◆ Monitor vital signs, pulse oximetry, and intake and output.
◆ Assess the patient's respiratory status.
◆ Assist during thoracentesis.
◆ Encourage deep-breathing exercises and use of incentive spirometer.
◆ Provide meticulous chest tube care.
◆ Maintain chest tube and monitor drainage.
◆ Provide wound care if indicated.
◆ Observe for signs and symptoms of complications.

PATIENT TEACHING
◆ Explain the disorder, diagnostic testing, and treatment plan.
◆ Teach about the administration, dosage, and possible adverse effects of prescribed medications.
◆ Describe signs and symptoms of complications and when to notify the practitioner.
◆ Teach wound care if appropriate.
◆ Provide a home health referral for follow-up care.
◆ Refer the patient to a smoking-cessation program if indicated.

Pleurisy

Overview

Pleurisy, also called *pleuritis,* is the inflammation of the visceral and parietal pleurae that line the inside of the thoracic cage and envelop the lungs.

CAUSES
- Cancer
- Certain drugs such as methotrexate or penicillin
- Chest trauma
- Dressler's syndrome
- Heart failure
- Human immunodeficiency virus
- Kidney disease
- Pathologic rib fractures
- Pneumonia
- Pneumothorax
- Pulmonary embolism
- Radiation therapy
- Rheumatoid arthritis
- Sickle cell disease
- Systemic lupus erythematosus
- Tuberculosis
- Viruses

PATHOPHYSIOLOGY
- The pleurae become swollen and congested.
- As a result, pleural fluid transport is hampered, and friction between the pleural surfaces increases, causing pain.

COMPLICATIONS
- Adhesions
- Pleural effusion
- Chronic pain or shortness of breath

Assessment

HISTORY
- Sudden dull, aching, burning, or sharp pain that worsens on inspiration
- One or more risk factors
- Cough
- Shortness of breath
- Fever

PHYSICAL FINDINGS
- Characteristic late-inspiration and early-expiration pleural friction rub
- Coarse vibration on palpation of the affected area

DIAGNOSTIC TEST RESULTS
- *Chest X-rays:* absence of pneumonia
- *Electrocardiography:* absence of ischemic heart disease

Treatment

- Treatment of symptoms
- Treatment of underlying cause
- Possible intercostal nerve block
- Bed rest
- Thoracentesis

MEDICATIONS
- Anti-inflammatory agents
- Analgesics
- Antibiotics (if infection is the cause)
- Oxygen therapy

Nursing interventions

◆ Give prescribed drugs.
◆ Monitor the patient's vital signs.
◆ Assess the patient's respiratory status and provide oxygen therapy.
◆ Assess the patient's pain level, administer analgesics, and evaluate their effects.
◆ Encourage deep breathing and coughing and use of an incentive spirometer.
◆ Assist the patient in splinting the affected side.
◆ Position the patient in high Fowler's position.
◆ Plan care to allow frequent rest periods.
◆ Assist with passive range-of-motion (ROM) exercises.
◆ Encourage active ROM exercises.
◆ Provide comfort measures.
◆ Assist with thoracentesis.
◆ Encourage the patient to verbalize his feelings and provide emotional support.

PATIENT TEACHING
◆ Explain the disorder, diagnostic testing, and treatment plan.
◆ Teach about the administration, dosage, and possible adverse effects of prescribed medications.
◆ Demonstrate how to perform splinting and deep-breathing exercises.
◆ Stress the importance of regular rest periods.
◆ Review signs and symptoms of possible complications and when to notify the practitioner.

Pneumonia

Overview

Pneumonia, which may be classified by etiology, location, or type, is an acute infection of the lung parenchyma that impairs gas exchange.

CAUSES

Aspiration pneumonia
◆ Caustic substance entering the airway

Bacterial and viral pneumonia
◆ Abdominal and thoracic surgery
◆ Alcoholism
◆ Aspiration
◆ Atelectasis
◆ Bacterial or viral respiratory infections
◆ Cancer
◆ Chronic illness and debilitation
◆ Chronic respiratory disease
◆ Endotracheal intubation or mechanical ventilation
◆ Exposure to noxious gases
◆ Immunosuppressive therapy
◆ Influenza
◆ Malnutrition
◆ Sickle cell disease
◆ Tracheostomy

RISK FACTORS
◆ Advanced age
◆ Nasogastric (NG) tube feedings
◆ Impaired gag reflex
◆ Poor oral hygiene
◆ Decreased level of consciousness
◆ Immobility
◆ History of smoking

PATHOPHYSIOLOGY
◆ A gel-like substance forms as microorganisms and phagocytic cells break down.
◆ This substance consolidates within the lower airway structure.
◆ Inflammation involves the alveoli, alveolar ducts, and interstitial spaces surrounding the alveolar walls.

◆ In lobar pneumonia, inflammation starts in one area and may extend to the entire lobe. In bronchopneumonia, it starts simultaneously in several areas, producing patchy, diffuse consolidation. In atypical pneumonia, inflammation is confined to the alveolar ducts and interstitial spaces.

COMPLICATIONS
◆ Septic shock
◆ Hypoxemia
◆ Respiratory failure
◆ Empyema
◆ Bacteremia
◆ Endocarditis
◆ Pericarditis
◆ Meningitis
◆ Lung abscess
◆ Pleural effusion

Assessment

HISTORY

Aspiration pneumonia
◆ Fever
◆ Weight loss
◆ Malaise

Bacterial pneumonia
◆ Sudden onset of pleuritic chest pain, cough, purulent sputum production, or chills

Viral pneumonia
◆ Nonproductive cough
◆ Constitutional symptoms
◆ Fever

PHYSICAL FINDINGS
◆ Fever
◆ Sputum production
◆ Dullness over the affected area
◆ Crackles, wheezing, or rhonchi
◆ Decreased breath sounds
◆ Decreased fremitus
◆ Tachypnea
◆ Use of accessory muscles

DIAGNOSTIC TEST RESULTS
◆ *Complete blood count:* leukocytosis
◆ *Blood cultures:* positive for causative organism
◆ *Arterial blood gas (ABG) values:* hypoxemia
◆ *Fungal or acid-fast bacilli cultures:* presence of etiologic agent
◆ *Assay for legionella soluble antigen in urine:* presence of antigen
◆ *Sputum culture, Gram stain, and smear:* presence of infecting organism
◆ *Chest X-rays:* generally, patchy or lobar infiltrates
◆ *Bronchoscopy or transtracheal aspiration specimens:* presence of etiologic agent
◆ *Pulse oximetry:* decreased oxygen saturation

Treatment

◆ Mechanical ventilation (positive end-expiratory pressure) for respiratory failure
◆ High-calorie, high-protein diet
◆ Adequate fluids
◆ Bed rest, initially, progressing to advancing activity as tolerated
◆ Drainage of parapneumonic pleural effusion or lung abscess

MEDICATIONS
◆ Antibiotics
◆ Oxygen therapy
◆ Antitussives
◆ Analgesics
◆ Bronchodilators

Nursing interventions

◆ Give prescribed drugs.
◆ Assess the patient's sputum production and appearance.
◆ Assess the patient's respiratory status and ABG results.
◆ Monitor the patient's vital signs, pulse oximetry, and intake and output.
◆ Give prescribed I.V. fluids and electrolyte replacement.
◆ Maintain a patent airway and adequate oxygenation.
◆ Give prescribed supplemental oxygen.
◆ Suction the patient as needed.
◆ Provide a high-calorie, high-protein diet of soft foods.
◆ Give supplemental oral feedings, NG tube feedings, or parenteral nutrition if needed.
◆ Provide a quiet, calm environment with frequent rest periods.
◆ Obtain daily weight.

PATIENT TEACHING
◆ Explain the disorder, diagnostic testing, and treatment plan.
◆ Teach about the administration, dosage, and possible adverse effects of prescribed medications.
◆ Stress the need for adequate fluid intake and adequate rest.
◆ Demonstrate deep-breathing and coughing exercises and chest physiotherapy.
◆ Describe signs and symptoms of complications and when to notify the practitioner.
◆ Teach about home oxygen therapy if required.
◆ Describe ways to prevent pneumonia.
◆ Refer the patient to a smoking-cessation program if indicated.

Pneumothorax

Overview

A pneumothorax, or collapsed lung, is caused by the accumulation of air or gas between the parietal and visceral pleurae. The amount of trapped air or gas determines the degree of lung collapse. The most common pneumothorax types are open, closed, and tension.

CAUSES

Open pneumothorax
- Central venous catheter insertion
- Chest surgery
- Penetrating chest injury
- Percutaneous lung biopsy
- Thoracentesis
- Transbronchial biopsy

Closed pneumothorax
- Barotrauma
- Blunt chest trauma
- Clavicle fracture
- Congenital bleb rupture
- Emphysematous bullae rupture
- Erosive tubercular or cancerous lesions
- Interstitial lung disease
- Rib fracture

Tension pneumothorax
- Chest tube occlusion or malfunction
- High positive end-expiratory pressures, causing rupture of alveolar blebs
- Lung or airway puncture from positive-pressure ventilation
- Mechanical ventilation after chest injury
- Penetrating chest wound

PATHOPHYSIOLOGY
- Air accumulates and separates the visceral and parietal pleurae.
- Negative pressure is eliminated, affecting elastic recoil forces.
- The lung recoils and collapses toward the hilus.

- In open pneumothorax, atmospheric air flows directly into the pleural cavity, collapsing the lung on the affected side.
- In closed pneumothorax, air enters the pleural space from within the lung, increasing pleural pressure and preventing lung expansion.
- In tension pneumothorax, air in the pleural space is under higher pressure than air in the adjacent lung. Air enters the pleural space from a pleural rupture only on inspiration. This air pressure exceeds barometric pressure, causing compression atelectasis. Increased pressure may displace the heart and great vessels and cause mediastinal shift.

COMPLICATIONS
- Pulmonary and circulatory impairment
- Death

Assessment

HISTORY
- Possibly no symptoms (with small pneumothorax)
- Sudden, sharp, pleuritic pain
- Pain that worsens with chest movement, breathing, and coughing
- Shortness of breath

PHYSICAL FINDINGS
- Asymmetrical chest wall movement
- Overexpansion and rigidity on the affected side
- Possible cyanosis
- Subcutaneous emphysema
- Hyperresonance on the affected side
- Decreased or absent breath sounds on the affected side
- Decreased tactile fremitus over the affected side

Tension pneumothorax
◆ Distended jugular veins
◆ Pallor
◆ Anxiety
◆ Tracheal deviation away from the affected side
◆ Weak, rapid pulse
◆ Hypotension
◆ Tachypnea
◆ Cyanosis

DIAGNOSTIC TEST RESULTS
◆ *Arterial blood gas analysis:* hypoxemia
◆ *Chest X-ray:* air in the pleural space; possibly, a mediastinal shift
◆ *Pulse oximetry:* decreased oxygen saturation

Treatment

◆ Conservative treatment of spontaneous pneumothorax with no signs of increased pleural pressure, less than 30% lung collapse, and no obvious physiologic compromise
◆ Chest tube insertion
◆ Needle thoracostomy
◆ Activity as tolerated
◆ Thoracotomy, pleurectomy for recurring spontaneous pneumothorax
◆ Repair of traumatic pneumothorax
◆ Doxycycline or talc installation into pleural space

MEDICATIONS
◆ Oxygen therapy
◆ Analgesics

Nursing interventions

◆ Provide oxygen therapy.
◆ Assess respiratory status.
◆ Give prescribed drugs.
◆ Assist with chest tube insertion.
◆ Provide comfort measures.
◆ Encourage deep-breathing and coughing exercises.
◆ Offer reassurance as appropriate.
◆ Monitor the patient's vital signs, pulse oximetry, and cardiac rhythm.
◆ Maintain the chest tube system and monitor drainage.
◆ Observe for signs and symptoms of complications.

PATIENT TEACHING
◆ Explain the disorder, diagnostic testing, and treatment plan.
◆ Teach about the administration, dosage, and possible adverse effects of prescribed medications.
◆ Explain need for chest tube insertion.
◆ Teach deep-breathing exercises.
◆ Describe the signs and symptoms of complications and when to notify the practitioner.
◆ Refer the patient to a smoking-cessation program if appropriate.

Pulmonary edema

Overview

Pulmonary edema, which may be chronic or acute, is the accumulation of fluid in the extravascular spaces of the lung and is a common complication of cardiovascular disorders. It causes gas exchange impairment and respiratory compromise.

CAUSES
♦ Heart disease or injury
♦ Lung disease or injury

RISK FACTORS
♦ Acute myocardial ischemia and infarction
♦ Arrhythmias
♦ Barbiturate or opiate toxicity
♦ Diastolic dysfunction
♦ Fluid overload
♦ Impaired pulmonary lymphatic drainage
♦ Inhalation of irritating gases
♦ Left atrial myxoma
♦ Left-sided heart failure
♦ Pneumonia
♦ Pulmonary veno-occlusive disease
♦ Valvular heart disease

PATHOPHYSIOLOGY
♦ Pulmonary edema results from either increased pulmonary capillary hydrostatic pressure or decreased colloid osmotic pressure. Normally, the two pressures are in balance.
♦ If pulmonary capillary hydrostatic pressure increases, the compromised left ventricle needs higher filling pressures to maintain adequate output; these pressures are transmitted to the left atrium, pulmonary veins, and pulmonary capillary bed.
♦ Fluids and solutes are then forced from the intravascular compartment into the lung interstitium. With fluid overloading the interstitium, some fluid floods peripheral alveoli and impairs gas exchange.
♦ If colloid osmotic pressure decreases, the pulling force that contains intravascular fluids is lost, and nothing opposes the hydrostatic force. Fluid flows freely into the interstitium and alveoli, causing pulmonary edema.

COMPLICATIONS
♦ Respiratory and metabolic acidosis
♦ Cardiac or respiratory arrest
♦ Death

Assessment

HISTORY
♦ One or more risk factors
♦ Persistent cough
♦ Dyspnea on exertion
♦ Paroxysmal nocturnal dyspnea
♦ Orthopnea

PHYSICAL FINDINGS
♦ Restlessness and anxiety
♦ Rapid, labored breathing
♦ Intense, productive cough
♦ Frothy, bloody sputum
♦ Mental status changes
♦ Jugular vein distention
♦ Sweaty, cold, clammy skin
♦ Wheezing
♦ Crackles
♦ Third heart sound
♦ Tachycardia
♦ Hypotension
♦ Thready pulse
♦ Peripheral edema
♦ Hepatomegaly

DIAGNOSTIC TEST RESULTS
♦ *Arterial blood gas (ABG) analysis:* hypoxemia, hypercapnia, or acidosis
♦ *Chest X-rays:* diffuse haziness of the lung fields, cardiomegaly, and pleural effusion
♦ *Pulse oximetry:* decreased oxygen saturation
♦ *Pulmonary artery catheterization:* increased pulmonary artery wedge pressures
♦ *Electrocardiography:* valvular disease and left ventricular hypokinesis or akinesis

Treatment

◆ Supportive measures for life-threatening signs and symptoms
◆ Treatment of underlying condition
◆ Sodium-restricted diet with fluid restriction
◆ Activity as tolerated
◆ Valve repair or replacement or myocardial revascularization, if appropriate, to correct the underlying cause

MEDICATIONS

◆ Oxygen therapy
◆ Diuretics
◆ Antiarrhythmics
◆ Morphine
◆ Preload-reducing agents
◆ Afterload-reducing agents
◆ Bronchodilators
◆ Positive inotropic agents
◆ Vasopressors

Nursing interventions

◆ Provide oxygen therapy and monitor ABG results.
◆ Position the patient in high Fowler's position.
◆ Assess the patient's respiratory status.
◆ Monitor the patient's vital signs, pulse oximetry, cardiac rhythm, and intake and output.
◆ Administer prescribed drugs.
◆ Restrict fluids and sodium intake.
◆ Promote rest and relaxation.
◆ Provide emotional support.
◆ Obtain daily weight.
◆ Observe for signs and symptoms of complications.

PATIENT TEACHING

◆ Explain the disorder, diagnostic testing, and treatment plan.
◆ Teach about the administration, dosage, and possible adverse effects of prescribed medications.
◆ Explain fluid and sodium restrictions.
◆ Describe signs and symptoms of fluid overload.
◆ Teach the patient strategies for conserving energy.
◆ Stress the need to avoid alcohol and smoking.
◆ Describe the signs and symptoms of complications and when to notify the practitioner.
◆ Refer the patient to a cardiac rehabilitation program if indicated.
◆ Refer the patient to a smoking-cessation program if indicated.

Pulmonary embolism

Overview

Pulmonary embolism is a thrombus that causes partial or complete obstruction of the pulmonary arterial bed when it lodges in the main pulmonary artery or branch. Most thrombi originate in the deep veins of the leg. A pulmonary embolism may not produce symptoms, but sometimes causes rapid death from pulmonary infarction.

CAUSES
◆ Deep vein thrombosis (DVT)
◆ Pelvic, renal, and hepatic vein thrombosis
◆ Rarely, other types of emboli, such as bone, air, fat, amniotic fluid, tumor cells, or a foreign body
◆ Right heart thrombus
◆ Upper extremity thrombosis
◆ Valvular heart disease

RISK FACTORS
◆ Various disorders and treatments (see *Who's at risk for pulmonary embolism?*)

PATHOPHYSIOLOGY
◆ Thrombus formation results from vascular wall damage, venous stasis, or blood hypercoagulability.
◆ Trauma, clot dissolution, sudden muscle spasm, intravascular pressure changes, or peripheral blood flow changes can cause the thrombus to loosen or fragmentize.
◆ The thrombus, which is now an embolus, floats to the heart's right side and enters the lung through the pulmonary artery. There, the embolus may dissolve, continue to fragmentize, or grow.
◆ By occluding the pulmonary artery, the embolus prevents alveoli from producing enough surfactant to maintain alveolar integrity. Alveoli collapse occurs and atelectasis develops.
◆ If the embolus enlarges, it may occlude most or all of the pulmonary vessels and cause death.

COMPLICATIONS
◆ Respiratory failure
◆ Pulmonary infarction
◆ Pulmonary hypertension
◆ Embolic extension
◆ Acute respiratory distress syndrome
◆ Massive atelectasis
◆ Right-sided heart failure
◆ Death

Assessment

HISTORY
◆ One or more risk factors
◆ Shortness of breath for no apparent reason
◆ Pleuritic pain or angina

PHYSICAL FINDINGS
◆ Tachycardia
◆ Low-grade fever
◆ Weak, rapid pulse
◆ Hypotension
◆ Productive cough, possibly with blood-tinged sputum
◆ Warmth, tenderness, and edema of the lower leg
◆ Restlessness
◆ Transient pleural friction rub
◆ Crackles
◆ Third and fourth heart sounds with increased intensity of the pulmonic component of the second heart sound
◆ Cyanosis, syncope, jugular vein distention (with a large embolus)

DIAGNOSTIC TEST RESULTS
◆ *Arterial blood gas (ABG) values:* hypoxemia
◆ *D-dimer level:* elevated
◆ *Spiral chest computed tomography scan:* central pulmonary emboli
◆ *Lung ventilation perfusion scan:* ventilation-perfusion mismatch
◆ *Pulmonary angiography:* pulmonary vessel filling defect, abrupt vessel ending, location and extent of pulmonary embolism

Treatment

- Supportive measures for life-threatening signs and symptoms
- Bed rest during the acute phase
- Vena caval interruption
- Vena caval filter placement
- Pulmonary embolectomy

MEDICATIONS

- Oxygen therapy
- Thrombolytics
- Anticoagulation
- Corticosteroids (controversial)
- Diuretics
- Antiarrhythmics
- Vasopressors for hypotension
- Antibiotics for septic embolus

Nursing interventions

- Provide oxygen therapy and monitor ABG results.
- Assess the patient's respiratory status.
- Monitor the patient's vital signs, pulse oximetry, cardiac rhythm, and laboratory values.
- Give prescribed drugs.
- Encourage active and passive range-of-motion exercises, unless contraindicated.
- Avoid massaging the lower legs.
- Apply antiembolism stockings.
- Provide adequate nutrition.
- Assist with ambulation as soon as the patient is stable.
- Encourage use of incentive spirometry.
- Observe for signs and symptoms of complications.

PATIENT TEACHING

- Explain the disorder, diagnostic testing, and treatment plan.
- Teach about the administration, dosage, and possible adverse effects of prescribed medications.
- Describe ways to prevent DVT and pulmonary embolism.
- Review signs and symptoms of complications.
- Explain how to monitor anticoagulant effects and the importance of follow-up care.
- Refer the patient to a weight-management program if indicated.

Who's at risk for pulmonary embolism?

Many disorders and treatments heighten the risk of pulmonary embolism. At particular risk are surgical patients. The anesthetic used during surgery can injure lung vessels, and surgery or prolonged bed rest can promote venous stasis, which compounds the risk.

Predisposing disorders

- Cardiac arrhythmia (especially atrial fibrillation)
- Lung disorders, especially chronic types
- Cardiac disorders
- Infection
- Diabetes mellitus
- History of thromboembolism, thrombophlebitis, or vascular insufficiency
- Sickle cell disease
- Autoimmune hemolytic anemia
- Polycythemia
- Osteomyelitis
- Long-bone fracture
- Manipulation or disconnection of central lines

Venous stasis

- Prolonged bed rest or immobilization
- Obesity
- Age older than 40
- Burns
- Recent childbirth
- Orthopedic casts

Venous injury

- Surgery, particularly of the legs, pelvis, abdomen, or thorax
- Leg or pelvic fractures or injuries
- I.V. drug abuse
- I.V. therapy

Increased blood coagulability

- Cancer
- Use of high-estrogen hormonal contraceptives

Pulmonary hypertension

Overview

Pulmonary hypertension, which occurs in a primary form (rare) and a secondary form, occurs when there's increased pressure in the pulmonary artery. With both forms, resting systolic pulmonary artery pressure (PAP) is above 30 mm Hg and mean PAP is above 20 mm Hg.

CAUSES

Primary pulmonary hypertension (PPH)
◆ Unknown
◆ Associated with portal hypertension
◆ Possible altered autoimmune mechanisms
◆ Possible hereditary factors

Secondary pulmonary hypertension
◆ Lung disease

RISK FACTORS

Secondary pulmonary hypertension
◆ Chronic obstructive pulmonary disease
◆ Congenital cardiac defects
◆ Diffuse interstitial pneumonia
◆ Hypoventilation syndromes
◆ Kyphoscoliosis
◆ Left atrial myxoma
◆ Malignant metastasis
◆ Mitral stenosis
◆ Obesity
◆ Pulmonary embolism
◆ Sarcoidosis
◆ Scleroderma
◆ Sleep apnea
◆ Use of some diet drugs
◆ Vasculitis

PATHOPHYSIOLOGY
◆ In PPH, the intimal lining of the pulmonary arteries thickens for no apparent reason. This thickening narrows the artery and impairs distensibility, increasing vascular resistance.
◆ Secondary pulmonary hypertension occurs from hypoxemia caused by conditions involving alveolar hypoventilation, vascular obstruction, or left-to-right shunting.

COMPLICATIONS
◆ Cor pulmonale
◆ Heart failure
◆ Cardiac arrest
◆ Death

Assessment

HISTORY
◆ Shortness of breath with exertion
◆ Weakness, fatigue
◆ Pain during breathing
◆ Near-syncope

PHYSICAL FINDINGS
◆ Ascites
◆ Jugular vein distention
◆ Peripheral edema
◆ Restlessness and agitation
◆ Mental status changes
◆ Decreased diaphragmatic excursion
◆ Apical impulse displaced beyond midclavicular line
◆ Right ventricular lift
◆ Reduced carotid pulse
◆ Hepatomegaly
◆ Tachycardia
◆ Systolic ejection murmur
◆ Widely split second heart sound
◆ Third and fourth heart sounds
◆ Hypotension
◆ Decreased breath sounds
◆ Tubular breath sounds

DIAGNOSTIC TEST RESULTS
◆ *Arterial blood gas (ABG) values:* hypoxemia
◆ *Ventilation-perfusion lung scan:* ventilation-perfusion mismatch
◆ *Pulmonary angiography:* pulmonary vasculature filling defects
◆ *Electrocardiography:* right-axis deviation
◆ *Pulmonary artery catheterization:* increased PAP with systolic pressure above 30 mm Hg, increased pulmonary artery

wedge pressure, decreased cardiac output, decreased cardiac index
◆ *Pulmonary function tests:* decreased flow rates, increased residual volume, reduced total lung capacity
◆ *Echocardiography:* valvular heart disease or atrial myxoma
◆ *Lung biopsy:* presence of tumor cells

Treatment

◆ Treatment of underlying disease
◆ Symptom relief
◆ Smoking cessation
◆ Low-sodium diet
◆ Fluid restriction with right-sided heart failure
◆ Bed rest during acute phase
◆ Heart-lung transplantation if indicated

MEDICATIONS
◆ Oxygen therapy
◆ Cardiac glycosides
◆ Diuretics
◆ Vasodilators
◆ Calcium channel blockers
◆ Bronchodilators
◆ Beta-adrenergic blockers
◆ Epoprostenol

Nursing interventions

◆ Administer prescribed drugs.
◆ Provide oxygen therapy and monitor ABG results.
◆ Assess the patient's respiratory status.
◆ Provide comfort measures and adequate rest periods.
◆ Offer emotional support.
◆ Monitor the patient's vital signs, cardiac rhythm, hemodynamic values, pulse oximetry, and intake and output.
◆ Obtain daily weight.
◆ Observe for signs and symptoms of complications.

PATIENT TEACHING
◆ Explain the disorder, diagnostic testing, and treatment plan.
◆ Teach about the administration, dosage, and possible adverse effects of prescribed medications.
◆ Review dietary restrictions.
◆ Stress the need for frequent rest periods.
◆ Describe the signs and symptoms of complications and when to notify the practitioner.
◆ Refer the patient to a smoking-cessation program if indicated.

Renal calculi

Overview

Renal calculi are stones formed anywhere in the urinary tract, most commonly in the renal pelvis or calyces. They vary in size and number.

Causes
◆ Unknown

Risk factors
◆ Dehydration
◆ Infection
◆ Urine pH changes
◆ Urinary tract obstruction
◆ Immobilization
◆ Metabolic factors
◆ Family member with history of renal calculi

Pathophysiology
◆ Calculi form when substances normally dissolved in the urine, such as calcium oxalate and calcium phosphate, precipitate.
◆ Large, rough calculi may occlude the opening to the ureteropelvic junction.
◆ The frequency and force of peristaltic contractions increase, causing pain.

Complications
◆ Renal parenchymal damage
◆ Renal cell necrosis
◆ Hydronephrosis
◆ Complete ureteral obstruction
◆ Recurrence of calculi
◆ Urinary tract infection

Assessment

History
◆ Classic renal colic pain, a severe pain that travels from the costovertebral angle to the flank and then to the suprapubic region and external genitalia
◆ Calculi in the renal pelvis and calyces, a relatively constant, dull abdominal pain
◆ Pain of fluctuating intensity; may be excruciating at its peak
◆ Nausea, vomiting
◆ Fever, chills
◆ Anuria (rare)

Physical findings
◆ Hematuria
◆ Abdominal distention
◆ Costovertebral tenderness on palpation
◆ Tachycardia
◆ Elevated blood pressure

Diagnostic test results
◆ *24-hour urine collection:* increased calcium oxalate, phosphorus, or uric acid excretion levels
◆ *Urinalysis:* increased urine specific gravity, hematuria, crystals, casts, pyuria
◆ *Kidney-ureter-bladder (KUB) radiography:* presence of renal calculi
◆ *Excretory urography:* calculi size and location
◆ *I.V. pyelography and abdominal computed tomography:* stones or obstruction of the ureter
◆ *Kidney ultrasonography:* obstructive changes and radiolucent calculi not seen on KUB radiography

Treatment

- Percutaneous ultrasonic lithotripsy
- Extracorporeal shock wave lithotripsy
- Vigorous hydration (more than 3 qt [2.8 L]/day)
- Dietary modification based on stone composition
- Cystoscopy
- Ureteral stent
- Percutaneous nephrostomy

MEDICATIONS

- Antibiotics
- Analgesics
- Diuretics
- Methenamine mandelate (Hiprex)
- Allopurinol (Zyloprim; for uric acid calculi)
- Ascorbic acid
- Ketorolac (Toradol), a nonsteroidal anti-inflammatory drug
- Desmopressin (DDAVP)

Nursing interventions

- Provide I.V. fluids as ordered; encourage fluids as needed.
- Strain all urine and save solid material for analysis.
- Encourage ambulation to aid spontaneous calculus passage.
- Monitor intake and output.
- Assess the patient's pain level, administer analgesics, and evaluate their effects.
- Observe for signs and symptoms of complications.

PATIENT TEACHING

- Explain the disorder, diagnostic testing, and treatment plan.
- Teach about the administration, dosage, and possible adverse effects of prescribed medications.
- Review the prescribed diet and the importance of compliance.
- Explain ways to prevent recurrences.
- Teach how to strain urine for stones.
- Instruct the patient to return to the hospital if fever, uncontrolled pain, or vomiting occur.
- Explain the importance of follow-up care.

Renal failure, acute

Overview

Acute renal failure (ARF), the sudden interruption of renal function resulting from obstruction, reduced circulation, or renal parenchymal disease, is usually reversible with medical treatment. If not treated, it may progress to end-stage renal disease, uremia, and death. ARF is classified as prerenal failure, caused by impaired blood flow; intrarenal failure (also called *intrinsic* or *parenchymal failure)*, which may occur after a severe episode of hypotension, which is commonly associated with hypovolemia; and postrenal failure, which usually occurs with urinary tract obstruction that affects the kidneys bilaterally such as in prostatic hyperplasia.

CAUSES
Prerenal failure
- Hemorrhagic blood loss
- Hypotension or hypoperfusion
- Hypovolemia
- Loss of plasma volume
- Water and electrolyte losses

Intrarenal failure
- Acute tubular necrosis
- Coagulation defects
- Glomerulopathies
- Malignant hypertension

Postrenal failure
- Bladder neck obstruction
- Obstructive uropathies (usually bilateral)
- Ureteral destruction

PATHOPHYSIOLOGY
- Three distinct phases normally occur: oliguric, diuretic, and recovery.

Oliguric phase
- This phase may last a few days or several weeks.
- Urine output is less than 400 ml/day.

- Excess fluid volume, azotemia, and electrolyte imbalances occur.
- Local mediators are released, causing intrarenal vasoconstriction.
- Medullary hypoxia causes cellular swelling and adherence of neutrophils to capillaries and venules.
- Hypoperfusion, cellular injury, and necrosis follow.
- Reperfusion causes reactive oxygen species to form, leading to further cellular injury.

Diuretic phase
- Renal function recovers.
- Urine output gradually increases.
- Glomerular filtration rate improves, although tubular transport systems remain abnormal.

Recovery phase
- Gradually, renal function returns to normal or near normal.
- It may take 3 to 12 months or longer to recover.

COMPLICATIONS
- Renal shutdown
- Electrolyte imbalance
- Metabolic acidosis
- Acute pulmonary edema
- Hypertensive crisis
- Infection

Assessment

HISTORY
- Predisposing disorder
- Recent fever, chills, or central nervous system problem
- Recent GI problem

PHYSICAL FINDINGS
- Oliguria or anuria
- Tachycardia
- Bibasilar crackles
- Irritability, drowsiness, or confusion

- Altered level of consciousness
- Bleeding abnormalities
- Dry, pruritic skin
- Dry mucous membranes
- Uremic breath odor

DIAGNOSTIC TEST RESULTS

- *Blood urea nitrogen, serum creatinine, and potassium levels:* elevated
- *Hematocrit, blood pH, bicarbonate, and hemoglobin levels:* decreased
- *Urine casts and cellular debris:* present
- *Specific gravity:* decreased
- *Proteinuria and urine osmolality:* close to serum osmolality level in glomerular disease
- *Urine sodium level:* less than 20 mEq/L from decreased perfusion in oliguria; greater than 40 mEq/L from an intrarenal problem in oliguria
- *Urine creatinine clearance:* glomerular filtration rate, number of remaining functioning nephrons
- *Kidney ultrasonography, kidney-ureter-bladder radiography, excretory urography renal scan, retrograde pyelography, computed tomography scan, and nephrotomography:* renal failure
- *Electrocardiography:* tall, peaked T waves, widening QRS complex, disappearing P waves if hyperkalemia present

Treatment

- Hemodialysis or continuous renal replacement therapy
- High-calorie, low-protein, low-sodium, and low-potassium diet
- Fluid restriction
- Rest periods when fatigued
- Insertion of vascular access for dialysis

MEDICATIONS

- Diuretics
- Hypertonic glucose-and-insulin infusions, sodium bicarbonate, or sodium polystyrene sulfonate for hyperkalemia

Nursing interventions

- Assist with dialysis.
- Monitor the patient's vital signs, cardiac rhythm, pulse oximetry, intake and output, and laboratory values.
- Give prescribed drugs.
- Provide emotional support.
- Obtain daily weight.
- Maintain the dialysis access site.

PATIENT TEACHING

- Explain the disorder, diagnostic testing, and treatment plan.
- Teach about the administration, dosage, and possible adverse effects of prescribed medications.
- Review recommended fluid allowance.
- Encourage compliance with the diet and drug regimen.
- Describe signs and symptoms of complications.
- Stress the importance of follow-up care with a nephrologist.

Renal failure, chronic

Overview

Chroninc renal failure (CRF) is the end result of gradually progressive loss of renal function. Symptoms are sparse until more than 75% of glomerular filtration is lost, worsening as renal function declines. CRF can be fatal unless treated; to sustain life, the patient may require maintenance dialysis or kidney transplantation.

CAUSES
◆ Chronic glomerular disease
◆ Chronic infections such as chronic pyelonephritis
◆ Collagen diseases such as systemic lupus erythematosus
◆ Congenital anomalies such as polycystic kidney disease
◆ Endocrine disease
◆ Nephrotoxic agents
◆ Obstructive processes such as calculi
◆ Vascular diseases

PATHOPHYSIOLOGY
◆ Nephron destruction eventually causes irreversible renal damage.
◆ The disease may progress through these stages: reduced renal reserve, renal insufficiency, renal failure, and end-stage renal disease.

COMPLICATIONS
◆ Anemia
◆ Peripheral neuropathy
◆ Lipid disorders
◆ Platelet dysfunction
◆ Pulmonary edema
◆ Electrolyte imbalances
◆ Sexual dysfunction

Assessment

HISTORY
◆ Predisposing factor
◆ Dry mouth
◆ Fatigue
◆ Nausea
◆ Hiccups
◆ Muscle cramps
◆ Fasciculations, twitching
◆ Infertility, decreased libido
◆ Amenorrhea
◆ Impotence
◆ Pathologic fractures

PHYSICAL FINDINGS
◆ Decreased urine output
◆ Hypotension or hypertension
◆ Altered level of consciousness
◆ Peripheral edema
◆ Cardiac arrhythmias
◆ Bibasilar crackles
◆ Pleural friction rub
◆ Gum ulceration and bleeding
◆ Uremic fetor
◆ Abdominal pain on palpation
◆ Poor skin turgor
◆ Pale, yellowish bronze skin color
◆ Thin, brittle fingernails and dry, brittle hair
◆ Growth retardation (in children)

DIAGNOSTIC TEST RESULTS
◆ *Blood urea nitrogen, serum creatinine, sodium, and potassium levels:* elevated
◆ *Arterial blood gas values:* decreased arterial pH and bicarbonate levels, metabolic acidosis
◆ *Complete blood count, hematocrit, and hemoglobin levels:* low; thrombocytopenia and platelet defects

◆ *Red blood cell (RBC) survival time:* decreased
◆ *Aldosterone secretion:* increased
◆ *Hyperglycemia and hypertriglyceridemia:* present
◆ *High-density lipoprotein levels:* decreased
◆ *Urine specific gravity:* 1.010 fixed
◆ *Urinalysis:* proteinuria, glycosuria, and urinary RBCs, leukocytes, casts, and crystals
◆ *Kidney-ureter-bladder radiography, excretory urography, nephrotomography, renal scan, and renal arteriography:* reduced kidney size
◆ *Renal biopsy:* underlying pathology
◆ *Electroencephalography:* metabolic encephalopathy

Treatment

◆ Hemodialysis or peritoneal dialysis
◆ Low-protein (high protein with peritoneal dialysis), high-calorie, low-sodium, low-phosphorus, and low-potassium diet
◆ Fluid restriction
◆ Rest periods when fatigued
◆ Creation of vascular access for dialysis
◆ Possible kidney transplantation

MEDICATIONS
◆ Loop diuretics
◆ Cardiac glycosides
◆ Antihypertensives
◆ Antiemetics
◆ Iron and folate supplements
◆ Erythropoietin
◆ Antipruritics
◆ Supplementary vitamins and essential amino acids

Nursing interventions

◆ Give prescribed drugs.
◆ Perform meticulous skin care.
◆ Encourage the patient to express his feelings.
◆ Provide emotional support.
◆ Monitor the patient's vital signs, intake and output, and laboratory values.
◆ Obtain daily weight.
◆ Observe for signs and symptoms of fluid overload.
◆ Assess the dialysis access site.
◆ Assist with the peritoneal dialysis regimen per facility policy.

PATIENT TEACHING
◆ Explain the disorder, diagnostic testing, and treatment plan.
◆ Teach about the administration, dosage, and possible adverse effects of prescribed medications.
◆ Review dietary recommendations and fluid restrictions.
◆ Teach dialysis site care as appropriate.
◆ Stress the importance of wearing or carrying medical identification.
◆ Stress the importance of complying with treatment and follow-up care.
◆ Refer the patient to resources and support services.

Respiratory acidosis and alkalosis

Respiratory acidosis and alkalosis are acid-base disorders characterized by abnormal levels of acid and bicarbonate (HCO_3^-) in the blood and may cause respiratory, metabolic, and renal responses that produce hypoventilation and other symptoms. Increased carbon dioxide levels are characteristic of respiratory acidosis; a loss of carbon dioxide is characteristic of respiratory alkalosis.

 Nursing alert

Severe or untreated respiratory acid-base disorders can be fatal.

CAUSES
♦ Respiratory or metabolic failure, causing a change in the carbon dioxide level

RISK FACTORS
♦ Airway obstruction
♦ Central nervous system trauma or depression
♦ Chronic bronchitis
♦ Chronic metabolic alkalosis (in respiratory acidosis)
♦ Chronic obstructive pulmonary disease
♦ Lung disorders
♦ Inadequate mechanical ventilation
♦ Anxiety (in respiratory alkalosis)
♦ Fever
♦ Metabolic acidosis (in respiratory alkalosis)
♦ Sepsis
♦ Hepatic failure

PATHOPHYSIOLOGY
Respiratory acidosis
♦ Depressed ventilation causes carbon dioxide retention.
♦ Hydrogen ion concentration increases.
♦ Respiratory acidosis results.

Respiratory alkalosis
♦ Increased pulmonary ventilation leads to excessive exhalation of CO_2, resulting in hypocapnia.
♦ Chemical reduction of carbonic acid occurs, along with excretion of hydrogen and bicarbonate ions, and elevated pH.

COMPLICATIONS
♦ Shock
♦ Respiratory failure or arrest
♦ Cardiac arrest

Assessment

HISTORY
♦ One or more risk factors
♦ Headache
♦ Shortness of breath
♦ Nausea and vomiting
♦ Increased rate and depth of respirations (in respiratory alkalosis)

PHYSICAL FINDINGS
♦ Diaphoresis
♦ Bounding pulses
♦ Rapid, shallow respirations
♦ Tachycardia and other arrhythmias
♦ Hypotension
♦ Papilledema
♦ Mental status changes
♦ Asterixis (tremor)
♦ Depressed deep tendon reflexes

DIAGNOSTIC TEST RESULTS
♦ *Arterial blood gas studies:* pH less than 7.35, $Paco_2$ above 35 mm Hg with respiratory acidosis; pH greater than 7.45, $Paco_2$ less than 35 mm Hg, normal HCO_3^- in the acute stage but less than normal in the chronic stage with respiratory alkalosis

◆ *Serum electrolyte studies:* metabolic disorders causing compensatory respiratory alkalosis; low in severe respiratory alkalosis

◆ *Chest X-ray:* lung disease or illness

◆ *Pulmonary function tests:* underlying respiratory disease

Treatment

◆ Supportive measures for life-threatening signs and symptoms

◆ Correction of the condition causing altered alveolar ventilation

◆ I.V. fluid administration

◆ Smoking cessation

◆ Bronchoscopy

MEDICATIONS

◆ Oxygen therapy

◆ Bronchodilators

◆ Antibiotics

◆ Sodium bicarbonate for respiratory acidosis

◆ Sedatives

◆ Electrolyte replacement therapy

◆ Drug therapy for the underlying condition

Nursing interventions

◆ Provide oxygen therapy and monitor ABG results.

◆ Monitor the patient's vital signs, pulse oximetry, cardiac rhythm, and intake and output.

◆ Give prescribed drugs.

◆ Provide adequate fluids.

◆ Maintain a patent airway.

◆ Perform tracheal suctioning as needed.

◆ Assess the patient's neurologic and respiratory status.

PATIENT TEACHING

◆ Explain the disorder, diagnostic testing, and treatment plan.

◆ Teach about the administration, dosage, and possible adverse effects of prescribed medications.

◆ Demonstrate how to perform coughing and deep-breathing exercises.

◆ Describe signs and symptoms of acid-base imbalance and when to notify the practitioner.

◆ Refer the patient for home oxygen therapy if indicated.

◆ Refer the patient to a smoking-cessation program if appropriate.

Salmonella infection

Overview

Salmonella infection, one of the most common intestinal infections in the United States, occurs as enterocolitis, bacteremia, localized infection, typhoid fever, or paratyphoid fever. Nontyphoid forms are usually mild to moderate illnesses with low mortality. Typhoid fever is the most severe form, usually lasting from 1 to 4 weeks and conferring lifelong immunity, although the patient may become a carrier.

CAUSES

◆ Gram-negative bacilli of the genus *Salmonella* (member of the *Enterobacteriaceae* family) including: *S. typhi* (typhoid fever), *S. enteritidis* (enterocolitis), and *S. choleresis* (bacteremia)

RISK FACTORS

◆ Ingestion of contaminated water or food or inadequately processed food, especially eggs, chicken, turkey, and duck (nontyphoidal infection)
◆ Contact with infected person or animal (nontyphoidal infection)
◆ Ingestion of contaminated dry milk, chocolate bars, or pharmaceuticals of animal origin (nontyphoidal infection)
◆ Consumption of water contaminated by excretions of a carrier (typhoid fever)
◆ Impaired gastric acidity and immunosuppression

Age considerations

Salmonella infection may be transmitted by the fecal-oral route in children younger than age 5. Patients older than age 60 are at risk for infection because of biliary sequestration of organisms.

PATHOPHYSIOLOGY

◆ Invasion occurs across the mucosa of the small intestine, which alters the plasma membrane and allows entry into the lamina propria.
◆ Invasion activates cell-signaling pathways, which alter electrolyte transport, and may cause diarrhea.
◆ Some *Salmonella* produce a molecule that increases electrolyte and fluid secretion.

COMPLICATIONS

◆ Dehydration
◆ Hypovolemic shock
◆ Abscess formation
◆ Sepsis
◆ Toxic megacolon

Assessment

HISTORY

◆ Possible eating of contaminated food 6 to 48 hours before symptoms develop (enterocolitis)
◆ Usually immunocompromised condition, especially acquired immunodeficiency syndrome (bacteremia)
◆ Possible ingestion of contaminated food or water, typically 1 to 2 weeks before symptoms develop (typhoid fever)

PHYSICAL FINDINGS

◆ Fever
◆ Abdominal pain
◆ Severe diarrhea (in enterocolitis)
◆ Headache, increasing fever, and constipation (in typhoid fever)

DIAGNOSTIC TEST RESULTS

◆ *Blood culture:* causative organism (typhoid fever, paratyphoid fever, and bacteremia)
◆ *Stool culture:* causative organism (typhoid fever, paratyphoid fever, and enterocolitis)
◆ *Urine, bone marrow, pus, and vomitus cultures:* causative organism
◆ *Stool culture (1 or more years after treatment):* S. typhi carrier (about 3% of patients)
◆ *Widal's test:* typhoid fever
◆ *Complete blood count:* transient leukocytosis (during first week of typhoidal *Salmonella* infection); leukopenia (during third week of typhoidal *Salmonella* infection); leukocytosis with local infection

Treatment

◆ Possible hospitalization for severe diarrhea
◆ Diet as tolerated with increased fluids and avoidance of milk products
◆ Activity as tolerated
◆ Surgical drainage of localized abscesses

MEDICATIONS

◆ I.V. fluids
◆ Electrolyte supplements
◆ Antipyretics
◆ Analgesics
◆ Antibiotics (possibly)

Nursing interventions

◆ Maintain enteric precautions until three consecutive stool cultures are negative.
◆ Assess the patient's hydration and nutritional status.
◆ Monitor vital signs and daily weight.
◆ Observe for signs and symptoms of complications.
◆ Administer I.V. fluid and electrolyte therapy as ordered.
◆ Provide skin and mouth care.
◆ Apply mild heat to relieve abdominal cramps.
◆ Report *Salmonella* cases to local public health officials.

PATIENT TEACHING

◆ Explain the disorder, diagnostic testing, and treatment plan.
◆ Teach about the administration, dosage, and possible adverse effects of prescribed medications.
◆ Stress the need for those in close contact with the patient to obtain a medical examination and treatment if cultures are positive.
◆ Explain how to prevent *Salmonella* infections.
◆ Stress the importance of proper hand washing.
◆ Explain the need to avoid preparing food for others until the *Salmonella* infection is eliminated.
◆ Arrange for follow-up with an infectious disease specialist or a gastroenterologist as needed.

Disorders

Seizure disorder

Overview

Seizure disorder, also known as *epilepsy*, is a neurologic condition characterized by recurrent seizure activity. In about 80% of patients, good seizure control can be achieved with strict adherence to prescribed treatment. Seizures may be partial (originating in one part of the brain) or generalized (involving electrical discharges throughout the entire brain).

CAUSES
◆ Idiopathic in 50% of cases

Nonidiopathic seizure disorder
◆ Anoxia
◆ Apparent familial incidence in some seizure disorders
◆ Birth trauma
◆ Brain tumors or other space-occupying lesions
◆ Genetic abnormalities (tuberous sclerosis and phenylketonuria)
◆ Ingestion of toxins, such as mercury, lead, or carbon monoxide
◆ Meningitis, encephalitis, or brain abscess
◆ Metabolic abnormalities (hypoglycemia, pyridoxine deficiency, hypoparathyroidism)
◆ Perinatal infection
◆ Perinatal injuries
◆ Stroke
◆ Traumatic injury

PATHOPHYSIOLOGY
◆ Seizures are paroxysmal events involving abnormal electrical discharges of neurons in the brain and cell membrane potential.
◆ On stimulation, the neuron fires, the discharge spreads to surrounding cells, and stimulation continues to one side or both sides of the brain, resulting in seizure activity.

COMPLICATIONS
◆ Anoxia
◆ Traumatic injury

Assessment

HISTORY
◆ Anoxia
◆ Seizure occurrence that's unpredictable and unrelated to activities
◆ Headache
◆ Head trauma
◆ Drug use
◆ Family history of seizure disorder
◆ Myoclonic jerking
◆ Description of an aura
◆ Unusual taste in the mouth
◆ Vision disturbance

PHYSICAL FINDINGS
◆ Related to underlying cause of the seizure
◆ Possibly normal findings while patient isn't having a seizure and when the cause is idiopathic

DIAGNOSTIC TEST RESULTS
◆ *EEG:* paroxysmal abnormalities
◆ *Computed tomography scan and magnetic resonance imaging:* internal structure abnormalities
◆ *Skull X-ray:* certain neoplasms within the brain substance, skull fractures
◆ *Brain scan:* malignant lesions
◆ *Cerebral angiography:* cerebrovascular abnormalities, such as aneurysm or tumor
◆ *Lumbar puncture:* abnormal cerebrospinal fluid pressure, indicating an infection

Treatment

- Airway protection during a seizure
- Vagus nerve stimulation
- Surgery, when indicated, in medically intractable patients screened for seizure type, frequency, site of onset, psychological functioning, and degree of disability
- Use of safety measures
- Removal of a demonstrated focal lesion
- Correction of the underlying cause (if applicable)

MEDICATIONS

- Anticonvulsants
- Lorazepam (Ativan) during a seizure

Nursing interventions

- Maintain a patent airway.
- Institute seizure precautions.
- Observe the patient for seizure activity; record the type and length of the seizure.
- Monitor the patient's vital signs.
- Give prescribed anticonvulsants and evaluate the patient's response.
- Protect the patient from injury during seizures.
- Promote the patient's self-esteem.
- Prepare the patient for surgery if indicated.

PATIENT TEACHING

- Explain the disorder, diagnostic testing, and treatment plan.
- Teach about the administration, dosage, and possible adverse effects of prescribed medications.
- Explain safety measures needed during seizure activity.
- Stress the importance of carrying a medical identification card or wearing medical identification jewelry.
- Refer the patient to the Epilepsy Foundation of America.
- Refer the patient to his state's motor vehicle department for information regarding driving.

Severe acute respiratory syndrome

Disorders

Overview

Severe acute respiratory syndrome (SARS) is a severe viral infection that may progress to pneumonia. Believed to be less infectious than influenza and having an estimated incubation period of 2 to 7 days (average, 3 to 5 days), it isn't highly contagious when protective measures are used.

CAUSES
◆ SARS-associated coronavirus (SARS-CoV)

RISK FACTORS
◆ Close contact with an infected person's exhaled droplets and bodily secretions
◆ Travel to endemic areas

PATHOPHYSIOLOGY
◆ Coronaviruses cause diseases in pigs, birds, and other animals.
◆ A coronavirus may have mutated, allowing infection of humans.

COMPLICATIONS
◆ Respiratory difficulties
◆ Severe thrombocytopenia (low platelet count)
◆ Heart failure
◆ Liver failure
◆ Death

Assessment

HISTORY
◆ Contact with a person known to have SARS
◆ Travel to an endemic area
◆ Flulike symptoms
◆ Headache
◆ Diarrhea
◆ Nausea and vomiting

PHYSICAL FINDINGS
◆ Nonproductive cough
◆ Rash
◆ High fever
◆ Respiratory distress in later stages

DIAGNOSTIC TEST RESULTS
◆ *Coronavirus antibodies:* presence of coronavirus antibodies
◆ *Sputum Gram stain and culture:* coronavirus identified
◆ *Platelet count:* low
◆ *Chest X-rays:* pneumonia or infiltrates
◆ *SARS-specific polymerase chain reaction test:* SARS-CoV ribonucleic acid
◆ *Enzyme-linked immunosorbent assay and immunofluorescent antibody test (a more sensitive test in development):* presence of coronavirus antibodies

Treatment

◆ Symptomatic treatment
◆ Isolation for hospitalized patients
◆ Strict respiratory and mucosal barrier precautions
◆ Quarantine of exposed people to prevent spread of the infection
◆ Global surveillance and reporting of suspected cases to national health authorities

MEDICATIONS
◆ Antivirals
◆ Combination of steroids and antimicrobials
◆ Oxygen therapy

Nursing interventions

◆ Provide oxygen therapy and monitor arterial blood gas results.
◆ Monitor the patient's vital signs, pulse oximetry, cardiac rhythm, and laboratory values.
◆ Maintain proper isolation technique.
◆ Give prescribed drugs.
◆ Assess the patient's respiratory, hydration, and nutritional status.
◆ Observe, record, and report the nature of rash.
◆ Observe for signs and symptoms of complications.

PATIENT TEACHING

◆ Explain the disorder, diagnostic testing, and treatment plan.
◆ Teach about the administration, dosage, and possible adverse effects of prescribed medications.
◆ Stress the importance of frequent hand washing and covering the mouth and nose when coughing or sneezing.
◆ Explain the need to avoid close personal contact with friends and family.
◆ Explain isolation needs, and the need to avoid sharing close personal objects or food.
◆ Refer the patient for follow-up care as needed.

Severe combined immunodeficiency disease

Overview

Severe combined immunodeficiency disease (SCID), also known as *graft-versus-host disease,* is a disorder that involves deficient or absent cell-mediated (T cell) and humoral (B cell) immunity. It predisposes infants to infection from all classes of microorganisms. SCID is classified as reticular dysgenesis (the most severe type), Swiss-type agammaglobulinemia, or enzyme deficiency.

CAUSES
◆ Failure of the thymus or bursa equivalent to develop normally
◆ Possible defect in the thymus and bone marrow, which are responsible for T- and B-cell development
◆ Possible enzyme deficiency
◆ Transmitted as autosomal recessive trait but may be X linked

RISK FACTORS
◆ Family history of SCID

PATHOPHYSIOLOGY
◆ With reticular dysgenesis, the hematopoietic stem cell fails to differentiate into lymphocytes and granulocytes.
◆ With Swiss-type agammaglobulinemia, the hematopoietic stem cell fails to differentiate into lymphocytes alone.
◆ With enzyme deficiency, such as adenosine deaminase deficiency, the buildup of toxic products in the lymphoid tissue causes damage and subsequent dysfunction.

COMPLICATIONS
◆ Death, if infection within 1 year of birth isn't treated
◆ Pneumonia
◆ Oral ulcers
◆ Failure to thrive
◆ Dermatitis

Assessment

HISTORY
◆ Extreme susceptibility to infection within the first few months after birth, but probably no sign of gram-negative infection until about age 6 months because of protection by maternal immunoglobulin G

PHYSICAL FINDINGS
◆ Emaciated appearance and failure to thrive
◆ Assessment findings dependent on the type and site of infection
◆ Signs of chronic otitis media and sepsis
◆ Signs of the usual childhood diseases such as chickenpox

DIAGNOSTIC TEST RESULTS
◆ *Defective humoral immunity:* difficult to detect before age 5 months
◆ *T-lymphocyte count:* severely decreased or absent T-cell number and function
◆ *Chest X-ray:* bilateral pulmonary infiltrates
◆ *Lymph node biopsy:* absence of lymphocytes
◆ *B-lymphocyte count:* decreased

Treatment

◆ Strict protective isolation
◆ Gene therapy (experimental)
◆ Activity as tolerated
◆ Histocompatible bone marrow transplantation
◆ Fetal thymus and liver transplantation
◆ Stem cell transplant

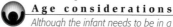 **Age considerations**
Although the infant needs to be in a germ-free environment, parent-child interactions and as much activity as possible are encouraged.

MEDICATIONS
◆ Immunoglobulin
◆ Antibiotics

Nursing interventions

◆ If infection develops, watch for adverse effects of drugs given.
◆ Avoid vaccinations, and give only irradiated blood products if a transfusion is ordered.
◆ Encourage parent-child interaction.
◆ Provide emotional support for the patient's family.
◆ Observe for signs and symptoms of infection, then provide prompt and aggressive drug therapy and supportive care as ordered.
◆ Evaluate the patient's growth and development.
◆ Assess the patient's respiratory status and skin integrity.
◆ Evaluate the patient's response to treatment.
◆ Observe for signs and symptoms of complications.

PATIENT TEACHING
◆ Explain the disorder, diagnostic testing, and treatment plan.
◆ Teach about the administration, dosage, and possible adverse effects of prescribed medications.
◆ Explain the proper technique for strict protective isolation.
◆ Describe the signs and symptoms of infection and when to notify the practitioner.
◆ Encourage the parents to seek genetic counseling.

Shock, cardiogenic

Overview

Cardiogenic shock, also called *pump failure,* is a condition of diminished cardiac output that severely impairs tissue perfusion. It's the most lethal form of shock and typically affects patients with a myocardial infarction (MI) involving 40% or more of left ventricular muscle mass (a group in which mortality may exceed 85%).

Causes
◆ Acute mitral or aortic insufficiency
◆ End-stage cardiomyopathy
◆ MI (most common)
◆ Myocardial ischemia
◆ Myocarditis
◆ Papillary muscle dysfunction
◆ Ventricular aneurysm
◆ Ventricular septal defect

Pathophysiology
◆ Left ventricular dysfunction initiates a series of compensatory mechanisms that attempt to increase cardiac output.
◆ As cardiac output decreases, aortic and carotid baroreceptors activate sympathetic nervous responses.
◆ These responses increase heart rate, left ventricular filling pressure, and peripheral resistance to flow to enhance venous return to the heart.
◆ The patient initially stabilizes but later deteriorates because of increased oxygen demands on the already compromised myocardium.
◆ These events consist of a cycle of low cardiac output, sympathetic compensation, myocardial ischemia, and even lower cardiac output.

Complications
◆ Multiple organ dysfunction
◆ Death

Assessment

History
◆ Disorder, such as MI or cardiomyopathy, that severely decreases left ventricular function
◆ Anginal pain

Physical findings
◆ Severe anxiety that may progress to decreased sensorium
◆ Pale, cold, clammy skin
◆ Rapid, shallow respirations
◆ Rapid, thready pulse
◆ Mean arterial pressure of less than 60 mm Hg in adults
◆ Gallop rhythm, faint heart sounds and, possibly, a holosystolic murmur
◆ Jugular vein distention
◆ Pulmonary crackles
◆ Urine output less than 20 ml/hour

Diagnostic test results
◆ *Serum enzyme measurements:* elevated levels of creatine kinase, lactate dehydrogenase, aspartate aminotransferase, and alanine aminotransferase
◆ *Troponin levels:* elevated
◆ *Cardiac catheterization and echocardiography:* cardiac tamponade, papillary muscle infarct or rupture, ventricular septal rupture, pulmonary emboli, venous pooling, and hypovolemia
◆ *Pulmonary artery pressure monitoring:* increased pulmonary artery pressure and pulmonary artery wedge pressure, increase in left ventricular end-diastolic pressure (preload), heightened resistance to left ventricular emptying (afterload), increased peripheral vascular resistance
◆ *Invasive arterial pressure monitoring:* systolic arterial pressure of less than 80 mm Hg
◆ *Arterial blood gas (ABG) analysis:* metabolic and respiratory acidosis and hypoxia
◆ *Electrocardiography:* injury pattern consistent with acute MI
◆ *Echocardiogram:* akinetic areas of ventricular wall function

Treatment

- Supportive measures for life-threatening signs and symptoms
- Intra-aortic balloon pump (IABP)
- Possible parenteral nutrition or tube feedings
- Bed rest
- Possible ventricular assist device
- Possible heart transplant

MEDICATIONS

- Oxygen therapy
- Vasopressors
- Inotropics
- Analgesics
- Sedatives
- Osmotic diuretics
- Vasodilators
- Antiarrhythmics

Nursing interventions

- Administer oxygen therapy and monitor ABG results.
- Monitor the patient's vital signs, cardiac rhythm, pulse oximetry, intake and output, and laboratory values.
- Assess the patient's cardiovascular and respiratory status.
- Assess the patient's pain level, administer analgesics, and evaluate their effects.
- Treat the underlying condition as ordered.
- Provide frequent rest periods.
- Follow IABP protocols and policies.
- Observe for signs and symptoms of complications.
- Provide emotional support.
- Reposition the patient every 2 hours and provide skin care.
- Apply sequential compression stockings while in bed.

PATIENT TEACHING

- Explain the disorder, diagnostic testing, and treatment plan.
- Teach about the administration, dosage, and possible adverse effects of prescribed medications.
- Explain the underlying cause and potential prognosis.
- Explain procedures and equipment.
- After recovery, stress the need for follow-up care.
- Refer the patient to cardiac rehabilitation as appropriate.

Shock, hypovolemic

Overview

Hypovolemic shock is a potentially life-threatening condition caused by a loss of blood, plasma, or fluids. It results in circulatory dysfunction and inadequate tissue perfusion.

CAUSES
◆ Acute blood loss (about one-fifth of total volume)
◆ Acute pancreatitis
◆ Ascites
◆ Burns
◆ Dehydration from excessive perspiration, severe diarrhea, protracted vomiting, diabetes insipidus, diuresis, or inadequate fluid intake
◆ Diuretic abuse
◆ Intestinal obstruction
◆ Peritonitis

PATHOPHYSIOLOGY
◆ When fluid is lost from the intravascular space, venous return to the heart is reduced.
◆ Ventricular filling decreases, which leads to a drop in stroke volume.
◆ Cardiac output falls, causing reduced perfusion to tissues and organs.
◆ Tissue anoxia prompts a shift in cellular metabolism from aerobic to anaerobic pathways.
◆ Lactic acid accumulates, resulting in metabolic acidosis.

COMPLICATIONS
◆ Acute respiratory distress syndrome
◆ Acute respiratory failure
◆ Acute tubular necrosis and renal failure
◆ Disseminated intravascular coagulation (DIC)
◆ Multiple organ dysfunction
◆ Death

Assessment

HISTORY
◆ Blood or fluid loss
◆ Trauma

PHYSICAL FINDINGS
◆ Pale, cool, clammy skin
◆ Decreased sensorium
◆ Rapid, shallow respirations
◆ Rapid, thready pulse
◆ Mean arterial pressure of less than 60 mm Hg in adults (in chronic hypotension, mean pressure possibly below 50 mm Hg before signs of shock)
◆ Orthostatic vital signs and tilt test results consistent with hypovolemic shock
◆ Urine output less than 20 ml/hour

DIAGNOSTIC TEST RESULTS
◆ *Hematocrit:* low
◆ *Hemoglobin levels, red blood cell and platelet counts:* decreased
◆ *Serum potassium, sodium, lactate dehydrogenase, creatinine, and blood urea nitrogen levels:* elevated
◆ *Urine specific gravity:* greater than 1.020
◆ *Urine osmolality:* increased
◆ *Partial pressure of arterial oxygen and pH:* decreased
◆ *Partial pressure of arterial carbon dioxide:* increased
◆ *Nasogastric tube aspiration of gastric contents:* internal bleeding.
◆ *Occult blood tests:* positive
◆ *Coagulation studies:* coagulopathy from DIC
◆ *Chest or abdominal X-rays:* internal bleeding sites
◆ *Gastroscopy:* internal bleeding sites
◆ *Invasive hemodynamic monitoring:* reduced central venous pressure, right atrial pressure, pulmonary artery pressure, pulmonary artery wedge pressure, and cardiac output

Treatment

◆ Supportive treatment of life-threatening signs and symptoms
◆ Blood transfusions
◆ Intra-aortic balloon pump, ventricular assist device, or pneumatic antishock garment in severe cases
◆ Direct application of pressure and related measures for bleeding control
◆ Possible parenteral nutrition or tube feedings
◆ Bed rest
◆ Surgery to correct the underlying problem if appropriate

MEDICATIONS
◆ I.V. fluids
◆ Positive inotropics
◆ Oxygen therapy

Nursing interventions

◆ Maintain a patent airway and adequate circulation, and provide oxygen therapy.
◆ Apply pressure to bleeding sites, if able.
◆ Administer I.V. fluids and blood products as ordered.
◆ Monitor the patient's vital signs, cardiac rhythm, pulse oximetry, intake and output, and laboratory values.
◆ Assess the patient's cardiovascular, respiratory status, hydration, and nutritional status
◆ Provide emotional support.

PATIENT TEACHING
◆ Explain the disorder, diagnostic testing, and treatment plan.
◆ Teach about the administration, dosage, and possible adverse effects of prescribed medications.
◆ Explain procedures and their purpose.
◆ Describe the risks associated with blood transfusions
◆ Explain the purpose of all equipment such as mechanical ventilation.
◆ Describe care of the underlying disorder as appropriate.

Shock, septic

Overview

Septic shock is a response to infections that release microbes or an immune mediator. It results in low systemic vascular resistance and an elevated cardiac output. Patients with septic shock exhibit evidence of systemic inflammatory response syndrome (SIRS), in which patients have two or more of these conditions: temperature greater than 100.4° F (38°C) or less than 96.8° F (36° C), heart rate greater than 90 beats/minute, respiratory rate greater than 20 breaths/minute, white blood cell count higher than 12,000/mm³ or lower than 4,000 mm³ with more than 10% of cells being immature.

CAUSES
◆ Any pathogenic organism
◆ Gram-negative bacteria, such as *Escherichia coli*, *Klebsiella pneumoniae*, Serratia, Enterobacter, and Pseudomonas (most common causes; up to 70% of cases)
◆ Gram-positive bacteria, such as *Staphylococcus aureus*, *Listeria*, *Clostridium*, and *Bacillus*

RISK FACTORS
◆ Impaired immunity
◆ Young or old age

PATHOPHYSIOLOGY
◆ Initially, the body's defenses activate chemical mediators in response to the invading organisms.
◆ The release of these mediators results in low systemic vascular resistance and increased cardiac output.
◆ Blood flow is unevenly distributed in the microcirculation, and plasma leaking from capillaries causes functional hypovolemia.
◆ Diffuse increase in capillary permeability occurs.
◆ Eventually, cardiac output decreases, and poor tissue perfusion and hypotension cause multisystem dysfunction syndrome and death.

COMPLICATIONS
◆ Disseminated intravascular coagulation
◆ Renal failure
◆ Heart failure
◆ GI ulcers
◆ Abnormal liver function
◆ Death

Assessment

HISTORY
◆ Immunosuppression-causing disorder or treatment
◆ Previous invasive tests or treatments, surgery, or trauma
◆ Fever and chills (although 20% of patients hypothermic)

PHYSICAL FINDINGS
Hyperdynamic (warm) phase
◆ Peripheral vasodilation
◆ Skin possibly pink and flushed or warm and dry
◆ Altered level of consciousness (LOC), evidenced by agitation, anxiety, irritability, and shortened attention span
◆ Rapid and shallow respirations
◆ Urine output below normal
◆ Rapid, full, bounding pulse
◆ Blood pressure normal or slightly elevated

Hypodynamic (cold) phase
◆ Peripheral vasoconstriction and inadequate tissue perfusion
◆ Pale skin and possible cyanosis
◆ Decreased LOC; possible obtundation and coma
◆ Respirations possibly rapid and shallow
◆ Urine output possibly absent or less than 25 ml/hour
◆ Rapid, weak, thready pulse
◆ Irregular pulse (if arrhythmias are present)
◆ Cold, clammy skin
◆ Hypotension
◆ Crackles or rhonchi if pulmonary congestion is present

DIAGNOSTIC TEST RESULTS

♦ *Blood cultures:* causative organism
♦ *Complete blood count:* presence or absence of anemia and leukopenia, severe or absent neutropenia, and usually thrombocytopenia
♦ *Blood urea nitrogen and creatinine levels:* increased
♦ *Creatinine clearance:* decreased
♦ *Prothrombin time and partial thromboplastin time:* abnormal
♦ *Serum lactate dehydrogenase levels:* elevated with metabolic acidosis
♦ *Urine studies:* increased specific gravity (more than 1.02), increased osmolality, and decreased sodium levels
♦ *Arterial blood gas (ABG) analysis:* increased blood pH and partial pressure of arterial oxygen, decreased partial pressure of arterial carbon dioxide with respiratory alkalosis in early stages
♦ *Invasive hemodynamic monitoring:* increased cardiac output and decreased systemic vascular resistance in hyperdynamic phase, decreased cardiac output and increased systemic vascular resistance in hypodynamic phase

Treatment

♦ Supportive measures for life-threatening signs and symptoms
♦ Removal or replacement of I.V., intra-arterial, or urinary drainage catheters if possible
♦ Reduction or discontinuation of drug therapy in immunosuppressed patients if possible
♦ Fluid volume replacement
♦ Possible parenteral nutrition or tube feedings
♦ Bed rest

MEDICATIONS

♦ I.V. fluids
♦ Oxygen therapy
♦ Antimicrobials
♦ Granulocyte transfusions
♦ Colloid or crystalloid infusions
♦ Diuretics
♦ Vasopressors
♦ Antipyretics
♦ Drotrecogin alfa (Xigris)

Nursing interventions

♦ Assess the patient's cardiovascular and respiratory status.
♦ Monitor the patient's vital signs, cardiac rhythm, pulse oximetry, intake and output, and laboratory values.
♦ Administer oxygen therapy and monitor ABG results.
♦ Give prescribed I.V. fluids and blood products.
♦ Remove or replace I.V., intra-arterial, or urinary drainage catheters, and send them to the laboratory for culture.
♦ Give prescribed drugs.
♦ Provide emotional support to the patient and his family.
♦ Reposition the patient every 2 hours and provide skin care.
♦ Apply sequential compression stockings.
♦ Observe for signs and symptoms of complications.

PATIENT TEACHING

♦ Explain the disorder, diagnostic testing, and treatment plan.
♦ Teach about the administration, dosage, and possible adverse effects of prescribed medications.
♦ Explain all procedures and equipment and their purpose.
♦ Describe signs and symptoms of complications.
♦ After recovery, stress the importance of follow-up care.

Stroke

Overview

Stroke, also known as *cerebrovascular accident* or *brain attack,* is the sudden impairment of blood circulation to the brain, which deprives brain cells of oxygen. It's the third most common cause of death in the United States and the most common cause of neurologic disability.

CAUSES

◆ Cerebral thrombosis (most common cause); site may be extracerebral or intracerebral
◆ Cerebral embolism resulting from cardiac arrhythmias, endocarditis, rheumatic heart disease, open heart surgery, posttraumatic valvular disease (second most common cause)
◆ Cerebral hemorrhage caused by arteriovenous malformation, cerebral aneurysms, or chronic hypertension (third most common cause)

RISK FACTORS

◆ History of transient ischemic attack
◆ Heart disease
◆ Smoking
◆ Familial history of cerebrovascular disease
◆ Obesity
◆ Alcohol use
◆ Cardiac arrhythmias
◆ Diabetes mellitus
◆ Hypertension
◆ Hormonal contraceptive use in conjunction with smoking and hypertension
◆ High red blood cell count
◆ Elevated cholesterol and triglyceride levels

PATHOPHYSIOLOGY

◆ The oxygen supply to the brain is interrupted or diminished, affecting cerebral cell function.
◆ In thrombotic or embolic stroke, neurons die from lack of oxygen.
◆ In hemorrhagic stroke, impaired cerebral perfusion causes infarction.

COMPLICATIONS

◆ Infections
◆ Sensory or motor impairment
◆ Aspiration
◆ Contractures
◆ Skin breakdown
◆ Deep vein thrombosis
◆ Pulmonary emboli
◆ Depression
◆ Seizures

Assessment

HISTORY

◆ Varying clinical features, depending on artery affected, severity of damage, and extent of collateral circulation
◆ Presence of one or more risk factors
◆ Sudden onset of hemiparesis or hemiplegia
◆ Gradual onset of dizziness, mental disturbances, or seizures
◆ Loss of consciousness
◆ Sudden difficulty speaking or swallowing
◆ Headache

PHYSICAL FINDINGS

◆ Left hemisphere stroke (signs and symptoms on the right side)
◆ Right hemisphere stroke (signs and symptoms on the left side)
◆ Stroke that causes cranial nerve damage (signs and symptoms on same side)
◆ Change in level of consciousness
◆ Anxiety with communication and mobility difficulties
◆ Hemiparesis or hemiplegia on one side of the body
◆ Hemianopsia on the affected side of the body
◆ Urinary incontinence
◆ Loss of voluntary muscle control
◆ Decreased deep tendon reflexes
◆ Problems with visuospatial relations in left-sided hemiplegia
◆ Sensory losses

Diagnostic test results

♦ *Anticardiolipin antibodies, antiphospholipid, factor V mutation, antithrombin III, protein S, and protein C tests:* evidence of conditions that increase the risk of thrombosis formation

♦ *Magnetic resonance imaging and angiography:* location and size of lesion

♦ *Cerebral angiography (cerebral blood flow test of choice):* location of cerebral circulation disruption

♦ *Computed tomography scan:* structural abnormalities

♦ *Positron emission tomography:* cerebral metabolism and cerebral blood flow changes

♦ *Transcranial Doppler studies:* decreased cerebral blood flow

♦ *Carotid Doppler studies:* carotid artery stenosis or occlusion

♦ *Two-dimensional echocardiography:* heart dysfunction

♦ *Cerebral blood flow studies:* blood flow to the brain

♦ *Electrocardiography:* possible arrhythmia, especially atrial fibrillation (a common risk factor for stroke)

Treatment

♦ Supportive measures for life-threatening signs and symptoms
♦ Physical, speech, and occupational rehabilitation
♦ Pureed dysphagia diet or tube feedings, if indicated
♦ Craniotomy
♦ Endarterectomy
♦ Extracranial-intracranial bypass
♦ Ventricular shunts

MEDICATIONS

♦ Oxygen therapy
♦ Tissue plasminogen activator when the cause isn't hemorrhagic (emergency care within 3 hours of onset of the symptoms)
♦ Antihypertensives
♦ Antiarrhythmics
♦ Anticoagulants
♦ Anticonvulsants

♦ Stool softeners
♦ Analgesics
♦ Antidepressants
♦ Antiplatelets
♦ Lipid-lowering agents

Nursing interventions

♦ Maintain a patent airway and oxygenation.
♦ Assess the patient's neurologic and respiratory status.
♦ Monitor the patient's vital signs, cardiac rhythm, pulse oximetry, intake and output, and laboratory values.
♦ Assess the patient's gag and swallowing ability.
♦ Assist with meals as appropriate; maintain aspiration precautions if indicated.
♦ Assist the patient with active and passive range-of-motion exercises.
♦ Establish and maintain patient communication.
♦ Provide psychological support.
♦ Set realistic, short-term goals.
♦ Protect the patient from injury and complications.
♦ Reposition the patient every 2 hours and provide skin care.
♦ Apply sequential compression stockings while in bed.
♦ Give prescribed drugs.
♦ Provide assistive devices as needed.
♦ Observe for signs and symptoms of complications.

PATIENT TEACHING

♦ Explain the disorder, diagnostic testing, and treatment plan.
♦ Teach about the administration, dosage, and possible adverse effects of prescribed medications.
♦ Review stroke prevention measures.
♦ Explain dietary needs and aspiration precautions as appropriate.
♦ Review safety measures, and demonstrate how to use assistive devices.
♦ Refer the patient to home care, outpatient, and speech and occupational rehabilitation programs as needed.

Syndrome of inappropriate antidiuretic hormone

Overview

Syndrome of inappropriate antidiuretic hormone is a disease of the posterior pituitary marked by excessive release of antidiuretic hormone (ADH) (vasopressin). Prognosis depends on the underlying disorder and response to treatment.

CAUSES
◆ Central nervous system disorders
◆ Drugs
◆ Miscellaneous conditions, such as myxedema and psychosis
◆ Neoplastic diseases
◆ Oat cell carcinoma of the lung
◆ Pulmonary disorders

PATHOPHYSIOLOGY
◆ Excessive ADH secretion occurs in the absence of normal physiologic stimuli for its release.
◆ Excessive water reabsorption from the distal convoluted tubule and collecting ducts results in hyponatremia and normal to slightly increased extracellular fluid volume.

COMPLICATIONS
◆ Water intoxication
◆ Cerebral edema
◆ Severe hyponatremia
◆ Heart failure
◆ Seizures
◆ Coma
◆ Death

Assessment

HISTORY
◆ Cerebrovascular disease
◆ Cancer
◆ Pulmonary disease
◆ Recent head injury
◆ Anorexia, nausea, vomiting
◆ Weight gain
◆ Lethargy, headaches, emotional and behavioral changes

PHYSICAL FINDINGS
◆ Tachycardia
◆ Disorientation
◆ Seizures and coma
◆ Sluggish deep tendon reflexes
◆ Muscle weakness

DIAGNOSTIC TEST RESULTS
◆ *Serum osmolality levels:* less than 280 mOsm/kg
◆ *Serum sodium levels:* less than 123 mEq/L
◆ *Urine sodium levels:* more than 20 mEq/L without diuretics
◆ *Renal function tests:* normal

Treatment

◆ Based primarily on symptoms
◆ Correction of the underlying cause
◆ Restricted water intake (500 to 1,000 ml/day)
◆ High-salt, high-protein diet or urea supplements to enhance water excretion
◆ Surgery to treat underlying cause such as cancer

MEDICATIONS
◆ Conivaptan (Vaprisol)
◆ Demeclocycline (Declomycin) or lithium (Eskalith) for long-term treatment
◆ Loop diuretics if the patient has fluid overload or a history of heart failure or resists treatment
◆ 3% sodium chloride solution if serum sodium level is less than 120 mEq/L or if the patient is having seizures

Nursing interventions

◆ Monitor the patient's vital signs, cardiac rhythm, intake and output, and laboratory values.
◆ Assess the patient's neurologic and respiratory systems.
◆ Restrict fluids as ordered.
◆ Provide a safe environment and reorient as needed.
◆ Institute seizure precautions as needed.
◆ Give prescribed drugs.
◆ Observe for signs and symptoms of complications.

PATIENT TEACHING
◆ Explain the disorder, diagnostic testing, and treatment plan.
◆ Teach about the administration, dosage, and possible adverse effects of prescribed medications.
◆ Stress fluid restriction and discuss methods to decrease discomfort from thirst.
◆ Describe signs and symptoms that require immediate medical intervention.
◆ Stress the importance of follow-up care.

Systemic lupus erythematosus

Overview

Systemic lupus erythematosus (SLE) is a chronic inflammatory autoimmune disorder that affects connective tissues. Discoid lupus erythematosus, another form of the disorder, only affects the skin.

CAUSES
◆ Unknown

RISK FACTORS
◆ Stress
◆ Streptococcal or viral infections
◆ Exposure to sunlight or ultraviolet light
◆ Injury
◆ Surgery
◆ Exhaustion
◆ Immunization
◆ Pregnancy
◆ Abnormal estrogen metabolism

PATHOPHYSIOLOGY
◆ The body produces antibodies, such as antinuclear antibodies (ANAs), against its own cells.
◆ The formed antigen antibody complexes suppress the body's normal immunity and damage tissues.
◆ Patients with SLE produce antibodies against many different tissue components, such as red blood cells (RBCs), neutrophils, platelets, lymphocytes, and almost any organ or tissue in the body.

COMPLICATIONS
◆ Pleurisy
◆ Pleural effusions
◆ Pericarditis, myocarditis, endocarditis
◆ Coronary atherosclerosis
◆ Renal failure
◆ Seizures and mental dysfunction

Assessment

HISTORY
◆ Fever, anorexia, weight loss, malaise, fatigue, abdominal pain, nausea, vomiting, diarrhea, constipation, rash, and polyarthralgia
◆ Drug use (25 different drugs can cause an SLE-like reaction.)
◆ Irregular menstruation or amenorrhea, particularly during flare-ups
◆ Chest pain and dyspnea
◆ Emotional instability, psychosis, organic brain syndrome, headaches, irritability, and depression
◆ Oliguria, urinary frequency, dysuria, and bladder spasms

PHYSICAL FINDINGS
◆ Joint pain
◆ Raynaud's phenomenon
◆ Skin eruptions provoked or aggravated by sunlight or ultraviolet light
◆ Tachycardia, central cyanosis, and hypotension
◆ Altered level of consciousness, weakness of the extremities, and speech disturbances
◆ Skin lesions
◆ Butterfly rash over nose and cheeks
◆ Patchy alopecia (common)
◆ Vasculitis
◆ Lymph node enlargement (diffuse or local and nontender)
◆ Pericardial friction rub

DIAGNOSTIC TEST RESULTS
◆ *ANA:* positive in most patients with active SLE
◆ *Complete blood count with differential:* anemia and reduced white blood cell (WBC) count, decreased platelet count, and elevated erythrocyte sedimentation rate
◆ *Serum electrophoresis:* hypergammaglobulinemia

- *Urine studies:* RBCs, WBCs, urine casts, sediment, and significant protein loss (more than 3.5 g in 24 hours)
- *Complement studies:* decreased serum complement levels (C3 and C4)
- *C-reactive protein level:* increased during flare-ups
- *Rheumatoid factor:* positive in 30% to 40% of patients
- *Chest X-rays:* pleurisy or lupus pneumonitis
- *EEG:* abnormal (central nervous system involvement in about 70% of patients)
- *Renal biopsy:* SLE progression and extent of renal involvement
- *Skin biopsy:* immunoglobulin and complement deposition in dermal-epidermal junction

Treatment

- Use of sunscreen with sun protection factor of at least 15
- Dietary restrictions (if renal failure occurs)
- Regular exercise program
- Possible joint replacement

MEDICATIONS
- Nonsteroidal anti-inflammatory drugs
- Topical corticosteroid creams
- Fluorinated steroids
- Antimalarials
- Corticosteroids
- Cytotoxic drugs
- Antihypertensives

Nursing interventions

- Apply heat packs to relieve joint pain and stiffness.
- Encourage regular exercise to maintain full range-of-motion (ROM).
- If the patient has Raynaud's phenomenon, warm and protect the patient's hands and feet.

- Observe for signs and symptoms of organ involvement, such as decreased urine output, seizures, and peripheral neuropathy.
- Monitor urine, stools, and GI secretions for blood.
- Assess the patient's scalp for hair loss and the skin and mucous membranes for petechiae, bleeding, ulceration, pallor, and bruising.
- Evaluate the patient's response to treatment.
- Assess the patient's nutritional status.
- Institute seizure precautions and observe for seizure activity.

PATIENT TEACHING
- Explain the disorder, diagnostic testing, and treatment plan.
- Teach about the administration, dosage, and possible adverse effects of prescribed medications.
- Demonstrate ROM exercises and describe body alignment and postural techniques.
- Discuss ways to avoid infection, such as avoiding crowds and people with known infections.
- Describe the signs and symptoms of complications and when to notify the practitioner.
- Stress the importance of eating a balanced diet and the restrictions associated with prescribed drugs.
- Stress the importance of follow-up care.
- Explain the need to wear protective clothing and use sunscreen.
- Arrange for a physical therapy and occupational therapy consultation if musculoskeletal involvement compromises mobility.

Thrombocytopenia

Overview

Thrombocytopenia, the most common cause of hemorrhagic disorders, is a deficient number of circulating platelets, which can cause inadequate hemostasis.

CAUSES
◆ Congenital or acquired
◆ Decreased or defective platelet production
◆ Increased platelet destruction outside the marrow caused by an underlying disorder, such as cirrhosis of the liver, disseminated intravascular coagulation, or severe infection
◆ Sequestration (hypersplenism, hypothermia) or platelet loss
◆ Transient occurrence after a viral infection or infectious mononucleosis
◆ Drugs

PATHOPHYSIOLOGY
◆ Four mechanisms are responsible for the lack of platelets: decreased platelet production, decreased platelet survival, pooling of blood in the spleen, and intravascular dilation of circulating platelets.
◆ Megakaryocytes are giant cells in bone marrow that produce the marrow. Platelet production decreases when the number of megakaryocytes is reduced or when platelet production becomes dysfunctional.

COMPLICATIONS
◆ Hemorrhage
◆ Death

Assessment

HISTORY
◆ Sudden onset of petechiae and ecchymoses or bleeding into mucous membranes (GI, urinary, vaginal, or respiratory)
◆ Malaise, fatigue, and general weakness, with or without accompanying blood loss
◆ Use of one or several offending drugs (in acquired form)
◆ Menorrhagia

PHYSICAL FINDINGS
◆ Petechiae and ecchymoses, along with slow, continuous bleeding from any injuries or wounds
◆ Blood-filled bullae in the mouth

DIAGNOSTIC TEST RESULTS
◆ *Platelet count:* diminished, less than 100,000/µl
◆ *Bleeding time:* prolonged
◆ *Prothrombin and partial thromboplastin times:* normal
◆ *Bone marrow study:* low number of megakaryocytes; rules out malignant disease process

Treatment

◆ Removal of the offending agents (in drug-induced thrombocytopenia)
◆ Treatment of underlying disorder
◆ Well-balanced diet
◆ Rest periods between activities; strict bed rest during active bleeding
◆ Splenectomy

MEDICATIONS
◆ Platelet transfusions
◆ Corticosteroids
◆ Immune globulin

Nursing interventions

◆ Monitor the patient's vital signs, pulse oximetry, intake and output, and laboratory values.
◆ Observe for signs of bleeding.
◆ Administer blood products as ordered.
◆ Provide emotional support.
◆ Provide rest periods between activities.
◆ Protect the patient from injury.
◆ Avoid invasive procedures if possible.
◆ Maintain strict bed rest during active bleeding.

PATIENT TEACHING

◆ Explain the disorder, diagnostic testing, and treatment plan.
◆ Teach about the administration, dosage, and possible adverse effects of prescribed medications.
◆ Explain signs and symptoms of complications.
◆ Review safety measures.
◆ Stress the importance of avoiding aspirin in any form and other drugs that impair coagulation.
◆ Demonstrate how to examine the skin for ecchymoses and petechiae.
◆ Explain the importance of wearing medical identification jewelry and receiving follow-up care.

Tuberculosis

Overview

Tuberculosis (TB) is an acute or chronic lung infection characterized by pulmonary infiltrates and the formation of granulomas with caseation, fibrosis, and cavitation. The prognosis is excellent with proper treatment and compliance.

CAUSES
- *Mycobacterium tuberculosis* exposure
- Exposure to other strains of mycobacteria

RISK FACTORS
- Close contact with newly diagnosed TB patient
- History of prior TB exposure
- Multiple sexual partners
- Recent immigration from Africa, Asia, Mexico, or South America
- Gastrectomy
- History of silicosis, diabetes, malnutrition, cancer, Hodgkin's disease, or leukemia
- Drug and alcohol abuse
- Residence in nursing home, mental health facility, or prison
- Immunosuppression and use of corticosteroids
- Homelessness

PATHOPHYSIOLOGY
- Multiplication of the bacillus *M. tuberculosis* causes an inflammatory process in affected areas.
- A cell-mediated immune response follows, usually containing the infection within 4 to 6 weeks.
- The T-cell response results in the formation of granulomas around the bacilli, making them dormant. This confers immunity to subsequent infection.

- Bacilli within granulomas may remain viable for many years, resulting in a positive purified protein derivative or other skin test for TB.
- Active disease develops in 5% to 15% of those infected.
- Transmission occurs when an infected person coughs or sneezes.

COMPLICATIONS
- Respiratory failure
- Bronchopleural fistulas
- Pneumothorax
- Pleural effusion
- Pneumonia
- Infection of other body organs by small mycobacterial foci
- Liver involvement secondary to drug therapy

Assessment

HISTORY
With primary infection
- May be asymptomatic after a 4- to 8-week incubation period
- Weakness and fatigue
- Anorexia, weight loss
- Low-grade fever
- Night sweats

With reactivated infection
- Chest pain
- Productive cough for blood, or mucopurulent or blood-tinged sputum
- Low-grade fever

PHYSICAL FINDINGS
- Dullness over the affected area
- Crepitant crackles
- Bronchial breath sounds
- Wheezes
- Whispered pectoriloquy

DIAGNOSTIC TEST RESULTS
- *Tuberculin skin test:* positive in active and inactive tuberculosis
- *Stains and cultures of sputum, cerebrospinal fluid, urine, abscess drainage, or*

pleural fluid: presence of heat-sensitive, nonmotile, aerobic, acid-fast bacilli
◆ *Chest X-rays:* presence of nodular lesions, patchy infiltrates, cavity formation, scar tissue, and calcium deposits
◆ *Computed tomography or magnetic resonance imaging:* presence and extent of lung damage
◆ *Bronchoscopy specimens:* presence of heat-sensitive, nonmotile, aerobic, acid-fast bacilli

Treatment

◆ Droplet precautions
◆ Negative pressure isolation room
◆ Well-balanced, high-calorie diet
◆ Rest, initially; then activity as tolerated

MEDICATIONS
◆ Oxygen therapy
◆ Antitubercular therapy for at least 6 months with daily oral doses of isoniazid (Nydrazid), rifampin (Rifadin), and pyrazinamide, plus ethambutol (Myambutol) in some cases
◆ Second-line drugs, such as capreomycin (Capastat), streptomycin, aminosalicylic acid (para-aminosalicylic acid) (Paser), and cycloserine (Seromycin)

Nursing interventions

◆ Maintain droplet precautions.
◆ Monitor the patient's vital signs, pulse oximetry, intake and output, and daily weight.
◆ Assess the patient's respiratory status.
◆ Give drugs as ordered.
◆ Isolate the patient in a negative pressure room.
◆ Properly dispose of secretions.
◆ Provide adequate rest periods.
◆ Provide well-balanced, high-calorie foods.
◆ Perform chest physiotherapy.
◆ Provide supportive care.
◆ Observe for signs and symptoms of complications.

PATIENT TEACHING
◆ Explain the disorder, diagnostic testing, and treatment plan.
◆ Teach about the administration, dosage, and possible adverse effects of prescribed medications.
◆ Explain the need for isolation.
◆ Demonstrate how to perform postural drainage, chest percussion, and coughing and deep-breathing exercises.
◆ Stress the importance of regular follow-up examinations.
◆ Describe the signs and symptoms of recurring TB.
◆ Review dietary recommendations.
◆ Refer the patient to the American Lung Association for education and support.
◆ Refer the patient to a smoking-cessation program if indicated.

Ulcerative colitis

Overview

Ulcerative colitis is an episodic inflammatory chronic disease that causes ulcerations of the mucosa in the colon. It begins in the rectum and sigmoid colon and may extend into the entire colon, although it rarely affects the small intestine, except for the terminal ileum. It produces congestion, edema (leading to mucosal friability), and ulcerations. Ulcerative colitis ranges from a mild, localized disorder to fulminant disease that causes many complications.

CAUSES
- Exact cause unknown
- May be related to an abnormal immune response in the GI tract, possibly associated with genetic factors

RISK FACTORS
- Stress (may increase severity of an attack)
- Family history
- Jewish ancestry

PATHOPHYSIOLOGY
- The disorder primarily involves the mucosa and the submucosa of the bowel.
- Crypt abscesses and mucosal ulceration may occur.
- The mucosa typically appears granular and friable.
- The colon becomes a rigid, foreshortened tube.
- In severe ulcerative colitis, areas of hyperplastic growth occur, with swollen mucosa surrounded by inflamed mucosa with shallow ulcers.
- The submucosa and the circular and longitudinal muscles may be involved.

COMPLICATIONS
- Nutritional deficiencies
- Perineal sepsis
- Anal fissure, anal fistula
- Perirectal abscess
- Perforation of the colon
- Hemorrhage, anemia
- Toxic megacolon
- Cancer
- Coagulation defects
- Erythema nodosum on the face and arms
- Pyoderma gangrenosum on the legs and ankles
- Uveitis
- Pericholangitis, sclerosing cholangitis
- Cirrhosis
- Cholangiocarcinoma
- Ankylosing spondylitis
- Strictures
- Pseudopolyps, stenosis, and a perforated colon leading to peritonitis and toxemia
- Arthritis

Assessment

HISTORY
- Remission and exacerbation of symptoms
- Mild cramping and lower abdominal pain
- Recurrent bloody diarrhea as often as 10 to 25 times daily
- Nocturnal diarrhea
- Fatigue and weakness
- Anorexia and weight loss
- Nausea and vomiting

PHYSICAL FINDINGS
- Liquid stools with visible pus, mucus, and blood
- Possible abdominal distention
- Abdominal tenderness
- Perianal irritation, hemorrhoids, and fissures
- Jaundice
- Joint pain

DIAGNOSTIC TEST RESULTS
- *Stool specimen analysis:* blood, pus, and mucus, but no pathogenic organisms
- *Serum chemistry:* decreased serum levels of potassium and magnesium

- *Complete blood count:* decreased hemoglobin level and leukocytosis
- *Albumin level:* decreased
- *Erythrocyte sedimentation rate:* elevated (correlates with attack severity)
- *Barium enema:* disease extent and complications, such as strictures and carcinoma (not performed with active signs and symptoms)
- *Sigmoidoscopy:* rectal involvement including mucosal friability, decreased mucosal detail, thick inflammatory exudates, edema, and erosions
- *Colonoscopy:* disease extent, areas of stricture and pseudopolyps (not performed with active signs and symptoms)
- *Biopsy during colonoscopy:* diagnosis confirmation

Treatment

- I.V. fluid replacement
- Blood transfusions if needed
- Nothing by mouth if severe
- Parenteral nutrition with severe disease
- Supplemental feedings
- Rest periods during exacerbations
- Surgery (treatment of last resort): proctocolectomy with ileostomy, pouch ileostomy, ileoanal reservoir with loop ileostomy, or colectomy (after 10 years of active disease)

MEDICATIONS
- Corticotropin and adrenal corticosteroids
- Sulfasalazine (Azulfidine)
- Mesalamine (Lialda)
- Antispasmodics and antidiarrheals
- Fiber supplements

Nursing interventions

- Assess the patient's GI status.
- Monitor the patient's stools and laboratory values.
- Encourage the patient to verbalize his feelings and provide support.
- Provide diet therapy.
- Administer drug therapy.
- Give blood transfusions as ordered.
- Provide frequent rest periods.
- Observe for signs and symptoms of complications.
- Provide wound care after surgery.

PATIENT TEACHING
- Explain the disorder, diagnostic testing, and treatment plan.
- Teach about the administration, dosage, and possible adverse effects of prescribed medications.
- Explain prescribed dietary changes.
- Stress the importance of avoiding GI stimulants, such as caffeine, alcohol, and smoking.
- Demonstrate stoma care after a proctocolectomy and ileostomy.
- Stress the importance of regular physical examinations.
- Refer the patient to a smoking-cessation program if indicated.
- Refer the patient to an enterostomal therapist if appropriate.

Urinary tract infection, lower

Disorders

Overview

A lower urinary tract infection (UTI) is a bacterial infection that occurs as cystitis, an infection of the bladder, or urethritis, an infection of the urethra. Recurring and resistant bacterial flare-ups during therapy are possible. Lower UTIs are nearly 10 times more common in females than in males (except elderly males), probably because a female's anatomic features facilitate infection.

CAUSES

◆ Ascending infection by a single gram-negative, enteric bacterium, such as *Escherichia coli*, Klebsiella, Proteus, Enterobacter, Pseudomonas, and Serratia
◆ Simultaneous infection with multiple pathogens

RISK FACTORS

◆ Natural anatomic variations
◆ Inadequate fluid consumption
◆ Trauma or invasive procedures
◆ Urinary catheter
◆ Urinary tract obstructions
◆ Vesicourethral reflux
◆ Urinary stasis
◆ Diabetes
◆ Bowel incontinence
◆ Immobility

PATHOPHYSIOLOGY

◆ Local defense mechanisms in the bladder break down.
◆ Bacteria invade the bladder mucosa and multiply.
◆ Bacteria can't be readily eliminated by normal urination.
◆ The pathogen's resistance to prescribed antimicrobial therapy usually causes bacterial flare-up during treatment.
◆ Recurrent lower UTIs result from reinfection by the same organism or a new pathogen.

COMPLICATIONS

◆ Damage to the urinary tract lining
◆ Infection of adjacent organs and structures

Assessment

HISTORY

◆ Urinary urgency and frequency
◆ Bladder cramps or spasms
◆ Pruritus
◆ Feeling of warmth during urination
◆ Nocturia or dysuria
◆ Urethral discharge (in men)
◆ Lower back or flank pain
◆ Malaise and chills
◆ Nausea and vomiting

PHYSICAL FINDINGS

◆ Pain or tenderness over the bladder
◆ Hematuria
◆ Fever
◆ Cloudy, foul-smelling urine

DIAGNOSTIC TEST RESULTS

◆ *Microscopic urinalysis:* red blood cell and white blood cell counts greater than 10 per high-power field
◆ *Bacterial count from clean catch:* more than 100,000/ml
◆ *Sensitivity testing:* identification of the organism, which guides antimicrobial therapy
◆ *Blood test or urethral discharge stained smear:* presence of sexually transmitted diseases
◆ *Voiding cystourethrography or excretory urography:* presence of congenital anomalies

Treatment

◆ Sitz baths or warm compresses
◆ Increased fluid intake

MEDICATIONS
◆ Antimicrobials

Nursing interventions

◆ Administer drug therapy.
◆ Encourage increased oral fluid intake unless contraindicated.
◆ Provide sitz baths or warm compresses as needed.
◆ Monitor the patient's intake and output.
◆ Evaluate urine characteristics and voiding patterns.

PATIENT TEACHING
◆ Explain the disorder, diagnostic testing, and treatment plan.
◆ Teach about the administration, dosage, and possible adverse effects of prescribed medications.
◆ Advise the patient to use warm sitz baths to relieve perineal discomfort.
◆ Teach about proper hygiene after toileting.

Vancomycin-resistant enterococci

Overview

Vancomycin-resistant enterococci (VRE) are mutations of common bacteria. Infection easily spreads by direct person-to-person contact.

CAUSES
◆ Direct contact with an infected or a colonized patient or a colonized health care worker
◆ Contact with a contaminated surface such as an overbed table.

RISK FACTORS
◆ Immunocompromised condition
◆ Old age
◆ Indwelling catheter
◆ Major surgery
◆ Open wounds
◆ History of taking vancomycin or a third-generation cephalosporin
◆ History of enterococcal bacteremia, often linked to endocarditis
◆ Organ transplantation
◆ Prolonged or repeated hospital admissions
◆ Chronic renal failure
◆ Exposure to contaminated equipment or a VRE-positive patient

PATHOPHYSIOLOGY
◆ Genes encode resistance and are carried on plasmids that transfer themselves from cell to cell.
◆ Resistance is mediated by enzymes that substitute a different molecule for the terminal amino acid so that vancomycin can't bind.

COMPLICATIONS
◆ Sepsis

Assessment

HISTORY
◆ Possible breach in the immune system, surgery, or condition predisposing the patient to the infection
◆ Multiple antibiotic use

PHYSICAL FINDINGS
◆ Carrier commonly asymptomatic

DIAGNOSTIC TEST RESULTS
◆ *Stool or a rectal swab*: presence of VRE

Treatment

◆ Contact isolation until the patient is culture-negative or discharged
◆ Rest periods when fatigued

MEDICATIONS
◆ Antimicrobials (VRE isolates not susceptible to vancomycin are generally susceptible to other antimicrobial drugs.)

Nursing interventions

◆ Consider grouping infected patients together and having the same nursing staff care for them.
◆ Institute contact isolation precautions.
◆ Ensure judicious and careful use of antibiotics. Encourage physicians to limit the use of antibiotics.
◆ Use infection-control practices, such as wearing gloves and employing proper hand-washing techniques, to reduce the spread of VRE.
◆ Monitor the patient's vital signs.
◆ Evaluate the patient's response to treatment.
◆ Observe for signs and symptoms of complications.

PATIENT TEACHING

◆ Explain the disorder, diagnostic testing, and treatment plan.
◆ Teach about the administration, dosage, and possible adverse effects of prescribed medications.
◆ Stress the importance of family and friends wearing personal protective equipment when visiting the patient.
◆ Explain proper protective equipment disposal and hand-washing techniques (see *Taking precautions at home*).

Taking precautions at home

Tell the caregivers of a patient infected with VRE to:
◆ wash their hands with soap and water after physical contact with the patient and before leaving the home
◆ use towels only once when drying hands after contact
◆ wear disposable gloves if they expect to come in contact with the patient's body fluids and to wash their hands after removing the gloves
◆ change linens routinely and whenever they become soiled
◆ clean the patient's environment routinely and when it becomes soiled with body fluids
◆ tell practitioners and other health care personnel caring for the patient that the patient is infected with an organism resistant to multiple drugs.

West Nile encephalitis

Overview

West Nile encephalitis, also called *West Nile virus,* is an infectious disease that's part of a family of vector-borne diseases that also includes malaria, yellow fever, and Lyme disease. The mortality rate ranges from 3% to 15% and is higher in the elderly population.

CAUSES
◆ A flavivirus commonly found in humans, birds, and other vertebrates in Africa, West Asia, and the Middle East

RISK FACTORS
◆ Recent chemotherapy
◆ Recent organ transplantation
◆ Immunocompromised state
◆ Pregnancy
◆ Advanced age
◆ Breast-feeding

PATHOPHYSIOLOGY
◆ The virus is transmitted to a human by the bite of an infected mosquito (mostly the Culex species).
◆ The virus has an incubation period of 5 to 15 days after exposure.
◆ Inflammation or encephalitis of the brain occurs.

COMPLICATIONS
◆ Neurologic impairment
◆ Seizures
◆ Bronchial pneumonia
◆ Death

Assessment

HISTORY
◆ Headache
◆ Myalgia
◆ Neck stiffness
◆ Possible recent exposure to bodies of water or dead birds, or recent mosquito bites
◆ Decreased appetite
◆ Nausea
◆ Vomiting
◆ Diarrhea

PHYSICAL FINDINGS
◆ Fever
◆ Rash
◆ Swollen lymph glands
◆ Stupor and disorientation
◆ Stiff neck
◆ Change in mental status
◆ Malaise
◆ Sore throat

DIAGNOSTIC TEST RESULTS
◆ *White blood cell (WBC) count:* normal or increased
◆ *Enzyme-linked immunosorbent assay (ELISA) and the IgM Antibody Capture ELISA:* positive for flavivirus
◆ *Serum or cerebrospinal fluid specimen analysis:* elevated WBC count and protein levels during acute illness

Treatment

◆ Respiratory support
◆ Increased fluid intake
◆ Rest periods when fatigued

MEDICATIONS
◆ Antipyretics
◆ Oxygen therapy

Nursing interventions

◆ Assess the patient's neurologic, hydration, and nutrition status.
◆ Assess the patient's respiratory status and provide oxygen therapy if needed.
◆ Administer I.V. fluids.
◆ Give prescribed medications.
◆ Follow standard precautions when handling blood or other body fluids.
◆ Report suspected cases of West Nile encephalitis to the state department of health.
◆ Monitor the patient's vital signs, pulse oximetry, intake and output, and laboratory values.
◆ Observe for signs and symptoms of complications.

PATIENT TEACHING

◆ Explain the disorder, diagnostic testing, and treatment plan.
◆ Teach about the administration, dosage, and possible adverse effects of prescribed medications.
◆ Discuss measures to prevent West Nile encephalitis (see *Preventing West Nile encephalitis*).
◆ Explain the expected course and outcomes of the illness.
◆ Stress the importance of drinking fluids to avoid dehydration.
◆ Refer the patient to an infectious disease specialist.

Preventing West Nile encephalitis

Advise patients to take these steps to reduce the risk of infection with West Nile encephalitis.
◆ Stay indoors at dawn and dusk and in early evening when mosquitoes are biting.
◆ Wear long-sleeved shirts and long pants when outdoors.
◆ Apply insect repellent sparingly to exposed skin. Effective repellents contain 20% to 30% DEET (N,N-diethyl-m-toluamide). DEET in high concentrations (greater than 30%) can cause adverse effects, particularly in children, and should be avoided. Repellant used on children should be applied by adults and should contain no more than 10% DEET.
◆ Don't place repellent under clothing.
◆ Don't apply repellent over cuts, wounds, sunburn, or irritated skin.
◆ Wash repellent off daily and reapply as needed
◆ Stop mosquitoes from breeding near the home by cleaning out birdbaths and wading pools at least weekly, cleaning roof gutters and downspout screens, eliminating any standing water, not allowing water to collect in trash cans, and turning over or removing containers in yards where rainwater collects.

II Treatments

Abdominal aortic aneurysm repair or resection

Overview

An abdominal aortic aneurysm (AAA), an abnormal widening of part of the aorta that's usually caused by inflammatory changes within the arterial walls, may be corrected with open surgical repair or endovascular repair. Open surgical repair involves resecting and replacing an aortic section with a vascular graft (patient's or donor's vein) or a synthetic polymer graft (polytetrafluoroethylene, Dacron, Teflon, or Gore-Tex). Endovascular grafting repair is performed under fluoroscopy with a local or regional anesthetic.

INDICATIONS
◆ Aneurysm greater than 4 cm in diameter
◆ Widening, leaking, or ruptured aneurysm

COMPLICATIONS
◆ Hemorrhage or hypovolemic shock from rupture
◆ Left-sided heart failure
◆ Arrhythmia
◆ Myocardial infarction
◆ Renal failure
◆ Lower extremity ischemia or embolization
◆ Infection
◆ Endovascular graft rejection or migration

Pretreatment care

◆ Verify that the patient signed an informed consent form, and complete a preoperative checklist.
◆ Ensure that the patient has a patent I.V. access.
◆ Assist with insertion of a pulmonary artery catheter and arterial pressure monitoring catheter if ordered.
◆ Assess baseline vital signs, cardiac rhythm, and peripheral pulses.
◆ Obtain baseline laboratory values, especially noting renal studies and complete blood count.
◆ Administer ordered medications.

PATIENT TEACHING
◆ Explain the surgery to the patient and his family and why it's being performed.
◆ Describe what the patient should expect after surgery, including factors such as being on a ventilator, having a nasogastric (NG) tube, and being connected to monitoring devices in the critical care unit.
◆ Show the client how to perform coughing and deep-breathing exercises and how to use an incentive spirometer.
◆ Answer all questions and provide emotional support.

Procedure

◆ Before elective surgery, medications such as I.V. nitroprusside (Nitropress) (to maintain blood pressure at 100 to 120 mm Hg systolic) and an analgesic (to relieve pain) may be required.

OPEN SURGICAL REPAIR
◆ Surgery requires general anesthesia.
◆ The surgeon makes an abdominal incision to expose the aneurysm.
◆ Clamps are applied to the aorta above and below the aneurysm.
◆ The aneurysm sac is opened and the aneurysm is resected.
◆ A prothetic graft is sewn into place and carefully tested for leakage.

ENDOVASCULAR REPAIR
◆ This type of surgery is appropriate for uncomplicated AAAs beginning below the left renal artery.
◆ The procedure is performed under fluoroscopy with a local or regional anesthetic.

◆ The access site in the femoral or iliac artery is prepared.
◆ A delivery catheter with an attached compressed graft is inserted over a guide wire.
◆ The delivery catheter is advanced to the aorta where it's positioned across the aneurysm.
◆ A balloon inside the graft expands the aorta and right femoral segments and affixes them to the vessel walls where they're sewn in place.

Posttreatment care

◆ Monitor cardiac rhythm, vital signs, pulse oximetry, and hemodynamic parameters per unit policy and clinical status.
◆ Assess cardiovascular and respiratory status every 2 hours or per clinical status.
◆ Measure hourly urine output and record intake and output.
◆ Maintain ventilator settings and alarms; perform pulmonary hygiene measures, including suctioning and chest physiotherapy.
◆ Reposition the patient every 2 hours, assess skin integrity, and provide skin care.
◆ Perform wound care as ordered and assess incision site for signs of infection.
◆ Maintain NG tube patency and assess GI status.
◆ Assess the patient's pain level, administer analgesics, and evaluate their effects.
◆ Administer medications as ordered.
◆ Provide deep vein thrombosis prophylaxis such as sequential compression stockings.

PATIENT TEACHING
◆ Reinforce instructions for controlling hypertension, including the importance of medication and diet therapy and the need for smoking cessation, if indicated.

◆ Teach about the administration, dosage, and possible adverse effects of prescribed medications.
◆ Review activity restrictions.
◆ Explain wound care needs and follow-up care.
◆ Review signs and symptoms of complications and when to seek medical care.

Treatments

Ablation therapy for arrhythmias

Overview

Ablation therapy, a nonsurgical procedure, is used to destroy heart tissue that's creating an arrhythmia, a heart beat originating outside the sinoatrial node (an ectopic foci) or permitting a foci's conduction. Ablations are generally done in an electrophysiology laboratory; the procedure used depends on the arrhythmia type and the presence of heart disease. (See *Types of cardiac ablation.*)

INDICATIONS
◆ Atrial fibrillation
◆ Atrial flutter
◆ Supraventricular tachycardia, including atrioventricular (AV) nodal reentry and Wolff-Parkinson-White syndrome, and certain types of ventricular tachycardia

COMPLICATIONS
◆ High-grade AV block, cardiac tamponade, coronary artery spasm or thrombosis, or pericarditis
◆ Retroperitoneal bleeding
◆ Hematoma at the insertion site
◆ Thromboembolism
◆ Transient ischemic attack or stroke
◆ Pneumothorax
◆ Acute pyloric spasm or gastric hypomotility
◆ Phrenic nerve paralysis
◆ Infection at the access site

Pretreatment care

◆ Verify that the patient signed an informed consent form.
◆ Obtain a 12-lead electrocardiogram (ECG), blood samples for a complete blood count, coagulation studies, and a complete chemistry panel if not done before admission.
◆ Confirm that cardiac drugs with electrophysiologic effects, such as beta-adrenergic blockers, calcium channel blockers, digoxin (Lanoxin), and class I and III antiarrhythmics, were reduced or discontinued as instructed. Verify that warfarin (Coumadin) therapy has also been stopped as ordered.
◆ Ensure that the patient had no food or fluids for a minimum of 6 hours before the procedure.

PATIENT TEACHING
◆ Explain the treatment and preparation to the patient and his family.
◆ Tell the patient that he'll be connected to monitors for ECG, heart rate, blood pressure, pulse oximetry and, possibly, hemodynamic monitoring.
◆ Explain to the patient that he may feel some discomfort or a burning sensation in the chest during the treatment, but that medication will be available if needed.

Procedure

◆ The patient's groin area is shaved and his neck, upper chest, arm, and groin are cleaned with antiseptic. Sterile drapes are placed over the patient.
◆ The practitioner numbs the insertion site with an anesthetic.
◆ Two to five electrode catheters are inserted via the femoral or internal jugular vein into the left side of the heart, the right side of the heart, or both. The coronary sinus may also be entered to evaluate for left-sided abnormal conduction.
◆ Anticoagulation with I.V. heparin is used to reduce the risk of thromboembolism.
◆ After the catheters are in place, the heart's conduction system is assessed and present rhythm confirmed.
◆ During traditional ablation, the practitioner uses a pacemaker to initiate the arrhythmia. Then the practitioner moves the catheters around the heart to determine the area of origin. When the practitioner

finds the area, energy is applied to ablate the source.

◆ Atrial fibrillation is commonly treated with pulmonary vein ablation where the tissue circling each entrance to the four pulmonary veins is ablated. Other ectopic foci for atrial fibrillation are also ablated.

◆ To facilitate the ablation process, three-dimensional electroanatomical mapping systems are projected on monitors. Intracardiac ECG may also be used.

◆ When the ablation is complete, the practitioner monitors the ECG to verify correction of the arrhythmic trigger.

◆ The practitioner removes the catheters from the groin and pressure is applied to the site.

Posttreatment care

◆ Enforce bed rest for 1 to 6 hours, as ordered, with the operative leg extended to prevent bleeding.

◆ Monitor the insertion site for signs of bleeding.

◆ Monitor telemetry for arrhythmias.

◆ Initiate aspirin therapy to prevent thromboembolic aftereffects.

PATIENT TEACHING

◆ Review insertion site care and tell the patient to call the practitioner if redness, swelling, or drainage at the incision site occurs.

◆ Instruct the patient to report to the practitioner signs and symptoms indicating that his arrhythmia is recurring. Inform him that postablation healing may take 6 to 8 weeks.

◆ Teach about the administration, dosage, and possible adverse effects of prescribed medications.

◆ Teach how to take a pulse and keep a record for the practitioner.

Types of cardiac ablation

Several commonly used cardiac ablation techniques are in use today.

◆ *The Maze or Cox-Maze III procedure* is considered the gold standard for certain arrhythmias. It's usually done via a small chest incision. Endoscopes guide the procedure.

◆ *Radiofrequency ablation* directs radio waves to the heart's ectopic foci, obliterating small portions of abnormal tissue with heat, creating scars that permanently block abnormal conduction.

◆ *Microwave and ultrasound ablation techniques* use microwave and high-frequency sound waves via peripheral access sites and specialized catheters and monitoring leads.

◆ *Laser ablation* uses small, focused laser beams that are placed through peripheral access sites or during cardiac surgery.

◆ *Cryoablation* uses a special, extremely cold catheter tip to freeze and destroy tiny amounts of abnormally conducting cardiac tissue through a peripheral access site or during other cardiac surgical procedures.

Angioplasty, percutaneous transluminal coronary

Overview

Percutaneous transluminl coronary angioplasty (PTCA), a nonsurgical alternative to coronary artery bypass surgery, uses a tiny balloon catheter to dilate a coronary artery that's been narrowed by atherosclerotic plaque. The expanding balloon compresses the plaque, expanding the arterial lumen and pressure gradients across the stenotic area. PTCA usually includes atherectomy and may include placement of a regular or drug-eluting stent.

INDICATIONS
◆ Documented myocardial ischemia and angina
◆ Proximal lesion in a single coronary artery
◆ Acute myocardial infarction (MI)
◆ Postthrombolytic therapy with high-grade stenosis
◆ Previous coronary artery bypass surgery
◆ Poor surgical candidate for coronary artery bypass surgery
◆ Stenosis that narrows the arterial lumen by 70% or more

COMPLICATIONS
◆ Arterial dissection
◆ Coronary artery rupture or spasm
◆ Cardiac tamponade
◆ MI or myocardial ischemia
◆ Abrupt reclosure of the affected artery (occurring within a few hours of the procedure)
◆ Arrhythmias
◆ Bleeding
◆ Hematoma
◆ Thromboembolism

Pretreatment care

◆ Ask the patient if he has had reactions to shellfish, iodine, contrast medium, aspirin products, or antiplatelet drugs in the past.
◆ Restrict food and fluid intake for at least 6 hours before the procedure.
◆ Obtain results of coagulation studies, complete blood count, serum electrolyte levels, blood urea nitrogen, and creatinine levels, and blood typing and crossmatching as ordered.
◆ Insert I.V. line and connect the patient to a cardiac monitor and pulse oximetry monitor.
◆ Locate, mark, and record the amplitude of bilateral distal pulses.
◆ Verify that an informed consent form was signed.
◆ Administer medications as ordered.

PATIENT TEACHING
◆ Explain the treatment and preparation.
◆ Explain that the contrast medium injection may cause a flushing sensation or transient nausea.
◆ Instruct the patient to tell the surgical team immediately if he has breathing difficulties, sweating, numbness, itching, nausea, vomiting, chills, or heart palpitations during the procedure.
◆ Tell the patient that he will be taken to the intensive care unit or to a postanesthesia care unit after the procedure for monitoring.
◆ Answer all questions and provide emotional support.

Procedure

◆ The catheter insertion site, usually femoral, is prepared and anesthetized.
◆ A guide wire is inserted into the femoral artery using a percutaneous or cutdown approach, and the catheter is guided fluoroscopically.
◆ The lesion is confirmed using angiography.
◆ Atherectomy may be performed before balloon insertion.
◆ A small, double-lumen, balloon-tipped catheter with or without a stent over the balloon is inserted over the guide wire and positioned properly. The balloon is inflated repeatedly with normal saline solution and contrast medium for 15 to 30 seconds, to a pressure of 6 atmospheres, until the residual gradient decreases to about 20% or until the pressure gradient measures less than 16 mm Hg. The stent is fixed to the vessel wall during this procedure.
◆ Angiography is repeated. The catheter may be left in place or removed.

Posttreatment care

◆ Monitor vital signs, pulse oximetry, cardiac rhythm, peripheral pulses, and neurovascular status of extremities.
◆ Administer an anticoagulant, I.V. nitroglycerin, and I.V. fluids as ordered.
◆ Keep the affected extremity straight, and elevate the head of the bed no more than 15 degrees as ordered.
◆ Monitor for hematoma formation, ecchymosis, or bleeding at the catheter insertion site. Report bleeding sites to the surgeon and apply direct pressure to them.

◆ If an expanding ecchymosis appears, mark the area, and obtain hemoglobin and hematocrit samples as ordered.
◆ After the sheath is removed, apply direct pressure to the insertion site until hemostasis occurs. Apply a dressing per facility policy.
◆ Report the results of electrocardiogram (ECG) monitoring and 12-lead ECGs, particularly changes in ST segments indicating ischemia or infarction.
◆ Assess the patient's pain level, administer analgesics, and evaluate their effects.

PATIENT TEACHING

◆ Teach about the administration, dosage, and possible adverse effects of prescribed medications.
◆ Discuss puncture site care, activity restrictions if applicable, and follow-up care and testing.
◆ Describe signs and symptoms of bleeding, infection, restenosis, or complications, and when to notify the practitioner.
◆ Teach the patient about appropriate lifestyle changes that may reduce the risk of recurrence.

Blood and plasma product transfusion

Overview

A transfusion is the administration of whole blood, packed red blood cells (RBCs), leukocyte-poor RBCs, RBCs removed of leukocytes, white blood cells (WBCs) or leukocytes, platelets, or fresh frozen plasma (FFP). A unit of whole blood or RBCs, which must be crossmatched to the patient's ABO blood group and Rh type before administration, has enough hemoglobin (Hb) to raise the Hb level in an average-sized adult by 1 g/dl (about 3%). Other blood products may be administered without a crossmatch, including albumin, factors VIII, II, VII, IX, and X complex (prothrombin complex).

INDICATIONS
Whole blood and packed RBCs
◆ Hemorrhage
◆ Chronic blood loss or anemia
◆ Sickle cell anemia

WBCs
◆ Sepsis unresponsive to antibiotics
◆ Granulocytopenia (granulocyte count usually less than 500/µl)

Platelets
◆ Thrombocytopenia

FFP
◆ Coagulation factor deficiency

Albumin
◆ Cirulating volume loss
◆ Hypoproteinemia (with or without edema)

Factor VIII
◆ Hemophilia A
◆ Uncontroled bleeding associated with factor VIII deficiency
◆ Decreased fibrinogen or deficient factor VIII

Factors II, VII, IX, and X complex
◆ Congenital factor V deficiency
◆ Bleeding disorders resulting from an acquired deficiency of factors II, VII, IX, and X

COMPLICATIONS
◆ Transfusion reaction (hemolytic, allergic, febrile, or pyogenic)
◆ Infectious disease transmission
◆ Circulatory overload
◆ Coagulation disturbances
◆ Citrate intoxication
◆ Hyperkalemia
◆ Acid-base imbalance

Pretreatment care

◆ Verify that the patient has signed an informed consent form.
◆ Obtain the blood sample for type and crossmatch if appropriate.
◆ Insert an appropriate size I.V. catheter.
◆ Record the patient's baseline vital signs.
◆ Obtain the blood product from the blood bank or pharmacy as appropriate.
◆ Perform a blood check per facility policy, which usually requires two qualified individuals to:
  ● compare the name and medical record number on the patient's wrist band with those on the component bag label
  ● check the expiration date on the component bag, and check for abnormal color, clumping, gas bubbles, and extraneous material
  ● check the component bag identification number, ABO blood group, and Rh compatibility
  ● compare the patient's blood bank identification number, if present, with the number on the blood bag
  ● sign the blood slip with their names, date, and time.

◆ Premedicate the patient with diphenhydramine (Benadryl) and acetaminophen (Tylenol) as prescribed.
◆ Obtain a blood sample for a coagulation assay before administration of factors II, VII, IX, and X complex and at suitable intervals during treatment.

PATIENT TEACHING
◆ Explain the procedure to the patient.
◆ Tell the patient to immediately report flushing, fever, chills, nausea, vomiting, faintness and headache, palpitations, difficulty swallowing or breathing, tingling in the fingers or muscle cramps, and intestinal colic, diarrhea, or muscle weakness to the nurse.

Procedure

◆ Put on gloves, a gown, and a face shield, as appropriate.
◆ Prepare a bag of normal saline solution to flush the line before and after transfusion or keep the vein open during a reaction or between transfusions.
◆ Set up an appropriate infusion set and filter.
◆ Obtain and set up an infusion pump or blood warmer, if ordered.
◆ Adjust the flow rate as appropriate for the component transfusion.
◆ Monitor the patient's vital signs, blood pressure, and facial color, and address patient complaints.
◆ If signs of a reaction develop, stop the transfusion and record the patient's vital signs. Infuse normal saline solution through a new I.V. line at a moderately slow infusion rate, and notify the practitioner. Return the blood product bag to the blood bank. Obtain a urine specimen and a blood sample and send them to the laboratory.

◆ If no signs of a reaction appear within 15 minutes, adjust the flow to the ordered infusion rate.

Posttreatment care

◆ Discard the used infusion equipment in the biohazard material receptacle.
◆ Return the empty component bag to the blood bank, or discard it in a biohazard material receptacle, per facility policy.
◆ Obtain and record the patient's vital signs.
◆ Obtain a blood sample for hemoglobin level and hematocrit as ordered and document the results.
◆ Monitor the patient for signs of circulatory overload.

PATIENT TEACHING
◆ Explain the need for follow-up laboratory studies and, possibly, additional blood products.

Bone grafting

Overview

Bone grafting, a surgical method of promoting new bone formation, is used during orthopedic procedures to stimulate bones to heal and to provide skeletal support by filling in gaps between two bones. A bone section is grafted where it's needed and, over time, it "remodels" and is replaced with new bone. An *autograft* or *autogenous bone graft* is when the bone comes from the patient's body; bone from someone else's body, such as an organ donor, is called an *allograft*. Artificial bone graft materials made from sea coral have also been used. Minimally invasive bone grafting involves injecting bone marrow, calcium phosphate cement, or processed allograft bone matrix gel.

INDICATIONS
◆ Fractures needing stimulation to heal
◆ Diseased joint or space between two bones that requires stimulation to heal (arthrodesis or fusion)
◆ Regeneration of bone that's lost or missing as a result of trauma, infection, or disease
◆ Improvement of bone healing response and regeneration of bone tissue around surgically implanted devices (such as artificial joint replacements or plates and screws)

COMPLICATIONS
◆ Nerve injury
◆ Infection
◆ Bleeding
◆ Fat embolism or thromboembolism
◆ Graft rejection (with allografts)

Pretreatment care

◆ Verify that the patient has signed an informed consent form.
◆ Make sure that prescribed preoperative tests and laboratory work have been completed.
◆ Confirm that the patient hasn't taken aspirin or nonsteroidal anti-inflammatory drugs (NSAIDs) within 1 week of the surgery.
◆ Confirm that the patient didn't eat or drink anything after midnight before the procedure.
◆ Start an I.V. line and administer fluids as ordered.
◆ Administer medications such as a prophylactic antibiotic as ordered.

PATIENT TEACHING
◆ Explain the treatment and preparation.
◆ Reassure the patient that pain medication will be available after the procedure.
◆ Review activity restrictions required after the procedure.

Procedure

◆ With an autogenous bone graft, the surgeon takes a small piece of bone from another area of the body (such as the pelvis or iliac crest) and attaches the bone graft to the graft site with a needle or by open, incisional surgery.
◆ With an allograft bone graft or biological products, such as bone graft extenders or bone graft replacements, the surgeon attaches the graft or product during surgery.
◆ Platelet gels may be used because they're easily removed from the patient's blood with few complications; however, they don't contain osteoinductive proteins and they aren't powerful enough stimulants to induce bone formation. They can

be used as graft extenders but not graft replacements.

◆ Bone morphogenetic proteins (such as BMP-2 and BMP-7) are produced and concentrated, and placed in the body in areas where bone formation is needed. They're powerful enough to stimulate bone formation without the patient's bone. Several of these proteins are found naturally in the body and play a role in bone formation.

◆ Minimally invasive bone graft material is injected with a large needle directly into the site where it's needed.

Posttreatment care

◆ Monitor the patient's vital signs and intake and output.

◆ Report laboratory results to the practitioner.

◆ Assess the patient for infection, hemorrhage, and severe combined immunodeficiency disease as indicated.

◆ Assist with the electrical stimulation device as indicated.

◆ Assess the patient's pain level and administer an analgesic as ordered.

◆ Provide cast care and incision care as indicated.

PATIENT TEACHING

◆ Teach about the administration, dosage, and possible adverse effects of prescribed medications.

◆ Explain activity restrictions.

◆ Explain wound care needs, cast care, and follow-up care as appropriate.

◆ Review signs and symptoms of complications and when to seek medical care.

◆ Advise the patient to avoid smoking, radiation therapy, chemotherapy, NSAIDs, and systemic corticosteroids, all of which slow bone healing.

Bowel resection

Overview

A bowel resection, the surgical removal of part of the bowel, may include the creation of an ostomy and stoma on the outer abdominal wall for feces elimination. Laparoscopic surgery may be used for a standard colostomy and end-ileostomy. A bowel resection with anastomosis (the preferred surgical technique for treating localized bowel cancer) is the resection of diseased intestinal tissue with the remaining segments connected or anastomosed.

INDICATIONS
Bowel resection with ostomy
♦ Inflammatory bowel disease
♦ Familial adenomatous polyposis
♦ Diverticulitis
♦ Advanced colorectal cancer

Bowel resection with anastomosis
♦ Localized obstructive disorders secondary to diverticulitis, intestinal polyps, adhesions, or malignant or benign intestinal lesions

COMPLICATIONS
♦ Hemorrhage
♦ Infection
♦ Ileus
♦ Fluid and electrolyte imbalance
♦ Skin excoriation
♦ Incompetent nipple valve (with a Kock ileostomy)
♦ Bleeding or leakage from the anastomosis site

Pretreatment care

♦ Verify that the patient has signed an informed consent form.
♦ Provide total parenteral nutrition as ordered.
♦ Administer an antibiotic and other medications as ordered.
♦ Monitor the patient's vital signs, nutritional status, fluid and electrolyte status, intake and output, and daily weight.

PATIENT TEACHING
♦ Explain preoperative and postoperative procedures and equipment to the patient and his family.
♦ Discuss postoperative analgesia.
♦ Tell the patient what to expect for fecal drainage and bowel movement control for the type of ostomy performed.
♦ Demonstrate coughing and deep breathing and splinting, and review how to use an incentive spirometer.

Procedure

♦ All procedures are performed under general anesthesia.

BOWEL RESECTION WITH OSTOMY
♦ The surgeon makes an incision in the abdominal wall based on the bowel area to be resected and type of ostomy required.
♦ The diseased bowel segment is resected, possibly along with several more inches of bowel.
♦ The surgeon creates a stoma.

ABDOMINOPERINEAL RESECTION
♦ A low abdominal incision is made and the sigmoid colon is divided.
♦ The proximal end of the colon is brought out through another, smaller abdominal incision to create an end-stoma.
♦ A wide perineal incision is made, and the anus, rectum, and distal portion of the sigmoid colon are resected.
♦ The abdominal wound is closed and abdominal drains are placed.
♦ The perineal wound may be left open, packed with gauze, or closed; several Penrose drains are placed.

ILEOSTOMY
♦ The surgeon resects all or part of the colon and rectum (proctocolectomy).
♦ A permanent ileostomy is created by bringing the end of the ileum out through a small abdominal incision in the right lower quadrant to create a stoma.

ILEOANAL RESERVOIR

◆ A colectomy is performed and an ileal loop or the distal ileum is used to create a stoma for a temporary ileostomy.
◆ The rectal mucosal layer is removed and an internal pouch is made with a portion of the ileum.
◆ A pouch-anal anastomosis is performed.
◆ The temporary ileostomy is usually closed after 3 to 4 months.

KOCK ILEOSTOMY

◆ The surgeon removes the colon, rectum, and anus, and closes the anus.
◆ A reservoir is constructed from a loop of the terminal ileum.
◆ A portion of the ileum is intussuscepted to form a nipple valve.
◆ The upper part of the sutured and cut ileum is pulled down and sutured to form a pouch.
◆ The nipple valve is used to create a stoma by pulling it through the abdominal wall and suturing it flush with the skin.
◆ A catheter is placed in the stoma.

BOWEL RESECTION WITH ANASTOMOSIS

◆ An abdominal incision is made, depending on location of the lesion.
◆ The diseased area and a wide margin of surrounding normal tissue are resected.
◆ Remaining bowel segments are anastomosed end-to-end or side-to-side.
◆ The incision is closed.
◆ A sterile dressing is applied.

Posttreatment care

◆ Assess the patient's pain level and administer analgesics as ordered.
◆ Monitor the patient's vital signs and intake and output.
◆ Provide appropriate wound and stoma care.
◆ Maintain nasogastric tube patency and assess drainage.
◆ After an abdominoperineal resection, irrigate the perineal area as ordered.

◆ For a patient with a Kock pouch with a catheter inserted in the stoma:
– Connect the catheter to low intermittent suction or to straight drainage as ordered.
● Check catheter patency regularly, and irrigate with 20 to 30 ml of normal saline solution as ordered.
● Assess pouch drainage and advance the patient's diet as ordered.
● Clamp and unclamp the pouch catheter to increase its capacity as ordered.
◆ Arrange for a consultation with an enterostomal therapist as appropriate.
◆ Assess stoma appearance and drainage. Look for skin irritation and excoriation.
◆ Monitor the patient for signs and symptoms of complications.
◆ Encourage deep-breathing and coughing exercises and use of incentive spirometry.
◆ Encourage splinting of the incision site as necessary.
◆ For anastomosis patients, encourage oral fluid intake and give stool softeners and laxatives as ordered.

PATIENT TEACHING

◆ Teach about the administration, dosage, and possible adverse effects of prescribed medications.
◆ Explain the ostomy type and function and review care of ostomy appliances.
◆ Teach stoma and skin care.
◆ Explain dietary restrictions and emphasize the importance of a high fluid intake.
◆ Explain the need to avoid alcohol, laxatives, and diuretics (unless approved by the practitioner).
◆ Review bowel retraining for appropriate ostomy patients.
◆ For patients who underwent abdominoperineal resection, teach about sitz bath use.
◆ Review the signs and symptoms of complications and when to notify the practitioner.
◆ Stress the importance of follow-up care.

Breast reconstruction

Overview

Breast reconstruction involves rebuilding the breast after mastectomy. The method used depends on the patient's needs and whether a flap or implant is used. For example, reconstruction under the skin or muscle is suitable only for women with small breasts. Additionally, reconstruction under the muscle can't be done in patients whose chest muscle was removed during radical mastectomy or in patients who have received radiotherapy because the muscles and skin are unlikely to stretch. The flap technique may be used when tissue expansion is unsuitable, such as when the patient has undergone previous radiotherapy or the breasts being reconstructed are large.

INDICATIONS
◆ Mastectomy

COMPLICATIONS
◆ Bleeding
◆ Fluid collection and swelling
◆ Bruising
◆ Excessive scar tissue
◆ Numbness or change in feeling
◆ Infection
◆ Capsular contracture (tightening of the scar or capsule around the implant)
◆ Complications with flap source site (limited movement)

Pretreatment care

◆ Verify that the patient has signed an informed consent form.
◆ Provide psychological support.
◆ Administer an antibiotic and other medications as ordered.
◆ Monitor the patient's vital signs, nutritional status, fluid and electrolyte status, intake and output, and daily weight.

PATIENT TEACHING
◆ Explain preoperative and postoperative procedures and equipment to the patient and her family.
◆ Discuss postoperative analgesia.
◆ Demonstrate coughing and deep breathing and splinting, and review how to use an incentive spirometer.

Procedure

◆ The patient is identified using two identifers. The procedure is verified and the correct breast to be reconstructed is identified by the patient and surgical team.

BREAST RECONSTRUCTION UNDER THE SKIN
◆ Breast tissue is removed but the skin and the nipple are preserved.
◆ The implant is placed beneath the skin to replace lost breast tissue.

BREAST RECONSTRUCTION UNDER THE MUSCLE
◆ The implant is placed beneath the muscles covering the chest.

BREAST RECONSTRUCTION INVOLVING TISSUE EXPANSION
◆ An expandable implant with a fill-valve is inserted beneath the skin and muscle to make use of the skin and muscle's ability to stretch.
◆ A sterile saline solution is injected over several months through a valve just under the skin of the armpit until the implant is slightly larger than the remaining breast.
◆ A permanent implant is made.

BREAST RECONSTRUCTION USING FLAPS
◆ Muscle and skin (known as flaps) are taken from the back (latissimus dorsi) or abdomen (rectus abdominis), which con-

Treatments

tain very large muscles, providing enough skin, fat, and muscle with a good blood supply to create the shape of a breast on the chest wall.

Posttreatment care

◆ Monitor the patient's vital signs and intake and output.
◆ Monitor drainage from the wound and provide skin care.
◆ Assess the patient for pain and provide an analgesic as ordered.
◆ Monitor the patient for infection, hemorrhage, and other signs of complications.
◆ Elevate the patient's arm on the operative side on a pillow and position it to facilitate drainage, ensuring that the patient is comfortable.
◆ Initiate flexion and extension arm exercises as ordered.
◆ Place a sign in the patient's room indicating that no blood pressure readings, injections, or venipunctures should be performed on the affected arm.

PATIENT TEACHING

◆ Advise the patient to stop smoking; nicotine can delay healing, resulting in conspicuous scars and prolonged recovery.
◆ Tell the patient that the surgical drain to remove excess fluids from the site will be removed within the 2 weeks after surgery. Most stitches are removed in 7 to 10 days.
◆ Teach about the administration, dosage, and possible adverse effects of prescribed medications.
◆ Tell the patient to report signs and symptoms of infection and increasing pain to the surgeon.
◆ Review exercises, as ordered, and wound care.
◆ Tell the patient that venipunctures, injections, and blood pressure measurements should be performed in the unaffected arm only.

Cardioversion, synchronized

Overview

Synchronized cardioversion, which is used to treat tachyarrhythmias, is the delivery of an electrical charge to the myocardium at the peak of the R wave. The electrical charge causes immediate depolarization, interrupting reentry circuits and allowing the sinoatrial node to resume control. Synchronized cardioversion may be performed by a nurse in the presence of a practitioner.

INDICATIONS
◆ Unstable supraventricular tachycardia due to reentry
◆ Atrial fibrillation
◆ Atrial flutter
◆ Unstable monomorphic ventricular tachycardia
◆ Arrhythmias that don't respond to vagal maneuvers or drug therapy

COMPLICATIONS
◆ Transient, harmless arrhythmias, such as atrial, ventricular, and junctional premature beats
◆ Serious ventricular arrhythmias such as ventricular fibrillation

Pretreatment care

◆ For nonemergency treatments, verify that the patient has signed an informed consent form.
◆ Check the patient's recent serum potassium and magnesium levels, arterial blood gas levels, and digoxin (Lanoxin) levels.
◆ Withhold food and fluids for 6 to 12 hours before the procedure.
◆ Obtain a 12-lead electrocardiogram (ECG) to serve as a baseline.
◆ Insert an I.V. catheter, or verify patency of an existing I.V. catheter.

◆ Provide emotional support.
◆ Connect the patient to a cardiac monitor and pulse oximeter and obtain vital signs.
◆ Have emergency cardiac medications and resuscitation equipment readily available at the patient's bedside.
◆ Administer prescribed medications.

PATIENT TEACHING
◆ Explain the procedure to the patient.
◆ Reassure the patient that sedation will be provided before administration of an electrical shock.
◆ Explain that the patient will have his heart rhythm monitored during and after the procedure.

Procedure

◆ Verify the patient's identity using two identifiers according to facility policy.
◆ Consider administering oxygen for 5 to 10 minutes before the cardioversion to promote myocardial oxygenation.
◆ Place the patient in a supine position and assess his vital signs, level of consciousness (LOC), cardiac rhythm, and peripheral pulses.
◆ Remove any oxygen delivery device just before cardioversion to avoid possible combustion.
◆ Press the POWER button to turn on the defibrillator.
◆ Push the SYNC button to synchronize the machine with the patient's QRS complexes. Make sure that the SYNC button flashes with each of the patient's QRS complexes. You should also see a marker on the monitor to signify correct synchronization.
◆ Turn the ENERGY SELECT dial to the ordered amount of energy and push the CHARGE button. Increase the second and subsequent shock doses as ordered.

◆ Place the defibrillator pads, conductive gel pads, or paddles in the same positions as you would to defibrillate.

◆ Make sure that everyone stands away from the bed, and move equipment that's touching the bed or patient.

◆ Discharge the current by pushing the DISCHARGE buttons of both paddles simultaneously or pressing the SHOCK button on the machine.

◆ Wait for the energy to be discharged— the machine has to synchronize the discharge with the QRS complex.

◆ Check the waveform on the monitor.

◆ If the arrhythmia fails to convert, repeat the procedure. Gradually increase the energy level to a maximum of 360 joules with each additional countershock.

Posttreatment care

◆ After the cardioversion, frequently assess the patient's LOC and respiratory status, including airway patency, respiratory rate and depth, and the need for supplemental oxygen.

◆ Carefully monitor the patient's blood pressure and respiratory rate until he recovers from the sedation.

◆ Record a postcardioversion 12-lead ECG, and monitor the patient's ECG rhythm.

◆ Check the patient's chest for electrical burns.

◆ Administer cardiac medications as ordered.

PATIENT TEACHING

◆ Review with the patient how to take his pulse and what abnormalities to report to the cardiologist.

◆ Teach about the administration, dosage, and possible adverse effects of prescribed medications.

◆ Emphasize the need for follow-up care.

Carpal tunnel release

Overview

Carpal tunnel syndrome, the most common nerve entrapment syndrome, is caused by median nerve compression in the wrist where it passes through the carpal tunnel, causing loss of movement and sensation in the wrist, hand, and fingers. Carpal tunnel release, the surgery that decompresses the median nerve to relieve pain and restore function, may be performed as open or endoscopic outpatient surgery using local anesthesia. Endoscopic carpal tunnel release may be single portal or double portal.

INDICATIONS
◆ Carpal tunnel syndrome

COMPLICATIONS
◆ Hematoma formation
◆ Infection
◆ Painful scar formation
◆ Tenosynovitis
◆ Nerve damage

Pretreatment care

◆ Explain to the patient that the affected arm will be shaved and cleaned and that he'll be given a local anesthetic. Assure him that although he may feel some pressure, the anesthetic will ensure a pain-free operation.
◆ Discuss postoperative care measures.
◆ Explain that analgesics will be available for pain control.
◆ Verify that the patient has signed an informed consent form.

PATIENT TEACHING
◆ Provide information on the disorder and the purpose of the planned surgery.
◆ Outline the steps of surgery and the expected recovery.
◆ Demonstrate the rehabilitative exercises that the patient will be asked to do.

Procedure

◆ Carpal tunnel release surgery can be performed in several ways, but the entire transverse carpal tunnel ligament must be transected to ensure adequate decompression of the median nerve.
◆ The surgeon makes an incision around the thenar eminence to expose the flexor retinaculum, which is transected to relieve pressure on the median nerve.
◆ If needed to free flattened nerve fibers and relieve tension and loosen surrounding adhesions, neurolysis may be performed to stretch the nerve.

ENDOSCOPIC CARPAL TUNNEL RELEASE
◆ The carpal tunnel is approached through small incisions that allow the passage of the endoscope along the ulnar border of the transverse carpal ligament.
◆ The ligament is sharply divided after transverse fibers are well visualized.
◆ The antebrachial fascia is divided proximally.

Posttreatment care

◆ Monitor the patient's vital signs and carefully assess circulation and sensory and motor functions in the affected arm and hand.
◆ Elevate the affected hand to reduce swelling and discomfort.
◆ Check the dressing often for unusual drainage or bleeding.
◆ Assess for pain and provide analgesics as needed.
◆ Encourage the patient to perform his wrist and finger exercises daily to improve circulation and enhance muscle tone. If these exercises are painful, have him perform them with his wrist and hand immersed in warm water.
◆ Assess the need for home care and assistance with activities of daily living, especially if the patient lives alone.

PATIENT TEACHING

◆ Teach about the administration, dosage, and possible adverse effects of prescribed medications.

◆ Teach appropriate wound care.

◆ Describe signs and symptoms of complications and when to notify the surgeon.

◆ Review recommended exercises and activity restrictions.

◆ Refer for occupational counseling if appropriate.

◆ Inform the patient that keeping the hand elevated is important to prevent swelling and stiffness of the fingers. Remind the patient not to walk with the hand dangling or to sit with the hand held in the lap.

◆ Emphasize the need for follow-up care.

◆ Refer the patient to appropriate resources and support services.

Cerebral aneurysm repair

Overview

Cerebral aneurysm repair involves clipping the cerebral aneurysm neck via craniotomy or an endovascular repair using detachable platinum coils that promote electrothrombosis within the aneurysm. The procedure used depends on the patient's condition and age and the aneurysm's location. (See *Common sites of cerebral aneurysms*.)

 Nursing alert

The coil procedure is contraindicated if the patient has a cerebral hematoma or an aneurysm with a wide opening.

INDICATIONS
◆ Cerebral aneurysm

COMPLICATIONS
◆ Infection
◆ Rupture of cerebral aneurysm
◆ Vasospasm
◆ Neurologic damage
◆ Hypothermia

Pretreatment care

◆ Check laboratory values, electrocardiogram, and chest X-rays as ordered; notify the surgeon or radiologist of abnormalities.
◆ Perform a neurologic examination.
◆ Verify that the patient has signed an informed consent form.
◆ Adminster medications as ordered.

PATIENT TEACHING
◆ Explain the planned surgical technique to the patient and his family, reinforcing the surgeon's explanations as necessary.
◆ Explain all tests, neurologic examinations, treatments, and procedures to the patient and his family.
◆ Describe the postoperative care that's expected.

Procedure

CLIPPING
◆ General anesthesia is given, and the area of the skull where the craniotomy will occur is shaved.
◆ The bone flap is removed and the various layers of tissue are cut away to expose the brain.
◆ Brain tissue is gently retracted back to expose the area containing the aneurysm.
◆ Surgical techniques performed through a microscope are then used to dissect the aneurysm away from the vessels feeding the aneurysm and expose the neck to receive the clip, which is usually made of titanium.
◆ The clip is placed on the neck of the aneurysm to stop the flow of blood into the aneurysm, causing it to deflate or obliterate.
◆ The brain tissue is carefully lowered back into place, the various layers are sutured closed, and the bone flap is reseated for healing.
◆ The skin and other outer layers are sutured closed.
◆ A postoperative magnetic resonance angiogram may be performed to confirm clip placement, total aneurysm obliteration, and continued blood flow through the neighboring vessels.

COILING
◆ A neurointerventionalist performs the procedure using fluoroscopic angiography.
◆ A microcatheter is threaded from the patient's femoral artery to the aneurysm. The catheter is used to place small platinum coils within the aneurysm using a delivery wire.
◆ After the coil has been maneuvered into place, an electrical charge is sent through the delivery wire that disintegrates the stainless steel of the coil, separating it

from the delivery wire, which is then removed from the body.

◆ Several coils may be necessary to block the neck of the aneurysm from the normal circulation and obliterate it.

◆ The coils act as a thrombogenic agent, causing blood to coagulate in the aneurysm, decreasing the risk of rupture.

Posttreatment care

◆ Monitor neurologic status and observe for signs of increased intracerebral pressure.

◆ Administer medications for vasospasm, anticoagulants, and I.V. fluids as ordered.

◆ Monitor vital signs, especially blood pressure, and notify the surgeon of a significant increase, especially in the systolic pressure.

◆ Administer oxygen as indicated and monitor pulse oximetry and arterial blood gas values.

◆ Apply elastic or compression stockings while the patient is in bed.

◆ Monitor laboratory values and intake and output.

◆ Monitor the incision site for signs and symptoms of infection.

PATIENT TEACHING

◆ Review signs of rebleeding to report, such as headache, nausea, vomiting, and changes in level of consciousness.

◆ Refer the patient to a home health care service or rehabilitation center as needed.

◆ Emphasize the importance of follow-up care.

Common sites of cerebral aneurysms

Cerebral aneurysms usually arise at the arterial bifurcation in the circle of Willis and its branches. This illustration shows the most common sites around this circle.

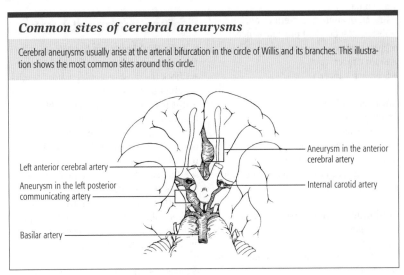

Aneurysm in the anterior cerebral artery

Left anterior cerebral artery

Aneurysm in the left posterior communicating artery

Internal carotid artery

Basilar artery

Chemotherapy

Overview

Chemotherapeutic drugs are administered to destroy or suppress the growth of cancer cells. They may be used alone or as an adjunct to surgery or radiation therapy. These drugs may be administered I.V. (most common route), orally, subcutaneously, I.M., intra-arterially, into a body cavity, through a central venous (CV) catheter, or through an Ommaya reservoir into the spinal canal, depending on the drug's pharmacodynamics and tumor's characteristics.

INDICATIONS
Alkylating agents
- Chronic and acute leukemias
- Non-Hodgkin's lymphoma
- Myeloma or multiple myeloma
- Sarcoma
- Breast, ovarian, and uterine cancers
- Testes, bladder, and prostate cancers
- Lung cancer
- Brain cancer
- Stomach cancer

Antimetabolites
- Acute leukemia
- Breast cancer
- GI tract adenocarcinomas
- Non-Hodgkin's lymphoma
- Squamous cell carcinomas of the head, neck, and cervix

Antibiotic antineoplastic agents
- Sarcomas
- Lymphomas
- Acute nonlymphoblastic or nonlymphocytic leukemia
- Breast cancer

Hormonal antineoplastic agents
- Hormone-dependent tumors
- Cancers of the prostate, breast, and endometrium

Tubulin-interactive agents
- Lymphomas
- Leukemias
- Sarcomas
- Breast and ovarian cancers

COMPLICATIONS
- Anorexia, nausea and vomiting
- Bone marrow suppression
- Intestinal irritation
- Stomatitis
- Hearing loss
- Anemia
- Alopecia
- Urticaria
- Esophagitis
- Diarrhea
- Constipation
- Extravasation, causing inflammation, ulceration, necrosis, and loss of vein patency

Pretreatment care

- Verify that the patient has signed an informed consent form.
- Check the most recent laboratory results for abnormalities.
- Instruct the patient to report adverse reactions during chemotherapy.
- Verify the drug, dosage, and administration route by checking the medication record against the oncologist's order.
- Administer pretreatment medications such as antiemetics.
- Insert an I.V. catheter, or access an existing central catheter and ensure its proper function. If administering a vesicant agent, avoid sites in the wrist or dorsum of the hand.
- Check for adverse reactions from previous chemotherapy administration.
- Provide emotional support to the patient and his family.

◆ Explain the specific treatment and preparation to the patient and his family.
◆ Review potential adverse effects and what to expect when treatment is completed.

Procedure

I.V. ADMINISTRATION

◆ The best site to administer the drug is determined based on drug compatibilities, frequency of administration, and the vesicant potential of the drug (see *Classifying chemotherapeutic drugs*). The facility's policy should be checked before administering a vesicant.
◆ Some facilities require two nurses to read the dosage order and to check the drug and the amount being administered.
◆ The patient's identity is verified using two patient identifiers according to facility policy.
◆ Special gloves are put on for use through all stages of handling the drug, including preparation, priming the I.V. tubing, and administration.
◆ The drug is administered as appropriate: nonvesicants by I.V. push or admixed in a bag of I.V. fluid; vesicants by I.V. push through a piggyback set connected to a rapidly infusing I.V. line. An infusion pump is used to ensure drug delivery within the prescribed time and rate.
◆ During administration, the patient is closely monitored for signs of a hypersensitivity reaction or extravasation.
◆ Adequate blood return from I.V. access is checked after 5 ml of the drug has been infused or according to the facility's guidelines.
◆ If extravasation is suspected, the infusion is immediately stopped. The I.V. catheter is left in place, and the oncologist is notified. A conservative method for treating extravasation involves aspirating

any residual drug from the tubing and I.V. catheter, instilling an I.V. antidote, and then removing the I.V. catheter. Afterward, heat or cold is applied to the site and the affected limb is elevated.
◆ After infusion of the medication, 20 ml of normal saline solution is infused between administrations of different chemotherapeutic drugs and before discontinuing the I.V. line.

Classifying chemotherapeutic drugs

Chemotherapeutic drugs may be classified as irritants, vesicants, or nonvesicants.

Irritants
◆ Carmustine (BiCNU)
◆ Dacarbazine (DTIC-Dome)
◆ Etoposide (Etopophos)
◆ Ifosfamide (Ifex)
◆ Streptozocin (Zanosar)
◆ Topotecan (Hycamtin)

Vesicants
◆ Dactinomycin (Cosmegen)
◆ Daunorubicin (Cerubidine)
◆ Doxorubicin (Adriamycin)
◆ Mechlorethamine (Mustargen)
◆ Mitomycin-C (Mutamycin)
◆ Mitoxantrone (Novantrone)
◆ Paclitaxel (Onxol)
◆ Vinblastine (Velban)
◆ Vincristine (Oncovin)

Nonvesicants
◆ Asparaginase (Elspar)
◆ Bleomycin (Blenoxane)
◆ Carboplatin (Paraplatin)
◆ Cisplatin (Platinol-AQ); if greater than 20 ml of 0.5 mg/ml, it's considered a vesicant
◆ Cyclophosphamide (Cytoxan)
◆ Cytarabine (Cytosar-U)
◆ Floxuridine (FUDR)
◆ Fluorouracil (Adrucil)

Treatments

Posttreatment care

◆ Dispose of used needles and syringes appropriately.
◆ Dispose of I.V. bags, bottles, gloves, and tubing in a properly labeled and covered trash container.
◆ Wash hands thoroughly with soap and warm water after giving any chemotherapeutic drug, even though gloves were worn.
◆ Observe the I.V. site frequently for signs of extravasation and allergic reaction (such as swelling, redness, and urticaria) if appropriate.
◆ Observe the patient for adverse reactions.
◆ Maintain a list of the types and amounts of drugs the patient has received, especially if he has received drugs that have a cu-mulative effect and that can be toxic to organs, such as the heart or kidneys.
◆ For 48 hours after drug administration, wear latex gloves when handling items contaminated with the patient's excreta.

PATIENT TEACHING

◆ Review the medications and adverse reactions with the patient.
◆ Discuss how to manage adverse reactions with the patient (see *Managing common adverse effects of chemotherapy*).
◆ Review the signs and symptoms of abnormal bleeding, infection, or bone marrow suppression.
◆ Advise the patient when to contact the practitioner.
◆ Stress the importance of follow-up care.
◆ Refer the patient to local resources or a home health care agency.

Managing common adverse effects of chemotherapy

Provide these instructions when teaching a patient how to manage the adverse effects of chemotherapy at home.

Adverse effect	Home care instructions
Bone marrow depression (leukopenia, thrombocytopenia, anemia)	◆ Immediately report fever, chills, sore throat, lethargy, unusual fatigue, or pallor. ◆ Avoid exposure to persons with infections during chemotherapy and for several months after the treatments have ended. ◆ Avoid receiving immunizations during or shortly after chemotherapy because an exaggerated reaction may occur. ◆ Avoid activities that could cause traumatic injury and bleeding. Report episodes of bleeding or bruising to the practitioner. ◆ Eat high-iron foods, such as liver and spinach. ◆ Make sure to schedule follow-up blood studies after completion of treatment.
Anorexia	◆ Have family supply favorite foods to help maintain adequate nutrition. ◆ Eat small, frequent meals.
Nausea and vomiting	◆ Use antiemetic suppositories. ◆ Take the drug on an empty stomach, with meals, or at bedtime. GI upset indicates that the drug is working. Report vomiting to the practitioner. ◆ Follow a high-protein diet.
Diarrhea and abdominal cramps	◆ Use antidiarrheals, and report diarrhea to the practitioner. ◆ Maintain adequate fluid intake and follow a bland, low-fiber diet. ◆ Perform good perianal hygiene to help prevent skin breakdown and infection.
Stomatitis	◆ Perform good mouth care. Rinse the mouth with 1 tsp of salt dissolved in 8 oz (237 ml) of warm water or hydrogen peroxide diluted to half strength with water. ◆ Avoid acidic, spicy, or extremely hot or cold foods. ◆ Report stomatitis to the practitioner, who may order a change in medication.
Alopecia	◆ Consider cutting hair short to make thinning hair less noticeable. ◆ Wash hair with a mild shampoo and avoid frequent brushing or combing. ◆ Wear a hat, scarf, toupee, or wig.

Treatments

Continuous renal replacement therapy

Overview

Continuous renal replacement therapy (CRRT) provides patients with continuous dialysis therapy, sparing them the destabilizing hemodynamic and electrolyte changes characteristic of intermittent hemodialysis (IHD). Types of CRRT include slow continuous ultrafiltration, continuous arteriovenous hemofiltration, continuous arteriovenous hemodialysis, continuous venovenous hemofiltration, and continuous venovenous hemodialysis. The type of CRRT performed is based on the patient needs.

INDICATIONS
◆ Acute renal failure
◆ Inability to tolerate traditional hemodialysis such as in those with hypotension

COMPLICATIONS
◆ Bleeding
◆ Hemorrhage
◆ Hemofilter occlusion
◆ Infection
◆ Hypotension
◆ Thrombosis
◆ Hypothermia
◆ Air embolism

Pretreatment care

◆ If a dialysis catheter will be inserted, confirm that the patient signed an informed consent form.
◆ Weigh the patient, take baseline vital signs, and make sure that all necessary laboratory studies have been done (such as electrolyte levels, coagulation factors, complete blood count, blood urea nitrogen, and creatinine studies). Monitor vital signs hourly or as indicated.
◆ Wash your hands. Assemble the equipment at the patient's bedside according to the manufacturer's recommendations and the facility's policy. Most facilities consult with dialysis centers to set up equipment for use.

PATIENT TEACHING
◆ Explain the reason for the treatment and what's involved in receiving the treatment.
◆ Review activity restrictions during treatment.

Procedure

◆ If necessary, assist with inserting the dialysis catheter into the femoral artery and vein, using strict sterile technique. An internal arteriovenous fistula or external arteriovenous shunt may sometimes be used instead of the femoral route.
◆ Put on sterile gloves and a mask. Clean the connection sites with povidone-iodine solution, and then connect them to the catheter ports.
◆ Turn on the hemofilter and monitor blood-flow rate through the circuit. The flow rate is typically 500 to 900 ml/hour.
◆ Inspect the ultrafiltrate during the procedure. It should remain clear yellow, with no gross blood. Pink-tinged or blood ultrafiltrate may signal a membrane leak in the hemofilter, which permits bacterial contamination. If a leak occurs, the hemofilter may need to be replaced.
◆ Calculate the amount of filtration replacement fluid every hour, as ordered, or according to the facility's policy. Infuse the prescribed amount and type of replace-

ment fluid through the infusion pump into the arterial side of the circuit.

◆ Monitor alarms and resolve indicated problems per recommended procedures.

◆ Infuse heparin as ordered and adjust the dose according to clotting values.

◆ Maintain intake and output records per facility policy.

Posttreatment care

◆ Assess all pulses in the affected leg every hour for the first 4 hours, then every 2 hours. Observe for signs of obstructed blood flow, such as coolness, pallor, and weak pulse.

◆ Monitor the groin area on the affected side for signs of bleeding.

◆ Maintain immobility of the affected leg.

◆ Monitor serum electrolytes as ordered.

◆ Inspect the site dressing every 4 to 8 hours for signs of infection and bleeding.

◆ Perform wound care at the catheter insertion sites every 48 hours, using sterile technique. Cover the sites with an occlusive dressing.

◆ Restart CRRT or assist with IHD as indicated.

PATIENT TEACHING

◆ Teach the patient about wound care as appropriate.

◆ Explain the need for IHD and what to expect during the treatment as appropriate.

◆ Explain the need for follow-up laboratory studies.

Coronary artery bypass grafting

Overview

Coroany artery bypass grafting, the grafting a blood vessel segment from another part of the body to the coronary vessels to restore normal myocardium blood flow, creates an alternate circulatory route that bypasses an occluded coronary artery. The saphenous vein or internal mammary artery is commonly used.

INDICATIONS
◆ Medically uncontrolled angina that adversely affects quality of life
◆ Left main coronary artery disease (CAD)
◆ Severe proximal left anterior descending coronary artery stenosis
◆ Three (or more)-vessel CAD with proximal stenoses or left ventricular dysfunction
◆ Three (or more)-vessel CAD with normal left ventricular function at rest, but with inducible ischemia and poor exercise capacity

COMPLICATIONS
◆ Cardiac arrhythmias
◆ Hypertension or hypotension
◆ Cardiac tamponade
◆ Thromboembolism
◆ Hemorrhage
◆ Postpericardiotomy syndrome
◆ Myocardial infarction
◆ Stroke
◆ Postoperative depression or emotional instability
◆ Pulmonary embolism
◆ Decreased renal function
◆ Infection

Pretreatment care

◆ Verify that an informed consent form has been signed.
◆ Monitor the patient's cardiac rhythm and vital signs.
◆ Assess the patient's pain level and administer analgesia as ordered.
◆ Administer cardiac medications as ordered.
◆ Have the patient shower with antiseptic soap as ordered.
◆ Restrict food and fluids after midnight as ordered.
◆ Provide sedation, as ordered, and assist with pulmonary artery catheterization and insertion of arterial lines.

PATIENT TEACHING
◆ Explain the reason for the treatment and preoperative preparation.
◆ Explain what to expect during the immediate postoperative period, and describe equipment that may be used, such as an endotracheal tube and a mechanical ventilator, a cardiac monitor, a nasogastric tube, a chest tube, an indwelling urinary catheter, an arterial line, epicardial pacing wires, and a pulmonary artery catheter.
◆ Demonstrate deep-breathing and coughing techniques and how to use an incentive spirometer.
◆ Review range-of-motion (ROM) exercises with the patient.

Procedure

◆ The patient receives general anesthesia, and the surgeon makes a series of incisions in the patient's thigh or calf to remove a saphenous vein segment for grafting; internal mammarian artery segments may also be removed.

◆ A medial sternotomy is done and the heart is exposed.

◆ Cardiopulmonary bypass is initiated; cardiac hypothermia and standstill are induced.

◆ The surgeon sutures one end of the venous graft to the ascending aorta and the other end to a patent coronary artery distal to the occlusion; this procedure is repeated for each artery that will be bypassed.

◆ After the grafts are in place, the surgeon flushes the cardioplegic solution from the heart, and cardiopulmonary bypass is discontinued.

◆ Epicardial pacing electrodes are implanted and a chest tube is inserted.

◆ The incision is closed and a sterile dressing is applied.

Posttreatment care

◆ Keep emergency resuscitative equipment immediately available.

◆ Monitor the patient's vital signs, cardiac rhythm, hemodynamic measurements, pulse oximetry, and intake and output.

◆ Monitor cardiovascular and respiratory status.

◆ Assess the patient's pain level, administer analgesics, and evaluate their effects.

◆ Maintain ventilator settings and alarms as ordered. Provide suctioning as needed.

◆ Administer medications as ordered.

◆ Assist with weaning the patient from the ventilator as appropriate.

◆ Maintain chest tube patency and observe and document the color and amount of drainage.

◆ Promote chest physiotherapy; encourage coughing, deep breathing, and incentive spirometry use.

◆ Assist the patient with ROM exercises. Encourage ambulation when permitted.

◆ Monitor the patient for complications.

◆ Assess surgical wounds and dressings.

◆ Monitor for electrolyte imbalances.

PATIENT TEACHING

◆ Teach about the administration, dosage, and possible adverse effects of prescribed medications.

◆ Review incentive spirometry therapy with the patient.

◆ Instruct the patient about how to care for the incision site.

◆ Tell the patient about the signs and symptoms of complications.

◆ Inform the patient how to identify and cope with postoperative depression.

◆ Review dietary restrictions with the patient.

◆ Teach the patient about activity restrictions, the need for adequate rest periods, and the prescribed exercise program.

◆ Provide information on smoking cessation programs as appropriate.

◆ Refer the patient for cardiac rehabilitation and home care as needed.

◆ Stress the importance of follow-up care.

◆ Refer the patient to the Mended Hearts Club and American Heart Association for information and support.

Craniotomy

Overview

A craniotomy is a surgical opening into the skull that exposes the brain for treatment. Supratentorial craniotomy involves frontal, parietal, temporal, occipital, or a combination of surgical approaches. An infratentorial craniotomy is an incision above the neck in the back of the skull.

INDICATIONS
- Ventricular shunt placement
- Tumor excision
- Abscess drainage
- Hematoma aspiration
- Aneurysm clipping

COMPLICATIONS
- Infection
- Vasospasm
- Hemorrhage
- Increased intracranial pressure (ICP)
- Diabetes insipidus
- Syndrome of inappropriate antidiuretic hormone
- Seizures
- Cranial nerve damage

Pretreatment care

- Verify that an informed consent form has been signed.
- Perform a complete neurologic assessment.
- Monitor the patient's vital signs.
- Provide support to the patient and his family.

PATIENT TEACHING
- Explain the reason for the treatment, how it's performed, and the preoperative preparation.
- Explain the intensive care unit and equipment the patient will see postoperatively.

Procedure

- The patient receives a general or local anesthetic.
- The surgeon marks an incision line and cuts through the scalp to the cranium, forming a scalp flap that's folded to one side.
- The surgeon then bores four or five holes through the skull in the corners of the cranial incision and cuts out a bone flap.
- After pulling aside or removing the bone flap, the surgeon incises and retracts the dura, exposing the brain; the surgeon then proceeds with the required surgery.
- The dura mater is closed, and a drain may be used.
- If swelling is anticipated, the bone flap usually isn't replaced.
- Periosteum and muscle are approximated. Skin closure is performed and dressings are applied.

Posttreatment care

- Maintain a patent airway.
- Administer prescribed oxygen, and monitor pulse oximetry.
- Monitor the patient's vital signs, intake and output, neurologic and respiratory status, ICP, heart rate and rhythm, and hemodynamic values.
- Take steps to protect the patient's safety.
- Administer medications as ordered.
- Position the patient with the head of the bed elevated 15 to 30 degrees; turn the patient carefully every 2 hours and provide skin care.
- Encourage careful deep breathing and coughing; suction gently as needed.
- Ensure a quiet, calm environment.
- Assist the patient with range of motion exercises.
- Maintain seizure precautions.

◆ Assess fluid and electrolyte balance, urine specific gravity, and daily weight.
◆ Monitor drain patency, the surgical wound and dressings, and drainage.
◆ Apply sequential compression stockings while the patient is in bed.
◆ Monitor the patient for complications.

PATIENT TEACHING
◆ Teach about the administration, dosage, and possible adverse effects of prescribed medications.
◆ Review care of the surgical wound with the patient.
◆ Review postoperative leg exercises and deep breathing with the patient.
◆ Instruct the patient on the use of antiembolism stockings.
◆ Review signs and symptoms of infection and other complications as well as when to notify the practitioner.
◆ Advise the patient to avoid alcohol and smoking.
◆ Emphasize follow-up care.

Deep brain stimulation

Overview

Deep brain stimulation (DBS) is the delivery of mild electrical stimulation that blocks signals from the thalamus, subthalamic nucleus, or globus pallidus to suppress tremors without destroying brain tissue. Target areas are identified by a computed tomography scan, magnetic resonance imaging, or microelectrode recording. Stimulation can be adjusted as symptoms change.

This procedure may be performed on one or both sides of the brain and is usually staged so that each side of the brain is treated on separate days.

INDICATIONS
◆ Essential tremor
◆ Parkinson's disease

COMPLICATIONS
◆ Infection
◆ Paresthesia
◆ Paralysis
◆ Ataxia
◆ Intracerebral hemorrhage
◆ Seizures
◆ Stroke
◆ Confusion

Pretreatment care

◆ Perform a complete neurologic assessment.
◆ Verify that the patient has signed an informed consent form.
◆ Tell the patient that his head may be shaved in the operating room.

PATIENT TEACHING
◆ Explain the treatment and preparation to the patient and his family.
◆ Tell the patient that headache and facial swelling may occur for 2 or 3 days after surgery.

◆ Review postoperative leg and deep-breathing exercises and use of antiembolism stockings or a pneumatic compression device.

Procedure

LEAD PLACEMENT
◆ The patient's scalp is anesthetized with local anesthetic. Occasional I.V. sedation is also used for patient comfort but generally the patient is awake during the lead placement.
◆ An incision is made on the top of the head behind the hairline and a small opening (burr hole) is made.
◆ The neurologist and neurosurgeon identify and mark the target sites, then a permanent DBS lead is inserted through the burr hole.
◆ The patient is asked to answer questions and perform some tasks during the procedure to test the stimulation and maximize symptom control.
◆ I.V. sedation is administered and the lead is anchored to the skull with a plastic cap and the scalp incision is sutured shut.

NEUROSTIMULATOR PLACEMENT
◆ The neurostimulator is generally placed at a later time than lead placement.
◆ This surgery is performed under general anesthesia.
◆ A small incision is made in the upper chest near the collar bone. A subcutaneous pocket is formed and the neurostimulator is implanted under the skin.
◆ The lead is attached to an extension cable which is passed under the skin of the scalp, neck, and shoulder and connected to the neurostimulator (see *Deep brain stimulation system*).
◆ Programming of the neurostimulator usually takes place 3 to 4 weeks after implantation.

Posttreatment care

◆ Monitor the patient's vital signs and closely observe neurologic status.
◆ Ensure a quiet, calm environment.
◆ Monitor fluid and electrolyte balance.
◆ Make sure dressings stay clean, dry, and intact.
◆ Assist with activities of daily living as appropriate.
◆ Administer medications as ordered.
◆ Observe for signs and symptoms of complications.

PATIENT TEACHING

◆ Teach about the administration, dosage, and possible adverse effects of prescribed medications.
◆ Review surgical wound care.
◆ Discuss the signs and symptoms of complications, and when to notify the practitioner.
◆ Tell the patient not to engage in light activities for 2 weeks after surgery and heavy activities for 4 to 6 weeks after surgery.
◆ Review how to activate and deactivate the neurostimulator, per practitioner recommendations.
◆ Explain the importance of follow-up care.

Deep brain stimulation system

The deep brain stimulation system consists of the stimulating lead (which is implanted to the desired target), the extension cable (which is tunneled under the scalp and soft tissues of the neck to the anterior chest wall), and the pulse generator (which is the programmable source of the electrical impulses). This illustration shows the placement of the stimulator in the patient's body.

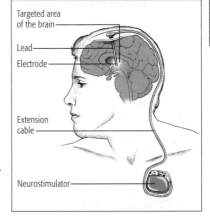

Targeted area of the brain

Lead

Electrode

Extension cable

Neurostimulator

Enhanced external counterpulsation

Overview

Enhanced external counterpulsation (EECP) is a noninvasive procedure that reduces the symptoms of chronic angina pectoris by increasing coronary blood flow in the heart's ischemic areas. The treatment involves using a sequential compression device that's modulated by events in the cardiac cycle via computer-interpreted electrocardiogram (ECG) signals to increase venous return and stimulate collateral circulation.

INDICATIONS
◆ Stable or unstable angina pectoris
◆ Patients considered at high risk for revascularization procedures
◆ Heart failure
◆ Cardiogenic shock

COMPLICATIONS
◆ Discomfort from the pulsatile movement and pressure on legs and buttocks

Pretreatment care

◆ At each visit and before treatment begins, take and record the patient's resting blood pressure, and measure and record the sitting pulse and respiratory rates.
◆ Examine the patient's legs for areas of redness, ecchymosis, and signs of other vascular problems.
◆ Advise the patient to urinate immediately before treatment.
◆ Ask the patient about symptoms of angina and review the patient's record.
◆ Place the patient in a comfortable position and give supplemental oxygen as indicated.
◆ Provide continuous cardiac monitoring as indicated.

PATIENT TEACHING
◆ Explain the underlying disorder and the reason for the treatment.
◆ Explain to the patient what to expect during and after the treatment.
◆ Tell the patient that discomfort from the pulsatile movement and pressure on legs and buttocks may be eliminated or minimized by using suitable protective clothing, such as tights or bicycle pants, during treatment.

Procedure

◆ The EECP device is placed on the patient's legs and set to inflate and deflate a series of compression cuffs wrapped around the patient's calves, lower thighs, and upper thighs (see *Enhanced external counterpulsation device*).
◆ At the start of treatment, external compression is progressively increased, as needed, to raise diastolic pressures gradually. Finger plethysmography is used to monitor correct timings.
◆ Inflation and deflation of the cuffs are modulated by events in the cardiac cycle via computer-interpreted ECG signals.
◆ During diastole, the cuffs inflate sequentially from the calves proximally, resulting in augmented diastolic central aortic pressure and increased coronary perfusion pressure. Rapid and simultaneous decompression of the cuffs at the onset of systole permits systolic unloading and decreased cardiac workload.
◆ Patients are treated with EECP 1 or 2 hours per day for a total of 35 hours over 7 weeks. The first week of treatment is limited to 1 hour daily to familiarize the patient with the procedure and to monitor the patient's tolerance. Two hours of treatment on the same day is usually separated by a rest period.

Posttreatment care

◆ Administer medications and monitor their effects as ordered.
◆ Monitor the patient's vital signs and intake and output as ordered.
◆ Provide support for the patient's family.

PATIENT TEACHING

◆ Review the signs and symptoms of heart failure.
◆ Advise the patient that if the pulsating sensation becomes uncomfortable, he should notify the treatment supervisor immediately to stop the treatment.
◆ Instruct the patient to record each anginal attack; its time of occurrence, duration, and severity; its relationship to precipitating factors; and the number of nitroglycerin tablets used to ease the attack. Check the patient's diaries for accuracy and completeness at each treatment visit.
◆ Emphasize the importance of follow-up care.

Enhanced external counterpulsation device

The enhanced external counterpulsation device is a series of compression cuffs that are placed on the patient's legs and set to inflate and deflate. This illustration shows the sequence of inflations: the calves are inflated first, then the thighs, then the buttocks.

SEQUENCE OF INFLATIONS

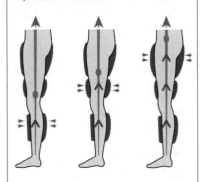

Femoral popliteal bypass

Overview

Femoral popliteal bypass is a surgical procedure performed to restore blood flow to a leg with a femoral or popliteal artery occlusion. A vein graft (usually from the saphenous vein) or a synthetic vein graft is transplanted into the leg to bypass the diseased vessel.

INDICATIONS

♦ Vessel damaged by an arteriosclerotic or thromboembolic disorder
♦ Arterial occlusive disease
♦ Limb-threatening acute arterial occlusion unresponsive to thrombolytic drug therapy
♦ Vessel trauma, infection, or congenital defect
♦ Vascular disease unresponsive to drug therapy or nonsurgical revascularization

COMPLICATIONS

♦ Vessel or nerve injury
♦ Thrombus or emboli formation
♦ Myocardial infarction
♦ Cardiac arrhythmias
♦ Hemorrhage
♦ Infection
♦ Leg edema
♦ Pulmonary edema
♦ Graft occlusion, narrowing, dilation, or rupture

Pretreatment care

♦ Verify that the patient has signed an informed consent form.
♦ Perform a complete neurovascular assessment; mark the location of distal peripheral pulses bilaterally, if present.
♦ Obtain baseline vital signs and obtain or verify the completion of the baseline 12-lead electrocardiogram and laboratory studies.
♦ Restrict food and fluids as ordered.
♦ Notify the surgeon if the patient is sensitive to or is allergic to any medications, latex, iodine, tape, contrast dyes, or local or general anesthetic agents.

♦ Make sure the surgeon marks the site where the procedure is to be performed.
♦ Complete the preoperative verification process.
♦ Initiate peripheral I.V. access; inform the patient that his heart rhythm will be monitored during the procedure.
♦ Administer medication as ordered.

PATIENT TEACHING

♦ Explain the underlying disorder and the reason for the treatment.
♦ Explain the treatment and preparation to the patient and his family.
♦ Explain postoperative care.
♦ Demonstrate how to perform coughing and deep-breathing exercises and how to use an incentive spirometer.

Procedure

♦ The procedure may be done under local or general anesthesia.
♦ The surgical area is shaved and thoroughly cleaned with an antiseptic solution.
♦ Immediately before starting the procedure, the surgical team takes a "time out" to verify the correct patient, procedure, and site.
♦ If the saphenous vein is used, an incision is made in the thigh and the other tissues are retracted until the vein can be seen. An appropriate length of the vein is excised for grafting and prepared (the vein is reversed so that the end that was originally located in the groin is now connected to the popliteal artery to eliminate hindrance of the valves).
♦ If the saphenous vein is inadequate, a synthetic vein graft is used.
♦ The saphenous access incision is closed and smaller incisions are made in the groin area to access the femoral artery, and behind the knee for the popliteal artery.
♦ One end of the vein graft is attached above the blockage femorally, and the free end of the graft is tunneled next to the artery to the popliteal site, where it's sutured in place.

Treatments

◆ Blood flow is initiated through the graft and the connections are assessed for leakage.

◆ A repeat arteriogram is performed to confirm that blood flow has been restored.

◆ The incisions are closed and dressings are applied.

Posttreatment care

◆ Monitor the patient's vital signs, heart rate and rhythm, and neurovascular status per facility policy. (Use Doppler ultrasonography if peripheral pulses aren't palpable.)

◆ Administer medications as ordered.

◆ Position the patient, as ordered, and encourage frequent turning, keeping pressure off the graft site.

◆ Provide comfort measures and analgesics as needed.

◆ Assist with initial transfers and ambulation when such movement is cleared by the practitioner, and explain recommended activity levels to the patient.

◆ Encourage frequent incentive spirometer use, coughing, and deep breathing.

◆ Assist with and teach the patient range-of-motion exercises.

◆ Assess incisions frequently for bleeding and infection, and provide care and dressing changes as ordered.

◆ Assess for complications, including abnormal bleeding, graft occlusion, signs of infection, chest pain, and breathing difficulty with embolism or pulmonary edema.

PATIENT TEACHING

◆ Review medications and possible adverse reactions with the patient.

◆ Teach the patient to monitor his lower extremities for changes in temperature, color, and sensation, and any return of preoperative symptoms, and to notify the surgeon of changes noted.

◆ Teach the patient how to care for the incision sites.

◆ Review the signs and symptoms of complications and when to notify the practitioner.

◆ Advise the patient to stop smoking, if appropriate, and encourage him to follow a low-cholesterol diet, exercise regularly per the practitioner's instructions, and have regular monitoring of his blood pressure and cholesterol levels.

◆ Stress the importance of follow-up care.

Gastric bypass

Overview

Gastric bypass, also called a *Roux-en-Y bypass,* is a procedure that creates a small stomach pouch attached to a portion of the jejunum to reduce the body's intake of calories, potentially resulting in significant weight loss. Postoperatively, the patient feels fuller faster because his stomach is smaller.

Before treatment is initiated, the patient undergoes a complete medical and psychological examination to evaluate his overall health and readiness for this lifestyle change. The patient also receives extensive nutritional counseling.

INDICATIONS

◆ Body mass index (BMI) of 40 or more (A patient with a BMI of 40 or more is at least 100 lb (45 kg) over his recommended weight; normal BMI is 18.5 to 25.)
◆ BMI of 35 or more plus a life-threatening illness that can be improved with weight loss, such as sleep apnea, type 2 diabetes, and heart disease

COMPLICATIONS

◆ Bleeding
◆ Infections
◆ Gallstones
◆ Gastritis
◆ Vomiting
◆ Iron or vitamin B_{12} deficiencies leading to anemia
◆ Calcium deficiency leading to osteoporosis
◆ Dumping syndrome (nausea, vomiting, diarrhea, dizziness, and sweating)
◆ Liver or renal failure

Pretreatment care

◆ Verify that the patient has signed an informed consent form.
◆ Obtain blood samples for hematologic and chemistry studies as ordered.
◆ Withhold food and fluids as ordered.
◆ Begin I.V. fluid replacement and total parenteral nutrition as ordered.
◆ Prepare the patient for abdominal X-rays as ordered.
◆ Monitor the patient's vital signs, intake and output, nutritional status, and laboratory test results.
◆ Complete the preoperative verification process.

PATIENT TEACHING

◆ Explain the treatment and preparation to the patient and his family.
◆ Explain postoperative care and equipment.
◆ Demonstrate coughing and deep-breathing exercises and how to use an incentive spirometer.

Procedure

GASTRIC BYPASS

◆ Immediately before starting the procedure, the surgical team takes a "time out" to verify the correct patient, procedure, and site.
◆ The surgery is performed under general anesthesia.
◆ The surgeon divides the stomach into a small upper section and a larger bottom section using staples similar to stitches.
◆ After the stomach has been divided, the surgeon connects a section of the small intestine (commonly the jejunum) to the upper section, or pouch.
◆ The surgeon then reconnects the base of the Roux limb with the remaining portion of the small intestines from the bottom of the stomach, forming a Y-shape.

Gastric bypass using a laparoscope

◆ Small incisions are made in the abdomen.

◆ Carbon dioxide is insufflated to separate the organs from one another.

◆ The surgeon passes slender surgical instruments through the incisions with a laparoscope to perform the procedure using video monitoring.

 Nursing alert

Gastric bypass with laparoscopy is contraindicated if the patient weighs more than 350 lb (159 kg) or if he has had previous abdominal surgery.

Posttreatment care

◆ Monitor the patient's vital signs, intake and output, and daily weight.

◆ Maintain I.V. replacement therapy as ordered.

◆ Keep the nasogastric tube patent, but don't reposition it.

◆ Encourage regular turning, coughing and deep-breathing exercises, and incentive spirometry use.

◆ Encourage splinting of the incision site with coughing and movement.

◆ Report signs of dehydration, peritonitis, sepsis, infection, or postresection obstruction.

◆ Administer medications as ordered.

◆ Assess the patient's pain level and administer analgesia as ordered.

◆ Administer medications as ordered.

◆ Assess GI status. After bowel sounds return, begin oral intake, providing six small feedings per day.

◆ Monitor laboratory test results.

◆ Provide wound care, and assess the type and amount of drainage.

◆ Monitor for complications of morbid obesity, such as pneumonia, thromboembolism, skin breakdown, and delayed wound healing.

Patient teaching

◆ Teach about the administration, dosage, and possible adverse effects of prescribed medications.

◆ Teach about vitamin supplements that may be required.

◆ Review the signs and symptoms of complications with the patient.

◆ Teach the patient wound care.

◆ Inform the patient about dumping syndrome (weakness, nausea, flatulence, and palpitations occurring within 30 minutes after a meal) and how to prevent it.

◆ Review recommended dietary restrictions and expected progress of weight loss.

◆ Advise the patient that he may need to separate fluid and food intake by at least 30 minutes and to sip fluids only.

◆ Review the recommended exercise program.

◆ Inform the patient that for the first year after surgery, physical and mental health status, change in weight, and nutritional needs will be reviewed during his follow-up visits.

Heart valve replacement

Treatments

Overview

Heart valve replacement, which can be done using a medial sternotomy or minimally invasive approach, is the replacement of a diseased heart valve with a prosthesis to improve cardiac output. Replacements may be mechanical valves, tissue valves, or homografts (valves from a human donor). (See *Replacement heart valves.*)

INDICATIONS

♦ Severe aortic valvular stenosis or insufficiency
♦ Severe mitral valvular stenosis or insufficiency
♦ Damage or disease from bacterial endocarditis, rheumatic fever, calcific degeneration, or congenital abnormalities

COMPLICATIONS

♦ Postpericardiotomy syndrome
♦ Cardiac arrhythmias
♦ Hemorrhage
♦ Coagulopathy
♦ Stroke
♦ Prosthetic valve endocarditis
♦ Valve dysfunction or failure
♦ Renal failure
♦ Pulmonary or thromboembolism
♦ Infection

Pretreatment care

♦ Verify that the patient has signed an informed consent form.
♦ Obtain results of chest X-ray, 12-lead electrocardiogram (ECG), and laboratory tests, including blood typing and cross-matching.
♦ Perform a preoperative assessment, and complete the preoperative verification process.
♦ Initiate cardiac monitoring and obtain baseline vital signs.

PATIENT TEACHING

♦ Explain the underlying disorder.

♦ Explain the procedure and preparation to the patient and his family.
♦ Explain postoperative care and equipment.
♦ Demonstrate how to perform coughing and deep-breathing exercises and how to use an incentive spirometer.

Procedure

♦ After the patient is anesthetized, a medial sternotomy is performed, and cardiopulmonary bypass is initiated.
♦ If using a minimally invasive approach, a small incision is made in the chest and the surgeon works between the ribs to reach the valve.
♦ For aortic valve replacement, the aorta is clamped above the right coronary artery; for mitral valve replacement, the left atrium is incised to expose the mitral valve.
♦ The diseased valve is excised.
♦ The surgeon sutures around the margin of the valve annulus.
♦ The suture is threaded through the sewing ring of the prosthetic valve.
♦ Using a valve holder, the prosthesis is positioned, and the sutures are secured.
♦ The patient is removed from the bypass machine.
♦ As the heart fills with blood, the surgeon vents the aorta and ventricle for air.
♦ Epicardial pacemaker leads and a chest tube are inserted.
♦ The incision is closed, and a sterile dressing is applied.

Posttreatment care

♦ Monitor the patient's vital signs, cardiac rhythm, pulse oximetry, and hemodynamic values.
♦ Monitor the patient's cardiovascular and respiratory status.
♦ Maintain ventilator settings, monitor arterial blood gas values, provide suctioning as needed, and assist with weaning measures.
♦ Administer medications as ordered.

- Assist with temporary epicardial pacing as indicated.
- Monitor the ECG for development of arrhythmias and ischemia.
- Maintain the chest tube system as ordered. Report a sudden change in the amount of drainage or an output of 200 ml/hour.
- Administer I.V. fluids and blood products as ordered.
- Encourage coughing, turning, deep breathing, and incentive spirometry use.
- Assist with early ambulation.
- Record and evaluate daily weight, sternal stability and drainage, and intake and output.
- Monitor for complications.
- Perform surgical wound care and dressing changes, as ordered, and monitor for signs of infection.

PATIENT TEACHING
- Review medications and possible adverse reactions with the patient.
- Teach the patient wound care.
- Tell the patient about the signs and symptoms of complications.
- Stress the importance of monitoring laboratory values while on anticoagulants.
- Review activity restrictions and need for adequate rest periods.
- Review dietary restrictions.
- Emphasize the importance of informing all health care providers of the valve surgery.
- Stress the importance of wearing medical identification at all times.
- Stress the need for follow-up care.

Replacement heart valves

The most commonly used prosthetic valves for replacing a patient's malfunctioning heart valve are the tilting-disk valve, bileaflet valve, porcine valve, and bovine valve.

Tilting-disk valve
The tilting-disk valve, developed as an alternative to the ball-in-cage valve, has a hingeless design and contains open-ended, elliptical struts that reduce the risk of thrombus formation, offer improved blood flow and cause minimal damage to blood cells. The most common tilting-disk valve is the Medtronic Hall prosthesis. (Photo courtesy of Medtronic, Inc.)

Bileaflet valve
The most commonly used prosthetic valve, a bileaflet valve consists of two semicircular leaflets that pivot on hinges, swing partially open, and close to permit an acceptable amount of regurgitant blood flow. In the United States, the St. Jude Medical Valve is the most commonly inserted bileaflet valve. (Photo courtesy of St. Jude Medical.)

Porcine valve
A porcine valve is the aortic valve of a pig that's sewn to a frame, called a stent, commonly made from a plastic composite that's covered with a polyester cloth. Porcine valves include the Carpentier-Edwards Duraflex Low-Pressure Bioprosthesis Valve and the Medtronic Hancock II Valve. (Photos courtesy of Edwards Lifesciences [top] and Medtronic, Inc. [middle].)

Bovine valve
A bovine valve is made from the pericardial tissue of a cow. The Carpentier-Edwards PERIMOUNT Pericardial Bioprosthesis Valve is widely used. (Photo courtesy of Edwards Lifesciences.)

Hemodialysis

Overview

Hemodialysis is a procedure used to extract toxic wastes from the blood, restore or maintain balance of the body's buffer system and electrolyte level, promote rapid return to normal serum values, and prevent uremia-associated complications. The process removes the blood from the body, circulates it through a purifying dialyzer, then returns it to the body. For long-term treatment, various access sites are used, including an arteriovenous (AV) fistula or shunt.

INDICATIONS
◆ Chronic end-stage renal disease
◆ Acute renal failure
◆ Acute poisoning
◆ Drug overdose

COMPLICATIONS
◆ Dialysis disequilibrium syndrome
◆ Hypotension
◆ Cardiac arrhythmias
◆ Cardiovascular disease
◆ Air embolism
◆ Thrombosis or stenosis of an AV fistula
◆ Bleeding
◆ Infection
◆ Electrolyte imbalance
◆ Fluid imbalance
◆ Anemia

Pretreatment care

◆ Prepare the hemodialysis equipment following the manufacturer's instructions and facility protocol.
◆ Test the dialyzer and dialysis machine for residual disinfectant after rinsing, and test all alarms.
◆ Maintain strict sterile technique to prevent introducing pathogens into the patient's bloodstream.
◆ Wear appropriate personal protective equipment throughout all procedures.
◆ Weigh the patient and record his weight.
◆ Record baseline vital signs.

◆ Assess the condition and patency of the access site.
◆ Auscultate for bruits and palpate for a thrill to confirm patency of the AV fistula or shunt before beginning and periodically throughout the procedure; notify the practitioner if bruits or a thrill is absent.
◆ Help the patient into a comfortable position (supine or sitting in recliner chair with feet elevated).
◆ Obtain blood samples from the patient, as ordered, before beginning hemodialysis; evaluate the results.

PATIENT TEACHING
◆ If the patient is undergoing hemodialysis for the first time, explain the procedure.

Procedure

◆ Place a clean drape under the access site, which may be located in the groin, arm, or chest.

HEMODIALYSIS WITH A DOUBLE-LUMEN CATHETER
◆ Make sure the extension tubing is clamped.
◆ Clean each catheter extension tube, clamp, and Luer-lock injection cap with povidone-iodine pads.
◆ Place a sterile gauze pad under the extension tubing, and place two 5-ml syringes and two sterile gauze pads on the drape.
◆ Prepare the anticoagulant regimen as ordered.
◆ Identify arterial and venous blood lines and place them near the drape.
◆ Remove catheter caps, attach syringes to each catheter port, open the clamp, aspirate 1.5 to 3 ml of blood, close the clamp, and flush each port with 5 ml of heparin flush solution.
◆ Remove the syringe from the arterial port and the line attached to it; administer heparin according to protocol.
◆ Grasp the venous blood line and attach it to the venous port; open the clamps on

the extension tubing and secure the tubing to the patient's extremity with tape.
- Start hemodialysis according to facility protocol.

HEMODIALYSIS WITH AN AV FISTULA OR SHUNT

- Flush the fistula needles, using attached syringes containing heparinized saline solution, and set them aside.
- Place a linen-saver pad under the patient's arm.
- Using sterile technique, clean the area of skin over the fistula or shunt with chlorhexidine gluconate.
- Apply a tourniquet above the fistula or shunt to distend the veins and facilitate venipuncture; avoid occluding the fistula or shunt.
- Put on clean gloves and remove the fistula or shunt needle guard and squeeze the wing tips firmly together. Insert the arterial needle above the anastomosis, being careful not to puncture the fistula or shunt.
- Release the tourniquet and flush the needle with heparin flush solution to prevent clotting.
- Clamp the arterial needle tubing with a hemostat, and secure the wing tips of the needle to the skin with adhesive tape.
- Perform another venipuncture with the venous needle a few inches above the arterial needle.
- Flush the venous needle with heparin flush solution.
- Clamp the venous needle tubing, and secure the wing tips of the venous needle with tape.
- Remove the syringe from the end of the arterial tubing, uncap the arterial line from the hemodialysis machine, and connect the two lines.
- Tape the connection securely to prevent separation during the procedure.
- Remove the syringe from the end of the venous tubing, uncap the venous line from the hemodialysis machine, and connect the two lines.

- Tape the connection securely.
- Release the hemostat and start hemodialysis.
- Monitor vital signs throughout hemodialysis at least hourly or as often as every 15 minutes, if indicated.
- Perform periodic tests for clotting time on patient's blood samples and samples from the dialyzer.
- Give necessary drugs during dialysis unless the drug would be removed in the dialysate.

Posttreatment care

- Monitor the patient's vital signs.
- Evaluate posttreatment laboratory values.
- Weigh the patient and record his weight; compare his current weight to his pretreatment weight.
- Observe the patient for adverse effects of treatment.
- Assess the catheter insertion site for signs of infection, such as purulent drainage, inflammation, and tenderness.
- Provide emotional support.

PATIENT TEACHING

- Tell the patient to notify the practitioner if pain, swelling, redness, or drainage occurs in the accessed arm.
- Provide the telephone number of the dialysis center.
- Remind the patient not to allow any treatments or procedures on the accessed arm, including blood pressure monitoring or needle punctures. Tell him to avoid putting excessive pressure on the arm.
- Review the dialysis schedule with the patient and his family. Make sure that they're aware of the next scheduled treatment.
- Review fluid and diet restrictions as needed.

Hypophysectomy

Overview

A hypophysectomy is the surgical excision of all or part of the pituitary gland. The most common approaches are transsphenoidal entry into the sella turcica from the inner aspect of the upper lip through the sphenoid sinus, and endoscopic transnasal entry into the sella turcica through a nostril and small opening into the sphenoid sinus.

INDICATIONS
◆ Pituitary tumor
◆ Palliative measure for metastatic breast or prostate cancer (rare)

COMPLICATIONS
◆ Diabetes insipidus
◆ Transient syndrome of inappropriate antidiuretic hormone
◆ Infection with possible brain abscess or meningitis
◆ Cerebrospinal fluid leakage
◆ Hemorrhage
◆ Vision defects
◆ Loss of smell and taste
◆ Nasal septum injury

Pretreatment care

◆ Verify that the patient has signed an informed consent form.
◆ Instruct the patient to fast after midnight before surgery.
◆ Arrange for a baseline visual field test and other appropriate tests and examinations as ordered.
◆ Administer antibiotics before the procedure as ordered.

PATIENT TEACHING
◆ Review the disorder and the reason for the procedure.
◆ Review the treatment and preparation with the patient and his family.
◆ Instruct the patient to begin taking hydrocortisone (Cortef) tablets the day before surgery as ordered, and explain what the drug is for, its adverse effects, and that it will be continued for a few days postoperatively.
◆ Explain postoperative care, including the presence of a nasal catheter and packing for 2 to 4 days after surgery following transsphenoidal approach.
◆ Explain to the patient that before preoperative magnetic resonance imaging is performed, he will have four or five marker, stick-on buttons applied to his skull. These marker buttons and the scan results are used to guide the surgery and should be left in place.

Procedure

TRANSSPHENOIDAL HYPOPHYSECTOMY
◆ After the patient receives general anesthesia, the surgeon makes an incision in the superior gingival tissue of the maxilla; membranes and tissues are dissected, and the nasal septum is removed.
◆ A speculum blade is placed slightly anterior to the sphenoid sinus.
◆ The deeper anatomy is evaluated using an operating microscope with binocular vision and high-power lighting.
◆ Using a microdrill, the surgeon penetrates the sphenoid bone to view the anterior sella floor and the tumor is resected and aspirated.
◆ Hemostatic agents, subcutaneous fat plug (from the abdomen or outer thigh), or a muscle plug (from the thigh as graft tissue) may be placed to control bleeding or leakage of cerebrospinal fluid and the sella floor may be sealed off with a small piece of bone or cartilage.
◆ The nasal septum is replaced.
◆ Nasal catheters are inserted, and petroleum gauze is packed around them.
◆ The initial incision is closed with stitches inside the inner lip.

Treatments

Endoscopic transnasal hypophysectomy

◆ After the patient receives general anesthesia, an endoscope is inserted into one nostril until the ostium (opening passageway) of the sphenoid sinus is visualized.

◆ The ostium is enlarged to allow passage of the endoscope into the sinus cavity.

◆ Using a microdrill, the surgeon penetrates the sphenoid bone to view the anterior sella floor and the tumor is resected and aspirated.

◆ Hemostatic agents or a fat plug may be used as needed.

◆ The endoscope is removed and a small mustache dressing is applied.

Posttreatment care

◆ Monitor vital signs, neurologic status, and intake and output.

◆ Administer medications and I.V. fluids as ordered.

◆ Elevate the head of the bed to facilitate drainage and reduce swelling.

◆ Maintain bed rest for 24 hours if ordered, then encourage ambulation (endoscopic transnasal approach may be done as same day surgery).

◆ Arrange for visual field testing as ordered.

◆ Obtain laboratory tests as ordered.

◆ Assess for complications.

Patient teaching

◆ Review medications and possible adverse reactions with the patient.

◆ Explain the signs and symptoms of complications and when to notify the practitioner.

◆ Review fluid restrictions as indicated.

◆ Advise the patient to avoid sneezing, coughing, blowing his nose, or bending over for several days after surgery.

◆ If the transsphenoidal approach was used, advise the patient to avoid brushing his teeth for 2 weeks, if directed by the practitioner; suggest he use a mouthwash instead.

◆ Inform the patient about the signs and symptoms of excessive or insufficient cortisol or thyroid hormone and to notify the practitioner of problems.

◆ Emphasize the importance of wearing medical identification if hormone replacements are required.

◆ Stress the need for follow-up care.

Implantable cardioverter-defibrillator

Overview

An implantable cardioverter-defibrillator (ICD) is an electronic device inserted into the body with electrodes that connect to the heart. This device monitors for bradycardia, ventricular tachycardia, and fibrillation; delivers shocks or paced beats when indicated; and stores information and electrocardiograms (ECGs) to track treatments and their outcomes. Settings are adjustable, and functions and battery status may be monitored, depending on the model used. (See *Types of ICD therapies*.) ICDs are implanted via transvenous approach, thoracotomy, subxiphoid approach, or median sternotomy.

INDICATIONS
◆ Cardiac arrhythmias refractory to drug therapy, surgery, or catheter ablation

COMPLICATIONS
◆ Infection
◆ Venous thrombosis and embolism
◆ Pneumothorax
◆ Pectoral or diaphragmatic muscle stimulation
◆ Arrhythmias
◆ Cardiac tamponade
◆ Cardiac arrest
◆ Myocardial infarction
◆ Lead dislodgment
◆ ICD malfunction

Pretreatment care

◆ Verify that an informed consent form has been signed.
◆ Obtain baseline vital signs and a 12-lead ECG.
◆ Evaluate the patient's radial and pedal pulses.
◆ Assess the patient's mental status.
◆ Restrict food and fluids before the procedure as ordered.
◆ If the patient is monitored, document and report arrhythmias.

◆ Administer medications as ordered, and prepare to assist with medical procedures, such as defibrillation if indicated.

PATIENT TEACHING
◆ Explain the underlying disorder and the reason for the treatment.
◆ Explain the treatment and preparation.
◆ Explain postoperative care.

Procedure

◆ The transvenous route with fluoroscopy, in which the leadwires are inserted into the heart via the subclavian vein, and the ICD device is implanted into a pocket under the skin, is the most commonly used ICD placement procedure.
◆ The thoracotomy approach, in which a thoracotomy is performed and the leadwires are sewn to the outside of the heart, may be used for patients who have mediastinal adhesions from previous sternal surgery.
◆ The subxiphoid approach is similar to a thoracotomy approach with the incision made slightly to the left of the sternum.
◆ A median sternotomy may be used if the patient requires other cardiac surgery such as revascularization.
◆ One or more leadwires are attached to the epicardium.
◆ A programmable pulse generator is inserted into a pocket made under the right or left clavicle.
◆ The device is programmed and checked for proper functioning.

Posttreatment care

◆ Monitor the patient's vital signs, intake and output, heart rate and rhythm, surgical incision, dressings, and drainage.
◆ Monitor for complications such as infection.
◆ Maintain the occlusive dressing for the first 24 hours.

◆ After the first 24 hours, begin passive range-of-motion exercises if ordered, and progress as tolerated.

◆ If the patient experiences cardiac arrest, initiate cardiopulmonary resuscitation (CPR) and advanced cardiac life support (wearing latex gloves to avoid experiencing an ICD shock).

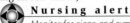 **Nursing alert**

Monitor for signs and symptoms of a perforated ventricle with resultant cardiac tamponade, distant heart sounds, pulsus paradoxus, hypotension accompanied by narrow pulse pressure, increased venous pressure, bulging jugular veins, cyanosis, decreased urine output, restlessness, and complaints of fullness in the chest. Notify the practitioner immediately of such findings, and prepare the patient for emergency surgery.

PATIENT TEACHING

◆ Teach about the administration, dosage, and possible adverse effects of prescribed medications.

◆ Describe signs and symptoms of possible complications and when to notify the practitioner.

◆ Provide written information on the ICD type and model, status (on or off), detection rates, and therapies to be delivered (such as pacing, antitachycardia pacing, cardioversion, and defibrillation).

◆ Instruct the patient to wear a medical identification that indicates placement of an ICD and to always carry information about the ICD.

◆ Advise the patient to avoid placing excessive pressure over the insertion site.

◆ Instruct the patient to follow activity restrictions as directed by the practitioner.

◆ Inform the patient about what to expect when the ICD discharges and to notify the practitioner after the ICD discharges.

◆ Tell the patient to inform airline personnel and health care workers who perform diagnostic tests (such as computed tomography scans and magnetic resonance imaging) of the presence of an ICD and possible disruption of the ICD by electrical or electronic devices.

◆ Stress the need for follow-up care.

◆ Advise the patient of what to do in an emergency, such as calling 911 and having a family member perform CPR if the ICD fails.

Types of ICD therapies

Implantable cardioverter-defibrillators (ICDs) can deliver a range of therapies, depending on the arrhythmia detected and how the device is programmed. Therapies include antitachycardia pacing, cardioversion, defibrillation, and bradycardia pacing. Some ICDs can also provide biventricular pacing.

Therapy	Description
Antitachycardia pacing	A series of small, rapid electrical pacing pulses are used to interrupt atrial arrhythmias or ventricular tachycardia and return the heart to its normal rhythm. Antitachycardia pacing isn't appropriate for all patients; it's initiated by the practitioner after appropriate evaluation of electrophysiology studies.
Cardioversion	A low- or high-energy shock (up to 34 joules) that's timed to the R wave to terminate atrial fibrillation or ventricular tachycardia and return the heart to its normal rhythm.
Defibrillation	A high-energy shock (up to 34 joules) to the heart to terminate atrial fibrillation or ventricular fibrillation and return the heart to its normal rhythm.
Bradycardia pacing	Electrical pacing pulses used when the natural electrical signals are too slow. ICD systems can pace one chamber (VVI pacing) of the heart at a preset rate or sense and pace both chambers (DDD pacing).

Intra-aortic balloon counterpulsation

Overview

Intra-aortic balloon counterpulsation (IABC) is a procedure that temporarily supports the heart's left ventricle by mechanically displacing blood by an intra-aortic balloon attached to an external pump console. It increases the supply of oxygen-rich blood to the myocardium, decreases myocardial oxygen demand, and can monitor myocardial perfusion and the effects of drugs on myocardial function and perfusion. It's usually inserted through the common femoral artery and positioned with its tip just distal to the left subclavian artery.

INDICATIONS

◆ Low cardiac output disorders, including refractory angina, ventricular arrhythmias, and cardiogenic shock
◆ Cardiac instability, including myocardial infarction and high-grade lesions
◆ Support measures, including bypass surgery, angioplasty, and cardiac catheterization

COMPLICATIONS

◆ Arterial embolism
◆ Extension or rupture of an aortic aneurysm
◆ Femoral or iliac artery perforation
◆ Femoral artery occlusion
◆ Sepsis
◆ Bleeding at the insertion site

Pretreatment care

◆ Depending on facility policy, a nurse or a perfusionist must balance the pressure transducer in the external pump console and calibrate the oscilloscope monitor to ensure accuracy.
◆ Verify that the patient has signed an informed consent form.
◆ Record the patient's baseline vital signs and hemodynamic results if available.
◆ Monitor the electrocardiogram (ECG) continuously in lead II.

◆ Obtain a baseline 12-lead ECG.
◆ Provide oxygen as needed.
◆ Maintain and monitor arterial line and pulmonary artery catheters.
◆ Insert an indwelling urinary catheter, and monitor intake and output.
◆ Assess the patient's left arm and peripheral leg pulses and document sensation, movement, color, and temperature of the arm and legs.
◆ Give the patient a sedative as ordered.
◆ Place a defibrillator, suction, temporary pacemaker, and emergency drugs nearby in case the patient develops complications, such as an arrhythmia, during insertion.

PATIENT TEACHING

◆ Explain the underlying disorder and the reason for the treatment.
◆ Explain the treatment and what the patient can expect during and after the procedure.
◆ Review activity restrictions necessary during the treatment.

Procedure

INSERTING THE INTRA-AORTIC BALLOON PERCUTANEOUSLY

◆ The cardiologist may insert the balloon percutaneously through the femoral artery into the descending thoracic aorta, using a modified Seldinger technique.
◆ The vessel is accessed with an 18G angiography needle, the inner stylet is removed, the guide wire is passed through the needle, and then the needle is removed.
◆ An introducer (dilator and sheath assembly) is passed over the guide wire into the vessel until 1″ (2.5 cm) remains above the insertion site.
◆ The inner dilator is removed, leaving the introducer sheath and guide wire in place.
◆ After passing the balloon over the guide wire into the introducer sheath, the cardiologist advances the catheter into position, $\frac{3}{8}$″ to $\frac{3}{4}$″ (1 to 2 cm) distal to the left sub-

clavian artery under fluoroscopic guidance.

◆ The balloon is then attached to the control system to start counterpulsation.

INSERTING THE INTRA-AORTIC BALLOON SURGICALLY

◆ The cardiologist may decide to insert the catheter through a femoral arteriotomy.

◆ After making an incision and isolating the femoral artery, the cardiologist attaches a Dacron graft to a small opening in the arterial wall and passes the catheter through this graft.

◆ Using fluoroscopic guidance, the catheter is advanced up the descending thoracic aorta and the catheter tip positioned between the left subclavian and renal arteries.

◆ The Dacron graft is sewn around the catheter at the insertion point and the other end is connected to the pump console.

◆ If the balloon can't be inserted through the femoral artery, the cardiologist may use the transthoracic method and insert it in an antegrade direction through the anterior wall of the ascending aorta.

◆ The balloon is positioned $3/8''$ to $3/4''$ beyond the left subclavian artery and the catheter brought out through the chest wall.

Posttreatment care

◆ Verify correct balloon placement with a chest X-ray.

◆ Monitor vital signs, cardiac rhythm, intake and output, pulse oximetry, and laboratory test results.

◆ Assess and record pedal and posterior tibial pulses as well as color, sensation, and temperature in the affected limb every 15 minutes for 1 hour and then hourly.

◆ Monitor the patient's arm pulses, arm sensation and movement, and arm color and temperature every 15 minutes for 1 hour after balloon insertion; repeat every 2 hours while the balloon is in place.

◆ If the control system malfunctions or becomes inoperable, don't let the balloon catheter remain dormant for more than 30 minutes. Inflate the balloon manually until another control system is available.

◆ Watch for signs of bleeding, especially at the insertion site.

◆ Adjust the heparin drip according to protocol to maintain partial thromboplastin time (PTT) at $1\frac{1}{2}$ to 2 times the normal value; monitor PTT according to facility policy.

◆ Measure pulmonary artery pressure and pulmonary artery wedge pressure every 1 or 2 hours.

◆ To begin weaning from IABC, gradually decrease the frequency of balloon augmentation to 1:2 and 1:4 as ordered.

◆ Assist frequency is usually maintained for 1 hour or longer, depending on facility policy. If the patient's hemodynamic status remains stable during this time, weaning may continue.

◆ Before the cardiologist removes the balloon, make sure PTT is within normal limits.

◆ Turn off the control system and disconnect the connective tubing from the catheter to ensure balloon deflation.

◆ After the cardiologist withdraws the balloon, apply pressure above the puncture site for 30 minutes or until bleeding stops, if facility policy permits.

◆ After balloon removal, provide wound care according to facility policy.

◆ Monitor and record the patient's pedal and posterior tibial pulses and the color, temperature, and sensation of the affected limb.

◆ Enforce bed rest, with the head of the bed elevated no more than 30 degrees, usually for 24 hours.

◆ Change the dressing at the balloon insertion site every 24 hours or as needed, using strict sterile technique.

Joint replacement, hip

Overview

Hip replacement surgery, a procedure to restore hip joint mobility and stability and relieve pain, involves the total or partial replacement of the hip joint with a synthetic prosthesis consisting of two major parts: the acetabular cup and femoral stem. Newer minimally invasive techniques include two-incision and mini-incision surgery, which use an incision one-third the size of the traditional incision and a metal prosthesis.

INDICATIONS
◆ Osteoarthritis
◆ Rheumatoid arthritis
◆ Trauma
◆ Avascular necrosis
◆ Ankylosing spondylitis

COMPLICATIONS
◆ Hip fracture or dislocation
◆ Stroke
◆ Myocardial infarction
◆ Fat embolism
◆ Infection
◆ Hypovolemic shock
◆ Pulmonary edema
◆ Arterial thrombosis
◆ Pseudoaneurysm
◆ Hematoma
◆ Fracture of the joint cement
◆ Displaced prosthetic head
◆ Heterotrophic ossification (mainly in men)

Pretreatment care

◆ Verify that the patient has signed an informed consent form.
◆ Make sure the patient's medical history and physical examination, laboratory studies, and diagnostic tests are completed; report abnormal results.
◆ Check for a history of allergies.

◆ Make sure blood typing and crossmatching are completed; verify if blood is to be kept on hold for the patient.
◆ Be aware that the affected limb must be marked by someone from the surgical team before surgery.

PATIENT TEACHING
◆ Explain the treatment and preparation to the patient and his family.
◆ Explain postoperative care.
◆ Demonstrate how to perform coughing and deep-breathing exercises and how to use an incentive spirometer.

Procedure

◆ After general or regional (spinal) anesthesia is administered, the orthopedic surgeon removes the head of the femur, exposing the marrow cavity of the femur's shaft.
◆ The femoral component of the prosthesis is inserted into the cavity so that its head articulates with the acetabular cup.
◆ The acetabular cup is attached to the pelvic bones.
◆ A cemented or noncemented technique is used. (See *Total hip replacement.*)

CEMENTED TECHNIQUE
◆ The orthopedic surgeon cements the head of the prosthesis into a position that allows articulation with a studded cup.
◆ The studded cup is then cemented into the deepened acetabulum.

NONCEMENTED TECHNIQUE
◆ In a porous-coated prosthesis, the smooth metal surface is studded with metal beads and sprayed with a bone-stimulating material.
◆ The coated beads are designed to stimulate bone growth between the beads to hold the prosthesis in place.

Posttreatment care

♦ Monitor the patient's vital signs and pulse oximetry.
♦ Monitor neurovascular status distal to the operative site.
♦ Assess the patient's pain level, administer analgesia, and evaluate the patient's response.
♦ Administer I.V. fluids and blood products as ordered.
♦ Monitor the surgical wound, dressings, and drainage.
♦ Maintain bed rest for the prescribed period, then assist with exercises.
♦ Maintain the hip in proper alignment, using a triangular abduction pillow.
♦ Reposition the patient every 2 hours and provide skin care.
♦ Apply sequential compression boots.
♦ Encourage frequent coughing and deep-breathing exercises.
♦ Assess for complications.
♦ Arrange for rehabilitation as appropriate.

PATIENT TEACHING
♦ Reinforce physical therapy teaching.
♦ Teach the patient about the signs and symptoms of complications.
♦ Teach the patient appropriate wound care.
♦ Stress the importance of maintaining hip abduction.
♦ Instruct the patient to avoid flexing his hips more than 90 degrees when rising from a bed or chair.
♦ Teach the patient the proper use of assistive devices.
♦ Stress the need for follow-up care.

Total hip replacement

To form a totally artificial hip, the surgeon cements a femoral head prosthesis in place to articulate with a cup, which he then cements into the deepened acetabulum. He may avoid using cement by implanting a prosthesis with a porous coating that promotes bony ingrowth.

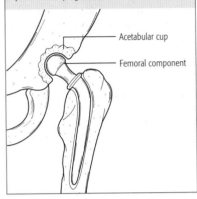

Acetabular cup

Femoral component

Joint replacement, knee

Overview

Knee replacement surgery, a procedure to restore knee joint mobility and stability and relieve pain, involves the total or partial replacement of the knee joint with a synthetic prosthesis. Newer minimally invasive techniques include two-incision and mini-incision surgery, which use an incision one-third the size of the traditional incision and a metal prosthesis.

INDICATIONS
◆ Severe chronic arthritis
◆ Degenerative joint disorders
◆ Extensive joint trauma
◆ Joint contractures
◆ Conditions that prohibit full extension or flexion

COMPLICATIONS
◆ Infection
◆ Hypovolemic shock
◆ Fat embolism
◆ Thromboembolism
◆ Pulmonary embolism
◆ Nerve compromise
◆ Prosthesis dislocation or loosening
◆ Heterotrophic ossification
◆ Avascular necrosis
◆ Atelectasis
◆ Pneumonia
◆ Deep vein thrombosis

Pretreatment care

◆ Verify that the patient has signed an informed consent form.
◆ Assure the patient that analgesics will be available as needed.
◆ Provide emotional support.
◆ Be aware that the affected limb must be marked by someone from the surgical team before the procedure.

PATIENT TEACHING
◆ Explain the treatment and patient preparation.
◆ Explain postoperative care.
◆ Demonstrate coughing and deep-breathing exercises and how to use an incentive spirometer.

Procedure

◆ After general anesthesia is administered, the orthopedic surgeon makes an incision over the affected knee.
◆ After the patella is moved, the prosthesis is placed, with adjustments made to the femur, tibia, and undersurface of the patella.
◆ Bone cement is used to secure the prosthesis. Then the area is sutured closed with a surgical drain in place.

Posttreatment care

◆ Monitor the patient's vital signs and intake and output.
◆ Monitor neurovascular status of the affected extremity.
◆ Assess the patient's pain level and provide analgesics as ordered.
◆ Administer medications as ordered.
◆ Maintain bed rest for the prescribed period.
◆ Maintain the affected joint in proper alignment.
◆ Apply sequential compression boots.
◆ Use a continuous passive motion (CPM) device as instructed.
◆ Monitor the surgical wound, dressings, and drainage, and change dressings as ordered.
◆ Reposition the patient every 2 hours and provide skin care.
◆ Encourage frequent coughing and deep-breathing exercises.

- Exercise the affected joint as ordered.
- If joint displacement occurs, notify the practitioner.
- If traction is used to correct joint displacement, periodically check the weights and other equipment.
- Assess for complications.

PATIENT TEACHING

- Review medications and possible adverse reactions with the patient.
- Tell the patient about the signs and symptoms of complications.
- Teach the patient appropriate wound care.
- Instruct the patient to follow the exercise program prescribed by the orthopedic surgeon and the physical therapist, including using a CPM device as ordered.
- Instruct the patient to follow the activity restrictions as directed by the orthopedic surgeon. Tell him to avoid contact sports, but that he can perform low-impact activities, such as swimming and golf, after he has recovered from surgery.
- Stress the need for follow-up care.

Lithotripsy

Overview

Lithotripsy, a procedure for removing obstructive renal calculi or gallstones, can be done as extracorporeal shock-wave lithotripsy (ESWL), a noninvasive, high-energy shock wave treatment, or percutaneous ultrasonic lithotripsy (PUL), an invasive procedure using ultrasonic shock waves at close range.

Nursing alert

Lithotripsy is contraindicated in patients with urinary or biliary tract obstruction distal to the calculi; with renal or gallbladder cancer; calculi that are fixed to the kidney, ureter, or gallbladder or located below the iliac crest level; or pacemakers; and in patients who are pregnant.

INDICATIONS
◆ Potentially obstructive calculi
◆ Emergency treatment for acute renal obstruction

COMPLICATIONS
◆ Hemorrhage
◆ Hematomas
◆ Obstruction (biliary or ureteral)

Pretreatment care

◆ Verify that the patient has signed an informed consent form.
◆ Arrange for the patient to see the ESWL device before treatment (if possible).
◆ Insert an I.V. catheter and place a cardiac monitor on the patient.
◆ Obtain baseline vital signs.

PATIENT TEACHING
◆ Review the underlying disorder, treatment and preparation with the patient and his family.
◆ Explain postprocedure care. If ESWL will be done for gallstones, explain that the patient may have mild pain afterward.

Procedure

◆ The patient receives I.V. or oral sedation, or a transcutaneous electrical nerve stimulator is used.

ESWL
◆ The patient is placed in a semi-reclining or supine position on the hydraulic stretcher of the ESWL machine on a water-filled cushion (or submerged in lukewarm water for gallstones) through which the shock waves are directed from the lithotriptor.
◆ The generator is focused on the calculi using biplane fluoroscopy confirmation.
◆ The generator is activated to direct high-energy shock waves through the cushion or water at the calculi.
◆ Shock waves are synchronized to the patient's R waves on the electrocardiogram and fired during diastole.
◆ The number of waves fired depends on the size, number, and composition of the calculi (500 to 2,000 shocks are delivered during a treatment).

PUL
◆ The patient receives local anesthesia or oral sedation.
◆ In addition to using ultrasound, gallstones may be broken up by using percutaneous fragmentation devices, such as laser pulses and electrohydraulics, which use electric sparks.
◆ Overall procedures for gallstones and renal calculi are similar, except for placement of the percutaneous device into the gallbladder or common bile duct versus the renal pelvis. (See *Understanding percutaneous ultrasonic lithotripsy.*)

Posttreatment care

◆ Monitor the patient's vital signs, intake and output, complications, and urine color and pH.
◆ Administer medications as ordered.
◆ Maintain a patent indwelling urinary catheter, if indicated, and an I.V. line.

◆ Strain urine for renal calculi fragments, and send the specimen to the laboratory.
◆ Report frank or persistent bleeding.
◆ Encourage ambulation as early as possible.
◆ Increase the patient's fluid intake as ordered.
◆ Provide comfort measures.
◆ Assess the patient for pain and provide an analgesic as ordered.
◆ Provide nephrostomy tube care as ordered.
◆ Prepare the patient for recurrent treatment with the same or other type of lithotripsy, or for surgical treatment if required.

PATIENT TEACHING
◆ Teach about the administration, dosage, and possible adverse effects of prescribed medications.
◆ Tell the patient about possible complications.

◆ Stress the importance of daily oral fluid intake of 3 to 4 qt (3 to 4 L) for about 1 month after treatment.
◆ Instruct the patient to strain urine for the first week after renal calculi removal, to save fragments in the container provided, and to bring the container to the first follow-up visit.
◆ Discuss expected adverse effects of ESWL, including pain in the treated side as fragments pass, slight redness or bruising on the treated side, blood-tinged urine for several days after treatment (after removal of renal calculi), and mild GI upset.
◆ Review activity recommendations.
◆ Stress the importance of complying with special dietary or drug regimens designed to reduce the risk of formation of new calculi.
◆ Discuss ways to prevent new calculi formation.
◆ Stress the need for follow-up care.

Understanding percutaneous ultrasonic lithotripsy

With percutaneous ultrasonic lithotripsy (PUL), an ultrasonic probe is inserted through a nephrostomy tube into the renal pelvis and ultrahigh-frequency sound waves are generated to shatter calculi, while continuous suctioning removes the fragments. (See the illustration below.)

Two stages
Some practitioners insert the nephrostomy tube and wait 1 or 2 days before doing the lithotripsy so that intrarenal bleeding has subsided and the calculi can be better visualized. The patient will have an excretory urography or lower abdominal X-rays 1 day before the procedure to locate the calculi.

Potential complications
PUL has many of the risks associated with surgery. In addition to possibly causing hemorrhage and infection, it may lead to renal damage from nephrostomy tube insertion and ureteral obstruction from incomplete passage of calculi fragments.

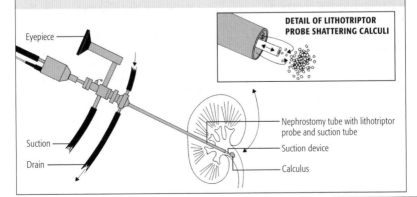

DETAIL OF LITHOTRIPTOR PROBE SHATTERING CALCULI

Eyepiece

Suction

Drain

Nephrostomy tube with lithotriptor probe and suction tube

Suction device

Calculus

Mechanical ventilation

Overview

Mechanical ventilation uses a machine that produces positive or negative pressure to generate a controlled flow of oxygen in and out of lungs. Positive-pressure ventilation causes inspiration while increasing tidal volume (VT). Negative-pressure ventilation pulls the thorax outward, allowing air to flow into lungs. Inspiratory cycles vary in volume, pressure, or time. Volume-cycled ventilation, the most commonly used, delivers a preset volume, regardless of the amount of lung resistance. Pressure-cycled ventilation generates flow until a preset pressure is reached. Time-cycled ventilation generates flow for a preset amount of time. High-frequency ventilation uses high respiratory rates and low VT to maintain alveolar ventilation.

INDICATIONS
Positive-pressure ventilation
◆ Central nervous system disorders, such as cerebral hemorrhage and spinal cord transection
◆ Acute respiratory distress syndrome
◆ Pulmonary edema
◆ Chronic obstructive pulmonary disease
◆ Flail chest
◆ Acute hypoventilation

Negative-pressure ventilation
◆ Neuromuscular disorders

COMPLICATIONS
◆ Ventilator-aquired pneumonia
◆ Tension pneumothorax
◆ Decreased cardiac output
◆ Oxygen toxicity
◆ Fluid volume excess
◆ Infection
◆ Stress ulcer

Pretreatment care

◆ Assist with endotracheal intubation as indicated.
◆ Note that, in most facilities, respiratory therapists set up and maintain the ventilator.
◆ Provide emotional support to reduce anxiety, even if the patient is unresponsive.

PATIENT TEACHING
◆ Explain the reason for mechanical ventilation to the patient and family.
◆ Describe the suctioning procedure and the need for arterial blood gas (ABG) and pulse oximetry monitoring.

Procedure

◆ The respiratory therapist or nurse puts on gloves and personal protective equipment.
◆ The ventilator is programmed with the prescribed settings and connected to the endotracheal tube.
◆ The respiratory therapist or nurse observes chest expansion and auscultates bilateral breath sounds.
◆ The patient's ABG values are monitored after initial ventilator setup (usually 20 to 30 minutes), after any changes in ventilator settings, and as the patient's clinical condition warrants.
◆ The ventilator settings are adjusted as ordered.
◆ Ventilator tubing is checked for condensation, drained into a collection trap and emptied. The condensate shouldn't be drained into the humidifier.
◆ The in-line thermometer is monitored to ensure that air is close to body temperature.

◆ Spontaneous and ventilator-delivered breaths are monitored along with vital signs.

◆ Ventilator tubing and equipment is changed, cleaned, or disposed of every 48 to 72 hours to reduce risk of bacterial contamination.

◆ When ordered, the patient is weaned from the ventilator.

Posttreatment care

◆ Monitor the patient's vital signs and cardiac rhythm and pulse oximetry.

◆ Assess the patient's respiratory status.

◆ Give a sedative or neuromuscular blocking drug as ordered. Monitor neuromuscular response when administering a neuromuscular blocking agent.

◆ If an alarm problem can't be immediately identified, disconnect the patient from the ventilator and use a handheld resuscitation bag to ventilate him.

◆ Unless contraindicated, turn the patient from side to side every 1 to 2 hours.

◆ Perform active or passive range-of-motion exercises.

◆ Position the patient at a 30- to 45-degree angle at all times if possible.

◆ Provide mouth care every hour. Suction as needed.

◆ Place the call bell within the patient's reach and provide an alternate communication method.

◆ Make sure that emergency equipment is readily available.

◆ Explain procedures and ensure patient safety.

◆ Make sure that the patient gets adequate rest and sleep.

◆ Observe for signs of hypoxia when weaning the patient.

◆ Provide endotracheal tube or tracheostomy care per facility policy.

PATIENT TEACHING

◆ When mechanical ventilation is being used at home, provide a teaching plan that covers ventilator care and settings, artificial airway care, suctioning, respiratory therapy, communication, nutrition, therapeutic exercise, signs and symptoms of infection, and troubleshooting minor equipment malfunctions.

◆ Have the caregiver demonstrate how to use the equipment.

◆ Refer the patient to a home health agency and durable medical equipment vendor.

◆ Refer the patient to community resources.

Treatments

Open reduction and internal fixation of fractures

Overview

Open reduction and internal fixation of fractures, also known as *surgical reduction*, involves using an implanted fixation device (consisting of nails, screws, pins, wires, or rods, possibly used with metal plates) to stabilize a fracture. It may be used to treat fractures of the face and jaw, spine, bones of the arms and legs, and joints (usually the hip). The device may remain in the body indefinitely unless the patient has adverse reactions after the healing process is complete. (See *Types of internal fixation devices.*)

INDICATIONS
◆ Fracture

COMPLICATIONS
◆ Wound infection
◆ Malunion or nonunion
◆ Fat or pulmonary embolism
◆ Neurovascular impairment
◆ Chronic pain

Pretreatment care

◆ Assess neurovascular status in the affected extremity.
◆ Verify that the patient has signed an informed consent form.

PATIENT TEACHING
◆ Explain the procedure to the patient.
◆ Explain postprocedure care and expected rehabilitation.
◆ Demonstrate deep-breathing and coughing exercises and how to use an incentive spirometer.

Procedure

◆ After the patient receives general anesthesia, the surgeon makes an incision at the fracture site or above and below the site, depending on the site and type of fracture.
◆ The surgeon manipulates the bone ends into their correct position and then fixes them with steel plates and screws. Rods may be inserted through the bone shaft to stabilize the fracture. This is called open reduction and internal fixation.
◆ A fine plastic drainage tube may be placed from the wound to drain any residual blood from the surgery.
◆ The skin wound is then closed with stitches.

Posttreatment care

◆ After the procedure, monitor the patient's vital signs every 2 to 4 hours for 24 hours, then every 4 to 8 hours, according to the facility's protocol.
◆ Monitor fluid intake and output every 4 to 8 hours.
◆ Perform neurovascular checks every 2 to 4 hours for 24 hours, then every 4 to 8 hours as appropriate. Assess color, motion, sensation, digital movement, edema, capillary refill, and pulses of the affected area.
◆ Apply an ice bag to the surgical site and elevate the extremity.
◆ Assess the patient's pain level, administer analgesics, and evaluate their effects.
◆ Give analgesics or opioids before exercising or mobilizing the affected area.
◆ Check surgical dressings for excessive drainage or bleeding.
◆ Observe for signs and symptoms of complications.

◆ Assist with range-of-motion and other muscle-strengthening exercises.
◆ Encourage coughing and deep breathing and incentive spirometer use.
◆ Apply elastic stockings and a sequential compression device as appropriate.

PATIENT TEACHING
◆ Review wound care.
◆ Describe the signs and symptoms of complications and when to notify the practitioner.

◆ Teach about the administration, dosage, and possible adverse effects of prescribed medications.
◆ Discuss activity restrictions.
◆ Teach the patient how to use crutches or a walker as appropriate.
◆ Stress the need for follow-up care.

Types of internal fixation devices

Choice of a specific internal fixation device depends on the fracture's location, type, and configuration.

In trochanteric or subtrochanteric fractures, the surgeon may use a hip pin or nail, with or without a screw plate. A pin or plate with extra nails stabilizes the fracture by impacting the bone ends at the fracture site

With an uncomplicated fracture of the femoral shaft, the surgeon may use an intramedullary rod. This device permits early ambulation with partial weight bearing.

Another choice for fixation of a long-bone fracture is a screw plate, shown here on the tibia.

With an arm fracture, the surgeon may fix the involved bones with a plate, rod, or nail. Most radial and ulnar fractures may be fixed with plates, whereas humeral fractures are commonly fixed with rods.

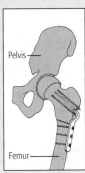
Pelvis
Femur

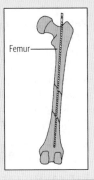
Femur

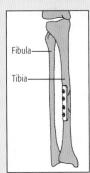
Fibula
Tibia

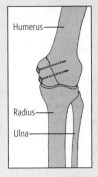
Humerus
Radius
Ulna

Pacemaker insertion

Overview

A pacemaker is a battery-operated generator that controls heart rate with timed electrical signals that trigger heart muscle contractions. Pacemakers can be temporary or permanent. A five-letter coding system describes their capabilities; however the first three letters of the system are more commonly used. The first letter identifies the heart chamber being paced (V [ventricle], A [atrium], D [dual, ventricle and atrium], or O [none]). The second letter identifies the heart chamber where the pacemaker senses intrinsic activity (V [ventricle], A [atrium], D [dual, ventricle and atrium], or O [none]). The third letter indicates pacemaker's mode of response to the intrinsic activity that it senses in the atrium or ventricle (T [triggered], I [inhibited], D [dual, triggered or inhibited], or O [none]). The fourth letter indicates the pacemaker's programmability (P [basic function programmability], M [multiprogrammable], C [communicating functions such as telemetry], R [rate responsiveness or modulation], or O [none]). The fifth letter denotes special tachyarrhythmia functions and identifies how the pacemaker will respond to a tachyarrhythmia (P [pacing ability], S [shock], D [dual, can shock and pace], or O [none]).

INDICATIONS
Temporary pacemaker
- Emergency treatment of symptomatic bradycardia
- Bridge to permanent pacemaker implantation or to determine the effect of pacing on cardiac function
- Open-heart surgery

Permanent pacemaker
- Symptomatic bradycardia
- Advanced symptomatic atrioventricular block
- Sick sinus syndrome
- Sinus arrest
- Sinoatrial block
- Stokes-Adams syndrome
- Tachyarrhythmias
- Arrhythmias caused by antiarrhythmic drugs

COMPLICATIONS
- Infection
- Venous thrombosis, embolism
- Pneumothorax
- Pectoral or diaphragmatic muscle stimulation from the pacemaker
- Arrhythmias
- Cardiac tamponade
- Heart failure
- Pacemaker malfunction
- Microshock (temporary)

Pretreatment care

- Verify that the patient or a responsible family member has signed an informed consent form.
- Obtain baseline vital signs and a 12-lead electrocardiogram (ECG).
- Restrict food and fluids as ordered.
- Establish an I.V. (if not already in place) so that emergency medications can be administered if needed.

PATIENT TEACHING
- Explain the underlying disorder and the reason for the treatment.
- Explain the treatment and preparation to the patient and his family.
- Explain any activity restrictions, based on the type of pacemaker used.
- Explain postoperative care.

Procedure

PERMANENT PACEMAKER
- The pacemaker is implanted using a transvenous endocardial approach (requiring local anesthesia).
- The patient is sedated and the chest or abdomen is prepared.
- A 3″ to 4″ (7.6- to 10-cm) incision is made in the selected site.

◆ The electrode catheter is inserted through a vein and guided by fluoroscopy to the heart chamber appropriate for the pacemaker type.

◆ Pacemaker leads are inserted.

◆ A pacing system analyzer is used to set the pulse generator to the proper stimulating and sensing thresholds.

◆ The pulse generator is attached to the leads and implanted into a pocket of muscle in the chest wall.

◆ The incision is closed, and a tight occlusive dressing is applied.

TEMPORARY PACEMAKER

◆ Insertion or application of a temporary pacemaker varies, depending on the device. (See *Types of temporary pacemakers*.)

Posttreatment care

For patients with a permanent pacemaker

◆ Monitor the patient's vital signs, cardiac rhythm, and intake and output.

◆ Administer medications as ordered.

◆ Document the type of pacemaker inserted, lead system, pacemaker mode, and pacing guidelines.

◆ If the patient requires defibrillation, place paddles at least 4″ (10.2 cm) from the pulse generator; avoid anteroposterior paddle placement.

◆ After the first 24 hours, begin passive range-of-motion exercises on the affected arm if ordered.

◆ Assess for complications, such as abnormal bleeding and infection.

◆ Assess the surgical wound and dressing.

◆ Monitor drainage.

◆ Assess pacemaker function (see *Assessing pacemaker function*, page 314).

For patients with a temporary pacemaker

◆ Assess the patient's vital signs, skin color, level of consciousness, and peripheral pulses to determine the effectiveness of the paced rhythm.

◆ Obtain a 12-lead ECG to serve as a baseline, and then obtain additional 12-lead ECGs daily or with clinical changes. Also, if possible, obtain a rhythm strip before, during, and after pacemaker placement;

Types of temporary pacemakers

Temporary pacemakers come in three types: transcutaneous, transvenous, and epicardial. They're used to pace the heart after cardiac surgery, during cardiopulmonary resuscitation, and when sinus arrest, symptomatic sinus bradycardia, or complete heart block occurs.

Transcutaneous pacemaker

Completely noninvasive and easily applied, a transcutaneous pacemaker proves especially useful in an emergency. To perform pacing with the device, the practitioner places pacing electrodes at heart level on the patient's chest and back and connects them to a pulse generator.

Transvenous pacemaker

This balloon-tipped pacing catheter is inserted via the subclavian or jugular vein into the right ventricle. The procedure can be done at the bedside or in the cardiac catheterization laboratory. A transvenous pacemaker offers better control of the heartbeat than a transcutaneous pacemaker. However, electrode insertion takes longer, limiting its usefulness in emergencies.

Epicardial pacemaker

Implanted during open-heart surgery, an epicardial pacemaker permits rapid treatment of postoperative complications. During surgery, the surgeon attaches the leads to the heart and runs them out through the abdominal wall. Afterward, the leads are coiled on the patient's chest, insulated, and covered with a dressing. If pacing is needed, the leads are simply uncovered and attached to a pulse generator. When pacing is no longer needed, the leads can be easily removed.

Assessing pacemaker function

After a pacemaker has been inserted, follow these steps to assess its function:
1. Determine the pacemaker's mode and settings.
2. Review the patient's 12-lead electrocardiogram (ECG).
3. Select a monitoring lead that clearly shows the pacemaker spikes.
4. Consider the pacemaker mode and whether symptoms of decreased cardiac output are present when evaluating the ECG.
5. Look for information that tells you which chamber is paced. Ask:
    – Is there capture?
    – Is there a P wave or QRS complex after each atrial or ventricular spike?
    – Do P waves and QRS complexes stem from intrinsic activity?
    – If intrinsic activity is present, what's the pacemaker's response?
6. Determine the rate by quickly counting the number of complexes in a 6-second ECG strip or, more accurately, by counting the number of small boxes between complexes and dividing by 1,500.

Pacemaker impulses are visible on an ECG tracing as spikes. Large or small, pacemaker spikes appear above or below the isoelectric line. The illustration shows an atrial and ventricular pacemaker spike.

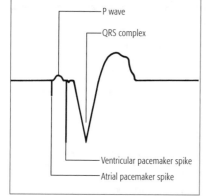

P wave

QRS complex

Ventricular pacemaker spike

Atrial pacemaker spike

any time pacemaker settings are changed; and whenever the patient receives treatment because of a complication caused by the pacemaker.

◆ Continuously monitor the ECG reading, noting capture, sensing, rate, intrinsic beats, and competition of paced and intrinsic rhythms. If the pacemaker is sensing correctly, the sense indicator on the pulse generator should flash with each beat.

◆ Watch for oversensing. If the pacemaker is too sensitive, it can misinterpret muscle movements or other events in the cardiac cycle as intrinsic cardiac electrical activity. Pacing won't occur when it's needed, and the heart rate and atrioventricular synchrony won't be maintained.

◆ When using a transcutaneous pacemaker, don't place the electrode over a bony area because bone conducts current poorly. With a female patient, place the anterior electrode under the patient's breast but not over her diaphragm.

◆ With a transvenous pacemaker, the practitioner inserts the electrode through the brachial or femoral vein and the patient's arm or leg is immobilized to avoid putting stress on the pacing wires.

◆ If the patient has epicardial pacing wires in place, clean the insertion site per facility policy and change the dressing daily. At the same time, monitor the site for signs of infection. Always keep the pulse generator nearby in case pacing becomes necessary.

◆ Institute precautions to prevent microshock including warning the patient not to use electrical equipment that isn't grounded, such as telephones, electrical shavers, televisions, or lamps.

◆ Place a plastic cover supplied by the manufacturer over the pacemaker controls to avoid an accidental setting change.

Treatments

Also, insulate the pacemaker by covering exposed metal parts, such as electrode connections and pacemaker terminals, with nonconducting tape, or place the pacing unit in a dry, rubber surgical glove.

PATIENT TEACHING

◆ Discuss the possible complications and when to notify the practitioner.

◆ Tell the patient about diet or activity restrictions ordered by the practitioner.

◆ Teach the patient how to monitor the heart rate and rhythm.

◆ Instruct the patient to avoid placing excessive pressure over the insertion site, making sudden moves, or extending his arms over his head for 4 weeks after discharge.

◆ Emphasize the importance of informing medical personnel of the implanted pacemaker before undergoing certain diagnostic tests.

◆ Stress the need for follow-up care.

◆ Advise the patient to notify the practitioner if he experiences signs of pacemaker failure, such as palpitations, a fast heart rate, a slow heart rate (5 to 10 beats less than the pacemaker's setting), dizziness, fainting, shortness of breath, swollen ankles or feet, anxiety, forgetfulness, or confusion.

◆ Provide the patient with an identification card that lists the pacemaker type and manufacturer, serial number, pacemaker rate setting, date implanted, and practitioner's name. Also instruct the patient in measures for daily care, safety and activity guidelines, and special precautions.

Paracentesis

Overview

Abdominal paracentesis is the aspiration of fluid from the peritoneal space through a needle or trocar and cannula that are inserted into the abdominal wall. This treatment relieves the pressure of ascites and helps determine the condition's cause. Abdominal paracentesis may precede other procedures, including radiography, peritoneal dialysis, and surgery.

INDICATIONS

♦ Massive ascites resistant to other therapy
♦ Intra-abdominal bleeding after traumatic injury
♦ To obtain a peritoneal fluid specimen for laboratory analysis

COMPLICATIONS

♦ Hypotension
♦ Oliguria
♦ Hyponatremia
♦ Perforation of abdominal organs
♦ Wound infection
♦ Peritonitis

Pretreatment care

♦ Verify that the patient has signed an informed consent form.
♦ Have the patient void before the procedure.
♦ If the patient can't void, insert an indwelling urinary catheter if ordered.
♦ Identify and record baseline values, including vital signs, weight, and abdominal girth. Indicate the abdominal area measured with a felt-tipped marking pen. Baseline data will be used to monitor the patient's status.
♦ Provide support to decrease the patient's anxiety during the procedure.

PATIENT TEACHING

♦ Explain the underlying disorder and the reason for the procedure.
♦ Explain the procedure and the preparation involved to the patient.
♦ Instruct the patient that he doesn't need to restrict fluid and food intake.

Procedure

♦ The patient is helped to sit up in bed, on the side of the bed, or in a chair so that fluid accumulates in the lower abdomen.
♦ The patient's abdomen is exposed from diaphragm to pubis.
♦ The patient is reminded to stay as still as possible during the procedure.
♦ The practitioner prepares the patient's abdomen with povidone-iodine solution, drapes the operative site with sterile drapes, and administers local anesthetic.
♦ A small incision may be made before the needle or trocar and cannula is inserted 1″ to 2″ [2.5 to 5 cm] below the umbilicus.
♦ A popping sound signifies that the needle or trocar has pierced the peritoneum.
♦ The nurse assists the practitioner in collecting specimens in proper containers.
♦ If the practitioner orders substantial drainage, the three-way stopcock and tubing are connected to the cannula.
♦ The other end of the tubing is connected to a large sterile Vacutainer, or the fluid is aspirated with a three-way stopcock and 50-ml syringe.
♦ If the patient shows signs of hypovolemic shock, the vertical distance is reduced between the needle or the trocar and cannula and the drainage collection container to slow the drainage rate. If necessary, the drainage is stopped.

◆ Vacutainer collection bottle suction is verified when it's connected to the drainage tubing. A macrodrip tubing without a backflow device is used.

◆ The patient is turned from side to side to enhance drainage.

◆ As the fluid drains, the patient's vital signs are monitored every 15 minutes.

◆ The incision may be sutured after the needle or trocar and cannula are removed.

◆ While wearing sterile gloves, dry, sterile pressure dressing and povidone-iodine ointment are applied to the site.

Posttreatment care

◆ Monitor the patient's vital signs and check the dressing for drainage every 15 minutes for 1 hour, every 30 minutes for 2 hours, every hour for 4 hours, and then every 4 hours for 24 hours to detect delayed reactions to the procedure.

◆ Note color, amount, and character of drainage.

◆ Label the Vacutainer specimen tubes, and send them to the laboratory with request forms. If the patient is receiving antibiotics, note this information on the request form.

◆ Remove and dispose of all equipment properly.

◆ After the procedure, observe for peritoneal fluid leakage; notify the practitioner if this develops.

◆ Maintain daily patient weight and abdominal girth records and compare these values with the baseline figures.

◆ Watch closely for signs and symptoms of complications.

PATIENT TEACHING

◆ Teach about the administration, dosage, and possible adverse effects of prescribed medications.

◆ Instruct the patient that he doesn't need to restrict food and fluids after the procedure.

◆ Explain that ascitic fluid may recur, thus the patient may require repeated procedures.

◆ Teach the patient with ascites to weigh himself daily and report sudden gains to the practitioner.

Pericardiocentesis

Overview

Pericardiocentesis is needle aspiration of pericardial fluid for analysis to confirm and identify the cause of pericardial effusion and determine therapy. It may be done for therapeutic and diagnostic purposes, but it's most useful as an emergency measure to relieve cardiac tamponade.

INDICATIONS
◆ Cardiac tamponade
◆ Pericardial effusion (see *Pericardial effusions: Transudates and exudates*)

COMPLICATIONS
◆ Laceration of a coronary artery or the myocardium (potentially fatal)
◆ Vasovagal arrest
◆ Infection
◆ Cardiac arrhythmias
◆ Myocardial perforation
◆ Respiratory distress

Pretreatment care

◆ Verify that an informed consent form has been signed.
◆ Tell the patient that he may feel pressure when the needle is inserted into the pericardial sac.
◆ Inform the patient that he'll be monitored closely during and after the procedure.
◆ Connect the patient to the bedside monitor, set to read lead V_1.
◆ Make sure that a defibrillator and emergency drugs are nearby.
◆ Place the patient in the supine position with his thorax elevated 60 degrees.
◆ Wash your hands and put on gloves and protective eyewear.
◆ Open the equipment tray on an overbed table, being careful not to contaminate the sterile field.

PATIENT TEACHING
◆ Explain the underlying disorder and the reason for the treatment.
◆ Explain the procedure to the patient and answer questions.
◆ Tell the patient that the anesthetic may cause brief burning and local pain.
◆ Instruct the patient to be still during the procedure; tell him that a sedative may be administered to help him relax.

Procedure

◆ The practitioner cleans the skin with sterile gauze pads soaked in povidone-iodine solution and an anesthetic is injected.
◆ The practitioner attaches a 50-ml syringe to one end of a three-way stopcock and the cardiac needle to the other.
◆ The V_1 lead (precordial leadwire) of the electrocardiogram (ECG) may be attached to the hub of the aspirating needle using the alligator clips to help determine if the needle is in contact with the epicardium during the procedure. An ECG may also be used to help guide needle placement.
◆ The practitioner inserts the needle through the chest wall into the pericardial sac, maintaining aspiration until fluid appears in the syringe.
◆ The needle is angled 35 to 45 degrees toward the tip of the right scapula between the left costal margin and the xiphoid process; doing so minimizes the risk of lacerating the coronary vessels or pleura.
◆ ST-segment elevation on the ECG tracing indicates that the needle has reached the epicardial surface and should be retracted slightly.
◆ After the needle is positioned, the practitioner attaches a Kelly clamp to the skin surface so it won't advance further.
◆ The specimen tubes are labeled and numbered, and the top of the tube used

Treatments

for culture and sensitivity is cleaned with povidone-iodine solution.

◆ A pericardial catheter may be connected to a drainage bag or to low-suction drainage.

◆ The insertion site is cleaned and dressed.

Posttreatment care

◆ If bacterial culture and sensitivity tests are scheduled, record on the laboratory request form any antimicrobial drugs the patient is receiving.

◆ If anaerobic organisms are suspected, consult the laboratory about proper collection technique to avoid exposing the aspirate to air.

◆ Send specimens to the laboratory immediately.

◆ Check blood pressure, pulse, respirations, oxygen saturation, and heart sounds every 15 minutes until stable, then every one-half hour for 2 hours, every hour for 4 hours, and every 4 hours thereafter. Some facilities may require more frequent monitoring.

◆ Monitor continuously for cardiac arrhythmias. Document rhythm strips according to facility policy.

◆ Dispose of equipment according to facility policy.

◆ Assess respiratory and cardiovascular status.

◆ Observe for signs and symptoms of complications.

PATIENT TEACHING

◆ Teach the patient the signs and symptoms of recurent effusion, infection, and cardiac arrhythmia to report to the practitioner.

◆ Teach about the administration, dosage, and possible adverse effects of prescribed medications.

Pericardial effusions: Transudates and exudates

Transudates are protein-poor effusions that usually arise from mechanical factors that alter fluid formation or resorption, such as increased hydrostatic pressure, decreased plasma oncotic pressure, or obstruction of the pericardial lymphatic drainage system by a tumor.

Most exudates result from inflammation and contain large amounts of protein. Inflammation damages the capillary membrane, allowing protein molecules to leak into the pericardial fluid.

Both effusion types occur in pericarditis, neoplasms, acute myocardial infarction, tuberculosis, rheumatoid disease, and systemic lupus erythematosus.

Treatments

Radiation therapy, external and internal

Overview

Radiation therapy delivers high levels of radiation to a specific body area. The radiation destroys the ability of cancer cells to grow and multiply by decreasing the mitosis rate or impairing synthesis of deoxyribonucleic or ribonucleic acid. Internal radiation therapy is also called *brachytherapy*; external radiation is also known as *external beam radiation* or *teletherapy*.

Various approaches are used to administer radiation therapy locally or systemically. The interstitial approach involves implanting a radioactive substance in the tumor or surrounding tissue or placing an applicator on top of a body surface. The intracavitary approach uses an unsealed radioactive substance for temporary radiation delivery into a hollow body cavity (such as the vagina, abdomen, or pleura). Intraoperative radiation delivers a large dose of external radiation to the tumor and surrounding tissue during surgery. Radiolabeled antibodies deliver radiation directly to the cancer site to actively seek out the cancer cells and destroy them, with potentially less risk of damage to healthy cells. Systemic radiation delivery involves giving radioactive material in a solution or colloidal suspension orally or I.V.

INDICATIONS
◆ Curative or palliative treatment for cancer
◆ Extensive skin disease (external)

COMPLICATIONS
◆ Local skin reactions
◆ Anorexia
◆ Fatigue
◆ Bone marrow suppression
◆ Stomatitis and esophagitis
◆ Pneumonitis, pericarditis
◆ GI distress
◆ Hemorrhage
◆ Neurologic dysfunction
◆ Leukemia and other cancers
◆ Cataracts
◆ Alopecia
◆ Xerostomia
◆ Thrombocytopenia
◆ Genetic mutation and sterility (if radiation is directed at gonads)

Pretreatment care

◆ Verify that the patient or responsible family member has signed an informed consent form.
◆ Obtain a thorough patient history.
◆ Obtain baseline white blood cell (WBC) and platelet counts.
◆ Obtain the patient's vital signs and temperature.

PATIENT TEACHING
◆ Explain the underlying disorder and the reason for treatment.
◆ Explain the treatment and preparation to the patient and his family.
◆ Evaluate the patient for possible problems in positioning, range of motion, and comfort.
◆ Prepare the patient for a temporary change in appearance if the implant is placed in a visible area, such as the neck or breast.

Procedure

◆ The proper precautions should be taken against radiation contamination.

INTERNAL RADIATION THERAPY
◆ The surgeon usually inserts the applicator for the radioactive source in the operating room, with the patient under anesthesia.
◆ To minimize exposure of facility personnel, the radioactive source is placed in the applicator after the patient returns to his room.

◆ If the radioactive source isn't permanent, it's left in place for 24 to 72 hours and then removed in the patient's room.
◆ If a remote afterloader is used, the patient is treated in an inpatient or outpatient department.
◆ I.V., oral, and intracavitary instillation of radiation is usually performed in the radiation therapy department.
◆ After intracavitary instillation of a suspension, the patient lies on a flat surface and is rotated every 15 minutes for 2 or 3 hours to distribute the suspension.

EXTERNAL RADIATION THERAPY
◆ External radiation treatments are given in the radiation department.
◆ The radiation oncologist may mark precise treatment areas on the patient's skin with tiny tattoo dots of semipermanent ink.
◆ The patient is placed on the treatment table and is instructed to lie immobile.
◆ A large machine directs radiation at the target site for the prescribed period, usually 1 or 2 minutes.

Posttreatment care

◆ Monitor the patient's vital signs and intake and output.
◆ Monitor for abnormal bleeding and signs of infection.
◆ Provide meticulous skin care.
◆ Provide comfort measures and supportive care.
◆ Monitor WBC and platelet counts.
◆ Assure the patient that normal activities can be resumed after the temporary radiation source has been removed or the permanent source has decayed.
◆ Report and properly store a dislodged radioactive implant according to facility policy.
◆ Follow facility policy regarding radiation precautions.

PATIENT TEACHING
◆ Teach about the administration, dosage, and possible adverse effects of prescribed medications.
◆ Teach about the home management of adverse effects, such as adequate fluid intake and not using creams or lotions on the affected skin.
◆ Tell the patient about possible complications and when to notify the practitioner.
◆ Inform the patient that the full benefits of treatment may not occur for several months.
◆ Stress the need for temporary isolation after ingestion or instillation of a radioactive source.
◆ Review activity restrictions related to applicator location as appropriate.
◆ Tell the patient that visits by children and pregnant women aren't allowed.
◆ Stress the importance of follow-up care.
◆ Refer the patient to support groups such as the American Cancer Society.

Radiofrequency ablation of tumors

Overview

Radiofrequency ablation (RFA) is a minimally invasive procedure that sends energy through a needle to destroy a tumor and is used when surgery isn't possible or if the patient is a poor surgical risk. It may be performed with laparoscopy or during open surgery; the percutaneous approach is preferred by most radiologists because it's less invasive and produces fewer complications.

INDICATIONS
◆ Liver tumors
◆ Kidney tumors
◆ Pain management for small bone cancer

COMPLICATIONS
◆ Injury to adjacent organs and tissues (such as gallbladder, bile ducts, diaphragm, and bowel loops) requiring surgical correction
◆ Shoulder pain
◆ Gallbladder inflammation
◆ Thermal damage to the bowel or adjacent tissues
◆ Postablation syndrome
◆ Bleeding

Pretreatment care

◆ Verify that an informed consent form has been signed.
◆ Ensure that the patient has taken nothing by mouth since midnight the evening before treatment.
◆ Medications may need to be restricted before treatment, such as aspirin (usually stopped 10 days before) or blood thinners (such as warfarin [Coumadin]).
◆ Have the patient void before the procedure.
◆ Identify and record baseline laboratory values.
◆ Perform a baseline nursing assessment.

PATIENT TEACHING
◆ Explain the underlying disorder and the reason for the treatment.
◆ Explain the procedure and the preparation involved to the patient.

Procedure

◆ A local anesthetic is injected into the site and the patient is sedated by I.V. injection.
◆ The physician guides a special needle through the skin and into the tumor by images from ultrasound or computed tomography (CT) scanning.
◆ When properly positioned, a plunger is advanced so that the electrodes extend from the needle tip. When fully extended, the electrodes resemble an open umbrella (see *Radiofrequency ablation*).
◆ Insulated wires to the needle electrodes and to the grounding pads are placed on the patient's back or thigh to connect the radiofrequency generator. The generator produces an alternating electric current in the range of radiofrequency waves.
◆ The needle sends a current from the hollow core of the needle to penetrate and destroy the tumor. Heat from the radiofrequency energy closes up small blood vessels, reducing the risk of bleeding.

Posttreatment care

◆ Monitor the patient's vital signs.
◆ Note the color, amount, and character of drainage.
◆ Monitor for complications.
◆ Assess the patient for pain and nausea as the sedation wears off.
◆ Make sure the patient has a CT scan or magnetic resonance imaging (MRI) scheduled within a few hours to 1 week after RFA to ensure that all tumor tissue has been destroyed and to detect complications.

Treatments

PATIENT TEACHING

◆ Review medications and possible adverse effects with the patient.

◆ Review care of the surgical wound with the patient.

◆ Tell the patient that a radiologist will interpret the CT scan or MRI and determine if the entire tumor appears to have been eliminated. Tell the patient that a repeat CT scan may be done every 3 months to check for new tumors.

◆ Discuss postablation syndrome, which produces flulike symptoms 3 to 5 days after the procedure and usually lasts 5 days, but can last a few weeks.

◆ Teach about possible complications and when to notify the practitioner.

◆ Stress the importance of follow-up care.

Radiofrequency ablation

A special needle shaped like an umbrella is used to ablate the tumor. When the needle is in place, the current is directed toward the tumor and the tumor is destroyed.

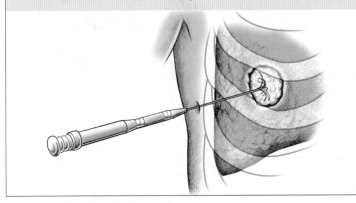

Restrictive gastric surgeries

Overview

Restrictive gastric surgery, which includes adjustable gastric banding and vertical banded gastroplasty, is a combination of procedures that use restriction and malabsorption methods to produce weight loss. The surgery results in a smaller stomach so the patient feels fuller faster, thus significantly reduces caloric intake.

Before treatment is initiated, the patient undergoes a complete medical and psychological examination to evaluate his overall health and readiness for this lifestyle change. The patient also receives extensive nutritional counseling.

INDICATIONS

◆ Body mass index (BMI) of 40 or more (A patient with a BMI of 40 or more is at least 100 pounds over his recommended weight; normal BMI is between 18.5 and 25.)
◆ A BMI of 35 or more along with a life-threatening illness that can be improved with weight loss, such as sleep apnea, type 2 diabetes, and heart disease

COMPLICATIONS

◆ Bleeding
◆ Infections
◆ Bowel obstruction
◆ Peritonitis
◆ Gallstones
◆ Gastritis
◆ Vomiting
◆ Dumping syndrome

Pretreatment care

◆ Verify that the patient has signed an informed consent form.
◆ Obtain blood samples for hematologic and chemistry studies as ordered.
◆ Withhold food and fluids as ordered.
◆ Begin I.V. fluid replacement and total parenteral nutrition as ordered.

◆ Prepare the patient for abdominal X-rays as ordered.
◆ Monitor the patient's vital signs, intake and output, nutritional status, and laboratory test results.
◆ Complete the preoperative verification process.

PATIENT TEACHING

◆ Explain the treatment and preparation to the patient and his family.
◆ Explain postoperative care and equipment.
◆ Demonstrate how to perform coughing and deep-breathing exercises and how to use an incentive spirometer.

Procedure

◆ The surgery is performed with the patient under general anesthesia.
◆ The small stomach pouch is created using bands (gastric banding), staples (stomach stapling), or a combination. The surgeon leaves a narrow passage in the newly created pouch so that food can still go through the remainder of the stomach and small intestines, except it does so more slowly. (See *Gastric banding and stapling.*)

Posttreatment care

◆ Monitor the patient's vital signs, intake and output, and daily weight.
◆ Maintain I.V. replacement therapy as ordered.
◆ Keep the nasogastric tube patent, but don't reposition it.
◆ Encourage regular turning, coughing and deep-breathing exercises, and incentive spirometry use.
◆ Encourage splinting of the incision site with coughing and movement.
◆ Report signs of dehydration, peritonitis, sepsis, infection, or postresection obstruction.

◆ Administer medications as ordered.
◆ Assess the patient's pain level and administer analgesia as ordered.
◆ Assess GI status. After bowel sounds return, begin oral intake, providing six small feedings per day.
◆ Monitor laboratory test results.
◆ Provide wound care, and assess the type and amount of drainage.
◆ Monitor for complications of morbid obesity, such as pneumonia, thromboembolism, skin breakdown, and delayed wound healing.

PATIENT TEACHING
◆ Teach about the administration, dosage, and possible adverse effects of prescribed medications.
◆ Discuss vitamin supplements that may be required.

◆ Review the signs and symptoms of complications.
◆ Teach the patient wound care.
◆ Inform the patient about dumping syndrome (weakness, nausea, flatulence, and palpitations occurring within 30 minutes after a meal) and how to prevent it.
◆ Inform the patient that he'll receive extensive nutritional counseling.
◆ Review recommended dietary restrictions and expected progress of weight loss.
◆ Advise the patient that he may need to separate fluid and food intake by at least 30 minutes and to sip fluids only.
◆ Review the recommended exercise regimen.
◆ Inform the patient that for the first year after surgery his physical and mental health status, change in weight, and nutritional needs will be reviewed during follow-up visits.

Treatments

Gastric banding and stapling

Adjustable gastric banding involves placing a band over the stomach to change its size. The band may be adjusted over time. Stomach stapling may also be done to reduce the size of the stomach.

Adjustable gastric banding
The stomach opening can be tightened or loosened over time to change the passage size.

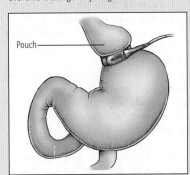

Pouch

Vertical banded gastroplasty
Band and staples create a smaller stomach pouch.

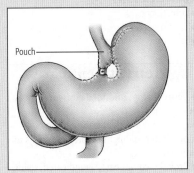

Pouch

Skin grafting

Overview

Skin grafting surgery uses healthy skin either from the patient (autograft), a donor (allograft), or an animal (xenograft) to repair an area damaged by burns, traumatic injury, or surgery. Grafting usually follows wound debridement—with enzymatic debridement performed 5 to 7 days after completion and surgical debridement performed the same day as surgery. Grafting techniques include pinch graft (one-quarter inch pieces of skin placed over wound sites not affected by poor blood supply); split-thickness graft (includes the epidermis and part of the dermis); full-thickness graft (includes the epidermis and entire dermis); and pedicle graft (full-thickness graft that also includes subcutaneous blood vessels with part of the donor site remaining attached to the donor area until blood supply is established at the recipient site.

INDICATIONS
◆ Burns
◆ Reconstructive surgical procedures requiring grafting
◆ Extensive wounds

COMPLICATIONS
◆ Infection
◆ Graft rejection
◆ Bleeding

Pretreatment care

◆ Verify that an informed consent form has been signed.
◆ Confirm the patient had nothing by mouth after midnight before surgery as appropriate.
◆ Provide wound care, as indicated, using sterile technique.

PATIENT TEACHING
◆ Explain the procedure to the patient and answer questions.
◆ Describe care performed after the procedure and the expected recovery period.
◆ Review activity restrictions if indicated.

Procedure

◆ Successful grafting depends on clean wound granulation with adequate vascularization, complete contact of the graft with the wound bed, sterile technique to prevent infection, adequate graft immobilization, and skilled care.
◆ The patient is usually given general anesthesia, but for minor grafting, local anesthesia and sedation may be given.
◆ The grafting donor site is predetermined before surgery; it's usually a site that's hidden under clothing. The skin must be healthy, with a good blood supply.
◆ The surgeon then cleans the wound site and removes dead tissue. Then he either injects epinephrine, or applies pressure to the area surrounding the wound to decrease blood flow to the area.
◆ The donor site is then marked 3% to 5% larger than the wound site and cleaned.
◆ For split-thickness grafts, the surgeon uses a dermatome to "shave" the donor tissue. The tissue may be applied as a sheet or a mesh (tissue is thinned and enlarged through the use of a special machine).
◆ For full-thickness grafts, a scalpel is used to cut the donor tissue; the tissue is then removed with a special hook and any fatty tissue is removed before attaching to the recipient site.
◆ The donor tissue is spread over the wound, then covered with a gentle pressure dressing. Small sutures may also be used to keep the graft intact.
◆ The donor site for split-thickness grafts is covered with a sterile, nonadherent dressing. The donor site for full-thickness grafts must be surgically closed.

Posttreatment care

◆ Monitor the patient's vital signs and pulse oximetry level.
◆ Monitor the patient's peripheral pulses; watch for signs of decreased tissue perfusion.
◆ Assess the patient's pain level, administer analgesics as ordered, and evaluate their effects.
◆ Provide adequate I.V. hydration as ordered.
◆ Administer medications as ordered.
◆ Provide emotional support.
◆ Monitor for signs and symptoms of complications.
◆ Provide wound care as ordered. (Graft dressings usually stay in place for 3 to 5 days after surgery to avoid disturbing the graft site.)
◆ If the graft becomes dislodged, apply sterile skin compresses to keep the area moist until the surgeon reapplies the graft.

◆ If the graft affects an arm or a leg, elevate the affected extremity to reduce postoperative edema and check for bleeding and signs of neurovascular impairment.
◆ Maintain bedrest or activity restrictions, as ordered, based on graft location.
◆ Inspect a sheet graft frequently for blebs and evacuate them carefully with a sterile scalpel if ordered (see *Evacuating fluid from a sheet graft*).
◆ Clean completely healed areas and apply a moisturizing cream to them to keep the skin pliable and to retard scarring.
◆ Provide donor graft site care.

PATIENT TEACHING
◆ Teach about the administration, dosage, and possible adverse effects of prescribed medications.
◆ Teach the patient how to perform skin graft care.
◆ Teach the patient about signs and symptoms to report.
◆ Stress the importance of follow-up care.

Treatments

Evacuating fluid from a sheet graft

When small pockets of fluid (called *blebs*) accumulate beneath a sheet graft, evacuate the fluid using a sterile scalpel and sterile cotton-tipped applicators.

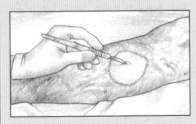

First, carefully perforate the center of the bleb with the scalpel.

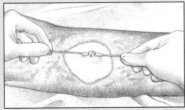

Gently express the fluid with the cotton-tipped applicators. Never express fluid by rolling the bleb to the edge of the graft. Doing so disturbs healing in other areas.

Stent placement

Overview

Stent placement is an invasive procedure in which a small, flexible tube made of medical grade plastic or wire mesh is implanted in a vessel or duct. A stent may be used to treat several medical conditions. It can open blocked or narrowed blood vessels caused by peripheral arterial disease or other conditions. Newer stents are coated with medications to prevent restenosis and are more effective than standard stents in preventing the artery from reoccluding. Two common stenting procedures are the cardiac stent and liver stent.

INDICATIONS
◆ Peripheral vascular disease or peripheral artery disease
◆ Renal procedures
◆ Hemodialysis access maintenance
◆ Carotid stenosis
◆ Coronary artery disease
◆ Abdominal aortic aneurysm
◆ Esophageal stricture
◆ Biliary disease
◆ Coronary artery blockage

COMPLICATIONS
◆ Bleeding or bruising at the catheter insertion site
◆ Restenosis of the artery
◆ Infection
◆ Stent migration
◆ Shunt failure or closure
◆ Death

Pretreatment care

◆ Ensure that preliminary evaluation is done as ordered, depending on the type of stent to be placed.
◆ Ensure that diagnostic testing has been completed, including computer tomography, magnetic resonance imaging, ultrasound, X-rays, or tests to check the patency of the vessels as ordered.
◆ Verify that an informed consent form has been signed.

◆ Review with the patient what to expect postoperatively.
◆ Perform a baseline assessment and verify pulse quality.
◆ Make sure the patient doesn't take anything by mouth after midnight before the procedure.
◆ Note if the patient has allergies or is taking any medications.

PATIENT TEACHING
◆ Explain the underlying disorder and the reason for the treatment.
◆ Review the procedure with the patient and answer any questions.
◆ Demonstrate how to perform coughing and deep-breathing exercises and how to use an incentive spirometer.

Procedure

◆ The patient receives anesthesia appropriate to the stent being placed. Local anesthesia is generally used with some analgesia; general anesthesia may be indicated in other conditions, especially if the procedure is anticipated to be painful.
◆ The procedure is done in a specially equipped suite with emergency equipment and staffing. The patient's electrocardiogram and oxygenation are monitored during the procedure.
◆ The interventional radiologist makes a pencil-tip–size incision in the skin. The stent, which is placed on the end of a catheter, is threaded under X-ray guidance to the area of treatment.

CARDIAC STENT
◆ Angioplasty is performed by a cardiologist who inserts a very small balloon attached to a catheter into a blood vessel through a small incision in the skin.
◆ The catheter is threaded under X-ray guidance to the site of the blocked artery.
◆ The balloon is inflated to open the artery.

◆ A small stent is inserted; it expands to hold the artery open and is usually placed at the narrowed section.

LIVER STENT

◆ A transjugular intrahepatic portosystemic shunt is inserted to treat portal hypertension.

◆ The interventional radiologist threads a catheter through a small incision in the skin near the neck and guides it to the blocked blood vessels in the liver.

◆ Under X-ray guidance, a tunnel is created in the liver through which the blocked blood can flow.

◆ A small metal stent is inserted to hold the tunnel open.

Posttreatment care

◆ Monitor the patient's vital signs, cardiac rhythm, pulse oximetry, and peripheral pulses.

◆ Assess the patient's cardiovascular and respiratory function.

◆ Maintain I.V. patency and provide hydration as ordered.

◆ Administer medications as ordered.

◆ Assess the surgical wound or catheter site for bleeding.

◆ Encourage the patient to breathe deeply and to cough as indicated; assist with incentive spirometry.

◆ Assist with ambulation as ordered.

◆ Monitor for signs of complications.

PATIENT TEACHING

◆ Teach about the administration, dosage, and possible adverse effects of prescribed medications.

◆ Review activity restrictions if indicated.

◆ Describe signs and symptoms of complications and what to report to the practitioner.

◆ Review appropriate lifestyle changes and the importance of compliance with treatment for coexisting disorders.

◆ Instruct the patient to notify the practitioner if pain, a warm feeling in the area where the catheter was inserted, or a change in the color of the leg occurs.

◆ Stress the importance of follow-up care.

Treatments

Stereotactic radiosurgery

Overview

Stereotactic radiosurgery (SRS) is the noninvasive delivery of a high dose of radiation to an area of the brain to treat abnormalities, tumors, or other functional disorders. Performed in a 1-day session, this approach may be the primary treatment for inaccessible tumors or an adjunct to other treatments for recurring or malignant tumors.

Particle-beam-based SRS (proton SRS) and cobalt-60-based SRS (gamma knife SRS) are used for small tumors. Linear accelerator-based SRS is used for larger tumors (greater than 1.4″ [3.5 cm]). It requires three-dimensional computer-aided planning and a high degree of immobilization to minimize radiation exposure to healthy brain tissue. Fractionated SRS is radiation administered over several days or weeks by the same procedure, using larger total radiation doses. (See *Types of stereotactic radiosurgery.*)

INDICATIONS
♦ Brain tumors (benign and malignant)
♦ Trigeminal neuralgia
♦ Essential tremor
♦ Parkinson's tremor or rigidity
♦ Arteriovenous malformations

COMPLICATIONS
♦ Headache
♦ Recurrence of tumor
♦ Nausea and vomiting
♦ Fatigue

Pretreatment care

♦ Verify that the patient has signed an informed consent form.
♦ Answer questions about pretreatment studies or the procedure and remind the patient that a stereotactic frame will be applied for the procedure but removed when the procedure is complete.
♦ Obtain baseline vital signs.
♦ Provide emotional support.

PATIENT TEACHING
♦ Review the underlying disorder and the reason for the treatment.
♦ Explain the treatment and preparation to the patient and his family.

Procedure

♦ Before SRS is performed, the patient is fitted with a stereotactic frame that allows for precise delivery of radiation to the required area. For fractionated radiotherapy, the frame is attached to a rigid plastic mask that contours to the patient's skeletal frame and is reused. The frame for single use is bolted to the patient's head with metal bolts.
♦ The patient doesn't require anesthesia, although local anesthesia may be used to attach the frame to the patient's head.
♦ Radiation is then aimed at the tumor from various directions. The amount of radiation required directly correlates to the exact size and location of the tumor as determined by magnetic resonance imaging and computed tomography scanning.
♦ The frame is detached when the procedure is complete.

Posttreatment care

◆ Monitor the patient's vital signs.
◆ Administer medications as ordered.
◆ Provide comfort measures and support-ive care.

PATIENT TEACHING
◆ Teach the patient how to manage ad-verse effects at home.

◆ Discuss possible complications with the patient and when to notify the practitioner.
◆ Stress the importance of follow-up care.
◆ Refer the patient to support groups such as the American Cancer Society.

Types of stereotactic radiosurgery

The three types of stereotactic radiosurgery differ in the type of instrument used and the source of radiation.

Gamma knife surgery
Gamma knife surgery is used to treat brain tumors of 1.4" (3.5 cm) or less, arteriovenous malformations, and other brain dysfunctions, such as trigeminal neuralgia and seizures. Gamma knife surgery uses 201 beams of highly focused gamma radiation that target the lesion, leaving surrounding tissue unharmed. One dose causes the lesion to slowly reduce in size and eventually dissolve.

Linear accelerator
Linear accelerator (LINAC) machines deliver high-energy photons or electrons in curving paths around the pa-tient's head. This type of radiation is effective on large tumors and may be used for fractionation of treatment. LINAC machines are also used for Intensity-Modulated Radiation Therapy (IMRT), an advanced type of high-precision radiotherapy that conforms to the shape of the target and uses higher radiation doses.

Proton beam radiosurgery
Proton beam radiosurgery uses the quantum wave properties of protons (through use of a cyclotron) to signifi-cantly reduce the amount of radiation to tissue surrounding the target. It can be used for unusually shaped tu-mors, skull base tumors, and vascular malformations of the brain.

Thoracentesis

Overview

Thoracentesis is an invasive procedure that relieves pulmonary compression and respiratory distress by removing accumulated air (pneumothorax) or fluid (hemothorax or pleural effusion) from the pleural space. It can also be used to instill chemotherapeutic agents or other drugs into the pleural space or to obtain a pleural fluid or tissue specimen for analysis.

INDICATIONS
♦ Excess pleural fluid or air due to trauma or other pulmonary disease
♦ Lung or pleural malignancy requiring local chemotherapy

COMPLICATIONS
♦ Pneumothorax
♦ Infection
♦ Pain
♦ Cough
♦ Failure to access the pleural air or fluid site
♦ Subcutaneous hematoma or laceration of intercostal artery
♦ Reexpansion pulmonary edema

Pretreatment care

♦ Verify that an informed consent form has been signed.
♦ Note and report the patient's allergies and record baseline vital signs.
♦ If the patient will receive sedation in addition to local anesthesia, restrict food and fluids as ordered.
♦ Explain to the patient that pleural fluid may be located by chest X-ray or ultrasound and that he'll receive a local anesthetic before the trocar is inserted.
♦ Instruct the patient to avoid coughing, deep breathing, or moving during the treatment.
♦ Explain chest tube drainage equipment and how to turn in bed safely with such devices to avoid kinking or obstructing the tubes.

PATIENT TEACHING
♦ Explain the underlying disorder and the reason for the treatment.
♦ Reinforce the practitioner's explanation of the procedure and describe the nursing care that will be provided.

Procedure

♦ The patient sits and leans forward on a support. If the patient can't sit up, he is positioned on the unaffected side with the arm on the affected side elevated.
♦ The practitioner determines the insertion site. For tension pneumothorax, the midclavicular second to third intercostal space is the usual insertion site because air rises to the top of the intrapleural space. For hemothorax or pleural effusion, the eighth to ninth posterior intercostal spaces are commonly used because fluid settles to the lower levels of the intrapleural space. For removal of air and fluid, chest tubes are inserted into a high and a low site. (See *Performing needle thoracentesis.*)
♦ The site is prepared and draped.
♦ A local anesthetic is injected into the subcutaneous tissue and the thoracentesis needle is inserted.
♦ When the needle reaches the pocket of fluid, it's attached to a 50-ml syringe or a vacuum bottle and the fluid is removed.
♦ During aspiration, the patient is monitored for signs of respiratory distress and hypotension.
♦ Pleural fluid characteristics and total volume are noted.
♦ After the needle is withdrawn, pressure is applied until hemostasis is obtained and then a small dressing is applied.
♦ Alternatively, one or more chest tubes may be inserted and connected to a thoracic drainage system, the tubes are sutured in place, and dressings are applied. Immediately after the drainage system is connected, the patient is instructed to take a deep breath, hold it momentarily, and slowly exhale to assist drainage of the pleural space and lung reexpansion.

◆ Fluid specimens are obtained and placed in proper containers, labelled appropriately, and sent to the laboratory immediately; pleural fluid for pH determination must be collected anaerobically, heparinized, kept on ice, and analyzed promptly.

Posttreatment care

◆ Monitor the patient's vital signs, pulse oximetry, and breath sounds.
◆ Elevate the head of the bed to facilitate breathing.
◆ Obtain a chest X-ray as ordered.
◆ Tell the patient to immediately report difficulty breathing or chest pain.
◆ Monitor the patient for complications.
◆ Observe the puncture site for drainage, inflammation or signs of infection, and change the dressings as ordered.
◆ If chest tubes are inserted, securely tape the junction of the chest tube and the drainage tube to prevent their separation. Connect to suction as ordered.
◆ Monitor and record the drainage in the drainage collection chamber.
◆ Place the rubber-tipped clamps at the bedside.
◆ If the drainage system cracks, or a tube disconnects, clamp the chest tube momentarily as close to the insertion site as possible, or submerge the distal end of the tube in a container of normal saline solution to create a temporary water seal while the drainage system is being replaced. Observe the patient closely for signs and symptoms of tension pneumothorax during the equipment repair. Follow facility policy.
◆ A chest tube is usually removed within 7 days of insertion to prevent infection in the tube tract.

PATIENT TEACHING
◆ Teach about the administration, dosage, and possible adverse effects of prescribed medications.
◆ Encourage the patient to perform coughing and deep-breathing exercises and to use an incentive spirometer until his usual lung function resumes.
◆ Teach the patient and his family how to use and read a finger pulse oximetry device at home, if ordered by the practitioner, and tell them which readings to report to the practitioner immediately.
◆ Refer the patient to appropriate resources and support services.

Performing needle thoracentesis

For a patient with life-threatening tension pneumothorax, needle thoracentesis temporarily relieves pleural pressure until a practitioner can insert a chest tube.

How needle thoracentesis works
A needle attached to a flutter valve is inserted into the affected pleural space. (If no flutter valve is available, one can be made from a perforated finger cot or glove attached with a rubber band.) When the patient exhales, trapped air escapes via the flutter valve instead of being retained under pressure. The flutter valve also prevents more air from entering the involved lung during inhalation.

How to perform the procedure
You may need to assist the practitioner in performing the procedure. Here's how to proceed:
◆ Clean the skin around the second intercostal space at the midclavicular line with antiseptic solution. Use a circular motion, starting at the center and working outward.
◆ The practitioner inserts a sterile 16G (or larger) needle over the superior portion of the rib and through the tissue covering the pleural cavity. The vein, artery, and nerve lie behind the rib's inferior border.
◆ Listen for a hissing sound. This sound signals the needle's entry into the pleural cavity.
◆ If a flutter valve is used, it's secured to the needle. The arrow on the valve indicates the direction of airflow. A sterile glove is placed on the distal end of the valve to collect drainage.
◆ The needle is left in place until a chest tube can be inserted.

Thoracotomy

Overview

Thoracotomy, a surgical incision into the thoracic cavity, usually is performed to remove part or all of a lung and to spare healthy lung tissue from disease. The procedure may involve a pneumonectomy, lobectomy, segmental resection, or wedge resection. An exploratory thoracotomy is used to examine the chest and pleural space for chest trauma and tumors. Decortication removes the fibrous membrane covering the visceral pleura and helps reexpand the lung in empyema. Video-assisted thoracotomy has replaced traditional thoracotomy for open pleural and lung biopsies.

INDICATIONS
◆ Diseased lung tissue requiring removal

COMPLICATIONS
◆ Hemorrhage
◆ Infection
◆ Tension pneumothorax
◆ Bronchopleural fistula
◆ Empyema
◆ Persistent air space that the remaining lung tissue doesn't expand to fill

Pretreatment care

◆ Verify that the patient has signed an informed consent form.
◆ Explain postoperative care.
◆ Arrange for laboratory studies and tests; report abnormal results.
◆ Withhold food and fluids as ordered.

PATIENT TEACHING
◆ Explain the underlying disorder and the reason the treatment is being done.
◆ Explain the treatment and preparation to the patient and his family.
◆ Demonstrate coughing and deep-breathing exercises and how to use an incentive spirometer.

Procedure

◆ The patient receives general anesthesia.
◆ In posterolateral thoracotomy, the incision begins in the submammary fold of the anterior chest, is drawn below the scapular tip and along the ribs, and then curves posteriorly and up to the scapular spine.
◆ In anterolateral thoracotomy, the incision begins below the breast and above the costal margins, extends from the anterior axillary line, and turns downward to avoid the axillary apex.
◆ In median sternotomy, a straight incision is made from the suprasternal notch to below the xiphoid process; the sternum must be transected with an electric or air-driven saw.
◆ After the incision is made, the surgeon may remove tissue for a biopsy.
◆ Bleeding sources are tied off.
◆ Injuries within the thoracic cavity are located and repaired.
◆ The ribs may be spread to expose the lung for excision.

PNEUMONECTOMY
◆ The surgeon ligates and severs the pulmonary arteries.
◆ The mainstem bronchus leading to the affected lung is clamped.
◆ The bronchus is divided and closed with nonabsorbable sutures or staples.
◆ The lung is removed.
◆ To ensure airtight closure, a pleural flap is placed over the bronchus and closed.
◆ The phrenic nerve is severed on the affected side.
◆ After air pressure in the pleural cavity stabilizes, the chest is closed.

LOBECTOMY
◆ The surgeon resects the affected lobe.
◆ Appropriate arteries, veins, and bronchial passages are ligated and severed.
◆ One or two chest tubes are inserted for drainage and lung reexpansion.

SEGMENTAL RESECTION

◆ The surgeon removes the affected lung segment.

◆ The appropriate artery, vein, and bronchus are ligated and severed.

◆ Two chest tubes are inserted to aid lung reexpansion.

WEDGE RESECTION

◆ The affected area is clamped, excised, and sutured.

◆ The surgeon inserts two chest tubes to aid lung reexpansion.

◆ After completing the procedure requiring the thoracotomy, the surgeon closes the chest cavity and applies a dressing.

Posttreatment care

◆ Monitor the patient's respiratory status, and assess breath sounds.

◆ Monitor the patient's vital signs, pulse oximetry, cardiac rhythm, and intake and output.

◆ Assess the patient's pain level, administer analgesics, and evaluate their effects.

◆ Administer medications as ordered.

◆ After pneumonectomy, position the patient on the operative side or his back until he's stabilized.

◆ Maintain chest tube function and assess amount and type of drainage.

◆ Encourage coughing, deep breathing, and incentive spirometry use.

◆ Have the patient splint the incision as needed.

◆ Perform passive range-of-motion (ROM) exercises, progressing to active ROM exercises.

◆ Perform wound care and assess type and amount of drainage.

◆ Assess for complications.

PATIENT TEACHING

◆ Review medications and possible adverse reactions with the patient.

◆ Encourage the patient to perform coughing and deep-breathing exercises and to use an incentive spirometer.

◆ Teach the patient appropriate wound care.

◆ Review the signs and symptoms of complications and when to notify the practitioner.

◆ Advise the patient to balance physical activity and rest as directed by the practitioner.

◆ Advise the patient to stop smoking and provide resources for assistance if appropriate.

◆ Arrange for home health care services if ordered and provide the patient with the agency's name and telephone number.

◆ Stress the importance of regular follow-up care.

Thrombolytic therapy

Overview

Thrombolytic therapy, the administration of a thrombolytic drug, such as streptokinase (Streptase), alteplase (Activase), tenecteplase (TNKase), or reteplase (Retavase), is used to rapidly correct acute and extensive thrombotic disorders by converting plasminogen to plasmin, which leads to lysis of thrombi, fibrinogen, and other plasma proteins.

INDICATIONS
◆ Acute myocardial infarction
◆ Failing or failed atrioventricular fistulas
◆ Thromboembolic disorders
◆ Deep vein thrombosis
◆ Peripheral arterial occlusion
◆ Acute pulmonary emboli
◆ Ischemic stroke
◆ Acute renal artery occlusion

COMPLICATIONS
◆ Bleeding
◆ Adverse reactions to the thrombolytic
◆ Streptokinase resistance (with repeated use of drug)
◆ Arrhythmias

Pretreatment care

◆ Make sure the patient has signed an informed consent form.
◆ Obtain samples for blood typing, cross-matching, and coagulation studies.
◆ Obtain a baseline electrocardiogram and serum electrolyte, arterial blood gas, blood urea nitrogen, creatinine, and cardiac enzyme levels as ordered.

PATIENT TEACHING
◆ Explain the underlying disorder and the reason for the treatment.
◆ Explain the treatment and preparation to the patient and his family.
◆ Explain posttreatment care.

Procedure

◆ Thrombolytic therapy may be administered in various settings, such as the interventional radiology department, intensive care unit, emergency department, or cardiac catheterization laboratory.
◆ Most thrombolytic agents are given by I.V. bolus, with I.V. infusion given at a specific rate in a separate I.V. line.
◆ Selected thrombolytics can be given by intracoronary infusion.
◆ Thrombolytics can also be given locally or directly into the thrombus (as in pulmonary embolism).

Posttreatment care

◆ Provide supplemental oxygen as ordered.
◆ Monitor the patient's vital signs and intake and output.
◆ Monitor the results of coagulation studies.
◆ Monitor heart rate and rhythm, and assess peripheral pulses.
◆ Assess the patient's motor and sensory function.
◆ Monitor the patient's respiratory status.
◆ Administer medications as ordered.
◆ Minimize I.M. injections.
◆ Administer anticoagulants as ordered.
◆ Provide comfort measures.
◆ Restrict physical activity as ordered.
◆ Assess for complications, such as hypersensitivity reactions and abnormal bleeding.

Treatments

PATIENT TEACHING

◆ Review medications and possible adverse reactions with the patient.

◆ Tell the patient to promptly report abnormal or prolonged bleeding to the practitioner.

◆ Review the signs and symptoms of thrombus formation and thromboembolic events with the patient.

◆ Instruct the patient to call the practitioner if he develops new irregular heartbeats, palpitations, or chest pain or discomfort.

◆ Teach the patient how to prevent thrombotic events.

◆ Encourage the patient to stop smoking.

◆ Stress the need for follow-up care.

Thyroidectomy

Overview

A thyroidectomy is the surgical removal of all or part of the thyroid gland.

INDICATIONS
- Hyperthyroidism
- Respiratory obstruction caused by goiter
- Thyroid cancer

COMPLICATIONS
- Hemorrhage
- Parathyroid damage
- Hypocalcemia
- Tetany
- Laryngeal nerve damage
- Vocal cord paralysis
- Thyroid storm

Pretreatment care

- Verify that the patient has signed an informed consent form.
- Inform the patient that he'll experience some hoarseness and a sore throat after surgery.
- Make sure the patient has followed the preoperative drug regimen as ordered.
- Collect blood samples for serum thyroid hormone measurement.
- Obtain a 12-lead electrocardiogram.

PATIENT TEACHING
- Explain the treatment and the preparation involved to the patient and his family.
- Explain postoperative care.

Procedure

- After the patient is anesthetized, the surgeon extends the patient's neck fully and determines the incision line by measuring bilaterally from each clavicle.
- The surgeon cuts through the skin, fascia, and muscle and raises skin flaps from the strap muscles.
- The muscles are separated at midline, revealing the isthmus of the thyroid.
- The thyroid artery and veins are ligated to help prevent bleeding.
- The surgeon locates and views the laryngeal nerves and parathyroid glands.
- He dissects and removes the thyroid tissue.
- A Penrose drain or a closed wound drainage device is inserted, and the wound is closed.

Posttreatment care

- Monitor the patient's vital signs, laboratory values, and intake and output.
- Monitor the patient's respiratory status.
- Keep the patient in high Fowler's position.
- Assess the patient's pain level, administer analgesics, and evaluate their effects.
- Administer medications as ordered.
- Evaluate the patient's speech for signs of laryngeal nerve damage.
- Keep a tracheotomy tray at the bedside for 24 hours after surgery.
- Provide surgical wound care and dressing changes as ordered.
- Maintain patency of drains and note type and amount of drainage.
- Assess for signs and symptoms of complications.

Patient teaching

◆ Review medications and possible adverse reactions with the patient.
◆ Review the signs and symptoms of complications.
◆ Explain the signs and symptoms of hypothyroidism and hyperthyroidism.
◆ Instruct the patient to take the prescribed thyroid hormone replacement therapy and return for annual blood testing once the dosage has been stabilized.
◆ Tell the patient to take calcium supplements as indicated.
◆ Teach the patient appropriate wound care.
◆ Stress the need for follow-up care.

Treatments

Tracheotomy

Overview

Tracheotomy, the surgical creation of an opening into the trachea through the neck, may be permanent or temporary and is usually performed to provide ventilation and oxygenation.

INDICATIONS
- Prolonged mechanical ventilation
- Aspiration prevention in an unconscious or paralyzed patient
- Upper airway obstruction caused by trauma, burns, epiglottitis, or tumors
- Removal of lower tracheobronchial secretions in patients who can't clear them

COMPLICATIONS
- Hemorrhage
- Edema
- Aspiration of secretions
- Pneumothorax
- Subcutaneous emphysema
- Infection
- Airway obstruction
- Hypoxia
- Arrhythmias

Pretreatment care

- Verify that the patient has signed an informed consent form.
- Obtain appropriate supplies or a tracheotomy tray.
- Devise an appropriate communication system with the patient to follow the procedure.
- Obtain samples for arterial blood gas analysis and other required diagnostic tests; report abnormal results.

PATIENT TEACHING
- Explain the underlying disorder and the reason for the treatment.
- Explain the treatment and the preparation involved to the patient and his family.

Procedure

- The technique varies with the type of tube used.
- In most instances, the patient receives general anesthesia. If a tracheotomy is done emergently, the patient is usually unconscious.
- A horizontal incision is made in the skin below the cricoid cartilage, and vertical incisions are made in the trachea.
- A tracheostomy tube is placed between the second and third tracheal rings (see *Comparing types of tracheostomy tubes*).
- Retraction sutures may be placed in the stomal margins.
- The tube cuff (if present) is inflated and tracheotomy ties are applied.
- Ventilation and suction are performed.
- Oxygen is administered. If an endotracheal tube was present, it's removed.

Posttreatment care

- Provide oxygen and humidification as ordered.
- Suction the airway as indicated and monitor the amount, color, and consistency of secretions.
- Monitor the patient's vital signs and pulse oximetry.
- Monitor the patient's respiratory status and assess breath sounds.
- Administer medications as ordered.
- Turn the patient every 2 hours and provide chest physiotherapy.
- Monitor cuff pressures as ordered (usually less than 25 cm H_2O [18 mm Hg]).
- Provide comfort measures.
- Perform tracheostomy care and dressing changes per facility policy.
- Keep a sterile tracheostomy tube with obturator (including a tube one size smaller) at the bedside.
- Observe for abnormal bleeding or other complications.

PATIENT TEACHING

♦ Teach about the administration, dosage, and possible adverse effects of prescribed medications.

♦ Teach the patient how to care for the tracheostomy site and tube.

♦ Reinforce the speech therapist's teaching about how to swallow.

♦ Remind the patient to protect the stoma from water.

♦ Tell the patient to use a foam filter over the stoma during winter.

♦ Review the signs and symptoms of complications and when to notify the practitioner.

♦ Teach proper disposal of expelled secretions with the patient.

♦ Advise the patient when to follow up with the practitioner.

Comparing types of tracheostomy tubes

Tracheostomy tubes are made of plastic or metal and are available in cuffed, uncuffed, or fenestrated varieties. Tube selection depends on the patient's condition and the practitioner's preference. Make sure you're familiar with the advantages and disadvantages of these commonly used tracheostomy tubes.

Tube type	Advantages	Disadvantages
Uncuffed (plastic or metal) 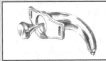	♦ Permits free flow of air around the tube and through the larynx ♦ Reduces the risk of tracheal damage ♦ Recommended for children because it doesn't require a cuff ♦ Allows mechanical ventilation in the patient with neuromuscular disease	♦ Lack of a cuff increases the risk of aspiration (in adults) ♦ Adapter may be necessary for ventilation
Plastic cuffed (low pressure and high volume) 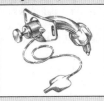	♦ Disposable ♦ Cuff bonded to the tube; won't detach accidentally inside the trachea ♦ Low cuff pressure, which is evenly distributed against the tracheal wall; no need to deflate periodically to lower pressure ♦ Reduces the risk of tracheal damage	♦ May be more costly than other tubes
Fenestrated 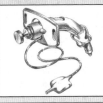	♦ Permits speech through the upper airway when the external opening is capped and the cuff is deflated ♦ Allows breathing by mechanical ventilation with an inner cannula in place and the cuff inflated ♦ Inner cannula can be easily removed for cleaning	♦ Possible occlusion of fenestration ♦ Possible dislodgment of inner cannula

Transcutaneous electrical nerve stimulation

Overview

Transcutaneous electrical nerve stimulation (TENS), the delivery of painless electrical current from a portable battery-powered device to peripheral nerves or directly to a painful area over relatively large nerve fibers, is used to change the patient's perception of pain by blocking painful stimuli traveling over smaller fibers. It's used with postoperative patients and those with chronic pain to reduce the need for analgesics based on the theory that painful impulses pass through a "gate" in the brain. TENS usually involves 3 to 5 days of treatment, but chronic pain may require intermittent treatments; certain conditions, such as phantom limb pain, may require continuous stimulation.

INDICATIONS
- Arthritis pain
- Bone fracture pain
- Bursitis pain
- Cancer-related pain
- Musculoskeletal pain
- Myofascial pain
- Pain from neuralgias and neuropathies
- Phantom limb pain
- Postoperative incision pain
- Pain from sciatica
- Whiplash pain

COMPLICATIONS
- Continued pain
- Skin irritation or allergy to electrode materials

Pretreatment care

- Obtain a commercial TENS kit that includes the stimulator, leadwires, electrodes, spare battery pack, and battery recharger.
- Clean the skin thoroughly where the electrode will be applied with an alcohol pad, then dry.
- If necessary, shave hair at the site where each electrode will be placed, taking care not to break the skin.

PATIENT TEACHING
- Explain the function of the unit and how it's applied.
- Demonstrate how the unit is used.

Procedure

- Apply electrode gel to the bottom of each electrode. Electrodes are adhesive and reusable as long as the adhesive remains intact.
- Place the ordered number of electrodes on the proper skin area, leaving at least 2″ (5 cm) between them. Some larger patches are designed to contain two electrodes, already separated, in one patch.
- Follow the practitioner's orders about electrode placement. Placement can be over or surrounding the affected area or can be higher in the nerve distribution to block signals to the affected area (as with phantom limb pain). If the patient's skin is moist, apply a special skin preparation agent to the skin before the electrodes are applied.

 Nursing alert

Alcohol pads should never be used before applying electrodes to the skin.

- Insert the leadwires into the electrodes. Make sure the control box controls are turned off, and insert the leadwire plug ends into the control box.
- Gradually increase the control settings within the parameters set by the practitioner. Usually, the pattern and intensity of the stimulation can be set separately.
- Set the controls to a level comfortable for the patient, which is when he feels a comfortable tingling sensation, generally between 60 and 100 Hz.
- Attach the TENS control box to part of the patient's clothing, such as a belt, pocket, or bra. Carefully place extra leadwire

into the patient's clothing so it doesn't dangle loosely.

◆ Monitor for signs of excessive stimulation, such as muscle twitches, and signs of inadequate stimulation, to make sure the device is working effectively.

◆ If TENS is used continuously for postoperative pain, remove the electrodes daily to check for skin irritation, to provide skin care, and to rotate sites of electrode placement.

Posttreatment care

◆ Turn off the controls and unplug the electrode leadwires, unless another treatment will be given soon, then leave the electrodes in place. If the electrodes must be moved during the procedure, first turn off the controls.

◆ Clean the electrodes with soap and water, and clean the patient's skin with alcohol pads. Check the patient's skin for reddening or other signs of allergy to the adhesive.

◆ Don't soak the electrodes in alcohol because it will damage the rubber. Place the electrodes back on the supplied silicone sheet to maintain gel freshness until the next application.

◆ Remove the battery pack and replace it with a charged battery pack.

◆ Recharge the used battery pack so it's always ready for use.

PATIENT TEACHING

◆ Review the operator's manual with the patient and reinforce where to locate trouble-shooting information.

◆ Teach the patient how to place the electrodes properly and how to take care of the TENS unit.

◆ Instruct the patient to report to the practitioner if the treatment becomes ineffective or causes skin irritation.

◆ Teach the patient about medications being taken, including administration and potential adverse reactions.

Transplantation, bone marrow

Overview

Bone marrow transplantation, the infusion of fresh or stored bone marrow into the bloodstream, is performed to replace blood cells destroyed by chemotherapy or radiation or to treat a blood disorder. The donated marrow cells migrate to the patient's bone marrow in 10 days to 4 weeks, and then begin proliferating. Autologous bone marrow donation involves harvesting bone marrow from the patient (before chemotherapy or radiation, or during remission) and freezing it for use up to 2 weeks later. Syngeneic bone marrow donation comes from a patient's identical twin. Allogenic bone marrow donation comes from a histocompatible individual.

INDICATIONS
- Aplastic anemia
- Severe combined immunodeficiency disease (SCID)
- Acute lymphocytic leukemia
- Myeloid leukemias
- Lymphoma
- Multiple myeloma
- Certain solid tumors
- Sickle cell anemia

COMPLICATIONS
During infusion
- Fluid volume overload
- Anaphylaxis
- Pulmonary fat embolism

After infusion
- Infection
- Abnormal bleeding
- Renal insufficiency
- Venous occlusive disease
- SCID (with allogenic donation)

Pretreatment care

- Verify that the patient has signed an informed consent form.
- Start an I.V. line, if needed, and administer I.V. fluids as ordered.
- Obtain an administration set with a special filter for debris.
- Administer medications as ordered.
- Obtain baseline vital signs.
- Assist with insertion of a central venous catheter if none is in place.

PATIENT TEACHING
- Explain the treatment and the necessary preparation to the patient.
- For an allogenic graft, discuss the immunosuppressant drugs that the patient will be taking, and explain their possible adverse effects. Remind the patient that these drugs increase his risk of infection.
- Instruct the patient and family members about measures used to control infection and minimize rejection after transplant.

Procedure

- The patient is treated at the bedside.
- An antihistamine or analgesic is administered as ordered.
- With syngeneic or allogenic donation, marrow is obtained in the operating room the same day as transplantation and is brought to the patient's room immediately.
- With autologous donation, the marrow is allowed to thaw before infusion.
- The practitioner infuses the marrow through the central venous catheter over 2 to 4 hours.
- The nurse obtains vital signs every 15 minutes for 1 hour, every 30 minutes for 2 hours, then every hour for 4 hours.

◆ The patient is monitored for fever, dyspnea, hypotension, bronchospasm, urticaria, chest pain, and back pain throughout the infusion.

◆ Diphenhydramine (Benadryl) or epinephrine (Adrenalin) is administered if necessary to manage transfusion reactions.

Posttreatment care

◆ Maintain asepsis.
◆ Institute safety measures.
◆ Administer transfusions and I.V. fluids as ordered.
◆ Obtain blood samples for laboratory analysis as ordered.
◆ Monitor vital signs and laboratory test results.
◆ Assess the patient for signs of infection, hemorrhage, and SCID

PATIENT TEACHING
◆ Teach about the administration, dosage, and possible adverse effects of prescribed medications.
◆ Review precautions against infection.
◆ Tell the patient how to avoid injury or bleeding.
◆ Teach the patient how to care for his central venous catheter if it's to remain in place for some time.
◆ Discuss the signs and symptoms of transplant failure and other complications of the procedure and when to notify the practitioner.
◆ Review when the patient should return to the surgeon and hematologist for follow-up care.
◆ Refer the patient and his family to support groups and local resources.

Transplantation, cerebral stem cell

Overview

Cerebral stem cell transplantation, the grafting of fetal or adult stem cells into the striatum of affected patients, is an experimental treatment in which gene-altered or virus-carrying cells are injected to stimulate dopamine production or other actions (called a *transfection procedure*).

INDICATIONS
◆ Neurologic disorders such as Parkinson's disease

COMPLICATIONS
◆ Infection
◆ Graft rejection
◆ Increased intracranial pressure (ICP)

Pretreatment care

◆ Check laboratory values, electrocardiogram, and chest X-rays as ordered, and notify the practitioner of abnormalities.
◆ Assess the patient's neurologic status and cardiopulmonary status and obtain baseline vital signs.
◆ Obtain stereotaxic X-rays as ordered for use during the procedure.
◆ Verify that the patient has signed an informed consent form.

PATIENT TEACHING
◆ Explain the underlying disorder and the reason for treatment.
◆ Review the explanation of the planned surgical technique with the patient.
◆ Explain what the patient can expect after he wakens from anesthesia, including the presence of I.V. lines, an indwelling urinary catheter, an arterial line and, possibly, a mechanical ventilator.
◆ Describe routine postoperative care, including frequent checks of vital signs, monitoring of intake and output, and respiratory therapy. Prepare him for postoperative pain, and assure him that analgesics will be available.
◆ Demonstrate how to perform coughing and deep-breathing exercises and, if ordered, incentive spirometry.
◆ Discuss the immunosuppressant drugs that the patient will take, and explain their possible adverse effects. Remind the patient that these drugs increase his risk of infection.
◆ Instruct the patient and family members about measures used to control infection and minimize rejection after transplant.

Procedure

◆ The patient is given general anesthesia and his head is shaved where the incision will be made.
◆ The neurosurgeon accesses selected brain tissue, such as in the cortex, hippocampus, or thalamus, with stereotaxic guidance via small burr holes in the skull and dural retraction.
◆ Genetically engineered cells, adrenal chromaffin cells, fetal neurons, or dopamine-producing tissues have been grafted experimentally.

Posttreatment care

◆ Administer oxygen as indicated, and suction and turn the patient.
◆ Assess the patient's neurologic status and report changes in trends; monitor for increased ICP.
◆ Monitor the patient's vital signs, intake and output, and laboratory test results.
◆ Apply elastic stockings or compression boots while the patient is in bed.
◆ Administer I.V. fluids as ordered.
◆ Observe for signs and symptoms of complications.

Treatments

PATIENT TEACHING

◆ Teach about the administration, dosage, and possible adverse effects of prescribed medications.

◆ Review precautions against infection.

◆ Tell the patient how to avoid injury or bleeding.

◆ Teach the patient and his family appropriate wound care.

◆ Teach the patient to care for his central venous catheter if it's to remain in place for some time.

◆ Discuss the signs and symptoms of transplant failure and other complications of the procedure and when to notify the practitioner.

◆ Review when the patient should return for follow-up care.

◆ Refer the patient and his family to support groups and local resources.

Transplantation, heart

Overview

Heart transplantation involves the replacement of a damaged heart with a donor or artificial heart.

INDICATIONS
◆ End-stage cardiac disease unresponsive to other therapies

COMPLICATIONS
◆ Graft rejection
◆ Infection
◆ Decreased cardiac output
◆ Arrhythmias

Pretreatment care

◆ Review necessary diagnostic tests such as antigen typing.
◆ Administer immunosuppressant agents as ordered.
◆ Verify that an informed consent form has been signed.
◆ Maintain oxygenation and hemodynamic stability with preexisting treatments as ordered.
◆ Provide emotional support to the patient and his family.

PATIENT TEACHING
◆ Reinforce the surgeon's explanation of the surgery, equipment, and procedures used in the cardiac care unit or postanesthesia care unit.
◆ Explain what the patient can expect after he wakens from anesthesia, including the presence of I.V. lines, an indwelling urinary catheter, and an arterial line. Remind the patient that he'll have a breathing tube in his throat, attached to a ventilator, until he can breathe independently (usually within 6 hours).
◆ Describe routine postoperative care. Prepare the patient for postoperative pain, and assure him that analgesics will be available.

◆ Demonstrate how to perform coughing and deep-breathing exercises and incentive spirometery.
◆ Review range-of-motion exercises to be used.
◆ Discuss the immunosuppressant drugs that the patient will be taking, and their possible adverse effects. Remind the patient that these drugs increase his risk of infection.
◆ Instruct the patient and family members about measures used to control infection.

Procedure

◆ The patient receives general anesthesia.
◆ Orthotopic heart transplantation involves removing most of the patient's (native) heart and retaining a large portion of the right and left atria. The donor heart is attached to the native atrial cusps, and direct end-to-end anastomoses of the aorta and pulmonary artery are created.
◆ The surgeon performs a median sternotomy and uses retractors to access the chest cavity.
◆ The patient is placed on cardiopulmonary bypass.
◆ Temporary epicardial pacemaker leadwires are placed because the transplanted heart is denervated and can't respond normally to stimuli from the autonomic nervous system.
◆ Heterotopic heart transplantation ("piggyback" heart transplantation) is less commonly performed and involves grafting a donor heart to a recipient heart without removing the recipient heart. The donor heart is used to assist the pumping ability of the native heart.

Posttreatment care

◆ Assess cardiopulmonary and hemodynamic status per unit protocol.
◆ Monitor cardiac rhythm. Keep in mind that the transplanted heart's electrocardiogram waveform appears different from that of the patient's native heart.
◆ Monitor vital signs, pulse oximetry, intake and output, nasogastric suction, and chest tube drainage.
◆ Monitor atrial and ventricular pacing if present, keeping the heart rate greater than 110 beats/minute.
◆ Institute strict infection control precautions; perform meticulous hand washing.
◆ Assist with extubating and administer supplemental oxygen as needed. Encourage coughing, deep breathing, incentive spirometry, and splinting; premedicate for pain as needed.
◆ Administer medications and titrate medication infusions as ordered.
◆ Prepare the patient for myocardial biopsy at about 7 days and 14 days postoperatively, and then as indicated by the surgeon.

PATIENT TEACHING

◆ Teach about the administration, dosage, and possible adverse effects of prescribed medications.
◆ Review precautions against infection.
◆ Tell the patient how to avoid injury or bleeding.
◆ Teach the patient and his family appropriate wound care.
◆ Teach the patient to care for his central venous catheter if it's to remain in place for some time.
◆ Review dietary and activity restrictions.
◆ Discuss the signs and symptoms of transplant failure and other complications of the procedure and when to notify the practitioner.
◆ Review when the patient should return for follow-up care.
◆ Refer the patient and his family to support groups and local resources.

Vacuum-assisted closure therapy

Overview

Vacuum-assisted closure (VAC) therapy, the application of localized subatmospheric pressure to draw the edges of a wound toward the center, is used to enhance delayed or impaired wound healing. A special sponge is placed in the wound and therapy is applied to remove fluids from the wound and stimulate growth of healthy granulation tissue. (See *Understanding VAC therapy.*)

 Nursing alert

VAC therapy is contraindicated in patients with fistulas that involve organs or body cavities, necrotic tissue with eschar, untreated osteomyelitis, and malignant wounds.

INDICATIONS
- Acute and traumatic wounds
- Pressure ulcers
- Chronic open wounds (such as diabetic ulcers, dehisced surgical wounds, meshed grafts, and skin flaps)

COMPLICATIONS
- Increased pain (temporary)
- Increased risk of infection
- Tissue damage or bleeding (with inappropriate application)

Pretreatment care

- Assemble the vacuum-assisted closure device at the bedside per the manufacturer's instructions.
- Set the negative pressure according to the practitioner's order (25 to 200 mm Hg).
- Premedicate the patient for pain as needed.
- Wash hands and, if necessary, put on a gown and goggles to protect from wound drainage and contamination.
- Position the patient to allow maximum wound exposure.
- Place the emesis basin under the wound to collect drainage.

- Remove the soiled dressing and discard it in a waterproof trash bag.

PATIENT TEACHING
- Explain the procedure to the patient.
- Explain that the treatment is continuous and the device can be moved with the patient.

Procedure

- Attach a 19G catheter to the 35-ml piston syringe and irrigate the wound thoroughly using normal saline solution.
- Clean the area around the wound with normal saline solution; wipe intact skin with a skin protectant wipe and allow it to dry.
- Remove and discard your gloves and put on sterile gloves.
- Use sterile scissors to cut the foam to the shape and measurement of the wound. More than one piece of foam may be needed to fit the wound accurately.
- Carefully place the foam in the wound, making sure not to exceed the edges of the wound.
- Place the transparent occlusive air permeable drape over the foam, enclosing the foam completely. Cut a small opening in the center of the occlusive dressing.
- Attach the adhesive patch with fenestrated tubing into the center of the foam, over the small opening.
- Attach the free end of the fenestrated tubing to the tubing that's connected to the evacuation canister.
- Turn on the vacuum unit and check that the sponge responds to the suction effect (it will be obvious if it's functioning correctly and there are no air leaks).

Treatments

Posttreatment care

◆ Make sure the patient is comfortably repositioned.
◆ Properly dispose of soiled dressings and drainage.
◆ Change the VAC dressing every 48 hours or as needed.
◆ Measure the amount of drainage every shift.
◆ Use audible and visual alarms to alert if the unit is tipped greater than 45 degrees (acute care model), the canister is full or occluded, the dressing has an air leak, or the canister becomes dislodged.
◆ Administer medications as ordered.
◆ Provide skin care.
◆ Provide emotional support.
◆ Monitor the patient's vital signs, intake and output, and peripheral pulses.

◆ Assess the patient for signs of decreased tissue perfusion and new or increasing infection.

PATIENT TEACHING
◆ Teach about the administration, dosage, and possible adverse effects of prescribed medications.
◆ Review the signs and symptoms of infection to report to the practitioner.
◆ If the patient is being discharged with the home care version of the device, teach him the correct procedures for caring for the device and his wound.
◆ Refer the patient to resources and support services.
◆ Refer the patient to home care and a wound care specialist, as indicated.

Understanding VAC therapy

Vacuum-assisted closure (VAC) therapy may be used when a wound fails to heal in a timely manner. It encourages healing by applying localized subatmospheric pressure at the site of the wound. This pressure reduces edema and bacterial colonization and stimulates the formation of granulation tissue.

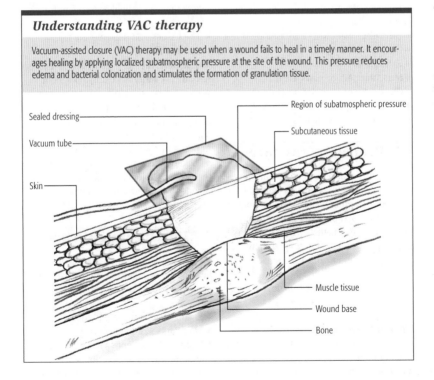

Sealed dressing

Vacuum tube

Skin

Region of subatmospheric pressure

Subcutaneous tissue

Muscle tissue

Wound base

Bone

Vagus nerve stimulation

Overview

Vagus nerve stimulation (VNS), the stimulation of widespread release of gamma-aminobutyric acid and glycine in the brain through use of a vagus nerve stimulator, is used to increase seizure threshold and to improve mood by stimulating serotonin and norepinephrine neurotransmitters and possibly specific brain structures involved in mood regulation. It's placed on the left vagus nerve because of the higher risk of cardiac arrhythmias with stimulation of the right vagus nerve.

INDICATIONS
◆ Partial seizures
◆ Treatment resistant depression
◆ Depression

COMPLICATIONS
◆ Hoarseness, throat pain, or voice alteration
◆ Difficulty swallowing and aspiration risk
◆ Coughing or dyspnea
◆ Paresthesia
◆ Muscular pain or nonspecific pain
◆ Chest pain or irregular heart rhythm
◆ Nausea, dyspepsia, or vomiting
◆ Infection at incision sites

Pretreatment care

◆ Make sure that presurgery medical evaluation and testing have been completed as ordered; this process may include monitoring seizures and performing electroencephalography, magnetic resonance imaging, or positron emission tomography.
◆ Verify that an informed consent form has been signed.
◆ Perform a baseline neurologic and mental status nursing assessment.

PATIENT TEACHING
◆ Review with the patient the procedure, nursing preparation, and postsurgical care, and answer any questions that he may have.

◆ Tell the patient that part of his head and chest may be shaved in the operating room.
◆ Explain to the patient that he'll be in the intensive care unit postoperatively and review the equipment he'll see when he awakens.

Procedure

◆ The patient is usually given general anesthesia.
◆ The left vagus nerve is isolated through a small incision, and a stimulating electrode is attached to it.
◆ A pulse generator with battery pack is positioned in the anterior chest wall through a small incision.
◆ A tunneling tool forms a channel under the subcutaneous tissue to thread the stimulating lead from the neck to the chest where the lead is hooked to the pulse generator.
◆ The tissues and incisions are replaced, sutured, and dressed.
◆ Generally, the pulse generator is then externally programmed using a magnetic wand. The pulse amplitude (maximum of 14 volts), pulse width, pulse frequency, and pulse on and off times are then set. Sometimes, however, the device is left off until the first postoperative day.
◆ Usually, the current output is adjusted to the patient's tolerance, and a pattern of 30 seconds "on" time and 5 minutes "off" time is set.

Posttreatment care

◆ Position the patient on his side with the head of the bed elevated 15 to 30 degrees; assist the patient with turning every 2 hours.
◆ Ensure a quiet, calm environment.
◆ Maintain seizure precautions.
◆ Monitor the patient's vital signs, intake and output, level of consciousness, respiratory status, heart rate and rhythm, and mental status.

◆ Monitor drainage and the surgical wound and dressings.
◆ Administer medications as ordered.
◆ Monitor for complications, particularly throat and voice changes, swallowing or breathing difficulties, and pain during stimulation; notify the practitioner of complications promptly.

PATIENT TEACHING

◆ Teach about the administration, dosage, and possible adverse effects of prescribed medications. Reinforce that some medications, prescribed for the original diagnosis, may be continued indefinitely or discontinued, based on response to the VNS therapy over time.
◆ Teach the patient appropriate wound care.
◆ Tell the patient that he may notice a slight bulge in the area under his collarbone (where the device is) and that the surgery will leave small scars on the side of his neck where the wire lead was placed and on his chest where the device was implanted.
◆ Stress the importance of appropriate psychiatric or neurologic follow-up care.
◆ Inform the patient that the VNS system isn't affected by microwave transmission, cellular phones, small electrical appliances, or airport security systems.
◆ Tell the patient that he must notify every health care provider or facility that he has an implanted VNS device because certain procedures may affect the device's functioning or aren't allowed, including any type of diathermy (special heat-based procedures), procedures involving certain electrical instruments (such as those used in surgery), certain types of magnetic resonance imaging (check with the imaging physician for safety), external defibrillation, and extracorporeal shockwave lithotripsy.
◆ Tell the patient that it may take several weeks to tune the pulse parameters to effective settings and up to 2 years to reach full benefit.

◆ Show the patient and his family how to use the supplied handheld magnet to activate a pulse at the onset of a seizure or aura by passing the magnet over the generator for a few seconds. Reinforce that keeping the magnet over the generator actually turns the generator off.
◆ Tell the patient that the battery needs to be replaced surgically every 1 to 16 years (depending on the patient's physiologic characteristics and usage), and to check it daily by activating one magnet stimulation each morning.
◆ Reinforce to the patient that the vagus nerve stimulator can begin working immediately, or as soon as the practitioner programs it, but that full effects develop over time.
◆ As a measure to prevent seizure or modify its severity, teach the patient how to use the handheld magnet to stimulate a pulse when he feels a seizure aura; instruct the patient to call the nurse for assistance as needed.

 Nursing alert
Tell the patient to stop stimulation and immediately call the nurse if it becomes painful or it triggers significant coughing, swallowing, or heart rate problems.

◆ Refer the patient to appropriate resources and support services.

Vena cava filter placement

Overview

Vena cava filter placement, the placement of a filter in the inferior vena cava to trap clots and prevent pulmonary embolism (PE), is used for prophylaxis and for treatment of thromboemboli.

INDICATIONS

◆ Deep vein thrombosis (DVT) or PE in patients who are unable to take or unresponsive to anticoagulants
◆ Frequently recurring thromboses
◆ Extension of a thromboembolism while on appropriate doses of anticoagulants
◆ Patients undergoing pulmonary embolectomy
◆ Prophylaxis for certain patients scheduled for elective orthopedic surgery, patients with major trauma, selected patients with malignancies or who are pregnant, and certain patients with serious heart or lung conditions

COMPLICATIONS

◆ Bleeding at the insertion site
◆ Damage to the vein during insertion
◆ Partial blockage of the vena cava

Pretreatment care

◆ Verify that a venacavogram report is available in the chart.
◆ If ordered, check that computed tomography scanning or magnetic resonance imaging of the trunk have been completed.
◆ Verify that an informed consent form has been signed.
◆ Check that preoperative laboratory studies, particularly bleeding studies, and an electrocardiogram have been completed if ordered.
◆ Administer preoperative sedation or a muscle relaxant as ordered.
◆ Complete a cardiovascular, pulmonary, and neurologic assessment and obtain baseline vital signs. Assess peripheral pulses.

PATIENT TEACHING

◆ Review the underlying disorder and the reason for the treatment.
◆ Review the procedure and nursing care with the patient.

Procedure

◆ Techniques vary based on the type of filter chosen (for example, Greenfield filter, Bird's Nest filter, Vena Tech LGM filter, or Simon Nitinol filter).
◆ Generally, a local anesthetic is administered near the femoral or jugular vein, where the catheter containing the filter will be inserted.
◆ A small incision is made over the selected site, and the catheter is inserted. Using X-ray equipment and fluoroscopy or ultrasound, the catheter is guided to the desired location in the vena cava.
◆ The filter is released from the catheter, allowing it to open and attach to the wall of the vena cava.
◆ The catheter is removed and the incision is closed and dressed.

Posttreatment care

◆ Place the patient in a comfortable position and give supplemental oxygen as indicated.
◆ Assess the incision site for bleeding or signs or symptoms of infection.
◆ Monitor peripheral pulses and check for circulation adequacy.
◆ Monitor the patient's vital signs, intake and output, and perform cardiac monitoring if ordered.
◆ Administer medications, including analgesics, and monitor their effects.
◆ Maintain the patency of I.V. tubes; maintain fluid restriction if ordered.
◆ Monitor the patient's hemodynamic status if ordered.
◆ Assess the patient for abnormal heart and breath sounds, and report changes immediately.

Treatments

◆ Monitor the results of ordered laboratory studies.

PATIENT TEACHING
◆ Teach about the administration, dosage, and possible adverse effects of prescribed medications.
◆ Instruct the patient to watch for signs of ongoing venous insufficiency, such as edema, darkened skin, tissue loss, and skin ulceration of the legs. Tell him to notify the practitioner of such signs immediately.
◆ Review the signs and symptoms of complications and when to notify the practitioner.
◆ Teach the patient about anticoagulant therapy, precautions, and monitoring if prescribed.
◆ Advise the patient to continue to use compression stockings as long as instructed by the practitioner.
◆ Reinforce basic precautions to prevent DVT.
◆ Encourage the patient to perform regular exercise and leg exercises as directed by the practitioner.
◆ Stress the importance of follow-up care.

Ventricular assist device

Overview

A ventricular assist device (VAD), an artificial pump implanted in the heart to divert blood from a ventricle to the pump, synchronizes to the patient's electrocardiogram (ECG) and functions as the ventricle, providing support to a failing heart as well as systemic and pulmonary support. A right VAD (RVAD) provides pulmonary support by diverting blood from a failing right ventricle to the VAD, which then pumps blood to the pulmonary circulation via the VAD connection to the pulmonary artery. With a left VAD (LVAD), blood flows from the left ventricle to the VAD, then the blood is pumped back to the body via the VAD connection to the aorta. Using both a RVAD and LVAD provides biventricular support.

INDICATIONS
- Ventricular failure
- Cardiac transplantation
- Refractory cardiogenic shock
- Cardiopulmonary bypass
- Respiratory failure
- Kidney failure
- Stroke

COMPLICATIONS
- Hemorrhage
- Air embolus
- Thrombus
- Infection
- Lethal arrhythmias

Pretreatment care

- Verify that an informed consent form has been signed.
- Provide emotional support.
- Monitor the patient's ECG, pulmonary artery and hemodynamic status, and intake and output.
- Administer ongoing medications as ordered.
- Before surgery, restrict food and fluid intake, and monitor cardiac function.

PATIENT TEACHING
- Review the purpose of the VAD and what to expect after its insertion.
- Demonstrate coughing and deep-breathing exercises and use of incentive spirometer.

Procedure

- The patient is given general anesthesia.
- An incision is made through the breastbone to expose the heart; heparin is administered to keep the blood from clotting.
- Cardiopulmonary bypass is initiated.
- An incision is made to form a pocket for the LVAD in the abdominal wall.
- Small incisions are placed through the diaphragm to allow placement of the tubes, which are used to channel blood from the ventricle to the LVAD and connect the pump to the aorta.
- An incision is also made through the abdominal wall to connect the VAD to an external power source.
- The surgeon cannulates the left ventricle with the inflow tube and the aorta with the outflow tube.
- When the pump is adequately supporting the heart, the patient is removed from the heart-lung machine.
- All incisions are sutured and dressings are applied.

Posttreatment care

- Assess the patient's cardiovascular and respiratory status.
- Monitor vital signs, pulse oximetry, hemodynamic parameters, cardiac rhythm, intake and output, and peripheral pulses.
- Keep the patient immobile to prevent accidental extubation, contamination, or disconnection of the VAD. When stable, turn the patient every 2 hours and begin range-of-motion exercises.
- Assess chest tube drainage and function. Notify the practitioner if drainage is greater than 150 ml/hour over 2 hours.

Treatments

◆ Obtain laboratory test results and report them to the practitioner.

◆ Administer medications as ordered and titrate medicated infusions per protocol.

◆ Give heparin as ordered, and observe for signs of bleeding.

◆ Monitor for signs and symptoms of complications.

◆ Provide wound care according to facility policy.

◆ Encourage coughing and deep breathing and incentive spirometer use.

PATIENT TEACHING

◆ Teach about the administration, dosage, and possible adverse effects of prescribed medications.

◆ Advise the patient about dietary and activity restrictions.

◆ Teach the patient wound care.

◆ Review with the patient the signs and symptoms of complications and when to notify the practitioner.

◆ Teach the patient how to care for the exit port and battery pack.

◆ Arrange for home care referral for follow-up care and teaching as indicated.

◆ Stress the need for regular follow-up care with his cardiologist.

III Procedures

Arterial pressure monitoring

Overview

Arterial pressure monitoring, also known as *intra-arterial pressure monitoring*, directly and continuously measures systolic, diastolic, and mean blood pressures through a catheter inserted in an artery. More accurate than indirect methods such as palpation and auscultation, which only measure blood flow, arterial pressure monitoring also reflects systemic vascular resistance. It's used in patients with low cardiac output and high systemic vascular resistance (when highly accurate or frequent blood pressure measurements are required), in patients with an intra-aortic balloon pump, when vasoactive medications are being titrated, or when frequent blood sampling is required for arterial blood gas or laboratory testing.

CONTRAINDICATIONS
◆ Severe injury to the extremity
◆ Positive Allen's test
◆ Injury proximal to vessel
◆ Local skin compromise

Preprocedure care for catheter insertion

◆ Explain the procedure to the patient.
◆ Verify that an informed consent form has been signed.
◆ Check the patient's history for allergy or hypersensitivity to iodine or the ordered local anesthetic.
◆ Wash your hands.
◆ Assemble the equipment, maintaining sterile technique.

Procedure for catheter insertion

Equipment: preassembled preparation kit (if available) ◆ sterile gloves ◆ sterile gown ◆ mask ◆ protective eyewear ◆ 16G to 20G arterial catheter (type and length depend on insertion site, patient's size,

and other anticipated uses of line) ◆ sterile drapes ◆ ordered local anesthetic ◆ sutures ◆ prepared pressure transducer system with flush solution (attached to bedside monitor) ◆ transparent dressing ◆ arm board ◆ optional: scissors to clip hair (if femoral artery is used)

◆ Set up and prime the monitoring system (see *Priming monitoring tubing*).
◆ Attach the tubing to the monitor's pressure module.
◆ Level the zeroing stopcock of the transducer with the phlebostatic axis, then zero the transducer system to atmospheric pressure.
◆ Set the alarms on the bedside monitor according to facility policy.
◆ Position the patient for easy access to the catheter insertion site.

Priming monitoring tubing

◆ Assemble the necessary equipment, including a pressure bag, 500 ml of normal saline solution or heparin flush (per facility policy or practitioner order), a pressure tubing kit, and an I.V. pole.
◆ Wash your hands.
◆ Inflate the pressure bag to 300 mm Hg, check it for air leaks, and then release the pressure.
◆ Prepare the I.V. flush solution.
◆ Open the bag of closed end caps.
◆ Close the control valve on the tubing.
◆ Attach the tubing to the flush solution and compress the drip chamber to partially fill it with solution.
◆ Turn the stopcock toward the end site of the tubing (where the tubing meets the patient).
◆ Open the control valve on the tubing and wait for fluid to flow through the tubing and the open end cap.
◆ Shut off the control valve and replace the open end cap with a closed one.
◆ Turn the stopcock toward the closed end cap, open the control valve, and allow fluid to flow to the end of the tubing, through the open end cap at the end of the tubing. Turn off the control valve and replace the open end cap with a closed one.
◆ Place the flush solution bag in a pressure bag and inflate it to 300 mm Hg of pressure, and hang the pressure bag on an I.V. pole.

- Place a sheet protector under the site.
- If the catheter will be inserted into the radial artery, perform Allen's test to assess the collateral circulation in the hand.
- Label all medication syringes, medication containers, and solution containers.
- Call a "time-out" to confirm the patient's identity using two patient identifiers, and verify the procedure according to facility policy.
- The practitioner prepares and anesthetizes the insertion site and covers the surrounding area with sterile drapes.
- The practitioner inserts the arterial catheter into the artery and attaches it to the fluid-filled pressure tubing.
- While the practitioner holds the catheter in place, activate the fast-flush release (flushing 1 to 3 seconds) to flush blood from the catheter.
- After each fast flush, observe the drip chamber to verify a correct continuous flush rate.
- Observe the pressure waveform on the monitor for the appropriate waveform (see *Recognizing abnormal waveforms*).
- The practitioner may suture the catheter in place or secure it with hypoallergenic tape.
- Cover the insertion site with a transparent dressing and mark it with the date and time.
- Place an arm board on the wrist for radial artery insertions.

Postprocedure care for catheter insertion

- Immobilize the insertion site according to facility policy.
- Check the transducer's zeroing stopcock level with the phlebostatic axis, then rezero the transducer system to atmospheric pressure.
- Activate monitor alarms as appropriate.
- Compare arterial readings with manual or automated cuff readings.

- Change the pressure tubing every 2 to 3 days according to facility policy.
- Change the catheter site dressing according to facility policy.

MONITORING

- Check the insertion site for bleeding, drainage, or signs of infection.
- Assess the arterial waveform.
- Note and record blood pressure readings as ordered or per facility policy.
- Regularly assess the amount of flush solution in the I.V. bag and maintain 300 mm Hg pressure in the pressure bag.
- Obtain blood samples per facility policy.

PATIENT TEACHING

- Review activity restrictions with the patient.
- Review the blood sampling procedure when appropriate.
- Explain all monitoring and care performed while the arterial catheter is in place.

DOCUMENTATION

- Document patient teaching provided and the patient's understanding of teaching.
- Document the date and time of system setup, tubing or flush changes, dressing changes, and site care.
- Record the systolic, diastolic, and mean blood pressure as ordered or per unit policy.
- Record manual or automated cuff blood pressure measurements every shift and as needed.
- Document the neurovascular status of the extremity distal to the site.
- Describe the appearance of the waveform and obtain a monitor strip every shift.
- Describe the insertion site's appearance every 4 to 12 hours.

Recognizing abnormal waveforms

Abnormal patterns and markings on waveforms may provide important diagnostic clues to the patient's cardiovascular status, or they may simply signal trouble in the monitor. Use this table to help you recognize and resolve waveform abnormalities.

Abnormality	Possible causes	Nursing interventions
Alternating high and low waves in a regular pattern 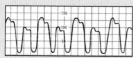	◆ Ventricular bigeminy	◆ Check the patient's electrocardiogram to confirm ventricular bigeminy. The tracing should reflect premature ventricular contractions every second beat.
Flattened waveform 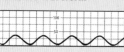	◆ Overdampened waveform or hypotensive patient	◆ Check the patient's blood pressure with a sphygmomanometer. If you obtain a reading, suspect overdampening. Correct the problem by trying to aspirate the arterial line. If you succeed, flush the line. If the reading is very low or absent, suspect hypotension.
Slightly rounded waveform with consistent variations in systolic height 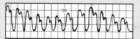	◆ Patient on ventilator with positive end-expiratory pressure	◆ Check the patient's systolic blood pressure regularly. The difference between the highest and lowest systolic pressure reading should be less than 10 mm Hg. If the difference exceeds that amount, suspect pulsus paradoxus, possibly from cardiac tamponade.
Slow upstroke 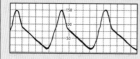	◆ Aortic stenosis	◆ Check the patient's heart sounds for signs of aortic stenosis. Also, notify the practitioner, who will document suspected aortic stenosis in his notes.
Diminished amplitude on inspiration 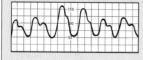	◆ Pulsus paradoxus, possibly from cardiac tamponade, constrictive pericarditis, or lung disease	◆ Note systolic pressure during inspiration and expiration. If inspiration pressure is at least 10 mm Hg less than expiratory pressure, call the practitioner. ◆ If you're also monitoring pulmonary artery pressure, observe for a diastolic plateau. This occurs when the mean central venous pressure (right arterial pressure), mean pulmonary artery pressure, and mean pulmonary artery wedge pressure are within 5 mm Hg of one another.

Preprocedure care for catheter removal

◆ Determine if you're permitted to perform this procedure according to facility policy.
◆ Obtain a manual or automated cuff blood pressure reading to establish a new baseline.
◆ Explain the procedure to the patient.
◆ Place a sheet protector under the site.
◆ Turn off the monitor alarms and the flow clamp to the flush solution.

Procedure for catheter removal

Equipment: gloves ◆ gown ◆ mask ◆ protective eyewear ◆ suture removal kit ◆ 2 to 6 sterile 4″ × 4″ gauze pads ◆ tape ◆ adhesive bandage ◆ sandbag (for femoral catheter removal) ◆ sterile scissors ◆ sterile specimen container ◆ laboratory labels (for culture)

◆ Carefully remove the dressing over the insertion site.
◆ Remove sutures using a suture removal kit.
◆ Withdraw the catheter using a gentle, steady motion, keeping the catheter parallel to the artery during withdrawal.
◆ Immediately apply pressure to the site with a sterile 4″ × 4″ gauze pad for at least 10 minutes (longer if bleeding or oozing persists) until hemostasis is obtained.
◆ If the patient has coagulopathy or is receiving anticoagulants, apply additional pressure to a femoral site.
◆ Cover the site with an appropriate dressing and secure it with tape.
◆ Make a pressure dressing for a femoral site by folding four sterile 4″ × 4″ gauze pads in half. Place the dressing over the femoral site, cover it with a tight adhesive bandage, and cover the bandage with a sandbag.
◆ If infection is suspected, obtain a culture of the catheter by cutting the tip so it falls into a sterile container. Label the specimen and send it to the laboratory.

Postprocedure care for catheter removal

◆ After femoral arterial line removal, have the patient remain on bed rest for 6 hours with the sandbag in place.

MONITORING
◆ Observe the site for bleeding.
◆ Assess the extremity distal to the site by evaluating color, pulses, and sensation every 15 minutes for the first 4 hours, every 30 minutes for the next 2 hours, and hourly for the next 6 hours.

PATIENT TEACHING
◆ Describe signs and symptoms of complications, such as bleeding or pain at the site, and when to notify the nurse.
◆ Review activity restrictions if appropriate.

DOCUMENTATION
◆ Document patient teaching provided and the patient's understanding of teaching.
◆ Record the time of catheter removal and document whether the catheter was intact.
◆ Describe the insertion site upon catheter removal.
◆ Record how long pressure was applied to the insertion site and if a sandbag was applied.
◆ Assess the extremity distal to the site, including color, pulses, and sensation.

Procedures

Autologous blood transfusion, perioperative

Overview

An autologous transfusion is the collection, filtration, and reinfusion of the patient's own blood. Its advantages over banked blood transfusions from other donors include a lack of transfusion reactions; prevention of disease transmission; decreased need for anticoagulants (except in postoperative autotransfusion, when acid citrate dextrose [ACD] or citrate phosphate dextrose [CPD] is added); and the presence of normal levels of 2,3-diphosphoglycerate, which increases tissue oxygenation. Autologous blood transfusions are done by preoperative blood donation or perioperative blood donation. Perioperative blood is collected during surgery or up to 12 hours afterward from chest tubes, mediastinal drains, or wound drains.

CONTRAINDICATIONS

◆ Malignant neoplasms, coagulopathies, excessive hemolysis, and active infections
◆ Antibiotic use
◆ Presence of blood that's contaminated by bowel contents
◆ Cardiovascular disease with compromised hemodynamic reserves

Preprocedure care

◆ Confirm the patient's identity using two patient identifiers according to facility policy.
◆ Explain the procedure to the patient.
◆ Ensure patency of a 20G or 18G I.V. catheter.
◆ Obtain and assemble the autologous transfusion system.
◆ Obtain the patient's vital signs.
◆ Check laboratory values obtained preoperatively for abnormalities.

Procedure

Equipment: autologous transfusion system (such as Davol or Pleur-evac systems) ◆ ACD or CPD collection bags ◆ vacuum source regulator ◆ suction tubing ◆ blood administration set with in-line filter ◆ 500 ml of normal saline solution ◆ optional: Hemovac and another autologous transfusion system

USING A DAVOL SYSTEM

◆ Open the transfusion unit onto the sterile field.
◆ Insert the drain tube from the patient to the connecting tube of the unit.
◆ Inject 25 to 35 ml of ACD or CPD into the injection port on top of the filter and wet the filter with anticoagulant to keep blood from clotting.
◆ Label the collection bag with the patient's name and time the transfusion was started so the reinfusion time is within 4 hours of obtaining the blood.

In the postanesthesia care unit or medical-surgical unit

◆ Note on the bag and on the postoperative sheet the amount of blood in the bag.
◆ Attach the tube from the suction source to the port on the suction control module.
◆ Adjust the suction source to between 80 and 100 mm Hg on the wall regulator.
◆ Start reinfusing the blood when 500 ml has been collected or as ordered.
◆ Discard drainage appropriately if the proportion of anticoagulant (administered in the operating room) to blood is too great to infuse.
◆ Remove the suction tube from the suction control unit.
◆ Clamp the connecting tubing above the filter.
◆ Detach the connecting tubing from the patient's tube and cap the patient's tube.

- Connect a closed-wound suction unit, such as a Hemovac, if you aren't going to collect more blood for reinfusion.
- If more than 500 ml of blood is collected in the first 4 hours, connect a new autologous transfusion unit to the patient.
- Reconnect the unit to suction, then monitor and record the drainage on the intake and output sheet.

To reinfuse blood
- Prime the blood filter with 500 ml of normal saline solution.
- Remove the suction control module.
- Remove the hanger assembly from the collection bag.
- Remove the clear cap from the top of the bag, and discard the cap and filter.
- Insert a spike adapter into the large port on top of the bottle.
- Expose the filtered vent and attach the blood to the Y-connector of the blood filter.
- Invert the bag and hang it.
- Start the infusion, following facility policy.

USING THE PLEUR-EVAC SYSTEM CONNECTED TO A CHEST TUBE
- Connect the patient's chest tube to Pleur-evac unit.
- Make sure all clamps are open and all connections are airtight.
- If prescribed, inject an anticoagulant through the red self-sealing port on the autologous transfusion connector using an 18G (or smaller) needle.
- Start collecting blood; open a replacement bag when the first is nearly full.
- Before removing the first collection bag from the drainage unit, reduce excess negativity with the high-negativity relief valve.
- Close the white clamp on the patient tubing.
- Close the two white clamps on top of the collection bag.
- Disconnect all connectors on the first bag.

- Attach the red (female) and blue (male) connector sections on top of the autologous transfusion bag.
- Using the red connectors, connect the collection tubing to the patient's chest drainage tube.
- Using the blue connectors, remove the protective cap from the replacement bag's suction tube and attach the tube to the Pleur-evac unit.
- Open all clamps and inspect the system for airtight connections.
- Spread the metal support arms and disconnect them.
- Remove the first bag from the drainage unit by disconnecting the foot hook.
- Use the foot hook and support arm to attach the replacement bag.
- Reinfuse blood from the original collection bag within 4 hours of the start of collection.
- Slide the bag off the support frame and invert it so the spike points upward.
- Remove the protective cap from the spike port and insert a filter.
- Close the clamp on the reinfusion line and remove residual air from the bag.
- Infuse the blood according to facility policy.

Postprocedure care

MONITORING
- Check the patient's laboratory data after infusion.
- Monitor the amount of blood drainage.

PATIENT TEACHING
- Explain the transfusion procedure when the patient is fully alert.
- Explain the need for laboratory testing.

DOCUMENTATION
- Record the amount of autologous blood the patient had reinfused.
- Describe how the patient tolerated each procedure, including vital signs.

Automated external defibrillation

Overview

An automated external defibrillator (AED) interprets the patient's cardiac rhythm and gives the operator step-by-step directions for administering an electrical current to the patient's heart if defibrillation is needed. Basic life support (BLS) and advanced cardiac life support (ACLS) training requires instruction on using an AED. However, automated external defibrillation may be performed to provide early cardiac arrest treatment even without a health care professional present.

CONTRAINDICATIONS

◆ Stable patient with a pulse
◆ Patient having a seizure
◆ Patient who has legal documentation requesting that he not be resuscitated
◆ Presence of immediate danger to rescuers because of environment, patient's location, or patient's condition

Preprocedure care

◆ After determining that the patient is unresponsive, has no pulse and is apneic, follow BLS and ACLS protocols for initiating cardiopulmonary resuscitation (CPR).
◆ Have someone bring the AED to the bedside.

Procedure

Equipment: AED ◆ 2 prepackaged electrodes (pads)
◆ After the AED arrives, open the packets containing the two electrode pads.
◆ Attach the white electrode cable connector to one pad and the red electrode cable connector to the other. If the electrodes don't have colored cables, use the illustrations provided on the pads or packaging to assure proper placement.
◆ Expose the patient's chest.
◆ Remove the plastic backing film from the electrode pads and place them on the pa-

tient's chest according to the illustrations provided on the pads.
◆ Firmly press the AED's ON button and wait while the machine performs a brief self-test.
◆ Most AEDs signal readiness by a computerized voice that says, "Push analyze" or by emitting a series of loud beeps.
◆ If the AED is malfunctioning, it will convey the message "Do not use the AED. Remove and continue cardiopulmonary resuscitation." Report AED malfunctions in accordance with facility procedure.
◆ Ask everyone to stand clear of the patient and press the ANALYZE button.

◆ Nursing alert

Don't touch or move the patient while the AED is in analysis mode. If you get the message "Check electrodes," make sure the electrodes are correctly placed and the patient cable is securely attached; then press the analyze button again.

◆ It will take 5 to 30 seconds for the AED to analyze the patient's rhythm.
◆ If a shock isn't needed, the AED will convey the message "No shock indicated" and you should then continue to follow ACLS protocol.
◆ If a shock is needed, the AED charges and will prompt you to press the shock button. (Some fully automatic AED models automatically deliver a shock within 15 seconds after analyzing the patient's rhythm.)
◆ Call out "stand clear" and check that no one is touching the patient or his bed.
◆ Press the shock button on the AED.
◆ After the shock, the AED will automatically reanalyze the patient's rhythm. If no additional shock is needed, check for a pulse. If no pulse is obtained, continue CPR.
◆ If the patient requires another shock, the AED will automatically begin recharging to deliver a second shock.
◆ Repeat the steps performed earlier before delivering a shock to the patient.

◆ According to the AED algorithm, the patient can receive up to three shocks at 360 joules, using a monophasic AED.

◆ The energy level delivered may be different when using a defibrillator that delivers biphasic shocks. Follow facility policy.

◆ Continue ACLS protocol and the algorithm sequence until the code team arrives to assume care of the patient.

Postprocedure care

◆ If the patient survives the event, assist with transport to the intensive care unit.

◆ Provide emotional support to the patient and family members as appropriate.

MONITORING

◆ Monitor the patient's cardiac rhythm, respiratory status, and vital signs.

PATIENT TEACHING

◆ Explain to the family and patient, if appropriate, the events that occurred, the procedure that was performed, and the patient's response.

DOCUMENTATION

◆ Note the time and condition in which the patient was found.

◆ Document when CPR was initiated, when the AED was used, and how many shocks the patient received.

◆ Note when the patient regained a pulse at any point.

◆ If the patient survived the event, note where and when the patient was transported.

◆ If the patient didn't survive the event, document time of death, post-arrest care and family notification.

◆ Document when the attending physician was notified.

◆ Make sure that a formal "code record" containing details about the treatment and the patient's response is placed on the patient's chart.

Bladder irrigation, continuous

Overview

Continuous bladder irrigation uses an irrigating solution to flush out small blood clots that form after prostate or bladder surgery. It helps prevent venous hemorrhage and urinary tract obstructions and may also be used to treat an irritated, inflamed, or infected bladder lining.

Preprocedure care

◆ Confirm the patient's identity using two patient identifiers according to facility policy.
◆ Explain the procedure to the patient and why it's necessary.
◆ Ensure that the patient has a three-way urinary catheter in place. If not, insert one according to facility policy using sterile technique.
◆ Double-check the irrigating solution against the practitioner's order.
◆ If the solution contains an antibiotic, check the patient's chart to make sure he isn't allergic to the drug.
◆ Assemble all equipment at the patient's bedside.

Procedure

Equipment: two 3,000-ml containers of irrigating solution (usually normal saline solution) or prescribed amount of medicated solution ◆ Y-type tubing made specifically for bladder irrigation ◆ alcohol or chlorhexidine pad ◆ large-capacity urinary drainage bag ◆ I.V. pole

◆ Wash your hands and put on gloves.
◆ Hang two containers of irrigating solution on the I.V. pole.
◆ Insert the spikes of the Y-type tubing into each container.
◆ Close the clamp on one container and keep the other clamp open.

◆ Squeeze the drip chamber on the spike of the tubing.
◆ Open the flow clamp and flush the tubing to remove air that could cause bladder distention.
◆ Close the clamp.
◆ Clean the opening to the inflow lumen of the catheter with an alcohol or a chlorhexidine pad.
◆ Insert the distal end of the Y-type tubing securely into the inflow lumen (third port) of the catheter using sterile technique.
◆ Make sure the catheter's outflow lumen is securely attached to the drainage bag tubing.
◆ Open the flow clamp under the container of the irrigating solution and set the drip rate as ordered.
◆ To prevent air from entering the system, don't allow the primary container to empty completely before replacing it.
◆ To prevent reflux of irrigation solution between containers, simultaneously close the flow clamp under the one that's nearly empty and open the flow clamp under the reserve container.
◆ Hang a new reserve container on the I.V. pole and insert the tubing, maintaining sterile technique.
◆ Empty the drainage bag as often as needed.

Postprocedure care

◆ Have the patient remain on bed rest throughout continuous bladder irrigation, unless ordered otherwise.
◆ Irrigate the catheter if clots occlude outflow, per facility policy or practitioner order.
◆ Infuse antibiotic solutions as ordered.
◆ Encourage oral fluid intake of 2 to 3 qt (2 to 3 L)/day unless contraindicated.

Monitoring

◆ Monitor the color of urine and the amount of clots present.
◆ Measure intake and output accurately.
◆ Monitor vital signs at least every 4 hours during irrigation, increasing the frequency if the patient becomes unstable.

Patient teaching

◆ Instruct the patient to notify the nurse if he experiences abdominal discomfort or bladder spasms.
◆ Review activity restrictions.

Documentation

◆ Document patient teaching performed and the patient's understanding of the teaching.
◆ Record the time when the procedure started and the type of solution used.
◆ Record intake and output accurately. Calculate true urine output by subtracting irrigation fluid infused from total output.
◆ Document the characteristics of the drainage.
◆ Record patient complaints.
◆ Record the time and date when irrigation is discontinued.

Procedures

Cardiac monitoring

Overview

A cardiac monitor converts electrical signals from electrodes placed on a patient's chest into tracings of cardiac rhythm on an oscilloscope. The monitor recognizes and counts abnormal heartbeats and changes, producing alarms when rhythms or rates need further attention or immediate treatment. With hardwire monitoring, the patient is connected at the bedside to a monitor that displays his cardiac rhythm. The monitor may also measure blood pressure, pulse oximetry, and other functions. With telemetry monitoring, a small transmitter that's connected to an ambulatory patient sends electrical signals to display heart rate and rhythm on a monitor at another location.

Preprocedure care

◆ Explain the procedure to the patient and why it's necessary.

Procedure

Equipment: cardiac monitor ◆ leadwires ◆ patient cable ◆ disposable pregelled electrodes ◆ alcohol pads ◆ 4″ × 4″ gauze pads ◆ hair clipping supplies and washcloth

Telemetry monitoring requires additional use of: transmitter with leads ◆ transmitter pouch ◆ telemetry battery pack

HARDWIRE MONITORING
◆ Plug the cardiac monitor into the electrical outlet and turn it on.
◆ Insert the cable with leadwires into the appropriate socket in the monitor.
◆ Connect an electrode to each leadwire immediately before applying, carefully checking that each leadwire is in its correct outlet.
◆ Wash your hands.
◆ Determine the electrode positions on the patient's chest based on the system and lead you're using.

◆ Avoid placing electrodes on bony prominences, hairy areas, areas where defibrillator pads will be placed, or areas for chest compression.
◆ If the leadwires and patient cables aren't permanently attached, verify that the electrode placement corresponds to the label on the patient cable.
◆ Clip the patient's hair in an area about 4″ (10 cm) in diameter around each electrode site if necessary.
◆ Clean the area with soap and water and dry the area completely to remove skin secretions that may interfere with electrode function. An alcohol pad may be used if skin is oily.
◆ Gently abrade the dried area by rubbing it briskly with a dry washcloth or gauze until it reddens; doing so promotes better electrical contact.
◆ Apply electrodes to the appropriate sites and press firmly to ensure a tight seal.
◆ Check for a tracing on the cardiac monitor.
◆ Compare the digital heart rate display with your count of the patient's heart rate.
◆ Use the "gain control" to adjust the size of the rhythm tracing.
◆ Set the upper and lower limits of the heart rate alarm based on unit policy, and turn the alarm on.

TELEMETRY MONITORING
◆ Put a new battery in the transmitter.
◆ Test the battery's charge and ensure the unit is operational by pressing the button at its top.
◆ If leadwires aren't permanently affixed to the telemetry unit, attach them securely.
◆ Tie the pouch strings around the patient's neck and waist, making sure the pouch fits snugly without causing discomfort.
◆ If no pouch is available, place the transmitter in the patient's bathrobe pocket.

Postprocedure care

◆ Obtain a rhythm strip by pressing the RECORD key on at the central station.
◆ Label the strip with patient's name, room number, date, and time; measure the intervals, and identify the rhythm.

MONITORING
◆ Monitor the patient's cardiac rhythm and rate and vital signs per facility policy.
◆ Assess skin integrity, and reposition electrodes every 24 hours or as necessary.

PATIENT TEACHING
For telemetry monitoring
◆ If the patient is being monitored by telemetry, show him how the transmitter works.
◆ If applicable, show the patient the button that will produce a recording of his electrocardiogram at the central station.
◆ Tell the patient to push the button whenever he has symptoms, which will cause the central console to print a rhythm strip.
◆ Tell the patient to remove the transmitter when he takes a shower or bath.
◆ Tell the patient to alert the nurse before removing the unit.

For hardwire monitoring
◆ Explain the reason for cardiac monitoring.
◆ Review activity restrictions.

DOCUMENTATION
◆ Document patient teaching performed and the patient's understanding of the teaching.
◆ Record date and time monitoring begins and which monitoring lead is used.
◆ Document a rhythm strip every shift and with changes in the patient's condition or according to facility policy.
◆ Label the rhythm strip with the patient's name, room number, date, and time.

Cardiac output measurement

Overview

Cardiac output measurement helps evaluate cardiac function by measuring the amount of blood ejected with a heartbeat. It can be calculated by multiplying the stroke volume by the heart rate. Methods for measuring cardiac output include bolus thermodilution (most widely used), the Fick method, and the dye dilution test. The bolus thermodilution method discussed here involves injecting a solution colder than the patient's blood into the right atrium via a pulmonary artery (PA) catheter port. The solution mixes with the blood as it travels through the right ventricle into the pulmonary artery, and the temperature change is measured by a thermistor on the catheter. A computer plots the temperature change over time as a curve and calculates flow based on the area under the curve. Normal range for cardiac output is 4 to 8 L/minute.

Preprocedure care

◆ Explain the procedure and why it's necessary.
◆ Tell the patient that he'll need to remain still during the procedure to obtain accurate measurements.
◆ Wash your hands and assemble the equipment at the bedside.

Procedure

Equipment: thermodilution PA catheter in position ◆ output computer and cables (or a module for the bedside cardiac monitor) ◆ closed or open injectant delivery system ◆ 10-ml syringe ◆ 500-ml bag of dextrose 5% in water or normal saline solution
◆ Insert the closed injectant system tubing into a 500-ml bag of I.V. solution.
◆ Connect the 10-ml syringe to the system tubing and prime the tubing with I.V. solution until it's free of air.
◆ Clamp the tubing.

◆ After clamping the tubing, connect the primed system to the stopcock of the proximal injectant lumen of the PA catheter.
◆ Connect the temperature probe from the cardiac output computer to the closed injectant system's flow-through housing device.
◆ Connect the cardiac output computer cable to the thermistor connector on the PA catheter and verify blood temperature reading.
◆ Turn on the cardiac output computer and enter the correct computation constant as provided by the catheter's manufacturer.
◆ Verify the appropriate PA waveform on the cardiac monitor. Obtain PA pressure, central venous pressure, and blood pressure.
◆ Unclamp the I.V. tubing and withdraw exactly 10 ml of solution.
◆ Reclamp the tubing.
◆ Turn the stopcock at the catheter injectant hub to open a fluid path between the injectant lumen of the PA catheter and the syringe.
◆ Press the start button on the cardiac output computer or wait for the "INJECT" message to flash.
◆ Inject the solution smoothly within 4 seconds, making sure it doesn't leak at the connectors.
◆ Analyze the contour of the thermodilution washout curve on a strip chart recorder for a rapid upstroke and a gradual, smooth return to baseline.
◆ Repeat these steps until three values are within 10% to 15% of the median value.
◆ Compute the average of three values and record the patient's cardiac output.
◆ Return the stopcock to the original position and make sure the injectant delivery system tubing is clamped.

Postprocedure care

◆ Verify the PA waveform on the cardiac monitor is normal. If it isn't normal, troubleshoot the catheter.

◆ Calculate the cardiac index (CI), which adjusts cardiac output for body size. To calculate the patient's CI, divide his cardiac output by his body surface area, a function of height and weight. Normal CI ranges from 2.5 to 4.2 L/minute/m² in adults and 3.5 to 6.5 L/minute/m² in pregnant women.

◆ Add the fluid volume injected for cardiac output determinations to the patient's total intake.

MONITORING

◆ Monitor the patient for signs or symptoms of inadequate perfusion, including restlessness, fatigue, changes in level of consciousness, decreased capillary refill time, diminished peripheral pulses, oliguria, and pale, cool skin.

◆ Monitor cardiac output and CI readings for changes after adding or discontinuing treatments and when titrating medications.

DOCUMENTATION

◆ Record the patient's cardiac output, CI, and other hemodynamic values and vital signs at the time of measurement.

◆ Note the patient's position during cardiac output measurement and when unusual occurrences, such as bradycardia or neurologic changes, occur.

Catheter, urinary (indwelling), insertion and removal

Overview

Also known as a *Foley* or *retention catheter*, an indwelling urinary catheter is a drainage tube that's inserted into the bladder and held in place with an inflated balloon at its distal end. It's used to relieve bladder distention caused by urine retention that may result from surgery, trauma, urinary tract obstruction, or neurogenic bladder paralysis. It's also used to monitor urine output, for bladder retraining of patients with neurologic disorders, such as stroke or spinal cord injury, and to determine post-void residual urine volume and the need for intermittent catheterization.

CONTRAINDICATIONS
◆ Urethral injury

Preprocedure care for catheter insertion

◆ Confirm the patient's identity using two patient identifiers according to facility policy.
◆ Explain the procedure and why it's being done to the patient.
◆ Check the practitioner's order on the patient's chart.
◆ Check whether the patient has an allergy to iodine.
◆ Wash your hands, and assemble equipment at the bedside.
◆ Provide privacy.
◆ Percuss and palpate the bladder to establish baseline data.

Procedure for catheter insertion

Equipment: sterile indwelling urinary catheter (latex or silicone #10 to #22 French; average adult sizes are #16 to #18 French) ◆ syringe filled with 5 to 8 ml of sterile water (normal saline solution is sometimes used) ◆ washcloth ◆ towel ◆ soap and water ◆ two linen-saver pads ◆ sterile gloves ◆ sterile drape ◆ sterile fenestrated drape ◆ sterile cotton-tipped applicators (or cotton balls and plastic forceps) ◆ povidone-iodine or other antiseptic cleaning agent ◆ urine receptacle ◆ sterile water-soluble lubricant ◆ sterile drainage collection bag ◆ intake and output sheet ◆ adhesive tape ◆ optional: urine-specimen container and laboratory request form, leg band with Velcro closure, gooseneck lamp or flashlight, pillows or rolled blankets or towels

◆ Put on gloves.
◆ Have a coworker hold a flashlight or place a lamp next to patient's bed.
◆ Place the linen-saver pads on the bed between the patient's legs and under the hips.
◆ Place the female patient in the supine position, with her knees flexed and separated and her feet flat on the bed, about 2′ (61 cm) apart.
◆ Place the male patient in the supine position with his legs extended and flat on the bed.
◆ Clean the patient's genital area and perineum thoroughly with soap and water.
◆ Dry the area with the towel.
◆ Remove your gloves and wash your hands.
◆ Open the prepackaged kit or equipment tray and place it between the female patient's legs or next to the male patient's hip.

- Put on sterile gloves (from tray).
- Place the sterile drape under the patient's hips.
- Drape the patient's lower abdomen with the sterile fenestrated drape so only the genital area remains exposed.
- Open the packet of povidone-iodine or other antiseptic cleaning agent and saturate sterile cotton balls or applicators.
- Open the packet of water-soluble lubricant and apply it to the catheter tip.
- Attach the drainage bag to the open end of the catheter if it isn't already attached.
- Inflate the catheter balloon with sterile water or normal saline solution and inspect for leaks.
- Deflate the balloon.
- Inspect the catheter for resiliency.

For the female patient
- Separate the labia with the thumb, middle, and index fingers of your nondominant hand. (This hand is now contaminated.)
- Identify the urinary meatus.
- Wipe one side of the urinary meatus with a sterile, cotton-tipped applicator with a single downward motion. Alternatively, use a sterile cotton ball held with the plastic forceps. Repeat this step on the other side with another sterile applicator or cotton ball.
- Wipe directly over the meatus with a third sterile applicator or cotton ball.
- Insert the lubricated catheter into the urinary meatus. Advance the catheter 2″ to 3″ (5 to 7.5 cm) until urine begins to flow.
- Attach the prefilled syringe to the luerlock and inflate the balloon.
- If the catheter is inadvertently inserted into the vagina, leave it there as a landmark, and then begin the procedure over again using new supplies.

For the male patient
- Hold the penis with your nondominant hand. (This hand is now contaminated.)
- If the patient is uncircumcised, retract the foreskin.
- Lift and stretch the penis to a 60- to 90-degree angle.
- Use your dominant hand to clean the glans with a sterile cotton-tipped applicator or a sterile cotton ball held in plastic forceps.
- Clean in a circular motion, starting at the urinary meatus and working outward.
- Repeat the procedure using another sterile applicator or cotton ball.
- Insert the lubricated catheter into the urinary meatus.
- To facilitate insertion by relaxing the sphincter, ask the patient to cough as you insert the catheter. Tell him to breathe deeply and slowly to further relax the sphincter.
- Hold the catheter close to its tip to ease insertion and control direction.
- Advance the catheter to the bifurcation 5″ to 7½″ (12.5 to 19 cm) and check for urine flow.
- Attach the prefilled syringe to the luerlock and inflate the balloon.
- Replace the retracted foreskin if appropriate.

Postprocedure care for catheter insertion

- Hang the collection bag below bladder level.
- Tape the catheter or attach a leg band to the patient's thigh.
- Dispose of all used supplies properly.
- If the practitioner orders a urine specimen, obtain it from the urine receptacle with a specimen collection container at the time of catheterization, and send it to the

laboratory with the appropriate laboratory request form.

◆ Provide catheter care per facility policy.
◆ Change catheter as ordered or per facility policy.

MONITORING

◆ Monitor the amount and characteristics of urine per unit protocol.
◆ Observe for signs and symptoms of infection.
◆ If necessary, provide the patient with detailed instructions for performing clean intermittent self-catheterization.

PATIENT TEACHING

◆ Review activity precautions to prevent dislodgment.
◆ If the patient will be discharged with long-term indwelling catheter, teach him and his family the aspects of daily catheter maintenance, including skin and urinary meatus care, signs and symptoms of urinary tract infection or obstruction, how to irrigate the catheter, if appropriate, importance of adequate fluid intake to maintain patency, and need for a home care nurse to visit every 4 to 6 weeks, or as needed, to change the catheter.

DOCUMENTATION

◆ Document patient teaching provided and the patient's understanding of the teaching.
◆ Record the date and time the catheter was inserted and the size and type of indwelling catheter used.
◆ Describe the amount, color, and other characteristics of urine emptied from the bladder.
◆ Describe the patient's tolerance of procedure.
◆ Record whether a urine specimen was sent for laboratory analysis.
◆ Document catheter care performed.

Preprocedure care for catheter removal

◆ Perform bladder retraining as ordered.
◆ Explain the procedure and why it's being done to the patient.
◆ Provide privacy.
◆ Wash your hands and bring equipment to the bedside.
◆ Place a linen-saver pad under the patient's buttocks.

Procedure for catheter removal

Equipment: gloves ◆ alcohol pad ◆ 10-ml syringe with a luer-lock ◆ bedpan ◆ linen-saver pad ◆ optional: clamp for bladder retraining

◆ Put on gloves.
◆ Place the linen-saver pad under the patient's buttocks.
◆ Attach the syringe to the luer-lock mechanism on the catheter.
◆ Pull back on the plunger of the syringe and aspirate the injected fluid to deflate the balloon.
◆ Grasp the catheter and pinch it firmly with your thumb and index finger to prevent urine from flowing back into the urethra.
◆ Gently pull the catheter from the urethra. Discard the catheter appropriately.
◆ If there's resistance, don't apply force; notify the practitioner.
◆ Measure and record the amount of urine in the collection bag before discarding.
◆ Remove and discard your gloves and the linen-saver pad, and wash your hands.

Procedures

Postprocedure care for catheter removal

◆ Provide perineal care.
◆ Report incidents of incontinence, urgency, dysuria, bladder spasm, or bladder distention to the practitioner.

MONITORING
◆ For the first 24 hours after catheter removal, note the time and amount of each voiding.

PATIENT TEACHING
◆ Review signs and symptoms of urinary tract infection and when to notify the practitioner.

DOCUMENTATION
◆ Document patient teaching provided and the patient's understanding of the teaching.
◆ Record the date and time of catheter removal and the patient's tolerance of the procedure.
◆ Report when and how much the patient voided after catheter removal and associated problems.

Central venous pressure monitoring

Overview

Central venous pressure (CVP) is an index of right ventricular function. Monitoring CVP helps assess cardiac function and evaluate venous return to the heart and indirectly gauges how well the heart is pumping. CVP is measured by a manometer or a monitor cable connected to a catheter that's inserted through a vein and advanced until its tip is in or near the right atrium. Because no major valves are at the vena cava and right atrium junction, pressure at end diastole reflects back to the catheter. Normal CVP ranges from 2 to 6 mm Hg. Higher values indicate increased circulating volume; lower values indicate decreased circulating volume.

The central venous line used in CVP monitoring also provides access to a large vessel for rapid, high-volume fluid or medication administration and allows easy blood withdrawal for laboratory samples.

CONTRAINDICATIONS
◆ Inability to insert catheter

Preprocedure care

◆ Explain the procedure and why it's necessary to the patient.
◆ Assist the practitioner with central venous catheter insertion.
◆ Assemble equipment and bring it to the bedside.

Procedure

INTERMITTENT CVP MONITORING WITH A WATER MANOMETER
Equipment: disposable CVP manometer set ◆ leveling device such as a rod from a reusable CVP pole holder or a carpenter's level or rule ◆ additional stopcock to attach the CVP manometer to the catheter ◆ extension tubing if needed ◆ I.V. pole ◆ I.V. solution ◆ I.V. drip chamber and tubing

◆ Position the patient flat or use semi-Fowler's position, per patient tolerance. Use the same degree of elevation for all subsequent measurements.
◆ Locate the right atrium level by identifying the phlebostatic axis with a leveling device.
◆ Align the right atrium (the zero reference point) with the zero mark on the manometer.
◆ Attach the manometer to an I.V. pole or place it next to the patient's chest. Make sure the zero reference point remains level with the right atrium.
◆ Verify that the manometer is connected to the I.V. tubing.
◆ Turn off the stopcock to the patient and slowly fill the manometer with I.V. solution until the fluid level is 10 to 20 cm H_2O higher than the patient's expected CVP value.
◆ Turn off the stopcock to the I.V. solution and open it to the patient. The fluid level in the manometer will drop.
◆ After the fluid level comes to rest, it will fluctuate slightly with respirations.
◆ Expect the fluid level to drop during inspiration and rise during expiration.
◆ Record CVP at the end of expiration, when intrathoracic pressure has a negligible effect.
◆ Depending on the type of manometer used, note the value either at the bottom of the meniscus or at the midline of the small floating ball.

CONTINUOUS CVP MONITORING WITH A PRESSURE MONITORING SYSTEM
Equipment: pressure monitoring kit with disposable pressure transducer ◆ leveling device ◆ bedside pressure module ◆ continuous I.V. flush solution ◆ pressure bag ◆ water manometer

◆ Make sure the central venous line or the proximal lumen of a pulmonary artery catheter is attached to the system.

◆ If the patient has a central venous line with multiple lumens, the distal lumen should be dedicated to continuous CVP monitoring and the others used for fluid administration.

◆ Set up a pressure transducer system.

◆ Connect the pressure tubing from the CVP catheter hub to the transducer.

◆ Connect the flush solution container to a flush device.

◆ Position the patient flat or use semi-Fowler's position, per patient tolerance. Use the same degree of elevation for all subsequent measurements.

◆ Locate the level of the right atrium by identifying the phlebostatic axis.

◆ Zero the transducer, leveling the transducer air-fluid interface stopcock with the right atrium.

◆ Read the CVP value from the digital display on the monitor and record the waveform.

Postprocedure care

◆ After obtaining the CVP value, turn the stopcock to resume the I.V. infusion, if necessary.

◆ Adjust the I.V. drip rate as required.

◆ Place the patient in a comfortable position.

◆ Arrange for daily chest X-rays to check catheter placement as ordered.

◆ Care for the insertion site according to facility policy.

MONITORING

◆ Observe for signs of infection, such as redness or drainage at the insertion site, and note patient complaints of tenderness.

◆ Obtain readings at 15-, 30-, and 60-minute intervals to establish a baseline. Then monitor readings according to facility policy or as ordered.

PATIENT TEACHING

◆ Review activity precautions to prevent line dislodgment.

DOCUMENTATION

◆ Record the time and date of central venous catheter insertion and verification of placement.

◆ Describe the patient's tolerance of the procedure.

◆ Record CVP readings every 4 hours or as ordered. Place a rhythm strip of the CVP waveform in the patient's chart.

Cerebral blood flow monitoring

Overview

Cerebral blood flow monitoring continuously evaluates cerebral blood flow in the capillary bed. A sensor placed on the cerebral cortex calculates the blood flow by thermal diffusion. Thermistors in the sensor detect the temperature differential between a heated and a neutral metallic plate, and the differential relates inversely to cerebral blood flow. As the differential decreases, cerebral blood flow increases; as the differential increases, cerebral blood flow decreases. Monitoring is indicated when cerebral blood flow alterations are anticipated, such as with subarachnoid hemorrhage or head trauma. It also provides information about the effects of interventions on cerebral blood flow and gives continuous, real-time values for cerebral blood flow that are essential in conditions in which compromised results may increase ischemia and infarction risks.

Preprocedure care

◆ Explain the procedure and why it's necessary to the patient and his family.
◆ Tell him that a sensor will be in place for about 3 days.
◆ Confirm informed consent has been obtained.
◆ Assemble at the bedside a monitor and a sensor cable with an attached sensor.
◆ Attach the distal end of the sensor cable from the patient's head to the sensor connect port on the monitor.
◆ When the sensor cable is securely in place, press the ON key to activate the monitor.
◆ Calibrate the system by pressing the CAL key. You should see the red light appear on the CAL key.
◆ Begin by calibrating the sensor to 00.0 by pressing the directional arrows.
◆ Sensor readouts of plus or minus 0.1 are acceptable.

Procedure

Equipment: special sensor that attaches to a computer data system
◆ The neurosurgeon places the sensor on the cerebral cortex in the operating room during or after a craniotomy or through a burr hole.
◆ The sensor is implanted far from major blood vessels, and the neurosurgeon verifies that the metallic plates have good contact with the brain surface (see *Inserting a cerebral blood flow sensor*).
◆ Press the RUN key to display the cerebral blood flow reading.
◆ Observe the monitor's digital display, and document the baseline value (see *Cerebral blood flow values*).

Inserting a cerebral blood flow sensor

Typically, the surgeon inserts a cerebral blood flow sensor during a craniotomy. He tunnels the sensor toward the craniotomy site and then carefully inserts the metallic plates of the thermistor to make sure that they continuously contact the surface of the cerebral cortex. After closing the dura and replacing the bone flap, he closes the scalp.

INSERTION SITE

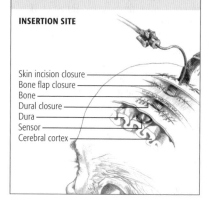

Skin incision closure
Bone flap closure
Bone
Dural closure
Dura
Sensor
Cerebral cortex

Procedures

Postprocedure care

◆ Give prophylactic antibiotics as ordered, and maintain a sterile dressing around the sensor insertion site.
◆ Perform insertion site care per facility policy.

MONITORING
◆ Record the cerebral blood flow hourly.
◆ Watch for trends and correlate sensor values with the patient's clinical status.
◆ Observe the insertion site for cerebrospinal fluid leakage.
◆ Observe for infections.

PATIENT TEACHING
◆ Review activity precautions to prevent sensor displacement.
◆ Review removal procedure when appropriate.

DOCUMENTATION
◆ Document the sensor readings every hour.
◆ Document insertion site care performed and the site's appearance.
◆ After sensor removal, report leakage from the site.

Cerebral blood flow values

Cerebral blood flow fluctuates with the brain's metabolic demands. It ranges from 60 to 90 ml/100 g/minute. The patient's neurologic condition dictates the acceptable range. For example, a patient in a coma may have a cerebral blood flow value of half the normal value. A patient in a barbiturate-induced coma may have a cerebral blood flow as low as 10 ml/100 g/minute.

Values less than 40 ml/100 g/minute may indicate vasospasm secondary to subarachnoid hemorrhage. Values greater than 90 ml/100 g/minute in a patient who is awake may indicate hyperemia.

Chest tube insertion and removal

Overview

Chest tube insertion allows drainage of air (pneumothorax) and fluid (hemothorax or pleural effusion) from the pleural space, which may help relieve intrapleural pressure and prevent partial or complete lung collapse. Insertion sites vary depending on the patient's condition and the practitioner's judgment. For hemothorax or pleural effusion, the fourth to sixth intercostal spaces are common sites because fluid settles to the lower levels of the intrapleural space. For pneumothorax, the second to third intercostal space is the usual site because air rises to the top of the intrapleural space. For removal of air and fluid, chest tubes are inserted into high and low sites. After insertion, chest tubes are usually connected to a thoracic drainage system that removes air, fluid, or both from the pleural space, promoting lung reexpansion.

Preprocedure care

♦ Confirm the patient's identity using two patient identifiers according to facility policy.
♦ Explain the procedure and why it's necessary to the patient.
♦ In a nonemergency situation, make sure the patient has signed an informed consent form.
♦ Assemble the equipment in the patient's room and set up the thoracic drainage system per manufacturer's recommendations.
♦ Record baseline vital signs and respiratory assessment.
♦ Position the patient.

Procedure

Equipment: two pairs of sterile gloves ♦ sterile drape ♦ povidone-iodine solution ♦ vial of 1% lidocaine ♦ 10-ml syringe ♦ alcohol pad ♦ 22G 1″ needle ♦ 25G ³/₈″ needle ♦ sterile scalpel (usually with #11 blade) ♦ sterile forceps ♦ two rubber-tipped clamps ♦ sterile 4″ × 4″ gauze pads ♦ two sterile 4″ × 4″ drain dressings ♦ 3″ or 4″ sturdy, elastic tape ♦ 1″ adhesive tape for connections ♦ chest tube of appropriate size (#16 to #20 French catheter for air or serous fluid; #28 to #40 French catheter for blood, pus, or thick fluid), with or without a trocar ♦ sterile Kelly clamp ♦ suture material (usually 2-0 silk with cutting needle) ♦ thoracic drainage system ♦ sterile Y-connector (for two chest tubes on the same side) ♦ petroleum gauze

♦ For pneumothorax, place the patient in high Fowler's, semi-Fowler's, or supine position for chest tube placement. (The chest tube will be inserted in the anterior chest at the midclavicular line in the second to third intercostal space.)
♦ For hemothorax, direct the patient to lean over the overbed table or straddle a chair with his arms dangling over the back for chest tube placement. (The chest tube will be placed in the fourth to sixth intercostal space at the midaxillary line.)
♦ The practitioner will prepare the insertion site by cleaning the area with povidone-iodine solution.
♦ Wipe the rubber stopper of the lidocaine vial with an alcohol pad.
♦ Invert the bottle and hold it for the practitioner to withdraw the anesthetic.
♦ After anesthetizing the site, the practitioner will make a small incision, insert the chest tube, and connect it to the thoracic drainage system.
♦ Immediately after the drainage system is connected, tell the patient to take a deep breath, hold it momentarily, and slowly exhale to assist drainage of the pleural space and lung reexpansion.
♦ Adjust the suction to obtain a steady bubbling in the suction chamber.
♦ The practitioner may secure the tube to the skin with a suture.
♦ Open the packages containing the petroleum gauze, 4″ × 4″ drain dressings, and gauze pads, and put on sterile gloves.

Procedures

- Place the petroleum gauze and two 4″ × 4″ drain dressings around the insertion site, one from the top and one from the bottom.
- Place several 4″ × 4″ gauze pads on top of the drain dressings.
- Tape the dressings, covering them completely.
- Securely tape the chest tube to the patient's chest distal to the insertion site to prevent accidental dislodgment.
- Securely tape the junction of the chest tube and the drainage tube to prevent separation.

Postprocedure care

- Make sure the tubing remains level with the patient and there are no dependent loops.
- Obtain a portable chest X-ray to check tube position and lung condition.
- During patient transport, keep the thoracic drainage system below chest level.
- Place the rubber-tipped clamps at bedside.
- If the chest tube comes out, cover the site immediately with 4″ × 4″ gauze pads and tape in place. Notify the practitioner and gather equipment needed to reinsert the tube, if appropriate.

MONITORING

- Check the patient's vital signs every 15 minutes for 1 hour, then as indicated.
- Monitor suction and check for air leaks every 4 hours.
- Monitor and record the drainage in the drainage collection chamber.
- Auscultate his lungs at least every 4 hours.
- Look for signs and symptoms of respiratory distress, an indication that air or fluid remains trapped in the pleural space.
- Chest tubes are usually removed within 7 days to prevent infection (see *Removing a chest tube*).

PATIENT TEACHING

- Review activity precautions to prevent tube dislodgment.

DOCUMENTATION

- Document the date and time of chest tube insertion.
- Document insertion site care provided and the condition of the insertion site.
- Indicate the drainage system used, amount of suction used, and if air leaks are present.
- Describe the amount and appearance of drainage.
- Record auscultation findings.

Removing a chest tube

After the patient's lung has reexpanded, you may assist the practitioner in removing a chest tube. First, check vital signs and perform a respiratory assessment. After explaining the procedure, give an analgesic, as ordered, 30 minutes before tube removal. Then follow these steps:
- Place the patient in semi-Fowler's position or on the unaffected side.
- Place a linen-saver pad under the affected side.
- Put on clean gloves, remove chest tube dressings—being careful not to dislodge the chest tube—and discard soiled dressings.
- The practitioner holds the chest tube in place with sterile forceps and cuts the suture anchoring the tube.
- Make sure the chest tube is securely clamped, then instruct the patient to perform Valsalva's maneuver by exhaling fully and bearing down. Valsalva's maneuver effectively increases intrathoracic pressure.
- The practitioner holds an airtight dressing, usually petroleum gauze, so he can cover the insertion site immediately after removing the tube.
- After the tube is removed and the site is covered, secure the dressing with tape. Cover the dressing completely to make it as airtight as possible.
- Dispose of the chest tube, soiled gloves, and equipment according to facility policy.
- Check vital signs as ordered, and assess depth and quality of respirations.
- Assess for signs and symptoms of pneumothorax, subcutaneous emphysema, or infection.

Closed-wound drain management

Overview

A closed-wound drain promotes healing and prevents swelling by suctioning serosanguineous fluid that accumulates at a wound site. Typically inserted during surgery in anticipation of substantial postoperative drainage, the perforated tubing's distal end lies inside the wound and usually exits from a site other than the primary suture line to preserve integrity of the surgical wound. A portable vacuum unit provides suction. The drainage must be emptied and measured frequently to maintain maximum suction and prevent strain on the suture line. Hemovac and Jackson-Pratt closed drainage systems are most commonly used.

Preprocedure care

◆ Explain to the patient how the closed-wound drain works and why it was placed.
◆ Explain activity precautions to prevent dislodgment.
◆ Wash your hands and assemble equipment at the bedside.

Procedure

Equipment: graduated biohazard cylinder ◆ sterile laboratory container if needed ◆ alcohol pads ◆ gloves ◆ gown ◆ face shield ◆ trash bag ◆ sterile gauze pads ◆ antiseptic cleaning agent ◆ prepackaged povidone-iodine swabs ◆ optional: label
◆ Put on personal protective equipment.
◆ Unclip the vacuum unit from the patient's bed or gown.
◆ Using sterile technique, release the vacuum by removing the spout plug on the collection chamber.
◆ The container expands completely as it draws in air.

◆ Empty the unit's contents into a graduated biohazard cylinder, and note the amount and appearance of drainage.
◆ If diagnostic tests will be performed on the specimen, pour the drainage directly into a sterile laboratory container, document the amount and its appearance, label the specimen pad, and send it to the laboratory.
◆ Clean the unit's spout and plug with an alcohol pad using sterile technique.
◆ To reestablish the vacuum that creates the drain's suction power, fully compress the vacuum unit.
◆ Compress the unit with one hand to maintain the vacuum and replace the spout plug (see *Using a closed-wound drainage system*).
◆ Ensure that the vacuum unit remains compressed when you release the manual pressure.
◆ Check the patency of equipment.

Postprocedure care

◆ Make sure the tubing is free of twists, kinks, and leaks.
◆ Fasten the vacuum unit to the patient's gown below wound level to promote drainage.
◆ Remove and discard personal protective equipment and wash your hands.
◆ Properly dispose of drainage, solutions, and the trash bag, and clean or dispose of soiled equipment and supplies according to facility policy.
◆ Perform wound care as ordered.

MONITORING

◆ Monitor the amount and characteristics of drainage.
◆ Observe for signs and symptoms of infection.

Procedures

PATIENT TEACHING

◆ Review activity precautions to prevent dislodgment.

DOCUMENTATION

◆ Record drainage color, consistency, type, and amount. If there's more than one closed-wound drain, number the drains and record the information for each drainage site.

◆ Describe the appearance of the drain site.

◆ Document equipment malfunctions that occur and subsequent nursing actions performed.

◆ Describe the patient's tolerance of the treatment.

◆ Record the time and date when the drain is discontinued.

Using a closed-wound drainage system

This system draws drainage from a wound site, such as the chest wall postmastectomy shown at left, by means of a Y-tube. To empty the drainage, remove the plug and empty the unit's contents into a graduated cylinder. To reestablish suction, compress the drainage unit against a firm surface to expel air and, while holding it down, replace the plug, as shown. The same principle is used for the Jackson-Pratt bulb drain, shown here (far right).

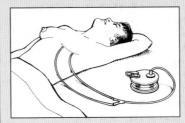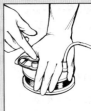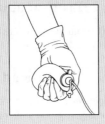

Procedures

Colostomy irrigation

Overview

Irrigation allows the patient with a descending or sigmoid colostomy to regulate bowel function and cleans the large bowel before and after tests, surgery, or other procedures. Irrigation may begin 7 to 10 days after surgery. A predictable elimination pattern is established after 4 to 6 weeks.

CONTRAINDICATIONS

◆ Bleeding from colostomy
◆ Prolapsed ostomy or peristomal hernia
◆ Chemotherapy
◆ Pelvic or abdominal radiation therapy
◆ Diarrhea

Preprocedure care

◆ Explain the procedure to the patient and why it's being done.

Procedure

Equipment: colostomy irrigation set containing irrigation drain or sleeve, ostomy belt to secure drain or sleeve if needed, water-soluble lubricant, drainage pouch clamp, irrigation bag with clamp, tubing, and cone tip ◆ 1,000 ml of tap water irrigant warmed to about 100° F (37.8° C) ◆ normal saline solution for cleansing enemas ◆ I.V. pole or wall hook ◆ washcloth and towel ◆ water ◆ ostomy pouching system ◆ linen-saver pad ◆ gloves ◆ optional: bedpan or chair, mild nonmoisturizing soap, rubber band or clip, small dressing or bandage, and stoma cap
◆ If irrigation is done with the patient in bed, place a bedpan beside the bed and elevate the head of the bed past 45 degrees.
◆ If irrigation is done in the bathroom, have the patient sit on the toilet or on a chair facing the toilet, whichever is more comfortable.
◆ Provide privacy and wash your hands.
◆ If the patient is in bed, place a linen-saver pad under him to protect the sheets.

◆ Set up the irrigation bag with tubing and cone tip.
◆ Fill the irrigation bag with warm tap water or normal saline solution, if the irrigation is for bowel cleaning.
◆ Hang the bag on the I.V. pole or wall hook.
◆ The bottom of the bag should be at the patient's shoulder level to prevent fluid from entering the bowel too quickly.
◆ Most irrigation sets also have a clamp that regulates flow rate.
◆ Prime the tubing with irrigant to prevent air from entering the colon and possibly causing cramps and gas pains.
◆ Put on gloves.
◆ Remove the ostomy pouch if the patient uses one.
◆ Place the irrigation sleeve over the stoma.
◆ If the sleeve doesn't have an adhesive backing, secure the sleeve with an ostomy belt.
◆ If the patient has a two-piece pouching system with flanges, snap off the pouch and save it.
◆ Snap on the irrigation sleeve.
◆ Place the open-ended bottom of the irrigation sleeve in the bedpan or toilet to promote drainage by gravity.
◆ If necessary, cut the sleeve so it meets the water level inside the bedpan or toilet.
◆ Lubricate your gloved little finger with water-soluble lubricant and insert it into the stoma. If you're teaching the patient, have him do this step to determine the bowel angle at which to insert the cone safely.
◆ Expect the stoma to tighten when the finger enters the bowel; it relaxes after a few seconds.
◆ Lubricate the cone with water-soluble lubricant to prevent it from irritating the mucosa.
◆ Gently insert the cone into the top opening of the irrigation sleeve, then into the stoma. Never force it in place.
◆ Angle the cone to match the bowel angle.

◆ Unclamp the irrigation tubing and allow the water to flow slowly.

◆ If you don't have a clamp to control the irrigant's flow rate, pinch the tubing to control the flow. The water should enter the colon over 10 to 15 minutes.

◆ Have the patient remain still for 15 to 20 minutes so the initial effluent can drain.

◆ If the patient is ambulatory, he can stay in the bathroom until all of the effluent empties, or he can clamp the bottom of the drainage sleeve with a rubber band or clip and return to bed.

◆ Suggest that the nonambulatory patient lean forward or massage his abdomen to stimulate elimination.

◆ Wait about 45 minutes for the bowel to finish eliminating the irrigant and effluent, and remove the irrigation sleeve.

◆ If the irrigation was intended to clean the bowel, repeat the procedure with warmed normal saline solution until the return solution appears clear, or per facility policy.

◆ Gently clean the area around the stoma using a washcloth, mild soap, and water.

◆ Rinse and dry the area thoroughly with a clean towel.

◆ Inspect the appearance of the skin and stoma.

◆ Apply a clean pouch or a small dressing, bandage, or commercial stoma cap (with regular elimination).

Postprocedure care

◆ Rinse a reusable irrigation sleeve and hang it to dry with the irrigation bag, tubing, and cone. Discard a disposable sleeve.

◆ If diarrhea develops, discontinue irrigations until stools form again.

MONITORING
◆ Observe the amount and characteristics of stool.

◆ Monitor the stoma for changes in appearance.

PATIENT TEACHING
◆ Explain the procedure to the patient and promote self-care.

◆ Review possible complications and when to notify the practioner.

◆ Review dietary and fluid recommendations.

DOCUMENTATION
◆ Record the date and time of irrigation and type and amount of irrigant used.

◆ Note the stoma's color and the character of drainage, including color, consistency, and amount.

◆ Document patient teaching provided and the patient's response to self-care instruction.

Endotracheal intubation, insertion

Overview

Endotracheal (ET) intubation establishes and maintains a patent airway, protects against aspiration by sealing the trachea off from the digestive tract, permits removal of tracheobronchial secretions in patients who can't cough effectively, and provides a route for mechanical ventilation for respiratory support in illness and during surgery. The procedure involves oral or nasal insertion of a flexible tube through the larynx into the trachea.

CONTRAINDICATIONS
Oral intubation
◆ Acute cervical spinal injury
◆ Degenerative spinal disorders

Nasal intubation
◆ Bleeding disorders
◆ Chronic sinusitis
◆ Nasal obstructions

Preprocedure care

◆ Explain the procedure and why it is necessary to the patient and his family (if able).
◆ Obtain baseline vital signs and pulse oximetry.
◆ Gather supplies or use a prepackaged intubation tray.
◆ Select an appropriately sized ET tube:
  ● Children age 8 and younger: 2.5 to 5.5 mm, uncuffed
  ● Adolescents ages 9 to 17: 7 to 8 mm
  ● Adults: 6 to 10 mm, cuffed (typically 7.5 mm for women or 9 mm for men)
  ● Nasal intubation: a slightly smaller tube
◆ Check the light in the laryngoscope for proper function.

Procedure

Equipment: gloves ◆ goggles ◆ handheld resuscitation bag ◆ oxygen source ◆ two ET tubes (one spare) ◆ stylet ◆ 10-ml syringe ◆ laryngoscope with a handle and various sized, curved and straight blades ◆ sedative ◆ local anesthetic spray ◆ mucosal vasoconstricting agent (for nasal intubation) ◆ water-soluble lubricant ◆ stethoscope ◆ carbon dioxide detector ◆ adhesive tape or Velcro tube holder ◆ suction equipment ◆ Magill forceps ◆ sterile saline solution ◆ sterile basin ◆ optional: prepackaged intubation tray, oral airway or bite block

◆ Attach the syringe to the port on the tube's exterior pilot cuff.
◆ Slowly inflate the cuff; watch for uniform inflation.
◆ A stylet may be used on oral intubations to stiffen the tube. Lubricate the stylet with normal saline solution and insert it into the tube until its distal tip is about $\frac{1}{2}''$ (1.3 cm) from the distal end of the tube.
◆ Attach the handheld resuscitation bag to the oxygen source and check that suction equipment is nearby and functioning.
◆ Wash your hands and put on gloves and goggles.
◆ Administer a sedative as ordered.
◆ Remove the patient's dentures or bridgework.
◆ Hyperventilate the patient using a handheld resuscitation bag until the tube is inserted.
◆ Place the patient supine in the sniffing position so his mouth, pharynx, and trachea are extended.
◆ Spray a local anesthetic into the throat or nasal passage.
◆ If necessary, suction the patient's pharynx before tube insertion.
◆ With your right hand, hold the patient's mouth open by crossing your index finger over your thumb and putting your thumb on his upper teeth and index finger on his lower teeth.
◆ Slide the blade of the laryngoscope into the right side of his mouth.
◆ Center the blade and push his tongue to the left.
◆ Advance the blade to expose the epiglottis. With a straight blade, insert the tip un-

Procedures

der the epiglottis; with a curved blade, insert the tip between the base of the tongue and the epiglottis.

◆ Lift the laryngoscope handle upward and away from your body to reveal the vocal cords. Avoid hitting the patient's teeth.

◆ Have an assistant apply pressure to the cricoid ring.

◆ For oral intubation, insert the ET tube into the right side of his mouth. When performing nasotracheal intubation, insert the tube through the nostril and into the pharynx; if necessary, use Magill forceps to guide the tube through the vocal cords.

◆ Guide the tube into the vertical openings of the larynx between the vocal cords; don't mistake the horizontal opening of the esophagus for the larynx.

◆ Advance the tube until the cuff disappears beyond the vocal cords.

◆ Remove the laryngoscope.

◆ Holding the ET tube in place, remove the stylet, if present.

◆ Inflate the tube's cuff with 5 to 10 cc of air until you feel resistance.

◆ Attach the carbon dioxide detector and observe for color change, indicating the presence of carbon dioxide.

◆ Watch for equal chest expansion and auscultate for bilateral breath sounds while providing breaths with a handheld resuscitation bag. Observe for condensation inside the tube.

◆ If you don't hear breath sounds, auscultate over the stomach while ventilating. (Stomach distention, belching, or gurgling indicates esophageal intubation.) Immediately deflate the cuff and remove the tube. After reoxygenating, repeat insertion using a sterile tube.

◆ If you don't hear breath sounds on both sides of the chest, deflate the cuff, withdraw the tube 1 to 2 mm, auscultate for bilateral breath sounds, and reinflate the cuff.

◆ Start mechanical ventilation; suction if indicated.

◆ Secure the tube with adhesive tape or a Velcro tube holder.

Postprocedure care

◆ Note the centimeter mark on the tube where it exits the patient's mouth or nose.

◆ Obtain a chest X-ray to verify the tube's position.

◆ Suction secretions through the ET tube as indicated to prevent mucus plugs.

◆ Adjust ventilator settings as ordered.

◆ Provide oral care per facility policy.

◆ Provide sedation or restraints as ordered and per facility policy.

MONITORING

◆ Monitor the patient's vital signs and pulse oximetry and arterial blood gas (ABG) values.

◆ Measure inflated cuff pressure at least every 8 hours.

PATIENT TEACHING

◆ Reassure the patient and provide a message board so he can communicate.

◆ Tell the patient that suctioning is needed before performing procedure.

◆ Review the weaning procedure when appropriate.

◆ Review activity restrictions to prevent dislodgment of ET tube.

DOCUMENTATION

◆ Note the date and time of procedure.

◆ Record the patient's vital signs and pulse oximetry and ABG values.

◆ Document the tube type and size and the centimeter mark at the lips or nostril.

◆ Document medication administration.

◆ Record ventilator settings and changes.

◆ Record the results of chest auscultation and chest X-rays.

◆ Note any complications and interventions performed.

Procedures

Feeding tube insertion and removal

Overview

A nasal or oral feeding tube in the stomach or duodenum allows the patient who can't or won't eat to receive nourishment, and it can provide supplemental feedings to a patient with high nutritional requirements. The nasal route is preferred, but the oral route may be used for the patient with a deviated septum or nose injury. Some tubes include tungsten weights to facilitate passage. Other tubes include a guide wire to prevent curling in the back of the throat. Radiopaque markings on the tube help estimate placement, and a water-activated coating provides a lubricated surface to ease insertion.

CONTRAINDICATIONS
◆ Absence of bowel sounds
◆ Suspected or confirmed intestinal obstruction
◆ Persistent vomiting

Preprocedure care for tube insertion

◆ Confirm the patient's identity using two patient identifiers according to facility policy.
◆ Explain the procedure and why it's necessary to the patient and his family.
◆ Assemble the equipment and bring it to the bedside.
◆ Provide privacy.
◆ Wash your hands and put on gloves.

Procedure for tube insertion

Equipment: feeding tube (#6 to #18 French, with or without guide) ◆ linen-saver pad ◆ gloves ◆ hypoallergenic tape ◆ water-soluble lubricant ◆ cotton-tipped applicators ◆ skin preparation ◆ facial tissues ◆ penlight ◆ small cup of water with straw or ice chips ◆ emesis basin ◆ 60-ml syringe ◆ pH test strip ◆ water ◆ stethoscope

◆ Assist the patient into semi-Fowler's or high Fowler's position.
◆ Place a linen-saver pad across his chest to protect him from spills.
◆ To determine the tube length needed to reach the stomach:
  ● Extend the tube's distal end from the tip of the patient's nose to his earlobe.
  ● Coil this portion of the tube so the end stays curved until it's inserted.
  ● Extend the uncoiled portion from the earlobe to the xiphoid process.
  ● Use hypoallergenic tape to mark the total length of the two portions.

NASAL INSERTION
◆ Assess the patient's history of nasal injury or surgery.
◆ Using the penlight, assess nasal patency. Inspect for a deviated septum, polyps, or other obstructions.
◆ Occlude one nostril, then the other, to determine which has better airflow.
◆ Lubricate the curved tip of the tube and the feeding tube guide, as needed, with water-soluble lubricant to ease insertion and prevent injury.
◆ Have the patient hold the emesis basin and facial tissues in case he needs them.
◆ Insert the curved, lubricated tip into the nostril and direct it along the nasal passage toward the ear on the same side.
◆ When it passes the nasopharyngeal junction, turn the tube 180 degrees to aim it downward into the esophagus.
◆ Instruct the patient to lower his chin to his chest to close the trachea.
◆ Ask him to swallow or sip water with a straw to ease the tube's passage.
◆ Advance the tube as he swallows.

ORAL INSERTION
◆ Have the patient lower his chin to close his trachea.
◆ Have him open his mouth.
◆ Place the tip of the tube at the back of his tongue; give water, and instruct him to swallow.

- Remind him to not clamp his teeth down on the tube.
- Advance the tube as he swallows.

POSITIONING THE TUBE
- Keep passing the tube until the tape marker reaches his nostril or lips.
- To check tube placement, attach the syringe to the end of the tube and try to aspirate gastric secretions.
- If no gastric secretions return, the tube may be in the esophagus. Advance the tube or reinsert it before proceeding.
- Examine the aspirate and place a small amount on a pH test strip.
- Probability of gastric placement is increased if the aspirate has a typical gastric fluid appearance (grassy green, clear and colorless with mucous shreds, or brown) and the pH is 5.0 or less.
- After confirming proper tube placement, remove the marker tape.
- Tape the tube to the patient's nose and remove the guide wire.
- Obtain an abdominal X-ray to verify tube placement.
- To advance the tube to the duodenum, especially a tungsten-weighted tube, position the patient on his right side to let gravity assist tube passage through the pylorus. Move the tube forward 2″ to 3″ (5 to 7.5 cm) hourly.
- Apply a skin preparation to the patient's cheek before securing the tube with tape to help the tube adhere to the skin and prevent irritation.
- Tape the tube securely to avoid excessive pressure on the nostrils.

Postprocedure care for tube insertion

- Check tube placement per facility policy.
- Flush the feeding tube every 8 hours with up to 60 ml of normal saline solution or water to maintain patency.
- Retape the tube daily and as needed. Alternate taping areas.
- Provide nasal hygiene daily.

- Assist with or provide oral care.

MONITORING
- Monitor the skin for redness and breakdown.
- Monitor feeding residuals and the patient's tolerance of feedings.

PATIENT TEACHING
- Make appropriate home care nursing referrals and teach the patient how to use and care for a feeding tube as needed.
- Tell the patient how to assemble equipment, insert and remove the tube, and prepare and store feeding formula.
- Teach how to solve problems with tube position and patency.

DOCUMENTATION
- Record the date, time, and tube type and size.
- Note the insertion site.
- Record confirmation of proper placement per facility policy.
- Document nasal care, skin condition, and oral care.
- Note the patient's tolerance of procedure.
- Document removal of the tube (see *Removing a feeding tube*).

Removing a feeding tube

Follow these steps to remove a feeding tube.
- Gather a linen saver pad, tube clamp, and bulb syringe and bring it to the patient's bedside.
- Explain the procedure and why it's necessary to the patient.
- Place a linen-saver over the patient's chest.
- Wash your hands and put on gloves.
- Flush the tube with air, then clamp or pinch it to prevent fluid aspiration.
- Withdraw the tube gently but quickly.
- Cover and discard the used tube.
- Document the date and time of tube removal.

Femoral compression device

Overview

A femoral compression device (an inflated plastic dome) provides individualized pressure to an arterial puncture site to maintain hemostasis after procedures such as cardiac catheterization or angiography. A trained technician or nurse monitors its use.

Preprocedure care

◆ Explain the procedure and why it's necessary to the patient.
◆ Assemble the equipment and bring it to the bedside.
◆ Provide privacy.
◆ Put on gloves and protective eyewear.
◆ Assess the condition of the puncture site, obtain vital signs, perform neurovascular checks, and assess pain according to facility policy.

Procedure

Equipment: femoral compression device strap ◆ compression arch with dome and three-way stopcock ◆ pressure inflation device ◆ sterile transparent dressing ◆ nonsterile and sterile gloves ◆ protective eyewear

◆ Check for a practitioner's order for the femoral compression device. Make sure the order includes the amount of pressure to be applied and length of time the device should remain in place.
◆ Place the device strap under the patient's hips before sheath removal, if a sheath is in place.
◆ After achieving hemostasis when the sheath is removed, put on sterile gloves and apply a sterile transparent dressing over the puncture site using sterile technique.
◆ With the assistance of another nurse, position the compression arch over the puncture site.

◆ Apply manual pressure over the dome area while the straps are secured to the arch.
◆ When the dome is properly positioned over the puncture site, connect the pressure inflation device to the stopcock.
◆ Turn the stopcock to the open position and inflate the dome with the pressure inflation device to the ordered pressure.
◆ Turn the stopcock off and remove the pressure inflation device.
◆ Assess the puncture site for proper placement of the device and for signs of bleeding or hematoma.
◆ Assess distal pulses and neurovascular condition according to facility policy.
◆ Confirm distal pulses after adjusting the device.

Postprocedure care

◆ Deflate the device hourly and assess the puncture site for bleeding or hematoma. Assess for proper placement of the dome over the puncture site.
◆ Reposition the compression arch and dome as necessary wearing gloves and protective eyewear.
◆ Observe for external bleeding or signs of internal bleeding.

Nursing alert

If internal or external bleeding develops, remove the device, apply pressure, and contact the practitioner.

◆ Remove the device as ordered or per facility policy.

MONITORING

◆ Assess the distal pulses, the puncture site, placement of the device, and ordered amount of pressure according to facility policy.
◆ After device removal, monitor for signs of bleeding at the puncture site and assess distal pulses.
◆ Change the dressing at the puncture site every 24 to 48 hours or according to facility policy.

◆ Inspect the site through the transparent dressing for bleeding, drainage, or hematoma.

PATIENT TEACHING
◆ Review activity restrictions.
◆ Describe signs and symptoms of bleeding that may occur when the device is removed.

DOCUMENTATION
◆ Document sheath removal and describe the puncture site.
◆ Document the date and time of device application and hourly deflations.
◆ Record the patient's tolerance of the procedure.
◆ Document the patient's vital signs.
◆ Describe the appearance of the puncture site.
◆ Record the date, time, and results of pulse assessments.
◆ Note neurovascular assessment findings.
◆ Document the length of time the device was in place.
◆ Document when the device was removed.
◆ Document patient and family teaching provided and their understanding of teaching.
◆ Note complications that occurred and interventions performed.

Hyperthermia-hypothermia blanket

Overview

A hyperthermia-hypothermia blanket raises, lowers, or maintains body temperature through conductive heat or cold transfer between the blanket and the patient. When used manually, the temperature on the unit is set and the blanket reaches and maintains a temperature independent of the patient's temperature. With automatic use, the patient's temperature is monitored by a rectal, skin or esophageal thermistor probe, and the unit alternates heating and cooling to achieve and maintain desired body temperature. The device is used to reduce high fever, maintain normal temperature during surgery or shock; induce hypothermia during surgery, reduce intracranial pressure; control bleeding and intractable pain in patients with amputations, burns, or cancer; and provide warmth in cases of severe hypothermia.

Preprocedure care

◆ Check for a practitioner's order.
◆ Explain the procedure and why it's necessary to the patient and his family.
◆ Assemble the equipment and bring it to the bedside.
◆ Take vital signs and assess the patient's level of consciousness, pupil reaction, limb strength, and skin condition.

Procedure

Equipment: hyperthermia-hypothermia control unit ◆ operation manual ◆ distilled water for control unit ◆ rectal, skin, or esophageal thermistor probe ◆ patient thermometer ◆ hyperthermia-hypothermia blanket ◆ disposable blanket covers, sheets, or bath blankets ◆ lanolin or a mixture of lanolin and cold cream ◆ adhesive tape ◆ towel ◆ sphygmomanometer ◆ gloves and gowns if necessary ◆ optional: protective wraps for the patient's hands and feet

◆ Wash your hands.
◆ Inspect the control unit and blankets for leaks and the plugs and connecting wires for broken prongs, kinks, or fraying.
◆ Connect the blanket to the control unit and set controls for manual or automatic operation and for ordered blanket or body temperature.
◆ Make sure the machine is properly grounded before plugging it into an outlet.
◆ Turn on the machine; add liquid to the unit reservoir, if necessary, as fluid fills the blanket.
◆ Allow the blanket to preheat or precool so the patient receives immediate thermal benefit.
◆ Place the blanket underneath the patient with a sheet or bath blanket as insulation between the patient and blanket as needed.
◆ Apply lanolin or cold cream to the patient's skin where it touches the blanket to help protect the skin from heat or cold sensation.
◆ With automatic operation, insert the thermistor probe appropriately and secure it with tape.
◆ Plug the other end of the probe into the unit's control panel.
◆ Place a sheet or, if ordered, the second hyperthermia-hypothermia blanket over the patient, increasing thermal benefit by trapping cooled or heated air.
◆ Wrap the patient's hands and feet to minimize chilling and promote comfort.

Postprocedure care

◆ Reposition the patient every 30 minutes to 1 hour, unless contraindicated.
◆ Keep the patient's skin, clothes, and blanket cover free from perspiration and condensation.
◆ When the patient's temperature stabilizes, remove the blanket.

MONITORING

◆ Monitor vital signs and neurologic activity every 5 minutes until the desired body temperature is reached, then every 15 minutes until the patient's temperature is stable.

◆ Check fluid intake and output hourly or as ordered.

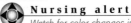 **Nursing alert**

Watch for color changes in the skin, lips, and nail beds and for edema, induration, inflammation, pain, or sensory impairment. If these problems occur, discontinue the procedure and notify the practitioner.

◆ Observe for excessive shivering; stop the procedure if it occurs.

◆ To gradually increase body temperature, especially in postoperative patients, the practitioner may order a disposable blanket warming system (see *Using a warming system*).

PATIENT TEACHING

◆ Explain to the patient the need for frequent monitoring and position changes.

DOCUMENTATION

◆ Record the date, time, and duration of blanket use.

◆ Note the type of hyperthermia-hypothermia unit used.

◆ Document manual or automatic temperature settings.

◆ Document vital signs, temperature, neurologic signs, fluid intake and output, and skin condition.

◆ Note the patient's tolerance of the procedure.

Using a warming system

Shivering, the compensatory response to falling body temperature, may use more oxygen than the body can supply, especially in a surgical patient. In the past, the caregiver would cover the patient with blankets to warm his body. Now, hospitals may supply a warming system such as the Bair Hugger patient-warming system.

This system helps to gradually increase body temperature. Similar to a large hair dryer, the warming unit draws air through a filter, warms the air to the desired temperature, and circulates it through a hose to a warming blanket placed over the patient.

When using the warming system, be sure to:
◆ use a bath blanket in a single layer over the warming blanket to minimize heat loss
◆ place the warming blanket directly over the patient with the paper side facing down and the clear tubular side facing up
◆ make sure the connection hose is at the foot of the bed
◆ take the patient's temperature during the first 15 to 30 minutes and at least every 30 minutes while the warming blanket is in use
◆ obtain guidelines from the patient's practitioner for discontinuing use of the warming blanket.

Procedures

Incentive spirometry

Overview

Incentive spirometry promotes deep breathing. The procedure increases lung volume, boosts alveolar inflation, and promotes venous return by hyperinflating the alveoli and preventing or reversing alveolar collapse that leads to atelectasis and pneumonitis. The device provides visual feedback to the patient while it measures respiratory flow or volume. Incentive spirometry benefits patients on prolonged bed rest, postoperative patients, those who smoke, those who are elderly, inactive, or obese, and those who have difficulty coughing effectively and expelling lung secretions.

CONTRAINDICATIONS

◆ Inability to cooperate or properly use the device
◆ Inability to deep-breathe effectively

Preprocedure care

◆ Explain the procedure and why it's necessary to the patient.
◆ Wash your hands.
◆ Help the patient into a comfortable sitting or semi-Fowler's position to promote optimal lung expansion.
◆ Auscultate the patient's lungs to provide a baseline for comparison with posttreatment auscultation.

Procedure

Equipment: incentive spirometer with sterile disposable tube and mouthpiece (the tube and mouthpiece are sterile on first use and clean on subsequent uses) ◆ stethoscope ◆ watch ◆ pencil ◆ paper
◆ Attach the sterile flow tube and mouthpiece to the device.
◆ Set the flow rate or volume goal as determined by the practitioner or respiratory therapist and based on the patient's preoperative performance.
◆ Instruct the patient to insert the mouthpiece and close his lips tightly around it.
◆ Tell the patient to exhale normally, then inhale as slowly and deeply as possible.
◆ Ask the patient to retain the entire volume of inhaled air for 3 seconds or, if using a device with a light indicator, until the light turns off.
◆ Note the tidal volume.
◆ Tell the patient to remove the mouthpiece and exhale normally.
◆ Allow the patient to relax and take several normal breaths before attempting another breath with the spirometer.
◆ Repeat this sequence five to ten times during every waking hour.

Postprocedure care

◆ Encourage the patient to cough after each effort because deep lung inflation may loosen secretions and facilitate their removal. Observe expectorated secretions.
◆ Auscultate the patient's lungs, and compare findings with the first auscultation.
◆ Place the mouthpiece in a plastic storage bag in between use, and label it and the spirometer with the patient's name.
◆ To prevent nausea, avoid performing incentive spirometry before the patient's mealtime.
◆ Give the patient paper and a pencil so he can note the times he uses the spirometer and the volumes.
◆ Immediately after surgery, encourage the patient to use the incentive spirometer frequently to ensure compliance and allow for assessment of his achievement.

MONITORING

◆ Note the number of inhalations and volume inhaled (see *Computing spirometry volume*).

Procedures

PATIENT TEACHING

◆ Explain the importance of recording times spirometry is used and the resulting volumes, so the patient can see improvement.

◆ Explain the importance of performing exercise regularly to maintain alveolar inflation.

◆ Instruct the patient to remove the mouthpiece, wash it in warm water, and shake it dry.

DOCUMENTATION

◆ Document patient teaching provided and the patient's understanding of the teaching.

◆ Document preoperative flow or volume levels.

◆ Record the date and time of the procedure, type of spirometer used, flow or volume levels achieved, and number of breaths taken.

◆ Note the patient's condition before and after the procedure, his tolerance of the procedure, and results of both auscultations.

Computing spirometry volume

To determine the volume a patient is able to inhale, multiply the incentive spirometer's setting by how long the patient keeps the ball or balls suspended. If a volume incentive spirometer is used, take the volume reading directly from the spirometer. For example, record 1,000 cc × 5 breaths.

Intracranial pressure monitoring

Overview

Intracranial pressure (ICP) monitoring measures pressure exerted by the brain, blood, and cerebrospinal fluid (CSF) against the inside of the skull and detects elevated ICP. The monitoring device is inserted by a neurosurgeon in the operating room, emergency department, or intensive care unit. It's used for patients with head trauma with bleeding or edema, overproduction or insufficient absorption of CSF, cerebral hemorrhage, and space-occupying brain lesions. ICP monitoring systems include the intraventricular catheter, subarachnoid bolt, epidural sensor, and intraparenchymal pressure monitor.

CONTRAINDICATIONS

◆ For intraventricular catheter monitoring, stenotic cerebral ventricles, cerebral aneurysms in path of catheter placement, and suspected vascular lesions

Preprocedure care

◆ Confirm the patient's identity using two patient identifiers according to facility policy.
◆ Explain the procedure and why it's necessary to the patient and his family.
◆ Check that the patient or a responsible family member has signed an informed consent form.
◆ Determine if the patient is allergic to iodine preparations.

Procedure

Equipment: monitoring unit and transducers ◆ 16 to 20 sterile 4″ × 4″ gauze pads ◆ linen-saver pads ◆ hair scissors ◆ sterile drapes ◆ povidone-iodine solution ◆ sterile gown ◆ surgical mask ◆ sterile gloves ◆ head-dressing supplies (two rolls of 4″ elastic gauze dressing, one roll of 4″ roller gauze, adhesive tape) ◆ optional: suction apparatus, I.V. pole, and yardstick

◆ Using sterile technique, set up monitoring units according to the type of system used and facility policy.
◆ Obtain baseline routine and neurologic vital signs.
◆ Place the patient in a supine position and elevate the head of the bed 30 degrees or as ordered.
◆ Place linen-saver pads under the patient's head.
◆ Clip the patient's hair at the site of insertion.
◆ Wash your hands thoroughly.
◆ Wear appropriate personal protection equipment throughout all procedures.
◆ Cover the patient with sterile drapes.
◆ Scrub the insertion site for 2 minutes with povidone-iodine solution.
◆ The practitioner puts on the sterile gown, mask, and gloves and opens the interior wrap of the sterile supply tray and proceeds with insertion of the catheter or bolt.
◆ Maintain the patient's head in a still position during the procedure by holding the patient's head with your hands or by attaching a long strip of 4″ roller gauze to one side rail and bringing it across the patient's forehead to the opposite rail.
◆ Talk to the patient frequently to assess his level of consciousness (LOC) and detect signs of deterioration.
◆ Watch for cardiac arrhythmias and abnormal respiratory patterns.
◆ After insertion, put on sterile gloves and apply a sterile dressing to the site.
◆ If not done by the practitioner, connect the catheter to the appropriate monitoring device, depending on the system used.
◆ If the practitioner has set up a ventriculostomy drainage system, attach the drip chamber to the headboard or bedside I.V. pole.

Postprocedure care

◆ Clean the insertion site and apply a fresh sterile dressing.
◆ If a skull-bone flap is surgically removed to provide room for the swollen brain to expand, keep the site clean and dry to prevent infection and maintain sterile technique when changing the dressing.

MONITORING

◆ Inspect the insertion site at least every 24 hours or according to facility policy for redness, swelling, and drainage.
◆ Assess the patient's status, evaluating routine and neurologic vital signs every hour or as ordered.
◆ Monitor waveforms and pressure parameters.
◆ Calculate cerebral perfusion pressure (CPP) hourly, using this equation: mean arterial pressure $-$ ICP $=$ CPP.
◆ Observe digital ICP readings and waves.
◆ Monitor the amount and appearance of CSF drainage.
◆ Watch for signs of decompensation, including unilateral or bilateral pupillary dilation; decreased pupillary response to light; decreasing LOC; rising systolic blood pressure and widening pulse pressure; bradycardia; slowed, irregular respirations; and, in late decompensation, decerebrate posturing.

PATIENT TEACHING

◆ Explain to the patient the ICP monitor and the nursing care involved in its use.
◆ Advise the patient of the importance of proper body positioning to reduce ICP.
◆ Explain to the patient that he must avoid Valsalva's maneuver and isometric muscle contractions and remain calm and quiet.
◆ Review the indications for removing the monitoring device and explain how the removal procedure is performed.

DOCUMENTATION

◆ Note the time and date of the insertion procedure.
◆ Document the patient's response to the procedure.
◆ Note the insertion site and type of monitoring system used.
◆ Record hourly ICP digital readings, waveforms, and CPP.
◆ Document factors that affect ICP
◆ Note vital signs hourly.
◆ Document patient teaching provided and the patient's understanding of the teaching.

Jugular venous oxygen saturation monitoring

Overview

Jugular venous oxygen saturation (Sjvo$_2$) monitoring measures the blood's oxygen saturation as the blood leaves the brain (after cerebral perfusion has taken place). This procedure helps determine if blood flow to the brain matches the brain's metabolic demand. The normal range is 55% to 70%; values higher than 70% indicate hyperperfusion. Values between 40% and 54% indicate relative hypoperfusion; values lower than 40% indicate ischemia. Criteria for monitoring include neurologic injury in which ischemia is a threat, such as with intra-operative monitoring, subarachnoid hemorrhage, and post-acute head injury involving increased intracranial pressure (ICP).

Preprocedure care

◆ Confirm the patient's identity using two patient identifiers according to facility policy.
◆ Explain the procedure and why it's necessary to the patient.
◆ Wash your hands and put on sterile gloves.

Procedure

Equipment: sterile towels ◆ sterile drapes ◆ surgical caps ◆ gowns ◆ sterile gloves ◆ masks ◆ povidone-iodine scrub ◆ povidone-iodine solution ◆ central venous catheter insertion kit ◆ 1% or 2% lidocaine without epinephrine ◆ 5- or 10-cc syringe with an 18G and 23G needle ◆ 5 French percutaneous introducer ◆ 4 French fiber-optic Sjvo$_2$ catheter ◆ oximetric monitor with cable ◆ 500 ml 0.9% sodium chloride solution (heparinized or nonheparinized based on facility policy) ◆ pressure tubing with continuous flush device ◆ pressure bag or device ◆ sterile occlusive dressing ◆ sterile marker ◆ sterile labels

◆ Using sterile technique, prime the pressure tubing system, removing all air bubbles and maintaining sterility.
◆ Follow the manufacturer's instructions for in vitro calibration of the catheter before insertion.
◆ Position the patient with his head elevated at 30 to 45 degrees and his neck in a neutral position. Document baseline ICP; note subsequent changes.
◆ Turn the patient's head laterally, away from the site chosen for catheter insertion.
◆ Follow dressing procedure guidelines for insertion of central lines.
◆ Put on new sterile gloves.
◆ Using sterile technique, open and prepare the central venous pressure insertion tray, and add a 5 French sterile introducer and a 4 French fiber-optic Sjvo$_2$ catheter.
◆ Label all medications, medication containers, and other solutions containers.
◆ The practitioner will scrub the insertion site with povidone-iodine scrub solution and position sterile drapes, exposing only the insertion site.
◆ Assist the practitioner during insertion as needed.
◆ Monitor the patient's neurologic status, vital signs, ICP, and pain during insertion.
◆ After the line is in place, attach pressure tubing and confirm the patency of both jugular catheter lumens by aspirating and flushing.
◆ Clean the insertion site with povidone-iodine solution and apply a sterile occlusive dressing.

Postprocedure care

◆ Obtain a lateral cervical spine or lateral skull X-ray to confirm catheter placement at the level of the jugular bulb.
◆ Draw a jugular vein blood gas sample and perform in vivo calibration according

Procedures

to the manufacturer's guidelines or facility policy.

◆ Assess the patient's neurologic status, vital signs, and ICP immediately after insertion.

◆ Record baseline measurements for continuously monitored $Sjvo_2$. Calculate arteriovenous oxygen content difference ($AVDO_2$), cerebral oxygen extraction (CEO_2) and oxygen extraction ratio (O_2ER) as a baseline.

◆ Verify the accuracy of the reading by drawing $Sjvo_2$ every 8 to 12 hours; the blood sample reading should be within 4% of reading shown on monitor.

◆ Calculate CEO_2 and O_2ER as indicated.

◆ Maintain a safe environment during monitoring to prevent catheter dislodgment.

◆ Provide sedation or analgesia as indicated.

◆ Provide insertion site care per facility policy.

◆ Change the I.V. solution and catheter tubing according to your facility's policy for central lines.

◆ If an $Sjvo_2$ catheter has low light intensity, it should be replaced.

◆ Check the fiber-optic catheter for obstruction or occlusion. Aspirate the catheter until blood can be freely sampled and normal light intensity is displayed.

◆ For an $Sjvo_2$ catheter with high light intensity (indicating vessel wall artifact), adjust the patient's head to ensure neutral neck position.

◆ Watch for low $Sjvo_2$ percentages and notify the practitioner if they occur.

MONITORING

◆ Record $Sjvo_2$ and ICP values hourly and note trends. Assess ICP in relation to $Sjvo_2$. Notify the practitioner of deviations.

◆ Assess for ICP changes.

◆ Monitor for complications, which are similar to those that can occur with any central line.

◆ After the monitor is removed, assess for signs of bleeding every 15 minutes for 1 hour, then every 30 minutes the next hour, then 1 hour later.

PATIENT TEACHING

◆ Explain activity restrictions as needed.

DOCUMENTATION

◆ Document the date and time of catheter insertion. Include the location of insertion and the depth (in centimeters) of the catheter.

◆ Record the patient's tolerance of the procedure.

◆ Document the ICP reading during insertion.

◆ Record the baseline $Sjvo_2$ reading.

◆ Note the initial CEO_2 and $AVDO_2$ calculations.

◆ Record $Sjvo_2$ and ICP hourly.

◆ Record CEO_2, $AVDO_2$, and O_2ER when indicated.

◆ Document findings from insertion site assessments.

◆ Record expected and unexpected outcomes and the interventions performed.

◆ Document patient and family education provided and their understanding of the teaching.

Latex allergy protocol

Overview

The latex allergy protocol is used to ensure that patients with latex allergies don't interact with latex. Patients at risk for latex allergy include those who undergo multiple surgical procedures, health care workers, latex product manufacturers, and those with a genetic predisposition to latex allergy. (See *Latex allergy screening*.) Signs and symptoms of a latex reaction include generalized itching, irritated eyes, sneezing and coughing, rash, hives, bronchial asthma, scratchy throat, difficulty breathing, anaphylaxis, and edema of face, hands, or neck. The three categories of latex sensitivity are a history of anaphylaxis or systemic reaction when exposed to a natural latex product; a history of nonsystemic allergic reaction; and no history of latex hypersensitivity but high risk because of associated medical condition, occupation, or allergy.

Preprocedure care

◆ Explain the procedure to the patient and why it's necessary.
◆ Assess for a latex allergy in all patients, including those admitted to the delivery room or short-procedure unit and those having a surgical procedure.
◆ Place the patient in a private room. If a private room isn't available, make the room latex-free to prevent spread of airborne particles from latex products used on the other patient.

Procedure

Equipment: latex allergy patient identification wristband ◆ latex-free equipment, including room contents ◆ anaphylaxis kit ◆ optional: latex allergy sign
◆ If the patient has a confirmed latex allergy, bring a cart with latex-free supplies into his room.

◆ Document that the patient has a latex allergy in his chart.
◆ Place a latex allergy identification bracelet on the patient if required by facility policy.
◆ If the patient will receive anesthesia, make sure that "latex allergy" is clearly visible on the front of his chart.
◆ Notify the circulating nurse in the surgical unit, the postanesthesia care unit nurses, and other team members that the patient has a latex allergy.
◆ If the patient is transported to another area, have the latex-free cart accompany him, and have all staff who come in contact with him wear latex-free gloves.
◆ Place a mask with cloth ties on the patient when he leaves his room to protect him from inhaling airborne latex particles.
◆ Make sure I.V. access is accomplished using all latex-free products.
◆ Post a "latex allergy" sign on the I.V. tubing to prevent access of the line using latex products.
◆ Flush I.V. tubing with 50 ml of I.V. solution to rinse the tubing out because of latex ports in the I.V. tubing.
◆ Place a warning label on I.V. bags that says, "Do not use latex injection ports."
◆ Use a latex-free tourniquet; if none are available, use a latex tourniquet over the patient's clothing.
◆ Remove the vial stopper to mix and draw up drugs.
◆ Use latex-free oxygen administration equipment; remove the elastic and tie equipment on with gauze.
◆ Wrap your stethoscope with a latex-free product to protect the patient.
◆ Wrap a clear dressing over the patient's finger before using pulse oximetry.
◆ Use latex-free syringes when administering drugs.

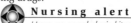 **Nursing alert**

Have an anaphylaxis kit readily available. If the pateint has an allergic reaction, you must act immediately.

Postprocedure care

MONITORING
◆ Monitor for signs and symptoms of latex allergy.

PATIENT TEACHING
◆ Explain what a latex allergy is to the patient.
◆ Discuss signs and symptoms of latex allergy.
◆ Inform the patient about the importance of wearing latex allergy identification.
◆ Explain the importance of informing all health care workers of the patient's latex allergy.
◆ Explain to the patient what to do if a hypersensitivity reaction occurs.
◆ Teach the patient measures to reduce latex exposure.

DOCUMENTATION
◆ Note the patient's history of allergies, including reactions to latex.
◆ Record signs and symptoms observed or reported by the patient.
◆ Document that other departments were notified of the patient's latex allergy.
◆ Document that an allergy identification bracelet was placed on wrist.
◆ Document that a latex allergy alert was placed on the medical record and in the patient's room.
◆ Document that a cart with latex-free items was placed in the patient's room.
◆ Record measures taken to prevent latex exposure.
◆ Note patient teaching performed and the patient's understanding of the teaching.

Latex allergy screening

To determine if your patient has a latex sensitivity or allergy, ask these screening questions:
◆ What's your occupation?
◆ Have you experienced an allergic reaction, local sensitivity, or itching following exposure to latex products, such as balloons or condoms?
◆ Do you have shortness of breath or wheezing after blowing up balloons or after a dental visit?
◆ Do you experience itching in or around your mouth after eating bananas, apricots, cherries, grapes, kiwis, passion fruit, avocados, chestnuts, tomatoes, or peaches?

If your patient answers "yes" to any of these questions, proceed with these questions:
◆ Do you have a history of allergies, dermatitis, or asthma? If so, what type of reaction do you have?
◆ Do you have congenital abnormalities? If yes, explain.
◆ Do you have food allergies? If so, what specific allergies do you have? Describe your reaction.
◆ If you experience shortness of breath or wheezing when blowing up latex balloons, describe your reaction.
◆ Have you had previous surgical procedures? Did you experience associated complications? If so, describe them.
◆ Have you had previous dental procedures? Did complications result? If so, describe them.
◆ Are you exposed to latex in your occupation? Do you experience a reaction to latex products at work? If so, describe your reaction.

Manual ventilation

Overview

Manual ventilation delivers oxygen or room air to the lungs through a handheld resuscitation bag attached to a face mask, an endotracheal tube (ET), or a tracheostomy tube. It's used when a patient can't breathe adequately by himself. It also maintains ventilation when a patient is disconnected temporarily from a mechanical ventilator, during transport, or before suctioning.

Preprocedure care

◆ Explain the procedure and why it's necessary to the patient, if able.
◆ Assemble the equipment and bring it to the bedside.
◆ Check that oxygen is available.
◆ Put on gloves and other personal protective equipment.
◆ Check the patient's upper airway for foreign objects. If any are present, remove them.
◆ Suction the patient to remove secretions that may obstruct the airway.

Procedure

Equipment: handheld resuscitation bag ◆ mask ◆ oxygen source (wall unit or tank) ◆ oxygen tubing ◆ nipple adapter attached to oxygen flowmeter ◆ gloves ◆ goggles ◆ optional: oxygen accumulator, positive end-expiratory pressure valve

◆ Attach one end of the tubing to the bottom of the handheld resuscitation bag and the other end to the nipple adapter on the flowmeter of the oxygen source.
◆ Turn on the oxygen, and adjust the flow rate according to the patient's condition.
◆ To increase the concentration of inspired oxygen, you can add an oxygen accumulator, which is also called an oxygen reservoir, to an adapter on the bottom of the bag, permitting a fraction of inspired oxygen of up to 1.0.

◆ If necessary, insert an oropharyngeal or nasopharyngeal airway to maintain airway patency.
◆ If the patient has a tracheostomy or ET tube in place, remove the mask on the resuscitation bag and attach the end to the tracheostomy or ET tube (see *How to use a bag-mask device*).
◆ Tilt the patient's head backward, if not contraindicated, and pull his jaw forward to move the tongue away from the base of the pharynx and prevent obstruction of the airway.
◆ Using your nondominant hand, apply downward pressure to seal the mask against the patient's face.
◆ For the adult patient, use your dominant hand to compress the bag every 6 to 7 seconds to deliver approximately 1 L of air.
◆ Deliver breaths with the patient's inhalations, if any are present. Don't attempt to deliver a breath as he exhales.
◆ Observe the patient's chest to make sure that it rises and falls with each compression.
◆ If ventilation fails to occur, check the fit of the mask and the patency of the patient's airway; if necessary, reposition his head and ensure patency with an oral airway.

Postprocedure care

◆ After ET tube insertion, attach it to a ventilator for automated ventilation.
◆ Keep the resuscitation mask close to the patient's bedside.

MONITORING
◆ Observe the patient for vomiting through the clear part of the mask.
◆ Monitor pulse oximetry.

PATIENT TEACHING
◆ Tell the patient why manual ventilation is being done, as necessary.

DOCUMENTATION

◆ Note the date and time of the procedure.
◆ Document complications and nursing actions performed.
◆ Note the patient's response to treatment according to facility protocol for respiratory arrest.

How to use a bag-mask device

Place the mask over the patient's face so the apex of the triangle covers the bridge of his nose and the base lies between his lower lip and chin.

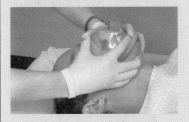

Make sure his mouth remains open underneath the mask. Attach the bag to the mask and the tubing leading to the oxygen source.

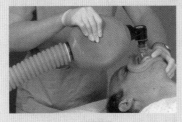

If the patient has a tracheostomy or endotracheal tube in place, remove the mask from the bag and attach the handheld resuscitation bag directly to the tube.

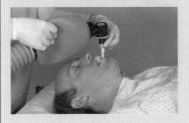

Mixed venous oxygen saturation

Overview

Mixed venous oxygen saturation ($S\bar{v}o_2$) uses a fiber-optic thermodilution pulmonary artery (PA) catheter to continuously monitor oxygen delivery to tissues as well as their oxygen consumption. The process, which allows rapid detection of impaired oxygen delivery, is used to evaluate the patient's response to drug therapy, endotracheal tube suctioning, and ventilator setting changes, as well as changes in positive end-expiratory pressure and fraction of inspired oxygen. $S\bar{v}o_2$ usually ranges from 60% to 80%; normal value is 75%.

Preprocedure care

◆ Confirm the patient's identity using two patient identifiers according to facility policy.
◆ Explain the procedure and why it's being done to the patient.

Procedure

Equipment: fiber-optic PA catheter ◆ co-oximeter (monitor) ◆ optical module and cable ◆ gloves
◆ Connect the optical module and cable to the monitor.
◆ Peel back the catheter wrapping just enough to uncover the fiber-optic connector.
◆ Attach the fiber-optic connector to the optical module; don't remove the rest of the catheter.
◆ Calibrate the fiber-optic catheter.
◆ Wash your hands and put on gloves.
◆ Assist with insertion of the fiber-optic catheter.
◆ After insertion, ensure correct positioning and function.
◆ Observe digital readout and record the $S\bar{v}o_2$ on graph paper (see *$S\bar{v}o_2$ waveforms*).

$S\bar{v}o_2$ waveforms

Mixed venous saturation ($S\bar{v}o_2$) waveforms vary based on factors such as patient activity, initiation of positive end-expiratory pressure (PEEP), and changes in fraction of inspired oxygen (Fio_2).

NORMAL $S\bar{v}o_2$ WAVEFORM

$S\bar{v}o_2$ WITH PATIENT ACTIVITIES

$S\bar{v}o_2$ WITH PEEP AND Fio_2 CHANGES

Postprocedure care

◆ Set alarms 10% above and 10% below the patient's current $S\bar{v}o_2$ reading.
◆ Recalibrate the monitor per facility policy (see *Recalibrating an $S\bar{v}o_2$ monitor*).
◆ If the patient's $S\bar{v}o_2$ drops below 60% or varies by more than 10% for 3 minutes or longer, reassess the patient.

MONITORING

◆ Repeat readings at least hourly to monitor and document trends.
◆ Recalibrate the monitor every 24 hours or whenever the catheter has been disconnected from the optical module.
◆ Monitor the $S\bar{v}o_2$ waveform. If abnormal, perform appropriate interventions to correct the problem.
◆ Monitor for signs and symptoms of infection, such as redness or drainage at the catheter site.

PATIENT TEACHING

◆ Explain activity precautions for preventing catheter dislodgment.

DOCUMENTATION

◆ Record the $S\bar{v}o_2$ value on a flowchart and attach a tracing.
◆ For comparison, note the $S\bar{v}o_2$ as measured by the fiber-optic catheter whenever a blood sample is obtained for laboratory analysis of $S\bar{v}o_2$.

Recalibrating an $S\bar{v}o_2$ monitor

To recalibrate a mixed venous oxygen saturation ($S\bar{v}o_2$) monitor:
◆ Draw a blood sample from the distal port of the pulmonary artery catheter and send it for laboratory analysis.
◆ Compare the laboratory's $S\bar{v}o_2$ reading with the fiber-optic catheter's reading.
◆ If the catheter values and monitor values differ by more than 4%, follow the manufacturer's instructions to enter the $S\bar{v}o_2$ value obtained by the laboratory into the oximeter.

Procedures

Nasal packing

Overview

Nasal packing, which generally is done by a practitioner, is the insertion of a device into the nasal cavity to create a tamponade effect on uncontrolled bleeding when routine therapeutic measures fail to control epistaxis.

CONTRAINDICATIONS

◆ Nasal trauma that might involve internal structure injury
◆ Coagulopathy
◆ Potential cerebrospinal fluid leak

Preprocedure care

◆ Confirm the patient's identity using two patient identifiers according to facility policy.
◆ Explain the procedure and why it's necessary to the patient.
◆ Wash your hands.
◆ Assemble all equipment at the patient's bedside.

Procedure

Equipment: gowns ◆ goggles ◆ masks ◆ sterile gloves ◆ emesis basin ◆ facial tissue ◆ patient drape ◆ nasal speculum and tongue depressors ◆ directed illumination source or fiber-optic nasal endoscope ◆ suction apparatus with sterile suction-connecting tubing and sterile nasal aspirator tip ◆ sterile bowl and sterile normal saline solution for flushing ◆ sterile towels ◆ sterile cotton-tipped applicators ◆ local anesthetic spray or solution, such as 2% lidocaine or 1% to 2% lidocaine with epinephrine (1:100,000) ◆ sedative or analgesic ◆ sterile cotton balls or cotton pledgets ◆ 10-ml syringe with 22G 1½" needle ◆ silver nitrate sticks ◆ electrocautery device ◆ topical vasoconstrictor ◆ absorbable hemostatic ◆ sterile normal saline solution (1-g container and 60-ml syringe with luer-

lock tip) ◆ hypoallergenic tape ◆ antibiotic ointment ◆ petroleum jelly
Additional equipment required for anterior packing: two packages of 1½" (4-cm) petroleum strips ◆ gauze (36" to 48" [0.9 to 1.2 m]) ◆ two nasal tampons
Additional equipment required for posterior packing: two #14 or #16 French catheters with 30-cc balloon or two single- or double-chamber nasal balloon catheters ◆ bayonet forceps
For assessment and bedside use after packing: tongue blades ◆ flashlight ◆ long hemostats or sponge forceps ◆ 60-ml syringe for deflating balloons if applicable
◆ Plug in and test the suction apparatus, and connect the tubing from the collection bottle to the suction source.
◆ Check the patient's vital signs, and observe for hypotension with postural changes.
◆ Monitor airway patency.
◆ If ordered, give a sedative or analgesic to reduce anxiety and pain and decrease sympathetic stimulation, which can exacerbate a nosebleed.
◆ Help the patient sit with his head tilted forward.
◆ Wash your hands and put on protective equipment.
◆ Clean the medication stopper and hold the vial so the practitioner can withdraw the anesthetic.
◆ Open the packages containing the sterile suction-connecting tubing and aspirating tip, and place them on the sterile field.
◆ Fill the sterile bowl with normal saline solution to flush the suction tubing.
◆ Thoroughly lubricate the anterior or posterior packing with antibiotic ointment.
◆ Test a balloon for leaks by inflating the catheter with normal saline solution.
◆ Turn on the suction apparatus and attach the connecting tubing.
◆ The practitioner uses a nasal speculum and an external light source or a fiber-optic nasal endoscope to inspect the nasal cavity.

◆ The practitioner uses suction or cotton-tipped applicators to remove collected blood and help visualize the bleeding vessel.

◆ The nose may be treated early with a topical vasoconstrictor such as phenylephrine to slow bleeding and aid visualization.

ANTERIOR NASAL PACKING

◆ After the practitioner applies a topical vasoconstrictor or uses chemical cautery to control bleeding, apply manual pressure to the nose for about 10 minutes.

◆ If bleeding persists, you may help insert an absorbable hemostatic nasal pack directly on the bleeding site.

◆ If these methods fail, prepare to assist with electrocautery or insertion of petroleum strip gauze.

POSTERIOR NASAL PACKING

◆ Wash your hands and put on sterile gloves.

◆ Lubricate the soft catheters to ease insertion.

◆ Instruct the patient to open his mouth and breathe normally.

◆ Help the practitioner insert the packing as directed.

◆ Help the patient assume a position with his head elevated 45 to 90 degrees.

Postprocedure care

◆ When using anterior packing, apply petroleum jelly to the patient's lips and nostrils while the packing is in place to prevent drying and cracking.

◆ If mucosal oozing persists, apply a moustache dressing.

◆ Change the pad when soiled.

◆ Provide supplemental humidified oxygen with a face mask if needed.

◆ Provide thorough mouth care often.

◆ Assist with removal of packing, usually in 2 to 5 days.

MONITORING

◆ Assess the patient for airway obstruction or respiratory changes.

◆ Monitor the patient's vital signs regularly.

PATIENT TEACHING

◆ Tell the patient his ability to smell and taste will likely decrease.

◆ After an anterior pack is removed, tell the patient to avoid picking, inserting any object into, or blowing his nose forcefully for 48 hours or as ordered.

◆ Advise the patient to eat soft foods because of impaired eating and swallowing functions.

◆ Instruct the patient to drink fluids or use artificial saliva to cope with dry mouth.

◆ Teach the patient how to prevent nosebleeds and to seek medical help if he can't stop bleeding.

DOCUMENTATION

◆ Note the type of pack used to ensure its removal at the appropriate time.

◆ Record estimated blood loss and all fluids given.

◆ Document the patient's vital signs.

◆ Note the patient's response to sedation or position changes.

◆ Record laboratory results.

◆ Document drugs given, including topical agents.

◆ Describe any complications.

◆ Document discharge instructions provided, clinical follow-up plans, and the patient's understanding of the instructions.

Procedures

Nasogastric tube insertion and removal

Overview

A nasogastric (NG) tube is usually inserted to decompress the stomach, but it may also be used to assess and treat upper GI bleeding, collect gastric contents for analysis, perform gastric lavage, aspirate gastric secretions, give drugs and nutrients, or prevent vomiting after major surgery. The most common tubes are the Levin tube, which has one lumen, and the Salem sump tube, with two lumens, one of which vents air to protect the gastric mucosa.

CONTRAINDICATIONS
◆ Facial or basilar skull fracture
◆ Hypothermia

Preprocedure care for insertion

◆ Confirm the patient's identity using two patient identifiers according to facility policy.
◆ Explain the procedure and why it's necessary to the patient.

Procedure for insertion

Equipment: tube (usually #12, #14, #16, or #18 French for a normal adult) ◆ towel or linen-saver pad ◆ facial tissues ◆ emesis basin ◆ penlight ◆ 1″ or 2″ hypoallergenic tape ◆ gloves ◆ water-soluble lubricant ◆ cup or glass of water with straw if appropriate ◆ pH test strip ◆ tongue blade ◆ catheter-tip or bulb syringe or irrigation set ◆ safety pin ◆ ordered suction equipment
◆ Put the patient in high Fowler's position unless contraindicated.
◆ Drape the towel or linen-saver pad over his chest.
◆ Have the patient blow his nose to clear his nostrils.
◆ Place the facial tissues and emesis basin within reach.

◆ Wash your hands and put on gloves.
◆ To determine how much of the NG tube to insert, hold the end of the tube at the tip of his nose, then extend the tube to his earlobe and down to the xiphoid process. Mark this distance on the tubing with tape.
◆ Using a penlight, inspect each nostril for a deviated septum or other abnormalities and assess airflow in both nostrils.
◆ Lubricate the first 3″ (7.6 cm) of the tube with a water-soluble gel.
◆ Instruct the patient to hold his head straight and upright.
◆ Grasp the tube with the end pointing downward, curve it if necessary, and carefully insert it into the more patent nostril.
◆ Aim the tube downward and toward the ear closer to the chosen nostril. Advance it slowly until you feel resistance.
◆ Instruct the patient to lower his head slightly to close the trachea and open the esophagus.
◆ Rotate the tube 180 degrees toward the opposite nostril.
◆ Unless contraindicated, direct the patient to sip and swallow water as you slowly advance the tube.
◆ Stop advancing the tube when the tape mark reaches the patient's nostril.
◆ If your patient is unconscious, tilt the chin toward his chest to close the trachea.
◆ Advance the tube between respirations.

ENSURING PROPER NG TUBE PLACEMENT
◆ Use a tongue blade and penlight to examine the patient's mouth and throat for signs of a coiled section of tubing.
◆ Attach a catheter-tip or bulb syringe and aspirate stomach contents.
◆ Examine the aspirate and place a small amount on the pH test strip.
◆ Correct gastric placement is likely if the aspirate has a typical gastric fluid appearance (grassy-green, clear and colorless

with mucus shreds, or brown) and the pH is 5 or less.

◆ If you still can't aspirate stomach contents, advance the tube 1" to 2" (2.5 to 5 cm), then inject 10 cc of air into the tube.

◆ If tests don't confirm proper tube placement, you'll need X-ray verification.

◆ Secure the NG tube to the patient's nose with hypoallergenic tape.

Postprocedure care for insertion

◆ Tie a slipknot around the tube with a rubber band, then secure the rubber band to the patient's gown with a safety pin.

◆ Attach the tube to suction equipment, if ordered, and set the designated suction pressure.

◆ Provide frequent nose and mouth care while the tube is in place.

MONITORING

◆ Monitor the amount and characteristics of drainage.

◆ Check tube placement every 4 hours or per facility policy.

PATIENT TEACHING

◆ Explain signs and symptoms to report as needed.

◆ Tell the patient to avoid food and drink while the tube is in place.

DOCUMENTATION

◆ Record the type and size of the NG tube.

◆ Note the date, time, and route of insertion.

◆ Note the patient's tolerance of the procedure.

◆ Document the type, color, odor, consistency, and amount of gastric drainage.

Preprocedure care for removal

◆ Explain the procedure to the patient.

◆ Assess bowel function by auscultating for peristalsis or flatus.

◆ Help the patient into semi-Fowler's position.

Procedure for removal

Equipment: stethoscope ◆ gloves ◆ catheter-tip syringe ◆ normal saline solution ◆ towel or linen-saver pad

◆ Wash your hands and put on gloves.

◆ Drape a towel or linen-saver pad across his chest.

◆ Using a catheter-tip syringe, flush the tube with 10 ml of normal saline solution.

◆ Untape the tube from the patient's nose and unpin it from his gown.

◆ Clamp the tube by folding it in your hand.

◆ Ask the patient to hold his breath then slowly withdraw the tube and place it on the towel or linen-saver pad.

◆ Cover and discard the tube.

Postprocedure care for removal

◆ Assist the patient with thorough mouth and skin care.

MONITORING

◆ Monitor for signs of GI dysfunction.

PATIENT TEACHING

◆ Tell the patient to notify the nurse if GI distress occurs.

DOCUMENTATION

◆ Document the date and time of tube removal.

◆ Document GI assessment findings.

◆ Record the patient's tolerance of the procedure.

Oronasopharyngeal suction

Overview

Oronasopharyngeal suction uses a catheter inserted through the mouth or nostril to remove secretions from the pharynx. This procedure maintains a patent airway for the patient who can't clear his airway effectively with coughing and expectoration. The procedure requires sterile equipment; however, clean technique may be used for a tonsil tip suction device, which an alert patient can use himself to remove secretions.

CONTRAINDICATIONS
- Deviated septum
- Nasal polyps
- Nasal obstruction
- Traumatic injury
- Epistaxis
- Mucosal swelling

Preprocedure care

- Explain the procedure and why it's necessary to the patient.
- Assemble the equipment and bring it to the bedside.
- Check the patient's vital signs.
- Evaluate the patient's ability to cough and deep-breathe.
- Check for a history of deviated septum, nasal polyps, nasal obstruction, traumatic injury, epistaxis, or mucosal swelling.

Procedure

Equipment: wall suction or portable suction apparatus ◆ collection bottle ◆ connecting tubing ◆ water-soluble lubricant ◆ normal saline solution ◆ disposable sterile container ◆ sterile suction catheter (#12 or #14 French for an adult, #8 or #10 French for a child, or pediatric feeding tube for an infant) ◆ sterile gloves ◆ clean gloves ◆ goggles ◆ overbed table ◆ waterproof trash bag ◆ soap ◆ water ◆ 70% alcohol for

cleaning catheters ◆ optional: nasopharyngeal or oropharyngeal airway (for frequent suctioning), tongue blade, tonsil tip suction device

- Wash your hands, and put on your personal protective equipment.
- Place the patient in semi-Fowler's or high Fowler's position.
- Turn on the suction from the wall or portable unit, and set the pressure according to facility policy, which usually is between 80 and 120 mm Hg.
- Write the date on the bottle of normal saline solution and open it.
- Open the waterproof trash bag.
- Using strict sterile technique, open the suction catheter kit or the packages containing the sterile catheter, container, and gloves.
- Put on the gloves; consider your dominant hand sterile and your nondominant hand nonsterile.
- Using your nondominant hand, pour the normal saline solution into the sterile container.
- With your nondominant hand, place a small amount of water-soluble lubricant on the sterile area.
- Pick up the catheter with your dominant hand, and attach it to the connecting tubing.
- Use your nondominant hand to control the suction valve while your dominant hand manipulates the catheter.
- Instruct the patient to cough and breathe slowly and deeply several times before beginning suction.

NASAL INSERTION
- Raise the tip of the patient's nose with your nondominant hand to straighten the passageway and facilitate insertion of the catheter.
- Without applying suction, gently insert the suction catheter.
- Roll the catheter between your fingers to help it advance through the turbinates.

◆ Continue to advance the catheter 5″ to 6″ (12.5 to 15 cm) until you reach the pool of secretions or the patient begins to cough.

ORAL INSERTION

◆ Without applying suction, gently insert the catheter into the patient's mouth.
◆ Advance it 3″ to 4″ (7.5 to 10 cm) along the side of the patient's mouth until you reach the pool of secretions or the patient begins to cough.
◆ Suction both sides of the patient's mouth and pharyngeal area.

INTERMITTENT SUCTION

◆ Withdraw the catheter with a continuous rotating motion to minimize invagination of the mucosa into the catheter's tip and side ports.
◆ Apply suction for only 10 to 15 seconds at a time to minimize tissue trauma.
◆ Between passes, wrap the catheter around your dominant hand to prevent contamination.
◆ Clear the lumen of the catheter by dipping it in water and applying suction.
◆ Repeat the procedure until gurgling or bubbling sounds stop and respirations are quiet.
◆ After completing suctioning, pull your sterile glove off over the coiled catheter and discard it and the nonsterile glove along with the container of water.
◆ Flush the connecting tubing with normal saline solution, replace the used items so they're ready for the next suctioning, and wash your hands.

Postprocedure care

◆ If the patient has no history of nasal problems, alternate suctioning between nostrils to minimize injury.
◆ If repeated oronasopharyngeal suctioning is required, the use of a nasopharyngeal or oropharyngeal airway will help

with catheter insertion, reduce traumatic injury, and promote a patent airway.
◆ To facilitate catheter insertion for oropharyngeal suctioning, depress the patient's tongue with a tongue blade.
◆ If the patient has excessive oral secretions, consider using a tonsil tip catheter.
◆ Let the patient rest after suctioning while you continue to observe him.

PATIENT TEACHING

◆ For the patient at home, instruct him to use clean technique for oronasopharyngeal suction rather than sterile technique.
◆ Instruct the patient that properly cleaned catheters can be reused.
◆ Instruct the patient to wash catheters in soapy water, then boil them for 10 minutes or soak them in 70% alcohol for 3 to 5 minutes.
◆ Tell the patient to rinse with normal saline solution or tap water.

DOCUMENTATION

◆ Record the date, time, reason for suctioning, and technique used.
◆ Note the amount, color, consistency, and odor of the secretions.
◆ Document the patient's respiratory status before and after the procedure.
◆ Record complications and nursing actions taken.
◆ Note the patient's tolerance of the procedure.
◆ Document patient teaching provided and the patient's understanding of the teaching.

Pain management

Overview

Pain management is used to distract the patient from the sensation of pain. Techniques for pain management include administering analgesics, providing emotional support or comfort measures, and using complementary and alternative therapies such as cognitive techniques. Sometimes, invasive measures, such as epidural analgesia or patient-controlled analgesia (PCA), are used. Pain is assessed based on the patient's subjective description and objective assessment tools.

Preprocedure care

◆ Explain to the patient that pain management aims to keep pain at a low level.

Procedure

Equipment: pain assessment tool or scale
◆ oral hygiene supplies ◆ nonopioid analgesic ◆ PCA device ◆ opioid
◆ Assess the patient's pain level using assessment tools or scales, or ask key questions about duration, severity, and location of pain (see *How to assess pain*).
◆ Note the patient's reaction to pain.
◆ Look for physiologic or behavioral clues to the pain's severity.
◆ Develop a nursing care plan with the patient, including prescribed drugs, emotional support, comfort measures, complementary and alternative therapies, and pain management education.
◆ Emphasize the importance of maintaining good bowel habits, respiratory functions, and mobility.

GIVING MEDICATIONS
◆ Confirm the patient's identity using two patient identifiers according to facility policy.
◆ Give a nonopioid analgesic if the patient is allowed oral intake.
◆ Give a mild opioid, as ordered, if relief isn't achieved with a nonopioid.

◆ Administer a strong opioid, as ordered, if the patient needs more relief.
◆ Check the appropriate drug information for each drug given.
◆ Teach the patient how to use a PCA device if ordered.

PROVIDING EMOTIONAL SUPPORT
◆ Spend time speaking with the patient.

PERFORMING COMFORT MEASURES
◆ Reposition the patient every 2 hours.
◆ Increase the angle of the bed to reduce pull on an abdominal incision.
◆ Elevate a limb to reduce swelling, inflammation, and pain.
◆ Splint or support abdominal and chest incisions with a pillow when coughing or changing position.
◆ Give a back massage, and provide hygiene as needed.
◆ Perform passive range-of-motion exercises.

PERFORMING COMPLEMENTARY AND ALTERNATIVE THERAPIES
◆ If the patient feels persistent pain, teach short, simple relaxation exercises, such as dimming the lights, removing restrictive clothing, and eliminating noise; having the patient recall a pleasant experience or focus his attention on an enjoyable activity; or having the patient close his eyes and concentrate on listening to music.

Guided imagery
◆ Guide the patient to concentrate on a peaceful, pleasant image
◆ Ask about its sight, sound, smell, taste, and touch
◆ Have the patient visualize the goal and picture himself taking action to achieve it.

Deep breathing
◆ Have the patient stare at an object and slowly inhale and exhale as he counts aloud.
◆ Ask him to concentrate on the rise and fall of his abdomen, and encourage him to

feel increasingly weightless with each breath.

Muscle relaxation
◆ Have the patient focus on a particular muscle group.
◆ Ask him to tense the muscles and note the sensation.
◆ After 5 to 7 seconds, tell him to relax his muscles and concentrate on the relaxed state.
◆ Have the patient describe the difference between the tense and relaxed states.
◆ After he tenses and relaxes one muscle group, have him proceed to another and another until he has covered his entire body.

Postprocedure care

◆ Reassess and alter your care plan as appropriate.
◆ Keep in mind that cultural beliefs affect behavioral responses to pain and treatment, so consider patient expectations when developing the care plan.
◆ If the patient has a preexisting drug addiction, make appropriate referrals to experts to develop an effective pain management plan.

MONITORING
◆ Evaluate the patient's response to pain management.

PATIENT TEACHING
◆ Teach about the administration, dosage, and possible adverse effects of prescribed medications.
◆ Reinforce the alternative therapy methods the patient has learned.

DOCUMENTATION
◆ Record subjective information from the patient, using his exact words.
◆ Note the location, quality, and duration of pain.
◆ Document the patient's rating of pain before and after interventions.

◆ Document precipitating and relieving factors.
◆ Note the pain-relief method selected.
◆ Note alternative treatments used and their effects.
◆ Record nursing interventions performed and the patient's response.
◆ Document complications of drug therapy.
◆ Document patient teaching provided and the patient's understanding of teaching.

How to assess pain

To assess pain, consider the patient's description and your observations of physical and behavioral responses. Start by asking the following questions and consider that the patient's responses will be shaped by his prior experiences, self-image, and beliefs about his condition:
◆ Where is the pain located?
◆ How long does it last?
◆ How often does it occur?
◆ Can you describe the pain?
◆ What triggers the pain?
◆ What relieves the pain or makes it worse?
  Ask the patient to rank his pain on a scale of 0 to 10, with 0 denoting no pain and 10 denoting the worst pain. This scale helps the patient verbally evaluate pain therapies.
  Observe the patient's behavioral and physiologic responses to pain. Physiologic responses may be sympathetic or parasympathetic.

Behavioral responses
Behavioral responses include altered body position, moaning, sighing, grimacing, withdrawal, crying, restlessness, muscle twitching, irritability, and immobility.

Sympathetic responses
Sympathetic responses are commonly associated with mild to moderate pain and include pallor, elevated blood pressure, dilated pupils, skeletal muscle tension, dyspnea, tachycardia, and diaphoresis.

Parasympathetic responses
Parasympathetic responses are commonly associated with severe, deep pain and include pallor, decreased blood pressure, bradycardia, nausea and vomiting, weakness, dizziness, and loss of consciousness.

Passive range-of-motion exercises

Overview

Passive range-of-motion (ROM) exercises move a patient's joints through as full of a range of movements as possible to improve or maintain joint mobility and help prevent contractures. These exercises are indicated for the patient with temporary or permanent loss of mobility, sensation, or consciousness. Performed by a nurse, physical therapist, or caregiver, passive ROM exercises require recognizing the patient's motion limitations and providing support of all joints during movement.

CONTRAINDICATIONS
◆ Septic joints
◆ Acute thrombophlebitis
◆ Severe arthritic joint inflammation
◆ Recent trauma with possible hidden fractures or internal injuries

Preprocedure care

◆ Confirm the patient's identity using two patient identifiers according to facility policy.
◆ Explain the procedure to the patient and why it's being done.
◆ Raise the bed to a comfortable working height.
◆ Determine which joints need ROM exercises.
◆ Consult the practitioner or physical therapist about limitations or precautions.

Procedure

Equipment: no specific equipment needed
◆ Perform appropriate exercises slowly, gently, and to the end of the normal ROM or to the point of pain, but no further. Repeat each exercise at least three times.

EXERCISING THE NECK
◆ Support the patient's head with your hands and extend the neck, flex the chin to the chest, and tilt the head laterally toward each shoulder.

◆ Rotate the patient's head from right to left.

EXERCISING THE SHOULDER
◆ Support the patient's arm in an extended, neutral position.
◆ Extend the forearm and flex it back.
◆ Abduct the arm outward from the side of the body.
◆ Adduct it back to the side.
◆ Rotate the shoulder so the arm crosses the midline; bend the elbow so the hand touches the opposite shoulder, then touches the bed for complete internal rotation.
◆ Return the shoulder to a neutral position; with the elbow bent, push the arm backward so the back of the hand touches the mattress for complete external rotation.

EXERCISING THE ELBOW
◆ Place the patient's arm at his side with his palm facing up.
◆ Flex and extend the arm at the elbow.

EXERCISING THE FOREARM
◆ Stabilize the patient's elbow, then twist the hand to bring the palm up (supination).
◆ Twist it back again to bring the palm down (pronation).

EXERCISING THE WRIST
◆ Stabilize the forearm, and flex and extend the wrist.
◆ Rock the hand sideways for lateral flexion, and rotate the hand in a circular motion.

EXERCISING THE FINGERS AND THUMB
◆ Extend the patient's fingers, and flex the hand into a fist.
◆ Repeat extension and flexion of each joint of each finger and thumb separately.
◆ Spread two adjoining fingers apart and then bring them together.
◆ Oppose each fingertip to the thumb, and rotate the thumb and each finger in a circle.

EXERCISING THE HIP AND KNEE
◆ Fully extend the patient's leg, and then bend the hip and knee toward the chest, allowing full joint flexion.
◆ Move the straight leg sideways, out and away from the other leg and then back, over, and across it.
◆ Rotate the straight leg internally toward the midline, and then rotate it externally away from the midline.

EXERCISING THE ANKLE
◆ Bend the patient's foot so the toes push upward, and then bend the foot so the toes push downward.
◆ Rotate the ankle in a circular motion.
◆ Invert the ankle so that the sole of the foot faces the midline, and evert the ankle so that the sole faces away from the midline.

EXERCISING THE TOES
◆ Flex the patient's toes toward the sole, and then extend them back toward the top of the foot.
◆ Spread two adjoining toes apart and bring them together.

Postprocedure care

◆ Place the patient in a comfortable position.

MONITORING
◆ Monitor the patient for pain or joint stiffness.
◆ Monitor for improved joint mobility or patient participation.

PATIENT TEACHING
◆ Teach and encourage active ROM exercises, or isometric exercises, if possible.
◆ Teach a family member or caregiver to perform passive ROM exercises, if appropriate.

DOCUMENTATION
◆ Record which joints were exercised.

◆ Record whether the patient experienced pain resulting from the exercises.
◆ Note limited or improved ROM.
◆ Record the patient's tolerance of the exercises.
◆ Document patient teaching provided and the patient's understanding of the teaching.

Peripheral I.V. line insertion and removal

Overview

Peripheral I.V. line insertion uses a catheter in a vein to administer fluids, medication, blood, and blood components. The device and site selected depend on the type of solution being administered; frequency and duration of infusion; patency and location of accessible veins; patient's age, size, and condition; and, if possible, the patient's preference. In emergency situations, the antecubital vein is the preferred access site.

CONTRAINDICATIONS

◆ Sclerotic vein
◆ Edematous or impaired arm or hand
◆ Postmastectomy arm
◆ Arteriovenous fistula

Preprocedure care

◆ Confirm the patient's identity using two patient identifiers according to facility policy.
◆ Explain the procedure and why it's necessary to the patient.
◆ Wash your hands.

Procedure

Equipment: alcohol pads or chlorhexidine ◆ gloves ◆ tourniquet ◆ I.V. access devices ◆ I.V. solution with attached and primed administration set ◆ I.V. pole ◆ transparent semipermeable dressing ◆ 1″ (2.5-cm) hypoallergenic tape
◆ Obtain the ordered I.V. solution or medication and prime the appropriate I.V. tubing.
◆ If using a winged infusion set, connect the adapter to the administration set, and unclamp the line until fluid flows from the open end of the needle cover.
◆ Put on gloves.
◆ Select an appropriate-gauge device.

◆ Apply a tourniquet 4″ to 6″ (10 to 15 cm).
◆ Lightly palpate the patient's veins with the index and middle fingers of your nondominant hand. If a vein feels hard or ropelike, select another.
◆ Stretch the skin to anchor the selected vein. Tell the patient to open and close his fist several times.
◆ Clean the site using a vigorous side-to-side motion. Allow the solution to dry.
◆ If using a winged infusion device, hold the short edges of the wings between the thumb and forefinger of your dominant hand, and squeeze the wings together.
◆ If you're using an over-the-needle cannula, grasp the plastic hub with your dominant hand, remove the cover, and examine the cannula tip.
◆ If the edge isn't smooth, discard it and replace the device.
◆ If using a through-the-needle cannula, grasp the needle hub with one hand, and unsnap the needle cover; rotate the access device until the bevel faces up.
◆ Using the thumb of your nondominant hand, pull the skin taut below the puncture site to stabilize the vein.
◆ Hold the needle bevel up, and enter the skin directly over the vein at a 0- to 15-degree angle.
◆ Push the needle through the skin and into the vein in one motion.
◆ Check the flashback chamber behind the hub for a blood return.
◆ Level the insertion device slightly by lifting the tip of the device to prevent puncturing the back wall of the vessel.
◆ If using a winged infusion device, advance the needle fully and hold it in place.
◆ Release the tourniquet, open the administration set, clamp slightly, and check for a free flow or an infiltration.
◆ If using an over-the-needle cannula, advance the device to at least half of its length to ensure that the cannula itself,

Procedures

not just the introducer needle, has entered the vein. Remove the tourniquet.

◆ Grasp the cannula hub to hold it in the vein, and withdraw the needle. As you withdraw it, press slightly on the catheter tip to prevent bleeding.

◆ Advance the cannula up to the hub or until you meet resistance.

◆ Using sterile technique, attach the I.V. tubing and begin the infusion.

◆ If you're using a through-the-needle cannula, remove the tourniquet, hold the needle in place, and grasp the needle through the protective sleeve.

◆ Slowly thread the cannula through the needle until the hub is within the needle collar.

◆ Withdraw the metal needle, split the needle along the perforated edge, carefully remove it, and dispose of the needle pieces appropriately.

◆ Remove the stylet and the protective sleeve, attach the administration set to the cannula hub, and open the administration set clamp.

◆ Use a transparent semipermeable dressing to secure the device.

◆ Loop the I.V. tubing on the patient's limb, and secure the tubing with tape.

◆ Label a piece of tape with the type and length of the cannula, the gauge of needle, the date and time of insertion, and your initials, and place it at the edge of the dressing covering the insertion site.

Postprocedure care

◆ Provide site care per facility policy.
◆ Rotate the I.V. site, usually every 72 hours or according to facility policy.
◆ Remove the catheter as ordered (see *Removing an I.V. catheter*).

MONITORING

◆ Monitor the insertion site for leakage and signs and symptoms of infiltration or infection.

◆ Monitor the infusion.

PATIENT TEACHING

◆ Teach the patient about movement restrictions.
◆ Tell the patient to call the nurse if pain occurs at the insertion site.

DOCUMENTATION

◆ Record the date, time, and location of I.V. access.
◆ Note the type, gauge, and length of the cannula or needle.
◆ Document the number of attempts at I.V. insertion.
◆ Document patient teaching provided and the patient's understanding of the teaching.

Procedures

Removing an I.V. catheter

To remove an I.V. catheter, follow these steps.
◆ Gather gloves, a gauze pad, an adhesive or pressure bandage, and normal saline solution.
◆ Clamp the I.V. tubing to stop the flow of solution.
◆ Put on gloves.
◆ Gently remove the transparent dressing and tape from the skin.
◆ Hold a sterile gauze pad over the puncture site with one hand; use the other to withdraw the cannula slowly, keeping it parallel to the skin.
◆ Inspect the cannula tip; if it isn't smooth, assess the patient immediately and notify the practitioner.
◆ Using the gauze pad, apply firm pressure over the puncture site for 1 to 2 minutes after removal or until bleeding stops.
◆ Clean the site with normal saline solution and apply the adhesive bandage or, if blood oozes, apply a pressure bandage.
◆ Tell the patient to restrict activity for about 10 minutes and to leave the dressing in place for at least 1 hour.
◆ If tenderness persists at the site, apply warm packs and notify the practitioner.

Pressure ulcer care

Overview

Pressure ulcer care involves relieving skin pressure, restoring circulation, promoting adequate nutrition, and resolving or managing related disorders. Care may require special pressure-reducing devices, such as beds, mattresses, mattress overlays, and chair cushions, decreasing risk factors, using topical treatments and dressings to support moist wound healing, wound cleansing, or debridement. Treatment effectiveness and duration depend on the pressure ulcer's characteristics.

Preprocedure care

♦ Explain the procedure to the patient and why it's necessary.
♦ Assemble equipment at the patient's bedside.

Procedure

Equipment: hypoallergenic tape or elastic netting ♦ overbed table ♦ piston-type irrigating system ♦ two pairs of gloves ♦ normal saline solution as ordered ♦ sterile 4″ × 4″ gauze pads ♦ sterile cotton swabs ♦ selected topical dressing ♦ linen-saver pads ♦ impervious plastic trash bag ♦ disposable wound-measuring device

♦ Cut the tape into strips.
♦ Wash your hands and put on gloves.
♦ Position the patient for comfort and easy access to site.
♦ Cover bed linens with a linen-saver pad to prevent soiling.
♦ Attach an impervious plastic trash bag to the overbed table.

CLEANING THE PRESSURE ULCER

♦ Pour normal saline solution carefully into a clean or sterile irrigation container and place the piston syringe in the container.
♦ Remove the old dressing and discard in the impervious plastic trash bag.

♦ Inspect the wound. Note the color, amount, and odor of any drainage or necrotic debris.
♦ Measure the wound perimeter with a disposable wound-measuring device.
♦ Apply full force of the piston syringe to irrigate the ulcer, remove necrotic debris, and decrease bacteria in the wound.
♦ Remove and discard your soiled gloves, and put on a fresh pair.
♦ Insert a gloved finger or sterile cotton swab into the wound to assess wound tunneling or undermining.
♦ Assess and note the condition of the clean wound and surrounding skin.
♦ Notify a wound care specialist if adherent necrotic material is present.
♦ Apply the appropriate topical dressing.
♦ After irrigating the wound, blot the surrounding skin dry.

APPLYING A MOIST SALINE GAUZE DRESSING

♦ Moisten the gauze dressing with normal saline solution.
♦ Gently place the dressing over the surface of the wound.
♦ To separate surfaces within the wound, gently place a dressing between opposing wound surfaces. Don't pack the gauze tightly.
♦ Change the dressing often enough to keep the wound moist.

APPLYING A HYDROCOLLOID DRESSING

♦ Choose a clean, dry, presized dressing, or cut one to overlap the pressure ulcer by about 1″ (2.5 cm).
♦ Remove the dressing from its package, remove the release paper, and apply the dressing to the wound. Carefully smooth wrinkles as you apply the dressing.
♦ If using tape to secure the dressing, apply a skin sealant to the intact skin around the ulcer.
♦ When dry, tape the dressing to the skin. Avoid tension or pressure.

♦ Change the hydrocolloid dressing every 2 to 7 days.
♦ Remove the dressing if signs of infection are present.

APPLYING A TRANSPARENT DRESSING
♦ Select a dressing to overlap the ulcer by 2″ (5 cm).
♦ Gently lay the dressing over the ulcer and press firmly on the edges of the dressing to promote adherence.
♦ Change the dressing every 3 to 7 days, depending on drainage.

APPLYING AN ALGINATE DRESSING
♦ Apply the alginate dressing to the ulcer surface. Cover it with a second dressing (such as gauze pads). Secure with tape or elastic netting.
♦ If drainage is heavy, change the dressing once or twice daily for the first 3 to 5 days.
♦ As drainage decreases, change the dressing less frequently—every 2 to 4 days or as ordered.
♦ When drainage stops or the wound bed looks dry, stop using the alginate dressing.

APPLYING A FOAM DRESSING
♦ Lay the foam dressing over the ulcer.
♦ Use tape, elastic netting, or gauze to hold the dressing in place.
♦ Change the dressing when the foam no longer absorbs the exudate.

APPLYING A HYDROGEL DRESSING
♦ Apply gel to the wound bed.
♦ Cover the area with a second dressing.
♦ Change the dressing as needed to keep the wound bed moist.
♦ If you choose a sheet form dressing, cut it to match the wound base.
♦ Hydrogel dressings also come in a prepackaged, saturated gauze to fill "dead space." Follow the manufacturer's directions for application.

Postprocedure care

♦ Provide measures to prevent formation of new pressure ulcers, or worsening of existing pressure ulcers, such as frequent repositioning of the patient and proper skin care.
♦ Follow prescribed wound care instructions.

MONITORING
♦ Assess the wound with each dressing change.
♦ Assess the dressing for drainage and intactness.

PATIENT TEACHING
♦ Teach the patient and family the importance of pressure ulcer prevention, position changes, and treatment. Teach the proper methods and encourage participation.
♦ Encourage the patient to follow a diet with adequate calories, protein, and vitamins.

DOCUMENTATION
♦ Record the date and time of initial and subsequent treatments.
♦ Document preventive strategies performed.
♦ Note the location, size (length, width, depth), color, and appearance of the ulcer.
♦ Record the amount, odor, color, and consistency of the drainage.
♦ Document the condition and temperature of surrounding skin.
♦ Reassess pressure ulcers at least weekly, and update the care plan.

Procedures

Prone positioning

Overview

Prone positioning, also known as *proning*, involves turning the patient from a supine to a face-down position. This positioning improves oxygenation and pulmonary mechanics by shifting blood flow to better ventilated regions of the lung and improving diaphragm movement by allowing the abdomen to expand more fully. The procedure, which is used for 6 or more hours per day for as long as 10 days, is used after acute onset of acute respiratory failure and for patients with acute lung injury, acute respiratory distress syndrome, or diffuse bilateral pulmonary infiltrates.

CONTRAINDICATIONS
♦ Increased intracranial pressure
♦ Spinal instability
♦ Unstable bone fractures
♦ Left-sided heart failure
♦ Shock
♦ Abdominal compartment syndrome
♦ Abdominal surgery
♦ Extreme obesity (weight greater than 300 lb [136 kg])
♦ Pregnancy
♦ Hemodynamic instability
♦ Inability to tolerate the face-down position

Preprocedure care

♦ Explain the procedure and why it's being done to the patient and his family.
♦ Check the practitioner's order.
♦ Assess the patient's hemodynamic and neurologic status.
♦ Wash your hands and put on gloves.

Procedure

Equipment: Vollman Prone Positioner or other prone-positioning device ♦ gloves
♦ Provide eye lubrication and taping of eyelid, if indicated.
♦ Protect the tongue with a bite block if edematous or protruding.

♦ Secure the endotracheal (ET) tube or tracheotomy tube.
♦ Perform anterior body wound care and dressing changes.
♦ Empty ileostomy or colostomy drainage bags.
♦ Reposition anterior electrocardiogram leads to the patient's back after he's prone.
♦ Engage the bed brake.
♦ Attach the surface of the prone positioner to the bed frame.

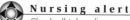 **Nursing alert**
Check all tubes, lines, and other equipment on the patient to prevent tangles.

♦ Stand on one side of the bed. Have other staff members stand on the other side of the bed and at the head of the bed.
♦ Position upper torso I.V. lines over the patient's right or left shoulder.
♦ Position chest tubes at the foot of the bed.
♦ Position lower torso lines at the foot of the bed.
♦ Turn the patient's face away from the ventilator, placing the ET tubing on the side of the patient's face that's turned away from the ventilator.
♦ Loop the remaining tubing above the patient's head.
♦ Place the straps under the patient's head, chest, and pelvic area.
♦ Attach the prone positioner by placing the frame on top of the patient.
♦ Position the chest piece to rest between the clavicles and sixth ribs.
♦ Adjust the pelvic piece so it rests ½″ (1.3 cm) above the iliac crest.
♦ Evaluate the distance between the chest and pelvic pieces to ensure suspension of the abdomen, while preventing bowing of the patient's back.
♦ Adjust the chin and forehead pieces to provide facial support in either a face-down or side-lying position without interfering with the ET tube.
♦ Fasten all adjustable straps on one side before tightening them on the opposite side. When secured, lift the positioner to ensure a secure fit.

- To help ensure a secure fit, look for cushion compression. If the frame isn't tightly secured, shear and friction injuries to the chest and pelvic area may occur.
- Lower the side rails.
- Move the patient with a draw sheet to the edge of the bed farthest from the ventilator.
- Tuck the straps to the center of the bed underneath the patient.
- Tuck the arm and hand, resting in the center of the bed, under the buttocks.
- Cross the leg closest to the edge of the bed over the opposite leg at the ankle.
- If the patient's arm can't be straightened and tucked under his buttocks, tuck the arm into the open space between the chest and pelvic pads.
- Turn the patient toward the ventilator at a 45-degree angle. Always turn the patient in the direction of the mechanical ventilator.
- The person on the side of the bed with the ventilator grasps the upper steel bar.
- The person on the other side grasps the lower steel bar or turning straps of the device.
- Lift the patient by the frame into the prone position.
- Move the patient's tucked arm and hand so they're comfortable.
- Loosen the straps if the patient is clinically stable.
- Support the patient's feet with a pillow or towel roll.
- Pad his elbows to prevent ulnar nerve compression.

RETURNING THE PATIENT TO SUPINE POSITION

- Fasten the positioning device straps securely.
- Position the patient on the edge of the bed closest to the ventilator.
- Adjust tubing and monitoring lines to prevent dislodgment.
- Straighten the patient's arms, and rest them on either side.
- Cross his leg closest to the edge of the bed over the opposite leg.
- Using the steel bars of the device, turn the patient to a 45-degree angle away from the ventilator, and then roll him to the supine position.
- Position the patient's arms parallel to his body.
- Unfasten the positioning device, and remove it from the patient.
- Discontinue prone positioning when the patient no longer demonstrates improved oxygenation with the position change as ordered.

Postprocedure care

- Obtain arterial blood gas values within $\frac{1}{2}$ hour of prone positioning and within $\frac{1}{2}$ hour before returning the patient to the supine position.
- Reposition the patient's head hourly.
- Perform range-of-motion exercises to shoulders, arms, and legs every 2 hours.
- Reposition the patient every 4 to 6 hours.
- Clean the prone positioner between turns and when discontinuing.

MONITORING

- Monitor the patient's vital signs, pulse oximetry, and mixed venous oxygen saturation.

PATIENT TEACHING

- Tell the patient to notify the nurse if he's unable to tolerate the procedure.

DOCUMENTATION

- Note the patient's response to the procedure.
- Record the patient's ability to tolerate the turning procedure.
- Document length of time prone positioning was used.
- Document the positioning schedule.
- Record monitoring findings, complications, and interventions performed.

Pulmonary artery pressure and pulmonary artery wedge pressure monitoring

Overview

Continuous pulmonary artery pressure (PAP) and intermittent pulmonary artery wedge pressure (PAWP) use a pulmonary artery (PA) catheter, also known as a *Swan-Ganz catheter,* to measure left ventricular function and preload. The PA catheter, which has up to six lumens, is inserted into the heart's right side with the distal tip lying in the pulmonary artery. PAP and PAWP monitoring is used to help diagnose conditions, refine assessments, guide interventions, and project patient outcomes. PAP monitoring is especially useful for patients with hemodynamic instability, shock, trauma, pulmonary or cardiac disease, or multiorgan disease, for patients who require multiple cardioactive drugs, and for fluid management and continuous cardiopulmonary assessment.

Preprocedure care

◆ Confirm the patient's identity using two patient identifiers according to facility policy.
◆ Explain the procedure and why it's being done to the patient.
◆ Confirm informed consent has been obtained.
◆ Check the patient's chart for heparin sensitivity, which contraindicates adding heparin to the flush solution.
◆ Assemble equipment and bring it to the patient's bedside.

Procedure

Equipment: introducer (one size larger than the catheter) ◆ sterile tray containing instruments for the procedure ◆ masks ◆ sterile gowns ◆ sterile gloves ◆ sterile drapes ◆ povidone-iodine ointment and solution ◆ sutures ◆ two 10-ml syringes ◆ anesthetic (1% to 2% lidocaine) ◆ one 5-ml syringe, 25G ½" needle ◆ balloon-tipped, flow-directed PA catheter ◆ prepared pressure transducer system ◆ I.V. solutions ◆ alcohol pads ◆ monitor and monitor cable ◆ I.V. pole with transducer mount ◆ emergency resuscitation equipment ◆ electrocardiogram (ECG) monitor ◆ ECG electrodes ◆ sterile 4" × 4" gauze pads, or other dry, occlusive dressing material ◆ small sterile basin ◆ sterile water ◆ optional: prepackaged introducer kit, dextrose 5% in water

◆ Obtain the necessary pressure modules and place them in the monitor.
◆ Prepare the pressure monitoring system (see *Priming monitoring tubing,* p. 360).
◆ Calibrate and zero the pressure monitoring system.
◆ Position the patient at the proper height and angle.
◆ When using the superior approach, place the patient in a flat, slight Trendelenburg position, and remove the pillow, then turn the patient's head to the side opposite the insertion site.
◆ When using the inferior approach, place the patient in a supine position.

INSERTING THE CATHETER
◆ Put on gloves and a mask.
◆ Clean the insertion site with a povidone-iodine solution, and drape it.
◆ Help the practitioner put on a sterile mask, gown, and gloves.
◆ Open the outer packaging of catheter, revealing the inner sterile wrapping.
◆ The practitioner opens the inner wrapping and picks up the catheter.
◆ Take the catheter lumen hubs as he hands them to you.
◆ Flush the catheter to remove air and verify patency, or flush the lumens with ster-

ile I.V. solution from sterile syringes attached to the lumens. Leave the filled syringes on during insertion.

◆ For multiple pressure lines, ensure the distal PA lumen hub is attached to the pressure line being monitored.

◆ Observe the diastolic values as the practitioner inserts the catheter.

◆ Set the scale on the monitor for lower pressures. A scale of 0 to 25 mm Hg or 0 to 50 mm Hg (more common) is preferred.

◆ To verify the integrity of the balloon, the practitioner inflates it with air (usually 1.5 cc) and submerges it in a small, sterile basin filled with sterile water.

◆ Attach it to the pressure monitoring system after it's handed to you.

◆ The practitioner injects lidocaine solution to the area where the catheter will be inserted.

◆ Assist the practitioner as he inserts the introducer to access the vessel.

◆ After the introducer is placed and the catheter lumens are flushed, the practitioner inserts the PA catheter through the introducer with the balloon deflated.

◆ As insertion begins, observe the bedside monitor for waveform variations.

◆ When the catheter exits the end of the introducer sheath and reaches the junction of the superior vena cava and right atrium at the 15- to 20-cm mark on the catheter shaft, the monitor shows oscillations that correspond to the patient's respirations.

◆ Inflate the balloon when directed as the practitioner advances it through the heart.

◆ Note right ventricle pressure. As the catheter is advanced into the pulmonary artery, note PAWP waveform, or wedge tracing, that appears when the catheter has been inserted 45 to 50 cm.

◆ Deflate the balloon as directed. The practitioner will secure the PA catheter with a suture.

◆ Apply a sterile occlusive dressing to the insertion site.

◆ Level and rezero the pressure monitoring system.

OBTAINING INTERMITTENT PAP VALUES

◆ After PA catheter insertion, record subsequent PAP values and monitor waveforms per facility policy or practitioner order.

◆ To ensure accurate values, make sure the transducer is properly leveled and zeroed.

◆ If possible, obtain PAP values at end expiration (when the patient completely exhales) to avoid respiratory interference.

◆ Obtain a printout of the digital readings over time and readings obtained during a full respiratory cycle.

◆ Use the averaged values obtained through the full respiratory cycle.

◆ To analyze trends accurately, record values at consistent times during the respiratory cycle.

TAKING A PAWP READING

◆ PAWP is recorded by inflating the balloon and letting it float in a distal artery.

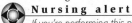 **Nursing alert**

If you're performing this procedure, do so with extreme caution, and make sure you're familiar with interpreting intracardiac waveforms.

◆ Verify that the transducer is properly leveled and zeroed.

◆ Detach the syringe from the balloon inflation hub.

◆ Draw 1.5 cc of air into the syringe, then reattach the syringe to the hub.

◆ Watching the monitor, inject the air through the hub slowly and smoothly.

♦ When you see a wedge tracing on the monitor, immediately stop inflating the balloon.

Nursing alert

Never inflate the balloon beyond the volume needed to obtain a wedge tracing. Overinflation may cause loss of elasticity or balloon rupture.

♦ Take the pressure reading at end expiration.

♦ Note the amount of air needed to change the pulmonary artery tracing to a wedge tracing, which is normally 1.25 to 1.5 cc.

♦ Detach the syringe from the balloon inflation port, and allow the balloon to deflate on its own.

Nursing alert

Never leave the balloon inflated; doing so may cause pulmonary infarction.

♦ Observe the waveform tracing, and make sure the tracing returns from the wedge tracing to the normal pulmonary artery tracing.

REMOVING THE CATHETER

♦ Only remove a PA catheter as permitted by facility policy.

♦ Inspect the chest X-ray for signs of catheter kinking or knotting.

♦ Obtain baseline vital signs and note the ECG pattern.

♦ Place the head of the bed flat, unless ordered otherwise.

♦ If the catheter was inserted using a superior approach, turn the patient's head to the side opposite the insertion site.

♦ Remove the dressing and any sutures securing the catheter.

♦ Turn off all stopcocks to the patient.

♦ You may turn on stopcocks to the distal port if you wish to observe waveforms. However, use caution because doing so may cause an air embolism.

♦ After verifying that the balloon is deflated, withdraw the catheter slowly and smoothly.

♦ If there's resistance, stop withdrawal.

♦ Watch the ECG monitor for arrhythmias.

♦ If the introducer was removed, apply pressure to the site, and check it frequently for signs of bleeding.

♦ Dress the site as necessary.

♦ If the introducer is left in place, observe the diaphragm for blood backflow, which verifies the integrity of the hemostasis valve.

♦ Turn off the bedside pressure modules but leave the ECG module on.

Postprocedure care

♦ Obtain a chest X-ray after catheter insertion to verify its position and to check for pneumothorax.

♦ Change the dressing whenever it's moist or every 24 to 48 hours; initial and date the dressings when changed.

♦ Re-dress the site and change tubing and flush solutions per facility policy.

MONITORING

♦ Monitor wave forms and readings per facility policy or practitioner order.

♦ Monitor for hemodynamic changes after treatment.

PATIENT TEACHING

♦ Advise the patient to use caution when moving in bed.

♦ Explain all procedures to the patient to lessen his anxiety.

DOCUMENTATION

♦ Record the date and time of catheter insertion.

♦ Document the name of the practitioner who performed the procedure.

♦ Document the location of the catheter insertion site.

♦ Record pressure waveforms and values for various heart chambers.

♦ Document the balloon inflation volume required to obtain a wedge tracing.

♦ Document arrhythmias that occurred during or after procedure.

◆ Record the type of flush solution used and its heparin concentration.
◆ Document the type of dressing applied.
◆ Document the patient's tolerance of the procedure.
◆ After catheter removal, document the patient's tolerance of the procedure, and note problems encountered.

Procedures

Pulse oximetry

Overview

A noninvasive technique, pulse oximetry uses a photodetector placed on the nailbed or ear to measure mixed venous oxygen saturation. It can be used intermittently or continuously to monitor arterial oxygen saturation (Sao_2). (See *How oximetry works.*) Normal Sao_2 levels for pulse oximetry are 95% to 100% for adults and 93.8% to 100% by 1 hour after birth for healthy, full-term neonates.

Preprocedure care

◆ Explain the procedure and why it's necessary.
◆ Assemble the equipment and bring it to the bedside.

Procedure

Equipment: oximeter ◆ finger or ear probe ◆ alcohol pads ◆ nail polish remover if necessary

USING A FINGER PROBE

◆ Select a finger (usually the index finger) for the test.
◆ Remove false fingernails and nail polish from the test finger.
◆ Place the photodetector probe over the patient's finger so the light beams and sensors oppose each other.
◆ Position the probe perpendicular to the finger.

◆ Turn on the power switch. If the device is working properly, a beep will sound, a display will light momentarily, and the pulse searchlight will flash.
◆ After four to six heartbeats, the pulse amplitude indicator will begin tracking the pulse.
◆ In a patient with continuous pulse oximetry monitoring, move the probe every 2 hours to decrease the risk of damaging the digits.

USING AN EAR PROBE

◆ Using an alcohol pad, massage the patient's earlobe for 10 to 20 seconds.
◆ Securely attach one end of the probe cord to the patient's earlobe or pinna and attach the other end of the cord to the monitor.
◆ After a few seconds, a saturation reading and pulse waveform will appear on the oximeter's screen.
◆ Leave the ear probe in place for 3 or more minutes.
◆ If ear pigment is a problem, reposition the probe, revascularize the site, or use a finger probe.

TROUBLESHOOTING

◆ Use the bridge of the nose if the patient has compromised circulation in his extremities.
◆ If light is a problem, cover the probes.
◆ If patient movement is a problem, move the probe or select a different probe.

Postprocedure care

◆ With intermittent readings or when discontinuing continuous readings, remove a nondisposable probe and clean it with an alcohol pad. Discard or recycle a disposable probe.
◆ Notify the practitioner of any significant change in the patient's condition.

MONITORING
◆ Monitor readings and arterial blood gas results as ordered.

PATIENT TEACHING
◆ Review activity precautions to prevent inaccurate readings.

DOCUMENTATION
◆ Note the date and time of the procedure, oxygen saturation, and nursing actions performed.
◆ Record the reading on appropriate flowcharts if indicated.

How oximetry works

The pulse oximeter allows noninvasive monitoring of a patient's arterial oxygen saturation (Sao_2) levels by measuring absorption of light waves as they pass through areas of the body that are highly perfused by arterial blood. Oximetry also monitors pulse rate and amplitude.

Light-emitting diodes in a transducer (photodetector) attached to the patient's body (shown below at right on the index finger) send red and infrared light beams through tissue. The photodetector records the relative amount of each color absorbed by arterial blood and transmits the data to a monitor, which displays the information with each heartbeat. If the Sao_2 level or pulse rate varies from preset limits, the monitor triggers visual and audible alarms.

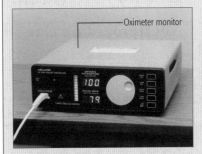

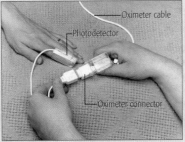

Rectal tube insertion and removal

Overview

A rectal tube relieves the discomfort of abdominal distention and flatus, which may result from various medical or surgical conditions, swallowed air, or use of medications such as atropine sulfate.

CONTRAINDICATIONS
◆ Recent rectal or prostate surgery
◆ Recent myocardial infarction
◆ Diseases of the rectal mucosa

Preprocedure care

◆ Confirm the patient's identity using two patient identifiers according to facility policy.
◆ Explain the procedure and why it's being done to the patient.
◆ Check for a practitioner's order.
◆ Bring all equipment to the patient's bedside, provide privacy, and wash your hands.

Procedure

Equipment: stethoscope ◆ linen-saver pads ◆ drape ◆ water-soluble lubricant ◆ commercial kit or #22 to #32 French rectal tube of soft rubber or plastic ◆ container, such as emesis basin, plastic bag, or water bottle with vent ◆ tape ◆ gloves ◆ drainage bag

◆ Check for abdominal distention.
◆ Using the stethoscope, auscultate for bowel sounds.
◆ Place the linen-saver pads under the patient's buttocks to absorb drainage that may leak from the tube.
◆ Position the patient in the left-lateral Sims' position to facilitate rectal tube insertion.

◆ Put on gloves.
◆ Drape the patient's exposed buttocks.
◆ Lubricate the rectal tube tip with water-soluble lubricant.
◆ Lift the patient's right buttock to expose the anus.
◆ Insert the rectal tube tip into the anus, advancing the tube 2″ to 4″ (5 to 10 cm) into the rectum. Direct the tube toward the umbilicus along the anatomic course of the large intestine.
◆ As you insert the tube, tell the patient to breathe slowly and deeply, or suggest that he bear down as he would for a bowel movement to relax the anal sphincter and ease insertion.
◆ Using tape, secure the rectal tube to the buttocks.
◆ Attach the tube to the drainage bag to collect possible leakage.
◆ Remove the tube after 15 to 20 minutes.
◆ If the patient reports continued discomfort or if gas wasn't expelled, repeat the procedure in 2 or 3 hours, if ordered.

Postprocedure care

◆ Clean the patient, and replace soiled linens and the linen-saver pad.
◆ Discard the disposable tube.
◆ If the tube isn't disposable, clean the tube and store it in the bedside cabinet.
◆ Repeat insertion periodically to stimulate GI activity.
◆ If the tube fails to relieve distention, notify the practitioner.

MONITORING
◆ Monitor GI status.

PATIENT TEACHING
◆ Inform the patient about each step of the procedure.
◆ Reassure the patient during the procedure to encourage cooperation and promote relaxation.

DOCUMENTATION
◆ Record the date and time that you insert the tube.
◆ Document the amount, color, and consistency of any evacuated matter.
◆ Document GI assessment findings from before and after the procedure.
◆ Document patient teaching provided and the patient's understanding of teaching.

Sequential compression therapy

Overview

Sequential compression therapy counteracts blood stasis and coagulation changes—two of the three major factors that promote deep vein thrombosis (DVT)—using noninvasive sequential compression sleeves and a sequential compression device. The sleeves massage the legs in a wavelike, milking motion that promotes blood flow and deters thrombosis, helping to empty pooled or static blood from the valve cusps of the femoral vein. Fibrinolytic activity increases, stimulating the release of a plasminogen activator. This therapy typically complements other preventive measures, such as antiembolism stockings and anticoagulant medications.

CONTRAINDICATIONS

◆ Acute DVT or DVT diagnosed within the past 6 months
◆ Severe arteriosclerosis or other ischemic vascular disease
◆ Massive leg edema resulting from pulmonary edema or heart failure
◆ Dermatitis
◆ Vein ligation
◆ Gangrene
◆ Recent skin grafting

Preprocedure care

◆ Explain the procedure and why it's necessary to the patient.
◆ Wash your hands.

Procedure

Equipment: measuring tape ◆ sizing chart for the sleeve brand ◆ pair of compression sleeves in correct size ◆ connecting tubing ◆ compression controller
◆ To determine the proper size of sleeve, measure the circumference of the upper thigh.

◆ Hold the tape snugly, but not tightly, under the patient's thigh at the gluteal furrow.
◆ Find the patient's thigh measurement on the sizing chart and locate the corresponding size of the compression sleeve.
◆ Remove the compression sleeves from the package and unfold them.
◆ Lay the unfolded sleeves on a flat surface with the cotton lining facing up.
◆ Position the sleeve at the appropriate ankle or knee landmark.

APPLYING THE SLEEVES

◆ Place the patient's leg on the sleeve lining; position the back of the knee over the popliteal opening.
◆ Make sure that the back of the ankle is over the ankle marking.
◆ Starting at the side opposite the clear plastic tubing, wrap the sleeve snugly around the patient's leg.
◆ Fasten the sleeve securely with the Velcro fasteners starting at the ankle and then moving to the calf and thigh.
◆ Check the fit by inserting two fingers between the sleeve and the patient's leg at the knee opening.
◆ Using the same procedure, apply the second sleeve.

OPERATING THE SYSTEM

◆ Connect both sleeves to the tubing leading to the controller.
◆ Line up the blue arrows on the sleeve connector with the arrows on the tubing connectors and push the ends together firmly.
◆ Listen for a click, signaling a firm connection. Make sure that the tubing isn't kinked.
◆ Plug the compression controller into the proper wall outlet. Turn on the controller.
◆ The controller automatically sets the compression sleeve pressure at 45 mm Hg, which is the midpoint of the normal range (35 to 55 mm Hg).

◆ The green light on the audible alarm key should be lit.

◆ The compression sleeves should function continuously (24 hours daily) until the patient is fully ambulatory.

◆ Check sleeves once each shift to ensure proper fit and inflation.

◆ Switch on cooling device for comfort measures or to help with increased temperature.

◆ Respond to instrument alarms appropriately and follow the manufacturer's recommendations.

TO REMOVE THE SLEEVES

◆ Depress the latches on each side of the connectors and pull the connectors apart.

◆ Store the tubing and compression controller according to facility protocol.

Postprocedure care

◆ Observe the patient to see how well he tolerated therapy.

MONITORING

◆ Monitor sleeve pressure.

◆ Assess skin every 4 hours or per facility policy.

◆ Monitor distal pulses.

◆ Observe for signs and symptoms of DVT.

PATIENT TEACHING

◆ Explain the importance of complying with sequential compression therapy.

◆ Tell the patient signs and symptoms of DVT and pulmonary embolism to report.

DOCUMENTATION

◆ Record the date and time the device and sleeves were applied.

◆ Note the type of sleeve used (knee- or thigh-length).

◆ Document the patient's response to and understanding of the procedure.

◆ Record the maximum sequential compression device inflation pressure and the patient's blood pressure.

◆ Note the reason for removing the sequential compression device along with the length of time it was removed.

◆ Document the status of the alarm and cooling settings.

◆ Document findings from assessing skin and lower extremity circulation, including distal pulses.

◆ Provide a rationale if only one leg sleeve is applied.

Skin staple and clip removal

Overview

Skin staples or clips are a quicker way than standard sutures to close lacerations or surgical wounds when cosmetic results aren't a prime consideration. They're made from surgical stainless steel to minimize tissue reaction. Proper placement of staples and clips distributes tension evenly along the suture line, minimizes tissue trauma and compression, promotes healing, and minimizes scarring.

CONTRAINDICATIONS

◆ Wound location requiring cosmetically superior results
◆ Incision site location that doesn't maintain a minimum of 5-mm distance between the staple and underlying bone, vessels, or internal organs

Preprocedure care

◆ Confirm the patient's identity using two patient identifiers according to facility policy.
◆ Explain the procedure and why it's being done to the patient.
◆ Check for patient allergies, especially to adhesive tape and povidone-iodine or other topical solutions or drugs.
◆ Assemble the equipment in the patient's room.

Procedure

Equipment: waterproof trash bag ◆ adjustable light ◆ clean gloves ◆ sterile gloves if needed ◆ sterile gauze pads ◆ sterile staple or clip extractor ◆ povidone-iodine solution or other antiseptic cleaning agent ◆ sterile cotton-tipped applicators ◆ optional: butterfly adhesive strips or adhesive strips
◆ Check the expiration date on each sterile package and inspect for tears.
◆ Open the waterproof trash bag and place it near the patient's bed.

◆ Position the bag to avoid reaching across the sterile field.
◆ Form a cuff by turning down the top of the bag to provide a wide opening.
◆ Position the patient to promote comfort and avoid undue tension on the incision. Have him recline to avoid nausea or dizziness.
◆ Adjust the light to shine directly on the incision.
◆ Wash your hands.
◆ Put on clean gloves and carefully remove the dressing, if present.
◆ Discard the dressing and gloves in the waterproof trash bag.
◆ Assess the patient's incision.
◆ Notify the practitioner of gaping, drainage, inflammation, and other signs of infection.
◆ Establish a sterile work area.
◆ Open the package containing the sterile staple or clip extractor.
◆ Put on sterile gloves.
◆ Remove surface encrustations by gently wiping the incision with sterile gauze pads soaked in an antiseptic cleaning agent or with sterile cotton-tipped applicators.
◆ Starting at one end of the incision, remove the staple or clip (see *Removing a staple*).
◆ Hold the extractor over the trash bag, and release the handle to discard the staple or clip.
◆ Repeat the procedure for each staple or clip.
◆ Apply a sterile gauze dressing if needed.
◆ Discard your gloves.
◆ Properly dispose of solutions, soiled supplies, and the trash bag, and clean soiled equipment.

Postprocedure care

◆ Make sure that the patient is comfortable.
◆ Inform the patient that he may shower in 1 or 2 days if the incision is dry and healing well.

◆ Butterfly strips or adhesive strips may be applied after removing staples or clips (even if the wound is healing normally) to give added support and prevent lateral tension from forming a wide scar.

MONITORING
◆ Monitor the wound.

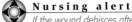

Nursing alert

If the wound dehisces after staples or clips are removed, apply butterfly adhesive strips or adhesive strips to approximate and support the edges, and call the practitioner immediately.

PATIENT TEACHING
◆ Teach the patient how to remove the dressing and care for the wound after staple removal.
◆ Instruct the patient to call the practitioner immediately if he observes wound discharge or other abnormal changes.
◆ Tell the patient that the redness surrounding the incision should gradually disappear and that, after a few weeks, only a thin line should show.

DOCUMENTATION
◆ Record the date and time of staple or clip removal.
◆ Note the number of staples or clips removed.
◆ Document the appearance of the incision and dressings or butterfly strips applied.
◆ Record signs of wound complications.
◆ Note the patient's tolerance of the procedure.
◆ Document patient teaching provided and the patient's understanding of the teaching.

Removing a staple

Position the extractor's lower jaws beneath the span of the first staple, as shown below.

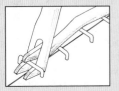

Squeeze the handles until they're completely closed, and then lift the staple away from the skin, as shown below. The extractor changes the shape of the staple and pulls the prongs out of the intradermal tissue.

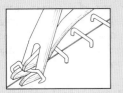

Procedures

ST segment monitoring

Overview

ST segment monitoring assesses the ST segment for changes that indicate cardiac distress or damage. This procedure is helpful for patients with acute coronary syndromes and those who have received thrombolytic therapy or undergone coronary angioplasty. It also allows early detection of reocclusion, and is useful for patients with a history of cardiac ischemia without chest pain, those who have difficulty distinguishing cardiac pain from pain associated with other sources, and those who have difficulty communicating.

ST segments are normally flat or isoelectric. A depressed ST segment may result from cardiac glycosides, myocardial ischemia, or a subendocardial infarction. An elevated ST segment suggests myocardial infarction.

Preprocedure care

◆ Explain the procedure and why it's being done to the patient.
◆ Plug the cardiac monitor into an electrical outlet.
◆ If the patient isn't already on a monitor, turn on the device and attach the cable.

Procedure

Equipment: electrocardiogram (ECG) electrodes ◆ gauze pads ◆ ECG monitor cable ◆ leadwires ◆ alcohol pads ◆ cardiac monitor programmed for ST segment monitoring ◆ indelible ink marker
◆ Select the sites for electrode placement and prepare the patient's skin.
◆ Attach the leadwires to the electrodes and position the electrodes on the patient's skin.
◆ Activate the cardiac monitor by pressing the MONITORING PROCEDURES key and then the ST key.

◆ Activate individual ST-segment parameters by pressing the ON/OFF PARAMETER key.
◆ Select the appropriate ECG to be monitored for each ST-segment channel by pressing the PARAMETERS key and then the ECG key.
◆ Press the CHANGE LEAD key to select the appropriate lead. Repeat this for all three channels.
◆ Adjust the ST-segment measurement points and baseline.
◆ Adjust the J point by pressing the J POINT key to move the cursor to the appropriate location.
◆ Adjust the ST point to 80 msec after the J point.
◆ Check facility policy for measuring the ST point. Some facilities recommend using 60 msec instead of 80 msec.
◆ Set the alarm limits for each ST-segment parameter by manipulating the high limit and low limit keys.
◆ Set the ST alarm parameter 1 to 2 mm above and below the patient's baseline ST-segment level, or as ordered by the practitioner, and measure ST-segment changes 60 msec beyond the J point of the ECG.
◆ Press the STANDARD DISPLAY key to return to the display screen.
◆ Assess the waveform shown on the monitor.

Postprocedure care

◆ Select the most appropriate lead by examining ECG tracings obtained during an ischemic episode.
◆ If monitoring only one lead, choose the lead most likely to show arrhythmias and ST-segment changes.
◆ Mark the electrode placement with an indelible ink marker.
◆ If the patient isn't being monitored continuously, remove the electrodes, clean the skin, and disconnect the leadwires from the electrodes.

MONITORING

◆ Evaluate the monitor for ST-segment depression or elevation (see *Understanding ST-segment changes*).

PATIENT TEACHING

◆ Answer the patient's questions as necessary.

DOCUMENTATION

◆ Record the leads being monitored.
◆ Document ST-segment measurement points.

Understanding ST-segment changes

Closely monitoring the ST segment can help detect ischemia or injury before infarction develops.

ST-segment elevation

An ST segment is considered elevated when it's 1 mm or more above the baseline. An elevated ST segment may indicate myocardial injury.

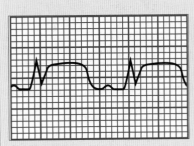

ST-segment depression

An ST segment is considered depressed when it's 0.5 mm or more below the baseline. A depressed ST segment may indicate myocardial ischemia or digoxin toxicity.

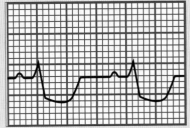

Procedures

Suture removal

Overview

Suture removal from a healed wound is a sterile procedure generally done 7 to 10 days after insertion. Removal timing depends on the shape, size, and location of the sutured incision; the absence of inflammation, drainage, and infection; and the patient's general condition. Removal techniques depend on the method of suturing and the ability to avoid damaging newly formed tissue.

CONTRAINDICATIONS
◆ Insufficient wound healing

Preprocedure care

◆ Confirm the patient's identity using two patient identifiers according to facility policy.
◆ Explain the procedure and why it's being done to the patient.
◆ Check the practitioner's order to confirm details of the procedure.
◆ If retention and regular sutures are in place, check the practitioner's order for the removal sequence.
◆ Check for patient allergies, especially to adhesive tape, povidone-iodine, or other topical solutions or drugs.
◆ Assemble equipment in the patient's room.

Procedure

Equipment: prepackaged, sterile suture-removal tray if available ◆ waterproof trash bag ◆ adjustable light ◆ clean gloves if the wound is dressed ◆ sterile gloves ◆ sterile forceps or sterile hemostat ◆ normal saline solution ◆ sterile gauze pads ◆ sterile curve-tipped suture scissors ◆ optional: adhesive butterfly strips or adhesive strips, compound benzoin tincture or other skin protectant
◆ Check the expiration date on each sterile package and inspect for tears.

◆ Open the waterproof trash bag, and place it near the patient's bed to avoid reaching across the sterile field or suture line when disposing of soiled articles.
◆ Turn down the top of the trash bag to provide a wide opening and prevent contamination of instruments or gloves by touching the bag's edge.
◆ Position the patient so he's comfortable without placing undue tension on the suture line.
◆ To avoid nausea or dizziness, have the patient recline.
◆ Adjust the light so it shines directly on the suture line.
◆ Wash your hands.
◆ Put on clean gloves and remove the dressing if present.
◆ Discard the dressing and gloves in the waterproof trash bag.
◆ Observe the wound for gaping, drainage, inflammation, signs of infection, or embedded sutures.
◆ Notify the practitioner if the wound has failed to heal properly.
◆ Establish a sterile work area with needed equipment and supplies.
◆ Open the suture removal tray if you're using one.
◆ Put on sterile gloves.
◆ Using sterile technique, clean the suture line, which moistens the sutures to ease removal.
◆ Soften the sutures further, if needed, with normal saline solution.
◆ Proceed according to the type of suture you're removing.
◆ Carefully clean the suture line before removing sutures to decrease the risk of infection when the visible, contaminated part of the stitch is too small to cut twice for sterile removal and must be pulled through the tissue.
◆ Cut sutures at the skin surface on one side.
◆ Lift and pull the visible end off the skin.
◆ If ordered, remove every other suture to maintain support for the incision, and then go back and remove remaining sutures.

Procedures

◆ After suture removal, wipe the incision with gauze pads soaked in normal saline solution.

◆ Apply a light, sterile gauze dressing if needed.

 Nursing alert

If the wound dehisces during suture removal, apply butterfly adhesive strips or adhesive strips to support and approximate the edges. Call the practitioner immediately to repair the wound.

◆ Discard your gloves.

◆ Properly dispose of the solutions and trash bag; clean or dispose of soiled equipment and supplies.

Postprocedure care

◆ Make sure that the patient is comfortable.

◆ According to the practitioner's preference, inform the patient that he may shower in 1 or 2 days if the incision is dry and heals well.

◆ Apply butterfly adhesive strips or adhesive strips after suture removal for added support of the incision line and prevention of wide scar formation.

MONITORING

◆ After removing mattress sutures, monitor the suture line for subsequent infection.

PATIENT TEACHING

◆ Before discharge, teach the patient how to remove the dressing and care for the wound.

◆ Instruct the patient to call the practitioner immediately if he observes wound discharge or other abnormal change.

◆ Tell the patient that the redness surrounding the incision should gradually disappear with only a thin line remaining after a few weeks.

DOCUMENTATION

◆ Record the date and time of suture removal.

◆ Note the type and number of sutures removed and the appearance of the suture line.

◆ Record signs of wound complications.

◆ Record whether dressings or butterfly strips were applied.

◆ Document the patient's tolerance of the procedure.

◆ Document patient teaching provided and the patient's understanding of the teaching.

Thoracic electrical bioimpedance monitoring

Overview

Thoracic electrical bioimpedance monitoring tracks hemodynamic status, providing information about a patient's cardiac index, preload, afterload, heart contractility, cardiac output, and blood flow. A noninvasive procedure, thoracic electrical bioimpedance monitoring eliminates the risk of infection, bleeding, pneumothorax, emboli, and arrhythmias associated with traditional invasive monitoring. Electrodes placed on the patient's thorax send harmless low-level electricity through the body and detect electrical signals from changes in the volume and velocity of blood as it flows through the aorta. A bioimpedance monitor interprets these signals as a waveform. Cardiac output is computed from the thoracic fluid content and the heart rate on the electrocardiogram (ECG). Monitoring accuracy is comparable to the thermodilution method of measuring cardiac output. (See "Cardiac output measurement," page 372.)

Preprocedure care

◆ Confirm the patient's identity using two patient identifiers according to facility policy.
◆ Explain the procedure and why it's necessary to the patient.
◆ Wash your hands and put on gloves.
◆ Plug the thoracic electrical bioimpedance unit into a power supply.
◆ Press the POWER button, and the initial display screen will appear.
◆ Press the RUN key on the display screen, and the patient data screen will appear.
◆ Enter patient data by pressing each patient data block on the screen. When you select metric or English for numbers, male or female, and adult or pediatric-neonate, a dot will appear beside your choice.
◆ To enter data for identification number, thoracic length, height, and weight, press the block that identifies the index desired; the numeric keypad screen will appear.
◆ Enter the actual value for the index by pressing the smaller blocks on the keypad, and then press ENTER to return to the patient data screen. Repeat for each index needed.
◆ Press the block on the patient data screen to call up the waveform screen to monitor patient status.
◆ The waveform screen displays an ECG and a pulmonary artery pressure waveform as well as six parameters that you choose by pressing PARAMETERS.
◆ When the parameter screen appears, press the blocks labeled with the parameters you wish to display on the waveform screen.
◆ Press the block at the bottom of the parameter screen to return to the waveform screen. All of the selected parameters will now appear on the waveform screen.

Procedure

Equipment: thoracic electrical bioimpedance unit ◆ patient harness with color-coded leadwires ◆ connecting cable ◆ four sets of thoracic electrical bioimpedance electrodes ◆ three ECG electrodes ◆ 3″ × 3″ or 4″ × 4″ gauze pads ◆ tape measure ◆ gloves
◆ Assist the patient onto his back and provide privacy.
◆ Expose the patient's chest.
◆ Wet the 4″ × 4″ or 3″ × 3″ gauze pads with warm water and clean the skin on each side of the patient's neck from the base to 2″ (5 cm) above the base. Clean the skin on both sides of his chest at the midaxillary line directly across the xiphoid process.
◆ Clean at least two fingerbreadths above and below the site.
◆ Place one electrode set vertically at the neck base below the ear with the arrow

end (containing the round electrode) pointing down.

◆ Place the bar electrode at least 2″ (5 cm) above the round electrode.

◆ If the two electrodes are an attached set, place the bar electrode directly above the round one.

◆ Place the second set of electrodes on the opposite side of the neck in line with the ear and about 180 degrees from the first set.

◆ Place the remaining two sets of electrodes on either side of the patient's chest.

◆ To determine the correct location, draw a line with your finger from the xiphoid process to the midaxillary line on one side of the chest. This is the site for the first chest electrode. Place the round electrode here with the arrow pointing up.

◆ Place the second (bar) electrode at least 2″ (5 cm) below the first. Alternatively, if you're using an attached set of electrodes, place the bar electrode directly below the round one.

◆ Place the final set of electrodes on the midaxillary line directly opposite the first set of electrodes.

◆ Attach the ECG electrodes and try different lead selections until you obtain a consistent QRS signal.

◆ Attach the leadwires of the bioimpedance harness to the thoracic electrical bioimpedance electrodes and the ECG electrodes.

◆ Attach the harness cable to the cable from the bioimpedance monitor.

◆ Measure the distance between the round electrode on one side of the patient's neck and the round electrode on the same side of his chest. This distance (thorax length) is the numeric value required by the monitor's computer to calculate accurate stroke volume.

◆ Call up the patient data screen and enter this value, and then return to the waveform screen.

Postprocedure care

◆ Answer any questions the patient may have.

 Nursing alert

Baseline bioimpedance values may be reduced in patients who have conditions characterized by increased fluid in the chest, such as pulmonary edema and pleural effusion. Bioimpedance values may be lower than thermodilution values in patients with tachycardia and other arrhythmias.

MONITORING

◆ Monitor values before and after treatment.

◆ Monitor waveform and hemodynamic values.

PATIENT TEACHING

◆ Review activity precautions.

DOCUMENTATION

◆ Note the waveforms and values on the monitor and document the values by pressing PRINT on the waveform screen.

◆ Place the printed strip on the patient's chart.

Procedures

Total parenteral nutrition administration

Overview

Total parenteral nutrition (TPN) is a nutrient solution that's administered through a central venous line inserted in the superior vena cava, or through a peripherally inserted central catheter. TPN is typically prescribed for a patient who is unable to absorb nutrients though the GI tract for more than 10 days. The solution contains protein, carbohydrates, electrolytes, vitamins, and trace minerals. A lipid emulsion may also be added to provide necessary fat.

CONTRAINDICATIONS
- Normally functioning GI tract
- Normal GI function to resume within 10 days
- Poor prognosis

Preprocedure care

- Confirm the patient's identity using two patient identifiers according to facility policy.
- Explain the procedure and why it's needed to the patient.
- Prepare the solution, patient, and equipment.
- Remove the solution from the refrigerator at least 1 hour before use to avoid pain, hypothermia, venous spasm, or venous constriction from chilled solution.
- Check the solution against the practitioner's order for correct patient name, expiration date, and formula components. Verify this information with another nurse.
- Observe the container for cracks and the solution for cloudiness, turbidity, and particles; if present, return the solution to the pharmacy.
- If giving a total nutrient admixture solution, look for a brown layer on the solution, which indicates that the lipid emulsion has "cracked," or separated from the

solution. If you see a brown layer, return the solution to the pharmacy.

Procedure

Equipment: bag or bottle of prescribed parenteral nutrition solution ◆ sterile I.V. tubing with attached extension tubing ◆ 0.22-micron filter (or 1.2-micron filter if solution contains lipids or albumin) ◆ reflux valve ◆ alcohol pads ◆ electronic infusion pump ◆ portable glucose monitor ◆ scale ◆ intake and output record ◆ sterile gloves ◆ optional: mask
- Verify the patient's name matches the name on the solution container.
- Put on gloves and, if specified by policy, a mask. Throughout the procedure, use strict sterile technique.
- In sequence, connect the pump tubing, the micron filter with attached extension tubing (if the tubing doesn't contain an in-line filter), and the reflux valve.
- Insert the filter as close to the catheter site as possible.
- If the tubing doesn't have luer-lock connections, tape all connections to prevent separation, which could lead to air embolism, exsanguination, and sepsis.
- Squeeze the I.V. drip chamber and, holding the drip chamber upright, insert the tubing spike into the I.V. bag or bottle.
- Release the drip chamber, and prime the tubing.
- Invert the filter at the distal end of the tubing, open the roller clamp, and let the solution fill the tubing and the filter. Tap it to dislodge air bubbles in the Y-ports.
- Record the date and time you hang the fluid, and initial the parenteral nutrition solution container.
- Attach the setup to the infusion pump, and prepare it according to the manufacturer's instructions. Remove and discard gloves.
- With the patient supine, flush the catheter with normal saline solution, ac-

cording to facility policy. Put on gloves and clean the catheter injection cap with an alcohol pad.

◆ If the container of parenteral nutrition solution is attached to a central venous line, clamp the central venous line before disconnecting it to prevent air from entering the catheter.

◆ Using sterile technique, attach tubing to the designated luer-locking port.

◆ After connecting the tubing, remove the clamp if applicable.

◆ Set the infusion pump at the ordered flow rate, and start the infusion.

Postprocedure care

◆ Check to make sure the catheter junction is secure; tag tubing with date and time of the tubing change.

◆ Record daily intake and output accurately, specifying volume and type of each fluid, and calculate daily caloric intake.

◆ Change the dressing over the catheter according to facility policy or whenever the dressing becomes wet, soiled, or nonocclusive.

Monitoring

◆ Monitor the patient's vital signs every 4 hours or more often, if necessary. Watch for increased temperature, an early sign of catheter-related sepsis.

◆ Check the patient's glucose level every 6 hours. Some patients may require supplementary insulin, either subcutaneously or added to the solution.

◆ Monitor results of routine laboratory tests; report abnormal findings to the practitioner.

◆ Obtain daily weight, monitoring for changes.

◆ Monitor the catheter site for swelling, which may indicate infiltration.

 Nursing alert

Extravasation of parenteral nutrition solution may lead to tissue necrosis.

Patient teaching

◆ Explain that long-term parenteral nutrition may be given at home and reduces the need for long hospitalizations.

◆ Teach the patient about potential adverse effects and complications, such as infiltration and infection.

◆ Encourage the patient to inspect his mouth regularly for signs of parotitis, glossitis, and oral lesions.

◆ Explain to the patient that he may have fewer bowel movements while receiving therapy.

◆ Encourage the patient to remain physically active to help his body use nutrients more fully.

Documentation

◆ Document verification of the TPN solution.

◆ Record the date and time of dressing, filter, and solution changes.

◆ Document the condition of the catheter insertion site.

◆ Document assessments of the patient's condition.

◆ Record complications and interventions performed.

Tracheal suction

Overview

Tracheal suction removes secretions from the trachea or bronchi by means of a catheter inserted through the mouth or nose, tracheal stoma, a tracheostomy tube, or an endotracheal (ET) tube. This procedure is performed as frequently as the patient's condition warrants and calls for strict sterile technique.

Preprocedure care

◆ Explain the procedure and why it's necessary to the patient.

Procedure

Equipment: oxygen source or handheld resuscitation bag ◆ 15-mm adapter or a positive end-expiratory pressure (PEEP) valve if indicated ◆ wall or portable suction apparatus ◆ collection container ◆ connecting tube ◆ suction catheter kit or a sterile suction catheter, sterile gloves, goggles, and a disposable sterile solution container ◆ 1 L bottle of sterile water or normal saline solution ◆ sterile water-soluble lubricant (for nasal insertion) ◆ syringe for deflating cuff of ET or tracheostomy tube ◆ waterproof trash bag

◆ Choose a suction catheter of appropriate size.
◆ Attach the collection container to the suction unit and the connecting tube to the collection container.
◆ Label and date the normal saline solution or sterile water.
◆ Open the waterproof trash bag.
◆ Assess the patient's vital signs, breath sounds, and appearance to establish a baseline.
◆ If performing nasotracheal suctioning, check for a deviated septum, nasal polyps, nasal obstruction, nasal trauma, epistaxis, or mucosal swelling.
◆ Wash your hands and put on protective equipment.

◆ Unless contraindicated, put the patient in semi-Fowler's or high Fowler's position.
◆ Remove the top from the normal saline solution or water bottle, and open the package containing the sterile solution container.
◆ Using strict sterile technique, open the suction catheter kit or individual supplies and put on gloves.
◆ Using your nondominant (nonsterile) hand, pour the normal saline solution or sterile water into the solution container.
◆ Place a small amount of water-soluble lubricant on the sterile area to facilitate passage of the catheter during nasotracheal suctioning.
◆ Using your dominant (sterile) hand, remove the catheter from its wrapper. Keep it coiled so it can't touch a nonsterile object. Using your other hand to manipulate the connecting tubing, attach the catheter to the tubing.
◆ Using your nondominant hand, set the suction pressure according to facility policy; typically between 80 and 120 mm Hg. Occlude the suction port to assess suction pressure.
◆ Dip the catheter tip in saline solution to lubricate the outside of the catheter. For nasal insertion, lubricate the catheter tip with the sterile, water-soluble lubricant.
◆ If the patient isn't intubated, instruct him to take three to six deep breaths.
◆ If he's being mechanically ventilated, preoxygenate him using either a handheld resuscitation bag or the ventilator.
◆ To use the resuscitation bag, set the oxygen flow meter at 15 L/minute, disconnect the patient from the ventilator, and deliver three to six breaths with the bag.
◆ To preoxygenate using the ventilator, adjust the fraction of inspired oxygen (F_{IO_2}) and tidal volume per facility policy.

SUCTIONING A NONINTUBATED PATIENT

◆ Disconnect the oxygen from the patient if applicable.

◆ Using your nondominant hand, raise the tip of the patient's nose.
◆ Insert the catheter into his nostril while rolling it between your fingers.
◆ As he inhales, quickly advance the catheter as far as possible.
◆ If the patient coughs as the catheter passes through the larynx, briefly hold the catheter still, then resume advancement when the patient inhales.

SUCTIONING AN INTUBATED PATIENT
◆ If you're using a closed system, the closed tracheal suctioning technique may be used.
◆ Using your nonsterile hand, disconnect the patient from the ventilator.
◆ Using your sterile hand, insert the suction catheter into the artificial airway.
◆ Advance the catheter, without applying suction, until you meet resistance.
◆ If the patient coughs, pause, and then resume advancement.
◆ Apply suction intermittently by removing and replacing the thumb of your nondominant hand over the control valve, being sure not to apply suction more than 10 seconds at a time.
◆ Simultaneously, use your dominant hand to withdraw the catheter as you roll it between your thumb and forefinger to prevent tissue damage.
◆ Use your nondominant hand to stabilize the ET tube tip as you withdraw the catheter.
◆ Resume oxygen delivery to hyperoxygenate the patient's lungs.
◆ Allow the patient to rest a few minutes before the next suctioning.
◆ Encourage the patient to cough between suctioning attempts.
◆ If secretions are thick, clear the catheter periodically by dipping the tip in the normal saline solution and applying suction.
◆ Observe the amount, color, and consistency of sputum.

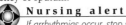
Nursing alert
If arrhythmias occur, stop suctioning and ventilate the patient.

AFTER SUCTIONING
◆ Hyperoxygenate the patient maintained on a ventilator with the handheld resuscitation bag or by using the ventilator's sigh mode and readjust the F_{IO_2}.
◆ After suctioning the lower airway, assess the need for upper airway suctioning.
◆ If the cuff of the ET or tracheostomy tube is inflated, suction the upper airway before deflating the cuff with a syringe.
◆ Discard the gloves and the catheter in the waterproof trash bag.
◆ Clear connecting tubing by aspirating the remaining normal saline solution or water.

Postprocedure care
◆ Wash your hands.
◆ Auscultate the lungs bilaterally and take vital signs, if indicated, to assess the procedure's effectiveness.

MONITORING
◆ Monitor cardiac rhythm, pulse oximetry, and respiratory status.

PATIENT TEACHING
◆ Tell the patient that suctioning usually causes transient coughing or gagging, but that coughing will help remove secretions.
◆ Teach deep-breathing and coughing exercises if appropriate.

DOCUMENTATION
◆ Record the date and time of the procedure, the technique used, and the reason for the procedure.
◆ Document the amount, color, consistency, and odor of secretions.
◆ Record complications and nursing actions performed.
◆ Document the patient's response to the procedure.

Procedures

Tracheostomy care

Overview

Tracheostomy care ensures airway patency by keeping the tracheostomy tube free of mucus buildup. It also maintains mucous membrane and skin integrity, prevents infection, and provides psychological support. Tracheostomy tubes may be uncuffed, cuffed, or fenestrated. An uncuffed plastic or metal tube allows air to flow freely around the tracheostomy tube and through the larynx, reducing risk of tracheal damage. A plastic cuffed tube is disposable, and the cuff and the tube won't separate inside the trachea because the cuff is bonded to the tube. This tube type doesn't require periodic deflating to lower pressure because cuff pressure is low and evenly distributed against the tracheal wall, reducing the risk of tracheal damage. A plastic fenestrated tube permits speech through the upper airway when the external opening is capped and the cuff is deflated. It also allows easy removal of the inner cannula for cleaning, but it may become occluded.

Preprocedure care

◆ Explain the procedure and why it's necessary to the patient.
◆ Wash your hands.

Procedure

ASEPTIC STOMA AND OUTER-CANNULA CARE

Equipment: waterproof trash bag ◆ two sterile solution containers ◆ sterile normal saline solution ◆ hydrogen peroxide ◆ sterile cotton-tipped applicators ◆ sterile 4″ × 4″ gauze pads ◆ sterile gloves ◆ prepackaged sterile tracheostomy dressing (or 4″ × 4″ gauze pad) ◆ supplies for suctioning and mouth care ◆ water-soluble lubricant or topical antibiotic cream ◆ materials for changing tracheostomy ties (see below)

ASEPTIC INNER-CANNULA CARE

Equipment: all preceding equipment plus a prepackaged commercial tracheostomy care set or sterile forceps ◆ sterile nylon brush ◆ sterile 6″ (15-cm) pipe cleaners ◆ clean gloves ◆ a third sterile solution container ◆ disposable temporary inner cannula (for a patient on a ventilator)

CHANGING TRACHEOSTOMY TIES

Equipment: 30″ (76.2-cm) length of tracheostomy twill tape ◆ bandage scissors ◆ sterile gloves ◆ hemostat

EMERGENCY TRACHEOSTOMY TUBE REPLACEMENT

Equipment: sterile tracheal dilator or sterile hemostat ◆ sterile obturator that fits the tracheostomy tube ◆ extra, appropriate-sized, sterile tracheostomy tube and obturator ◆ suction equipment and supplies

CUFF PROCEDURES

Equipment: 5- or 10-ml syringe ◆ padded hemostat ◆ stethoscope
◆ Check the expiration date on each sterile package and inspect for tears.
◆ Place the open waterproof trash bag next to you to avoid reaching across the sterile field or the patient's stoma when discarding soiled items.
◆ Establish a sterile field near the patient's bed and place equipment and supplies on it.
◆ Pour normal saline solution, hydrogen peroxide, or a mixture of equal parts of both solutions into one of the sterile solution containers; pour normal saline solution into the second sterile container for rinsing.
◆ For inner-cannula care, use a third sterile solution container to hold the gauze pads and cotton-tipped applicators saturated with cleaning solution.
◆ If replacing the disposable inner cannula, open the package containing the new inner cannula while maintaining sterile technique.

◆ Obtain or prepare new tracheostomy ties if indicated.

◆ Keep supplies in full view for easy emergency access. Consider taping a wrapped, sterile tracheostomy tube to the head of the bed for emergencies.

◆ Place the patient in semi-Fowler's position, unless contraindicated, to decrease abdominal pressure on the diaphragm and promote lung expansion.

◆ Remove the humidification or ventilation device.

◆ Using sterile technique, suction the entire length of the tracheostomy tube to clear the airway of secretions that may hinder oxygenation.

◆ Reconnect the patient to the humidifier or ventilator if necessary.

CLEANING A STOMA AND OUTER CANNULA

◆ Put on sterile gloves.

◆ With your dominant hand, saturate a sterile gauze pad or cotton-tipped applicator with the cleaning solution.

◆ Squeeze out excess liquid to prevent accidental aspiration.

◆ Wipe the patient's neck under the tracheostomy tube flanges and twill tapes.

◆ Saturate a second pad or applicator, and wipe until the skin surrounding the tracheostomy is cleaned. Use additional pads or cotton-tipped applicators to clean the stoma site and the tube's flanges.

◆ Rinse debris and peroxide, if used, with one or more sterile 4″ × 4″ gauze pads dampened in normal saline solution.

◆ Dry the area thoroughly with additional sterile gauze pads, and then apply a new sterile tracheostomy dressing. Remove and discard your gloves.

CLEANING A NONDISPOSABLE INNER CANNULA

◆ Put on sterile gloves. Using your nondominant hand, remove and discard the patient's tracheostomy dressing.

◆ With the same hand, disconnect the ventilator or humidification device, and unlock the tracheostomy tube's inner cannula by rotating it counterclockwise.

◆ Place the inner cannula in the container of hydrogen peroxide.

◆ Working quickly, use your dominant hand to scrub the cannula with the sterile nylon brush.

◆ If the brush doesn't slide easily into the cannula, use a sterile pipe cleaner.

◆ Immerse the cannula in the container of normal saline solution, and agitate it for about 10 seconds to rinse it.

◆ Inspect the cannula for cleanliness. Repeat the cleaning process if necessary.

◆ When the cannula is clean, tap it against the inside edge of the sterile container to remove excess liquid and prevent aspiration.

◆ Reinsert the inner cannula into the patient's tracheostomy tube.

◆ Lock it in place and make sure it's positioned securely. Reconnect the mechanical ventilator. Apply a new sterile tracheostomy dressing.

◆ If the patient can't tolerate being disconnected from the ventilator for the time it takes to clean the inner cannula, replace the existing inner cannula with a clean one and reattach the mechanical ventilator. Then clean the cannula just removed and store it in a sterile container for the next time.

CARING FOR A DISPOSABLE INNER CANNULA

◆ Put on clean gloves. Using your dominant hand, remove the inner cannula.

◆ After evaluating the secretions in the cannula, discard it properly.

◆ Pick up the new inner cannula, touching only the outer locking portion. Insert the cannula into the tracheostomy and, following manufacturer's instructions, lock it securely.

CHANGING TRACHEOSTOMY TIES

♦ Get help from another nurse or a respiratory therapist to avoid accidental tube expulsion. Patient movement or coughing may dislodge the tube.

♦ Wash your hands, and put on sterile gloves if you aren't already wearing them.

♦ If you aren't using commercially packaged tracheostomy ties, prepare new ties from a 30″ (76.2 cm) length of twill tape by folding one end back 1″ (2.5 cm) on itself and then, with bandage scissors, cutting a ½″ (1.3-cm) slit down the center of the tape from the folded edge.

♦ Prepare the other end of the tape the same way.

♦ Hold both ends together and cut the resulting circle of tape so one piece is about 10″ (25.5 cm) long and the other is about 20″ (51 cm) long.

♦ After your assistant puts on gloves, instruct her to hold the tracheostomy tube in place to prevent expulsion during replacement of the ties. (If performing without assistance, fasten the clean ties in place before removing the old ties to prevent tube expulsion.)

♦ With the assistant's gloved fingers holding the tracheostomy tube in place, cut the soiled tracheostomy ties with bandage scissors or untie them and discard.

♦ Thread the slit end of one new tie a short distance through the eye of one tracheostomy tube flange from the underside; use the hemostat, if needed, to pull the tie through. Thread the other end of the tie completely through the slit end and pull it taut so it loops firmly through the flange. Doing so avoids knots that can cause throat discomfort, tissue irritation, pressure, and necrosis.

♦ Fasten the second tie to the opposite flange in the same manner.

♦ Instruct the patient to flex his neck while you bring the ties around to the side, and tie them together with a square knot. Flexion produces the same neck circumference as coughing and helps prevent an overly tight tie.

♦ Have your assistant place one finger under the tapes as you tie them to ensure they're tight enough to avoid slippage but loose enough to prevent choking or jugular vein constriction.

♦ Place the closure on the side to allow easy access and prevent pressure necrosis at the back of the neck when the patient is recumbent.

♦ After securing the ties, cut off excess tape with scissors and have your assistant release the tracheostomy tube.

DEFLATING AND INFLATING A TRACHEOSTOMY CUFF

♦ Read the cuff manufacturer's instructions; cuff types and procedures vary.

♦ Suction the oropharyngeal cavity to prevent pooled secretions from descending into the trachea after cuff deflation.

♦ Release the padded hemostat clamping the cuff inflation tubing if a hemostat is present.

♦ Insert a 5- or 10-ml syringe into the cuff pilot balloon and slowly withdraw all air from the cuff. Leave syringe attached to tubing for cuff reinflation.

♦ Slow deflation allows positive lung pressure to push secretions upward from the bronchi. Cuff deflation may also stimulate the cough reflex, producing additional secretions.

♦ Remove the ventilation device and suction the lower airway through the existing tube to remove all secretions.

♦ Reconnect the patient to the ventilation device.

♦ Maintain cuff deflation for the prescribed time.

♦ Observe for adequate ventilation, and suction as necessary.

♦ If the patient has difficulty breathing, reinflate the cuff immediately by depressing the syringe plunger very slowly.

♦ Use a stethoscope to listen over the trachea for the air leak, then inject as little air as necessary to achieve an adequate tracheal seal.

◆ When inflating the cuff, you may use the minimal-leak technique or the minimal occlusive volume technique to help gauge the proper inflation point.

◆ If you're inflating the cuff using cuff pressure measurement, don't exceed 25 mm Hg to prevent tissue damage.

◆ After you've inflated the cuff, if the tubing doesn't have a one-way valve at the end, clamp the inflation line with a padded hemostat and remove the syringe.

◆ Check for a minimal-leak cuff seal. You shouldn't feel air coming from the patient's mouth, nose, or tracheostomy site, and a conscious patient shouldn't be able to speak.

◆ Be alert for air leaks from the cuff itself.

◆ Note the exact amount of air used to inflate the cuff to detect tracheal malacia if more air is consistently needed.

Postprocedure care

◆ Provide oral care as needed because the oral cavity can become dry and malodorous or develop sores from encrusted secretions.

◆ Observe soiled dressings and suctioned secretions for amount, color, consistency, and odor. Properly clean or dispose of equipment, supplies, solutions, and trash. Remove and discard your gloves.

◆ Make sure the patient is comfortable and can reach the call button easily.

◆ Make sure necessary supplies are readily available at the bedside.

◆ Repeat the procedure at least once every 8 hours or as needed.

◆ Change the dressing as often as necessary.

◆ Follow facility policy if a tracheostomy tube is expelled or the outer cannula becomes blocked. If breathing is obstructed, call the appropriate code and provide manual resuscitation with a handheld resuscitation bag or reconnect the patient to the ventilator. Don't remove the tracheostomy tube; the airway may close completely. Use caution when reinserting, to avoid tracheal trauma, perforation, compression, and asphyxiation.

MONITORING

◆ Monitor skin around stoma for signs of breakdown.

◆ Monitor pulse oximetry while performing tracheostomy care.

PATIENT TEACHING

◆ If the patient will be discharged with a tracheostomy, start self-care teaching as soon as he's receptive.

◆ Teach the patient how to change and clean the tube.

◆ If the patient is being discharged with suction equipment, make sure he and his family are knowledgeable and comfortable about using the equipment.

DOCUMENTATION

◆ Record the date and time the procedure was performed.

◆ Describe the amount, consistency, color, and odor of secretions.

◆ Document the condition of the stoma and skin.

◆ Document that the practitioner changed the tracheostomy tube.

◆ Record the duration of cuff deflation.

◆ Document the amount of cuff inflation.

◆ List complications and nursing actions performed.

◆ Document patient and family teaching performed and their understanding of teaching.

◆ Record the patient's tolerance of the treatment.

Transcranial Doppler monitoring

Overview

Transcranial Doppler monitoring monitors blood flow in the intracranial vessels, specifically the circle of Willis, using a continuous waveform obtained by a Doppler unit. A noninvasive procedure, Transcranial Doppler monitoring helps detect intracranial stenosis, vasospasm, and arteriovenous malformations and assess collateral pathways in patients who have experienced cerebrovascular disorders, such as stroke, head trauma, or subarachnoid hemorrhage. It can also be used for intraoperative monitoring of cerebral circulation, monitoring the effect of intracranial pressure changes on cerebral circulation, evaluating patient response to various drugs, evaluating carbon dioxide reactivity (which may be impaired or lost from arterial obstruction or trauma), and confirming brain death.

Preprocedure care

◆ Confirm the patient's identity using two patient identifiers according to facility policy.
◆ Explain the procedure and why it's necessary to the patient and his family.
◆ Assemble the equipment and bring it to the bedside.
◆ Place the patient in the proper position (usually supine).
◆ Remove head dressings over the test site.

Procedure

Equipment: transcranial Doppler unit ◆ transducer with an attachment system ◆ terry cloth headband ◆ ultrasonic coupling gel ◆ marker
◆ Turn the Doppler unit on and watch as it performs a self-test.
◆ Enter the patient's name and identification number in the unit; additional information, such as diagnosis or practitioner's name, may also need to be entered.

◆ Indicate the vessel you wish to monitor (usually the right or left middle cerebral artery [MCA]) and set the approximate depth of the vessel within the skull (50 mm for the MCA).
◆ Use the keypad to increase the power level to 100% to initially locate the signal. You can later decrease the level as needed, depending on skull thickness.
◆ Visualize the three windows of the transtemporal access route: posterior, middle, and anterior.
◆ Apply ultrasonic gel at the level of the temporal bone between the tragus of the ear and the end of the eyebrow, over the area of the three windows.
◆ Place a transducer on the posterior window, angling it slightly in an anterior direction, slowly moving in a narrow circle (the "flashlighting" technique).
◆ During flashlighting, slowly move the transducer forward across the temporal area, listening for the audible signal with the highest pitch. This sound corresponds to the highest velocity signal of the vessel you're assessing.
◆ Headphones allow you to better evaluate the audible signal and provide the patient privacy.
◆ After locating the highest-pitched signal, draw a circle around the transducer head on the patient's temple.
◆ Note the angle of the transducer so you can duplicate it after the transducer attachment system is in place.
◆ Place the plate of the transducer attachment system over the patient's temporal area, matching the circular opening in the plate exactly with the circle on his head.
◆ Holding the plate in place, encircle the patient's head with the straps attached to the system.
◆ Tighten the straps so the transducer attachment system stays in place.
◆ Fill the circular opening in the plate with the ultrasonic gel.
◆ Place the transducer in the gel-filled opening in the attachment system plate.

♦ Using plastic screws provided, loosely secure the two plates together to hold the transducer in place, while allowing it to rotate for the best angle.

♦ Adjust the transducer's position and angle until you again hear the highest-pitched audible signal.

♦ On the monitor you should see a clear waveform with a bright white line (an envelope) at its upper edge. The envelope exactly follows the contours of the waveform.

♦ If the envelope doesn't follow the waveform's contours, adjust the gain setting.

♦ If the signal is wrapping around the screen, use the scale key to increase the scale and the baseline key to drop the baseline.

♦ When you have the strongest, highest-pitched signal and the best waveform, lock the transducer in place by tightening the plastic screws. The tightened plates will hold the transducer at the angle you've chosen.

♦ Disconnect the transducer handle.

♦ Place a wide terry cloth headband over the transducer attachment system, and secure it around the patient's head to provide additional stability for the transducer.

♦ You should be able to see a waveform on the monitor and read the numeric values of the peak, mean velocities, and pulsatility index above the displayed waveform. The shape of the waveform reveals more information.

Postprocedure care

♦ Establish a baseline for the mean velocity; as velocity increases or decreases, the value (%) will change negatively or positively from the baseline.

♦ Be aware that emboli appear as high-intensity transients occurring randomly during the cardiac cycle, making a distinctive "clicking," "chirping," or "plunking" sound.

♦ You may set up an emboli counter to count either the total number of emboli aggregates or the rate of embolic events per minute.

♦ Various screens may be stored on the system's hard drive and may be recalled or printed.

MONITORING
♦ Monitor vital signs during the procedure.

PATIENT TEACHING
♦ Review activity restrictions during the test.

DOCUMENTATION
♦ Record the date and time monitoring began and which artery was monitored.

♦ Document patient teaching provided as well as the patient's understanding of the teaching.

Tube feedings

Overview

Tube feedings involve delivering a liquid formula directly to the stomach (known as *gastric gavage*), duodenum, or jejunum. They're indicated for the patient who can't eat normally because of dysphagia or oral or esophageal obstruction or injury. Duodenal or jejunal feedings decrease the risk of aspiration because the formula bypasses the pylorus. Jejunal feedings reduce pancreatic stimulation, so they may require an elemental diet.

CONTRAINDICATIONS
◆ Absent bowel sounds
◆ Suspected intestinal obstruction

Preprocedure care

◆ Confirm the patient's identity using two patient identifiers according to facility policy.
◆ Explain the procedure and why it's necessary to the patient and his family.
◆ Check the practitioner's order.
◆ Confirm the correct formula on the container and note the delivery rate.

Procedure

GASTRIC FEEDINGS
Equipment: feeding formula ◆ graduated container ◆ 120 ml of water ◆ gavage bag with tubing and flow regulator clamp ◆ towel or linen-saver pad ◆ 60-ml syringe ◆ pH test strip ◆ adapter to connect gavage tubing to feeding tube ◆ optional (for continuous administration): infusion controller and tubing set

DUODENAL OR JEJUNAL FEEDINGS
Equipment: feeding formula ◆ enteral administration set containing a gavage container, drip chamber, roller clamp or flow regulator, and tube connector ◆ I.V. pole ◆ 60-ml syringe with adapter tip ◆ water ◆ Y-connector ◆ pump administration set (optional, for an enteral infusion pump)

◆ Shake the container well to mix the formula thoroughly, and allow the formula to warm to room temperature before administering it.
◆ Pour 60 ml of water into the graduated container.
◆ After closing the flow clamp on the administration set, pour the appropriate amount of formula into the gavage bag or attach administration set to the infusion bottle.
◆ Open the flow clamp on the administration set to remove air from the lines.
◆ If the patient has a nasal or oral tube, cover his chest with a towel or linen-saver pad.
◆ Assess his abdomen for bowel sounds and distention.
◆ Elevate the bed to semi-Fowler's or high Fowler's position.

DELIVERING A GASTRIC FEEDING
◆ Check the feeding tube for proper placement and patency. Remove the cap or plug from the feeding tube, and attach the syringe.
◆ Gently aspirate gastric secretions.
◆ Examine the aspirate and place a small amount of it on the pH test strip. Proper placement of the gastric tube is likely if the aspirate has a typical gastric fluid appearance (grassy-green, clear and colorless with mucus shreds, or brown) and a pH of 5 or less.
◆ To assess gastric emptying, aspirate and measure residual gastric contents. Hold feedings if residual volume is greater than the predetermined amount specified in the practitioner's order (usually 50 to 100 ml). Reinstill any aspirate obtained.
◆ Connect the gavage bag tubing to the feeding tube.
◆ If using a bulb or catheter-tip syringe, remove the bulb or plunger and attach the syringe to the pinched-off feeding tube to prevent excess air from entering the patient's stomach, causing distention.
◆ If using an infusion controller, thread the tube from the formula container through

Procedures

the controller according to the manufacturer's directions, and attach it to the feeding tube.

◆ Open the regulator clamp on the gavage bag tubing and adjust the flow rate appropriately.

◆ When using a bulb syringe, fill the syringe with formula and release the feeding tube to allow formula to flow through it, typically 200 to 350 ml over 15 to 30 minutes, depending on the patient's tolerance and the practitioner's order. The height at which you hold the syringe will determine flow rate. Continue to fill the syringe until the dose is complete.

◆ If you're using an infusion controller, set the flow rate according to the manufacturer's directions.

◆ After giving the appropriate amount of formula, flush the tubing by adding about 60 ml of water to the gavage bag or bulb syringe, or manually flush it using a barrel syringe.

◆ To discontinue gastric feeding (depending on the equipment), close the regulator clamp on the gavage bag tubing, disconnect the syringe from the feeding tube, or turn off the infusion controller.

◆ Cover the end of the feeding tube with its plug or cap to prevent leakage and contamination.

Postprocedure care

◆ Leave the patient in semi-Fowler's or high Fowler's position for at least 30 minutes after delivering a feeding.

◆ If you're giving a continuous feeding, flush the feeding tube every 4 hours. A needle catheter jejunostomy tube may require flushing every 2 hours to prevent formula buildup inside the tube.

◆ Rinse reusable equipment with warm water. Dry and store equipment in a convenient place for the next feeding. Change equipment every 24 hours or according to facility policy.

◆ Provide or assist with oral care every 4 hours.

MONITORING

◆ Monitor gastric emptying every 4 hours.

◆ Assess the patient's hydration status; increase fluid intake as ordered.

◆ Monitor the flow rate of a blended or high-residue formula to determine if the formula is clogging the tubing as it settles. To prevent such clogging, squeeze the bag frequently to agitate the solution.

◆ Monitor the patient's blood glucose levels to assess glucose tolerance.

◆ Monitor electrolytes, blood urea nitrogen, glucose, and osmolality to determine response to therapy and assess hydration status.

◆ Monitor stools and GI status.

PATIENT TEACHING

◆ Teach the patient about the infusion control device to maintain accuracy, use of the syringe or bag and tubing, care of the tube and insertion site, and formula-mixing.

◆ Teach family members signs and symptoms to report to the practitioner or home care nurse as well as measures to take in an emergency.

DOCUMENTATION

◆ On the intake and output sheet, record the date and the volume of formula and volume of water used.

◆ Record abdominal assessment findings; amount of residual gastric contents; verification of tube placement; amount, type, and time of feeding; and tube patency.

◆ Note the result of blood and urine tests, hydration status, and drugs given through the tube.

◆ Record the date and time of administration set changes and oral and nasal hygiene.

◆ Record laboratory results of specimen collections.

Venipuncture

Overview

Venipuncture uses a needle to pierce a vein to collect a blood sample into a syringe or an evacuated tube. Laboratory personnel or nurses with proper training perform the procedure on a vein in the antecubital fossa, dorsal forearm, dorsum of the hand or foot, or other accessible location.

Preprocedure care

◆ Confirm the patient's identity using two patient identifiers according to facility policy.
◆ Explain the procedure and why it's being done to the patient.
◆ Assemble the equipment and bring it to the bedside.
◆ Ask the patient if he's ever felt faint, sweaty, or nauseated when having blood drawn. If he's on bed rest, ask him to lie supine with his head slightly elevated and his arms at his sides.
◆ Ask the ambulatory patient to sit in a chair and support his arm securely on an armrest or table.

Procedure

Equipment: tourniquet ◆ gloves ◆ syringe or evacuated tubes and needle holder ◆ alcohol or povidone-iodine pads ◆ 20G or 21G needle for the forearm or 25G needle for the wrist, hand, and ankle and for children ◆ color-coded collection tubes containing appropriate additives ◆ labels ◆ laboratory request form ◆ 2″ × 2″ gauze pads ◆ adhesive bandage
◆ Wash your hands and put on gloves.
◆ If you're using evacuated tubes, open the needle packet, attach the needle to its holder, and select the appropriate tubes.
◆ If you're using a syringe, attach the appropriate needle to it.
◆ Choose a syringe large enough to hold all the blood required for the test.

◆ Label all collection tubes clearly with the patient's name and room number, the practitioner's name, and date and time of collection.
◆ Assess the patient's veins to determine the best puncture site.
◆ Tie a tourniquet 2″ (5 cm) proximal to the area chosen.
◆ Observe the skin for the vein's blue color, or palpate the vein for a firm rebound sensation.
◆ If the tourniquet fails to dilate the vein, have the patient open and close his fist a few times. Then ask him to close his fist as you insert the needle and open it again when the needle is in place.
◆ Clean the venipuncture site with an alcohol or povidone-iodine pad using a side-to-side motion.
◆ If you use alcohol, apply it with friction for 30 seconds, or until the final pad comes away clean.
◆ Allow the skin to dry before performing the venipuncture.
◆ Press just below the venipuncture site with your thumb and draw the skin taut. Ask the patient to form a fist.
◆ Position the needle holder or syringe with the needle bevel up and the shaft parallel to the path of the vein and at a 30-degree angle to the arm.
◆ Insert the needle into the vein. Ask the patient to release his fist.
◆ If using a syringe, blood will appear in the hub; withdraw the blood slowly, pulling the plunger of the syringe gently to create steady suction until you obtain the required sample. Pulling the plunger forcibly may collapse the vein.
◆ If using a needle holder and an evacuated tube, grasp the holder securely to stabilize it in the vein; push down on the collection tube until the needle punctures the rubber stopper. Blood will flow into the tube automatically.
◆ Remove the tourniquet as soon as blood flows adequately to prevent stasis and hemoconcentration, which can impair test results.

◆ Continue to fill the required tubes, removing one and inserting another.

◆ Rotate each tube as you remove it to help mix the additive with the sample.

◆ After you've obtained enough blood, place a gauze pad over the puncture site, and slowly remove the needle from the vein.

◆ When using an evacuated tube, remove it from the needle holder to release the vacuum before withdrawing the needle from the vein.

◆ Apply gentle pressure to the puncture site for 2 or 3 minutes or until bleeding stops, then apply an adhesive bandage.

◆ If you've used a syringe, transfer the sample to a collection tube.

◆ Detach the needle from the syringe, open the collection tube, and empty the sample into the tube, being careful to avoid foaming, which can cause hemolysis.

◆ Discard syringes, needles, and used gloves in appropriate containers.

Postprocedure care

◆ Send the blood samples to the laboratory.

MONITORING

◆ Check the venipuncture site again; apply pressure if the site shows signs of bleeding.

PATIENT TEACHING

◆ Tell the patient to notify the nurse if he detects signs of rebleeding from the venipuncture site.

DOCUMENTATION

◆ Record the date, time, and site of venipuncture.

◆ Note the name of the test and the time the sample was sent to the laboratory.

◆ Document adverse reactions to the procedure.

Wound irrigation

Overview

Wound irrigation cleans tissues and flushes cell debris and drainage from an open wound. This procedure helps a wound heal properly from the inside tissue layers outward to the skin surface and prevents premature surface healing over an abscess pocket or infected tract. Strict sterile technique is required. After irrigation, open wounds are usually packed to absorb additional drainage.

Preprocedure care

◆ Confirm the patient's identity using two patient identifiers according to facility policy.
◆ Explain the procedure to the patient and why it's necessary.
◆ Check the practitioner's order, and assess the patient's condition.
◆ Identify the patient's allergies, especially to povidone-iodine or other topical solutions or drugs.
◆ Assemble the equipment in the patient's room.

Procedure

Equipment: waterproof trash bag ◆ linen-saver pad ◆ emesis basin ◆ clean gloves ◆ sterile gloves ◆ goggles ◆ gown, if indicated ◆ prescribed irrigant such as sterile normal saline solution ◆ sterile water ◆ soft rubber or plastic catheter ◆ sterile container ◆ materials as needed for wound care ◆ sterile irrigation and dressing set ◆ 35-ml piston syringe with 19G needle or catheter ◆ skin protectant wipe
◆ Using sterile technique, dilute the prescribed irrigant to the correct proportions with sterile water or normal saline solution if necessary.
◆ Position the waterproof trash bag to avoid reaching across the sterile field or the wound when disposing of soiled items. Turn down the top of the trash bag to pro-

vide a wide opening, preventing contamination by touching the bag's edge.
◆ Place the linen-saver pad under the patient.
◆ Wash your hands and put on gloves, goggles, and gown.
◆ Place the emesis basin below the wound so irrigating solution flows from the wound into the basin.
◆ Remove the soiled dressing; discard the dressing and your gloves in the trash bag.
◆ Establish a sterile field with the equipment and supplies you'll need for irrigation and wound care.
◆ Pour the prescribed amount of irrigating solution into a sterile container.
◆ Put on sterile gloves.
◆ Fill the syringe with irrigating solution; connect the catheter to the syringe.
◆ Instill a slow, steady stream of irrigating solution into the wound until the syringe empties.
◆ Make sure the solution reaches all areas of the wound and flows from the clean to the dirty area of the wound to prevent contamination of clean tissue.
◆ Refill the syringe, reconnect it to the catheter, and repeat irrigation.
◆ Continue to irrigate the wound until you've given the prescribed amount of solution or until the solution returns clear.
◆ Remove and discard the catheter and syringe.
◆ Keep the patient positioned to allow further wound drainage into the basin.
◆ Clean the area around the wound with normal saline solution; wipe intact skin with a skin protectant wipe and allow it to dry to help prevent skin breakdown and infection.
◆ Pack the wound, if ordered, and apply a sterile dressing.
◆ Remove and discard your gloves and gown.
◆ Properly dispose of drainage, solutions, and the trash bag, and clean or dispose of soiled equipment and supplies.

Postprocedure care

◆ Try to coordinate wound irrigation with the practitioner's visit so he can inspect the wound.

MONITORING
◆ Monitor the wound's appearance and the amount and characteristics of drainage.

PATIENT TEACHING
◆ If the wound must be irrigated at home, teach the patient or a family member how to do it using strict sterile technique. Provide written instructions, and ask for a return demonstration of the proper technique.
◆ Arrange for home health supplies and nursing visits as appropriate.
◆ Urge the patient to call his practitioner if he detects signs of infection.

DOCUMENTATION
◆ Record the date and time of irrigation and the amount and type of irrigant used.
◆ Describe the characteristics of the wound and sloughing tissue or exudate.
◆ Document the amount of solution returned.
◆ Record skin care performed around the wound and the type of dressings applied.
◆ Document the patient's tolerance of the treatment.

Procedures

IV Diagnostic tests

Angiography

Overview

Angiography, also known as *arteriography* or an *angiogram*, involves radiographic examination of vasculature after injecting an intra-arterial contrast medium.

PURPOSE
◆ To detect vascular abnormalities
◆ To evaluate vascular displacement caused by tumor, hematoma, edema, herniation, vasospasm, increased intracranial pressure, or hydrocephalus

PRECAUTIONS
◆ Check whether the patient is allergic to iodine or other contrast media; notify the practitioner of allergies.
◆ Angiography is contraindicated in patients with severe renal or thyroid disease, recent anticoagulation therapy, and recent thrombotic or embolic events.

Test

PREPARATION
◆ Confirm the patient's identity using two patient identifiers and verify the procedure to be done according to facility policy.
◆ Explain the purpose of the test and how it's done.
◆ Tell the patient who will perform the test and where it will be done.
◆ Make sure the patient has signed an informed consent form.
◆ Have the patient fast for 8 to 10 hours before the test.
◆ Initiate an I.V. access; give I.V. fluids as ordered.
◆ Tell the patient that he'll need to lie still during the procedure.
◆ Explain to the patient that he'll receive sedation and a local anesthetic.
◆ Warn the patient that nausea, warmth, or burning may occur with the contrast injection.
◆ Inform the patient that the test takes about 2 to 4 hours.

KEY STEPS
◆ The patient is placed in a supine position on a radiographic table.
◆ The access site is prepared and draped, and a local anesthetic is injected.
◆ The artery is punctured with the appropriate needle and catheterized under fluoroscopic guidance.
◆ Contrast medium is injected.
◆ X-rays are taken and reviewed.
◆ The patient's vital signs and neurologic status are monitored continuously.
◆ The catheter is removed, firm pressure is applied to the access site until bleeding stops, and a pressure dressing is applied.

POSTPROCEDURE CARE
◆ Enforce bed rest and apply an ice bag to the puncture site as ordered.
◆ If active bleeding or expanding hematoma occurs, apply firm pressure to the puncture site and inform the practitioner immediately.
◆ Monitor the patient's vital signs, intake and output, and the neurovascular status of the extremity distal to the access site.
◆ If the femoral approach was used, keep the involved leg straight at the hip for 6 hours or longer and routinely check pulses distal to the site.
◆ If the carotid artery was used, watch for dysphagia, respiratory distress, disorientation, weakness, or numbness in the extremities.

Interpretation

NORMAL RESULTS
◆ Normal vasculature
◆ Opacified superficial and deep arteries and arterioles during arterial phase of perfusion
◆ Opacified superficial and deep veins during the venous phase

ABNORMAL RESULTS
◆ Vessel displacement, suggesting a possible tumor
◆ Vessel occlusion or narrowing

Arterial blood gas analysis

Overview

Arterial blood gas analysis measures partial pressure of arterial oxygen (Pao_2), partial pressure of arterial carbon dioxide ($Paco_2$), the pH of an arterial sample, oxygen content (O_2CT), arterial oxygen saturation (Sao_2), and bicarbonate (HCO_3^-) values.

Purpose
◆ To evaluate pulmonary gas exchange efficiency
◆ To determine blood acid-base level
◆ To monitor respiratory therapy

Precautions
◆ Exposing the sample to air interferes with accurate results.

Test

Preparation
◆ Confirm the patient's identity using two patient identifiers and verify the test to be done according to facility policy.
◆ Explain the purpose of the test and how it's done.
◆ Warn the patient that he may experience a brief cramping or throbbing pain at the puncture site.
◆ Wait at least 20 minutes before drawing arterial blood when starting, changing, or discontinuing oxygen therapy.
◆ Perform the Allen test before puncturing the radial artery.

Key steps
◆ Use a heparinized blood gas syringe to draw the sample.
◆ Perform an arterial puncture, or draw blood from an arterial line.
◆ Eliminate air from the sample and prepare to transport it to the laboratory for analysis.
◆ Note the oxygen therapy flow rate and delivery method.
◆ Note the patient's temperature.

Postprocedure care
◆ Apply pressure to the puncture site for 3 to 5 minutes or until bleeding has stopped, then tape a gauze pad firmly over the site.
◆ Observe for indications of circulatory impairment, such as swelling, discoloration, pain, numbness, and tingling in the bandaged arm.

Interpretation

Normal results
◆ pH levels: 7.35 to 7.45 (SI, 7.35 to 7.45)
◆ Pao_2: 80 to 100 mm Hg (SI, 10.6 to 13.3 kPa)
◆ $Paco_2$: 35 to 45 mm Hg (SI, 4.7 to 5.3 kPa)
◆ O_2CT: 15% to 23% (SI, 0.15 to 0.23)
◆ Sao_2: 94% to 100% (SI, 0.94 to 1)
◆ HCO_3^-: 22 to 25 mEq/L (SI, 22 to 25 mmol/L)

Abnormal results
◆ Decreased Pao_2, O_2CT, and Sao_2 levels and increased $Paco_2$ levels, possibly indicating impaired respiratory functions, such as respiratory muscle weakness or paralysis, respiratory center inhibition (from head injury, brain tumor, or drug abuse), and airway obstruction
◆ Decreased Pao_2, O_2CT, and Sao_2 levels, possibly from bronchiole obstruction; from an abnormal ventilation-perfusion ratio caused by partially blocked alveoli or pulmonary capillaries; or from alveoli that are damaged or filled with fluid because of disease, hemorrhage, or near drowning
◆ Insufficient oxygen levels, decreased Pao_2, O_2CT, and Sao_2 levels, and normal Pao_2 levels of inspired air, indicating pneumothorax, impaired diffusion between alveoli and blood, or an arteriovenous shunt
◆ Low O_2CT with normal Pao_2, Sao_2, and, possibly, $Paco_2$ values, indicating possible severe anemia, decreased blood volume, or reduced hemoglobin oxygen-carrying capacity

Arthrocentesis

Overview

Arthrocentesis involves inserting a needle under sterile conditions into a joint space, most commonly the knee, to obtain a synovial fluid specimen.

PURPOSE
◆ To analyze synovial fluid
◆ To aid in the diagnosis of arthritis
◆ To identify joint effusion
◆ To relieve pain and distention from joint effusion
◆ To administer drugs locally
◆ To help diagnose joint infection

PRECAUTIONS
◆ Send the specimen to the laboratory immediately.

Test

PREPARATION
◆ Confirm the patient's identity using two patient identifiers and verify the procedure to be done according to facility policy.
◆ Explain the purpose of the test and how it's done.
◆ Tell the patient who will perform the test and where it will be done.
◆ Make sure the patient has signed an informed consent form.
◆ Document and report allergies.
◆ If glucose testing of synovial fluid is ordered, tell the patient to fast for 6 to 12 hours before the test.
◆ Give the patient a sedative as ordered.
◆ Warn the patient that transient pain may occur when the needle penetrates the joint capsule.

KEY STEPS
◆ The patient is positioned and told to maintain the position.
◆ The skin over the puncture site is cleaned and prepared.
◆ A local anesthetic is given, and then an aspirating needle is inserted quickly into the joint space.

◆ Fluid is aspirated into the syringe.
◆ The needle is withdrawn, and pressure is applied to the puncture site until bleeding stops.
◆ A sterile dressing is applied.
◆ A venipuncture is performed to obtain a specimen for blood glucose analysis, if synovial fluid glucose is being measured.
◆ The labeled specimens are sent to the laboratory immediately.

POSTPROCEDURE CARE
◆ Apply ice to the affected joint for 24 to 36 hours after aspiration.
◆ Use pillows to support the joint.
◆ Have the patient resume normal activities after the procedure.
◆ Warn the patient to avoid excessive use of the joint for a few days after the test.
◆ Watch for and immediately report increased pain, swelling, and fever.

Interpretation

NORMAL RESULTS
◆ Clear or colorless to pale yellow synovial fluid specimens
◆ Synovial fluid volumes of 0.3 to 3.5 ml (in knee)
◆ pH levels of 7.2 to 7.4
◆ Good mucin clot
◆ Synovial fluid glucose within 10 mg/dl of the serum glucose value

ABNORMAL RESULTS
◆ Sodium urate in the specimen, indicating gout
◆ Calcium pyrophosphate crystals, indicating pseudogout
◆ Red blood cells, possibly indicating traumatic aspiration or hemarthritis
◆ Cloudy specimen with white blood cell (WBC) count of greater than 50,000 × 10^6/L, possibly indicating bacterial infection or rheumatoid arthritis; WBC of greater than 100,000 × 10^6/L, possibly indicating septic arthritis

Arthroscopy

Overview

Arthroscopy is the use of a fiber-optic endoscope to visually examine the interior of a joint. It also permits concurrent surgery or biopsy.

PURPOSE
◆ To evaluate joint disease
◆ To provide an alternative to open surgery and separate biopsy
◆ To detect, diagnose, treat, and monitor ligament, meniscal, patellar, condylar, extrasynovial, and synovial diseases

PRECAUTIONS
◆ Arthroscopy is contraindicated in patients with local skin or wound infections and in patients with fibrous ankylosis with flexion less than 50 degrees.

Test

PREPARATION
◆ Confirm the patient's identity using two patient identifiers and verify the procedure and its site according to facility policy.
◆ Explain the purpose of the test and how it's done.
◆ Tell the patient who will perform the test and where it will be done.
◆ Make sure the patient has signed an informed consent form.
◆ Document and report allergies.
◆ Instruct the patient to fast after midnight before the procedure.
◆ Warn the patient that he may feel discomfort from the injection of the anesthetic and tourniquet pressure.
◆ Explain that the patient may feel a thumping sensation as the cannula is inserted into the joint.

KEY STEPS
◆ Give the patient a sedative.
◆ A local or regional anesthetic is given by the practitioner.
◆ A cannula is passed through a small incision and positioned in the joint cavity.

◆ The arthroscope is inserted through the cannula and the knee structures are visually examined.
◆ A synovial biopsy or appropriate surgery is performed, if indicated.
◆ The joint is irrigated and pressure is then applied to remove the irrigating solution.
◆ An adhesive strip and compression bandage are applied to the site.

POSTPROCEDURE CARE
◆ Monitor the extremity for neurovascular impairment.
◆ Elevate the leg and apply ice for the first 24 hours.
◆ Monitor for fever, bleeding, drainage, redness, swelling, or pain in the joint.
◆ Advise the patient to limit weight bearing per practitioner orders.
◆ Apply an immobilizer, if ordered.

Interpretation

NORMAL RESULTS
◆ Diarthrodial joint lined with synovial membrane surrounded by muscles, ligaments, cartilage, and tendons
◆ Smooth and white articular cartilage
◆ Cablelike, silvery ligaments and tendons
◆ Smooth synovium marked by a fine vascular network

ABNORMAL RESULTS
◆ Meniscal abnormalities
◆ Patellar abnormalities, suggesting chondromalacia, dislocation, subluxation, fracture, or parapatellar synovitis
◆ Condylar abnormalities, suggesting degenerative articular cartilage, osteochondritis dissecans, or loose bodies
◆ Extrasynovial abnormalities, suggesting torn anterior cruciate or tibial collateral ligament, Baker's cyst, or ganglion cyst
◆ Synovial abnormalities, suggesting synovitis, rheumatoid arthritis, or degenerative arthritis
◆ Foreign bodies, suggesting gout, pseudogout, or osteochondromatosis

Biopsy

Overview

A biopsy is a procedure used to obtain cells for histologic examination. It may be done by fine needle aspiration under local anesthesia or by surgical excision under general anesthesia (open biopsy). A biopsy is performed when a mass or deformity is found on a bone scan, computed tomography (CT) scan, X-ray, arteriography, or magnetic resonance imaging.

PURPOSE
◆ To distinguish between benign and malignant tumors

PRECAUTIONS
◆ Send the specimen to the laboratory immediately.
◆ Perform the procedure cautiously in patients with coagulopathies.

Test

PREPARATION
◆ Confirm the patient's identity using two patient identifiers, and verify the procedure to be done and the site to be used according to facility policy.
◆ Explain the purpose of the test and how it's done.
◆ Explain who will perform the test and where it will be done.
◆ Make sure the patient has signed an informed consent form.
◆ Document and report allergies.
◆ If the patient is having an open biopsy, tell him to fast after midnight the night before the test.
◆ Warn the patient that he'll experience some discomfort and pressure when the biopsy needle is inserted.

KEY STEPS
Needle biopsy
◆ The biopsy site is shaved and prepared as needed. After a local anesthetic is given, the practitioner inserts the needle into the lump or mass.

◆ The cells are aspirated with the needle and spread on a glass slide.
◆ Pressure is applied to the biopsy site until bleeding stops, then a dressing or bandage is applied.
◆ A CT scan or ultrasound may be used with needle biopsy to target the suspicious mass.

Open biopsy
◆ After the patient is anesthetized, the biopsy site is shaved and prepared. An incision is made, and the practitioner removes a piece of the suspected mass or bone and sends it to the laboratory for immediate histologic analysis.
◆ The incision is closed, and a sterile dressing is applied.

POSTPROCEDURE CARE
◆ Give the patient an analgesic as ordered.
◆ Resume the patient's usual diet after he fully recovers from anesthesia.
◆ Monitor the patient's vital signs.
◆ Monitor the biopsy site for signs and symptoms of infection.

Interpretation

NORMAL RESULTS
◆ Well-circumscribed and nonmetastasizing lesions, suggesting benign tumors

ABNORMAL RESULTS
◆ Irregularly and rapidly spreading lesions, suggesting malignant tumors
◆ Presence of malignant cells

Diagnostic tests

Blood culture

Overview

A blood culture involves inoculating a culture medium with a blood sample, incubating it for isolation, and identifying the causative pathogens of bacteremia and septicemia. About 67% of pathogens are identified within 24 hours, up to 90% within 72 hours; anaerobic organisms may take longer to grow. Sample collection depends on the type of suspected bacteremia and whether drug therapy needs to start regardless of test results.

PURPOSE
◆ To confirm a diagnosis of bacteremia
◆ To identify the causative organism in bacteremia and septicemia
◆ To determine the cause of fever with an unknown origin

PRECAUTIONS
◆ Maintain standard precautions while collecting the samples.
◆ Send each sample to the laboratory within 30 minutes after collection.
◆ Collect blood cultures before giving antimicrobials, if possible.

Test

PREPARATION
◆ Confirm the patient's identity using two patient identifiers and verify the test to be done according to facility policy.
◆ Explain the purpose of the test and how it's done.
◆ Explain to the patient that the test requires two blood samples and that he may feel transient discomfort from the tourniquet and the needle punctures.
◆ Tell the patient that the test usually takes less than 5 minutes.

KEY STEPS
◆ Clean the venipuncture site, first with an alcohol swab and then with a povidone-iodine swab, using a side-to-side motion.
◆ Wait at least 1 minute for the skin to dry.

◆ Perform a venipuncture, and draw 10 to 20 ml of blood for an adult or 2 to 6 ml for a child.
◆ Clean the diaphragm tops of the culture bottles with alcohol or povidone-iodine, and change the needle on the syringe.
◆ Inoculate the anaerobic bottle first if both anaerobic and aerobic cultures are needed.
◆ If using broth medium, add blood to each bottle until achieving a 1:5 or 1:10 dilution. (For example, add 10 ml of blood to a 100-ml bottle.) The size of the bottle may vary depending on hospital protocol.
◆ If using a special resin, add blood to the resin in the bottles according to facility protocol. Invert the bottle gently to mix the substances.
◆ Draw the blood directly into a special collection and processing tube, if using the lysis-centrifugation technique (Isolator).
◆ Document the current or recent antimicrobial therapy on the laboratory request form.
◆ Send each sample to the laboratory immediately.

 Nursing alert
Improper collection technique may contaminate the sample and alter test results.

POSTPROCEDURE CARE
◆ Apply pressure to the venipuncture site until bleeding stops.
◆ Monitor the venipuncture site for bleeding and signs of infection.

Interpretation

NORMAL RESULTS
◆ No growth or organisms

ABNORMAL RESULTS
◆ Presence of bacteria and sensitivities, allowing for more accurate antibiotic treatment

Bone marrow aspiration

Overview

Bone marrow aspiration is the collection of a soft tissue specimen from the medullary canals of long bone and interstices of cancellous bone for biopsy and histologic and hematologic examination.

PURPOSE
◆ To diagnose thrombocytopenia, leukemias, granulomas, anemias, and primary and metastatic tumors
◆ To determine causes of infection
◆ To help stage diseases such as Hodgkin's disease
◆ To evaluate chemotherapy
◆ To monitor myelosuppression

PRECAUTIONS
◆ Bone marrow aspiration is contraindicated in patients with bleeding disorders.

Test

PREPARATION
◆ Confirm the patient's identity using two patient identifiers and verify the test to be done according to facility policy.
◆ Explain the purpose of the test and how it's done.
◆ Explain who will perform the test and when it will be done.
◆ Make sure the patient has signed an informed consent form.
◆ Document the patient's allergies.
◆ Give the patient a mild sedative 1 hour before the test.
◆ Explain to the patient that he'll feel pressure when the biopsy needle is inserted and a brief, pulling pain when bone marrow is removed.

KEY STEPS
◆ Position the patient and instruct him to remain as still as possible.
◆ The aspiration site is prepared and draped, and a local anesthetic is injected. A needle is inserted through the skin, sub-cutaneous tissue, and bone cortex, using a twisting motion.
◆ The stylet is removed from the aspiration needle, and a 10- to 20-ml syringe is attached. Bone marrow is aspirated, and the needle is withdrawn.
◆ If the aspiration specimen is inadequate, the needle may be repositioned within the bone marrow cavity or removed and reinserted in another anesthetized site. If the second attempt fails, a needle biopsy may be necessary.

POSTPROCEDURE CARE
◆ Monitor the aspiration site for signs and symptoms of infection.
◆ Enforce bedrest for 30 to 60 minutes after the procedure.

Interpretation

NORMAL RESULTS
◆ Fat cells and connective tissue in yellow bone marrow
◆ Hematopoietic cells, fat cells, and connective tissue in red bone marrow
◆ A +2 level in the iron stain, which measures hemosiderin (storage iron)
◆ Negative Sudan black B stain, which shows granulocytes
◆ Negative periodic acid–Schiff (PAS) stain, which detects glycogen reactions

ABNORMAL RESULTS
◆ Decreased hemosiderin levels in an iron stain, suggesting a true iron deficiency
◆ Positive iron stain, suggesting differentiation of acute myelogenous leukemia from acute lymphoblastic leukemia (negative stain) or granulation in myeloblasts
◆ Increased hemosiderin levels, suggesting other types of anemias or blood disorders
◆ Positive PAS stain, suggesting acute or chronic lymphocytic leukemia, amyloidosis, thalassemia, lymphoma, infectious mononucleosis, iron deficiency anemia, or sideroblastic anemia

Bone scan

Overview

A bone scan involves injecting a radioactive tracer compound (radioactive technetium diphosphonate) I.V. and using a scanning camera to produce images of the skeleton. Increased tracer concentrations collect in bone tissue at abnormal metabolism sites, appearing as hot spots that are commonly detectable months before radiography reveals a lesion.

PURPOSE
◆ To detect malignant bone lesions
◆ To rule out suspected bone lesions
◆ To detect occult bone trauma associated with pathologic fractures
◆ To monitor degenerative bone disorders
◆ To detect infection
◆ To evaluate unexplained bone pain
◆ To assist in staging cancer

PRECAUTIONS
◆ A bone scan is contraindicated during pregnancy or lactation.
◆ Avoid scheduling additional radionuclide tests for the following 24 to 48 hours.

Test

PREPARATION
◆ Confirm the patient's identity using two patient identifiers and verify the test to be done according to facility policy.
◆ Explain the purpose of the test and how it's done.
◆ Explain who will perform the test and when it will be done.
◆ Make sure the patient has signed an informed consent form.
◆ Document the patient's allergies.
◆ Explain the importance of holding still during scanning.
◆ Explain that the scan is painless and that the radioactive isotope emits less radiation than a standard radiography machine.
◆ Ensure a functional peripheral I.V. access.
◆ Tell the patient that the test will take about 1 hour.

KEY STEPS
◆ The I.V. tracer and imaging agent are given by the technician 3 hours before the scan.
◆ Encourage increased fluid intake for the next 1 to 3 hours to facilitate the renal clearance of circulating free tracer that isn't picked up by bone.
◆ Instruct the patient to urinate immediately before the scan, or insert a urinary catheter to empty the bladder.
◆ After the patient is positioned on the scanner table, the scanner moves over the patient's body, detects low-level radiation emitted by the skeleton and translates this into a two-dimensional picture.
◆ The scanner takes as many views as needed to cover the specified area.
◆ The patient may be repositioned as needed during the test to obtain adequate views.

POSTPROCEDURE CARE
◆ Instruct the patient to drink additional fluids and to empty his bladder frequently for the next 24 to 48 hours.
◆ Monitor the patient for signs and symptoms of infection at the injection site.
◆ Monitor intake and output.

Interpretation

NORMAL RESULTS
◆ Symmetrical and uniform tracer uptake
◆ Tracer concentrations at sites of new bone formation or increased metabolism
◆ High concentration (hot spots) at the epiphyses of growing bone

ABNORMAL RESULTS
◆ Increased tracer uptake at bone formation sites compared with surrounding bone, suggesting bone cancer, infection, fracture, or additional disorders, when used along with the patient's medical and surgical history, radiographic findings, and laboratory test results

Bronchoscopy

Overview

Bronchoscopy is the direct visualization of the larynx, trachea, and bronchi using a rigid or fiber-optic bronchoscope.

PURPOSE

♦ To diagnose bronchogenic carcinoma, tuberculosis, interstitial pulmonary disease, and fungal or parasitic pulmonary infections
♦ To obtain specimens for microbiologic and cytologic examination
♦ To locate bleeding sites in the tracheobronchial tree
♦ To visualize and remove foreign bodies, malignant or benign tumors, mucus plugs, and excessive secretions from the tracheobronchial tree
♦ To administer brachytherapy
♦ To identify vocal cord paralysis

PRECAUTIONS

♦ Failure to observe dietary restrictions before the test may result in aspiration.

Test

PREPARATION

♦ Confirm the patient's identity using two patient identifiers and verify the procedure to be done according to facility policy.
♦ Explain the purpose of the test and how it's done.
♦ Explain who will perform the test and when it will be done.
♦ Make sure the patient has signed an informed consent form.
♦ Document the patient's allergies.
♦ Instruct the patient to fast for 6 to 12 hours before the test.
♦ Administer an I.V. sedative as ordered.
♦ Remove the patient's dentures.
♦ Explain that the test takes 45 to 60 minutes.

KEY STEPS

♦ Local anesthetic is sprayed into the patient's mouth and throat to suppress the gag reflex.

♦ The bronchoscope is inserted through the mouth or nose.
♦ Tissue specimens are obtained from suspect areas.
♦ A suction apparatus may remove foreign bodies or mucus plugs.
♦ Bronchoalveolar lavage may remove thickened secretions or may diagnose infectious causes of infiltrates.
♦ Specimens are prepared and immediately sent to the laboratory.

POSTPROCEDURE CARE

♦ Observe the patient for signs of laryngospasm or bronchospasm, fever, or hypoxemia.
♦ Resume the patient's usual diet, beginning with sips of clear liquid or ice chips, when the gag reflex returns.
♦ Monitor the patient's vital signs and respiratory status and assess sputum characteristics.

Interpretation

NORMAL RESULTS

♦ Bronchi appearing structurally similar to the trachea
♦ Right bronchus slightly larger and more vertical than left bronchus
♦ Smaller segmental bronchi branching off the main bronchi

ABNORMAL RESULTS

♦ Structural abnormalities in the bronchial wall, indicating inflammation, ulceration, tumors, and enlargement of submucosal lymph nodes
♦ Structural abnormalities of endotracheal origin, suggesting stenosis, compression, ectasia, strictures, and diverticula
♦ Structural abnormalities in the trachea or bronchi, suggesting calculi, foreign bodies, masses, and paralyzed vocal cords
♦ Tissue and cell study abnormalities, suggesting interstitial pulmonary disease, infection, carcinoma, and tuberculosis

Cardiac catheterization

Overview

Cardiac catheterization evaluates heart function by passing a catheter into the heart. Left-sided catheterization checks patency and left ventricle function of the coronary arteries; right-sided catheterization checks pulmonary artery pressures.

PURPOSE

◆ To evaluate valvular insufficiency or stenosis, septal defects, congenital anomalies, myocardial function, myocardial blood supply, and cardiac wall motion
◆ To help diagnose left ventricular enlargement, aortic root enlargement, ventricular aneurysms, and intracardiac shunts
◆ To evaluate previous cardiac surgery

PRECAUTIONS

◆ Left bundle-branch block contraindicates catheterization of the right side of the heart.

Test

PREPARATION

◆ Confirm the patient's identity using two patient identifiers and verify the procedure to be done according to facility policy.
◆ Explain the purpose of the test and how it's done.
◆ Explain who will perform the test and when it will be done.
◆ Make sure the patient has signed an informed consent form.
◆ Stop anticoagulants, as ordered.
◆ Document the patient's allergies.
◆ Instruct the patient to fast for at least 6 hours before the test.
◆ Insert an I.V. catheter.
◆ Warn the patient that a transient hot, flushing sensation, or nausea may occur.
◆ Tell him that the test will take 1 to 2 hours.

KEY STEPS

◆ The patient is placed in a supine position on a padded table, and his heart rhythm and vital signs are monitored throughout the test.
◆ The insertion site is shaved and cleaned.
◆ A local anesthetic is injected at the insertion site and a small incision is made into the artery or vein, depending on whether the test is for the left or right side.
◆ When the catheter is in place, contrast medium is injected.
◆ Pressures are recorded through the catheter, and computers assist with cardiac function measurements. Images are rapidly taken and reviewed during and after the procedure.
◆ After catheter removal, direct pressure is applied to the incision site until bleeding stops and a sterile dressing is applied.

POSTPROCEDURE CARE

◆ Keep the affected extremity straight for 3 to 6 hours.
◆ Monitor the insertion site for signs of bleeding, and apply pressure if bleeding occurs.
◆ Monitor the patient's peripheral vascular status distal to the puncture site.

Interpretation

NORMAL RESULTS

◆ Normal heart valve function, chamber size, pressures, configuration, wall motion or thickness, and blood flow
◆ Smooth and regular outline of coronary arteries

ABNORMAL RESULTS

◆ Coronary artery narrowing greater than 70%, suggesting significant coronary artery disease
◆ Narrowing or occlusion of vessels, suggesting the need for revascularization surgery
◆ Impaired wall motion, suggesting myocardial incompetence
◆ Retrograde flow across the valves, indicating valvular incompetence

Diagnostic tests

Colonoscopy

Overview

Colonoscopy is the visualization of the large intestine's lining using a flexible fiber-optic video endoscope.

PURPOSE
- To detect or evaluate inflammatory and ulcerative bowel disease
- To locate the origin of lower GI bleeding
- To help diagnose colonic strictures and benign or malignant lesions
- To evaluate postoperatively for recurrence of polyps and malignant lesions

PRECAUTIONS
- The test is contraindicated in pregnant women near term, in patients who have had recent abdominal surgery, and in those with peritonitis, colitis, or a perforated viscus.

Test

PREPARATION
- Confirm the patient's identity using two patient identifiers and verify the test to be done according to facility policy.
- Explain the purpose of the test and how it's done.
- Tell the patient who will perform the test and where it will be done.
- Make sure the patient has signed an informed consent form.
- Document the patient's allergies.
- Insert an I.V. line and administer sedation as ordered.
- Tell the patient to maintain a clear liquid diet for 24 to 48 hours before the test and to take nothing by mouth after midnight the night before the test.
- Instruct the patient regarding the appropriate bowel preparation.
- Inform the patient that the test will take about 30 to 60 minutes.

KEY STEPS
- Position the patient on his left side with knees flexed.

- Obtain baseline vital signs and monitor cardiac rhythm and pulse oximetry during the procedure.
- The practitioner palpates the mucosa of the anus and rectum and inserts the lubricated colonoscope through the patient's anus into the sigmoid colon under direct vision.
- A small amount of air is insufflated to locate the bowel lumen and then the scope is advanced through the rectum.
- Abdominal palpation or fluoroscopy may be used to help guide the colonoscope through the large intestine.
- Suction may be used to remove blood and secretions that obscure vision.
- Biopsy forceps or a cytology brush may be passed through the colonoscope to obtain specimens for histologic or cytologic examination; an electrocautery snare may be used to remove polyps.
- Send specimens to the laboratory immediately after collection.

POSTPROCEDURE CARE
- Observe the patient for signs of bowel perforation or bleeding.
- Check the patient's vital signs and document them accordingly.
- Encourage fluid intake.

Interpretation

NORMAL RESULTS
- Light pink-orange mucosa of the large intestine beyond the sigmoid colon marked by semilunar folds and deep tubular pits
- Visible blood vessels beneath the intestinal mucosa

ABNORMAL RESULTS
- Inflamed tissue, indicating proctitis, Crohn's disease, and malignant or benign lesions
- Changes in the mucosal lining, suggesting diverticular disease, ulcerative colitis, or ulceration that may cause lower GI bleeding

Diagnostic tests

Computed tomography scan

Overview

A computed tomography scan combines radiologic and computer technology to produce cross-sectional images of various layers of tissue in areas such as the pelvis, chest, and head.

PURPOSE

◆ To evaluate soft tissue and organs of the abdomen, pelvis, and retroperitoneal space
◆ To evaluate inflammatory disease
◆ To help stage neoplasms
◆ To evaluate trauma
◆ To detect tumors, cysts, hemorrhage, or edema
◆ To evaluate response to chemotherapy

PRECAUTIONS

◆ Check the patient's history for hypersensitivity to iodine or contrast media used in other diagnostic tests.
◆ Check the patient's laboratory studies for abnormal renal function. If present, the contrast shouldn't be given, the test may not be done, or the practitioner may order medications and hydration before the test.
◆ The test is contraindicated during pregnancy because of potential risk to the fetus.

Test

PREPARATION

◆ Confirm the patient's identity using two patient identifiers and verify the test to be done according to facility policy.
◆ Explain the purpose of the test and how it's done.
◆ Tell the patient who will perform the test and when it will be done.
◆ Make sure the patient has signed an informed consent form.
◆ Document and report allergies.
◆ If the patient will receive a contrast medium, instruct him to fast for 4 hours before the test.
◆ Ensure adequate peripheral I.V. access.

◆ Stress the need to remain still during testing because movement may limit the test's accuracy.
◆ Warn the patient about transient discomfort from the needle puncture and a warm or flushed feeling or metallic taste if an I.V. contrast medium is used.
◆ Inform the patient that the test takes about 35 to 40 minutes.

KEY STEPS

◆ Assist the patient into a supine position with his arms above his head.
◆ An I.V. contrast agent may be injected into a vein to help define certain tissues.
◆ The table advances slightly between each scan.
◆ Cross-sectional images are obtained and reviewed.

POSTPROCEDURE CARE

◆ Instruct the patient to resume his normal diet and activities unless ordered otherwise.

Interpretation

NORMAL RESULTS

◆ Organs normal in size and position
◆ No masses or other abnormalities

ABNORMAL RESULTS

◆ Well-circumscribed or poorly defined areas of slightly lower density than normal parenchyma, suggesting possible primary and metastatic neoplasms
◆ Relatively low-density, homogeneous areas, usually with well-defined borders, suggesting possible abscesses
◆ Sharply defined round or oval structures, with densities less than that of abscesses and neoplasms, suggesting cysts
◆ Dilatation of the biliary ducts, suggesting obstructive disease from a tumor or calculi

Cystometry

Overview

Cystometry measures the pressure and volume of fluid in the bladder during filling, storing, and voiding, and assesses neuromuscular bladder function.

PURPOSE
◆ To evaluate detrusor muscle function and tonicity
◆ To determine the cause of bladder dysfunction or detect the cause of involuntary bladder contractions and incontinence
◆ To measure bladder reaction to thermal stimulation

PRECAUTIONS
◆ The test is contraindicated in patients with acute urinary tract infections (UTIs).
◆ Tell the patient not to strain at voiding; doing so could cause ambiguous readings.

Test

PREPARATION
◆ Confirm the patient's identity using two patient identifiers and verify the test to be done according to facility policy.
◆ Explain the purpose of the test and how it's done.
◆ Tell the patient who will perform the test and when it will be done.
◆ Document and report any allergies.
◆ Check the patient's medication history for drugs that may affect test results.
◆ Have the patient void before the test.
◆ Tell the patient he may feel a strong urge to urinate during the test.
◆ Ask the patient to report pain, flushing, sweating, or nausea during the procedure.

KEY STEPS
◆ Assist the patient into the supine position on an examination table.
◆ A catheter is passed into the bladder to measure residual urine.
◆ To test the response to thermal sensation, 1 oz (30 ml) of room-temperature normal saline solution is instilled into the bladder. Then an equal volume of warm fluid is instilled.
◆ Fluid is drained from the bladder and the catheter is connected to the cystometer.
◆ Normal saline solution, sterile water, or gas (usually carbon dioxide) is slowly introduced into the bladder.
◆ When the bladder reaches its full capacity, the patient is asked to void.
◆ Related pressures and volumes are automatically plotted on a graph.
◆ If results are abnormal, medication may be injected and the study repeated in 20 to 30 minutes.

POSTPROCEDURE CARE
◆ Encourage oral fluid intake.
◆ Monitor for hematuria.
◆ Give the patient a prescribed antibiotic.
◆ Monitor the patient's vital signs and intake and output.
◆ Monitor for signs of infection.

Interpretation

NORMAL RESULTS
◆ Micturition started and stopped with no residual urine
◆ Positive vesical sensation
◆ First urge to void at 150 to 200 ml
◆ Bladder capacity at 400 to 500 ml
◆ No bladder contractions and low intravesical pressure
◆ Positive bulbocavernosus reflex and saddle sensation test
◆ Positive ice water test and anal reflex
◆ Heat sensation and pain

ABNORMAL RESULTS
◆ Inability to stop or start micturition, absent or early first urge to void, absent vesical sensation, decreased bladder capacity, bladder contractions, increased intravesical pressure, positive bethanechol sensitivity test, increased bulbocavernosus reflex, negative saddle sensation test, absent heat sensation, pain, and abnormal anal reflex, suggesting neurogenic bladder

Cystourethroscopy

Overview

Cystourethroscopy, which combines the endoscopic techniques of cystoscopy and urethroscopy, allows visual examination of the bladder, urethra, ureter orifice, ureters, and prostate in males.

PURPOSE
◆ To diagnose and evaluate urinary tract disorders
◆ To facilitate biopsy, lesion resection, removal of calculi or foreign objects, and dilation of a constricted urethra
◆ To help coagulate bleeding areas
◆ To implant radium seeds into a tumor

PRECAUTIONS
◆ The test is contraindicated in acute forms of urethritis, prostatitis, or cystitis and in bleeding disorders.

Test

PREPARATION
◆ Confirm the patient's identity using two patient identifiers and verify the test to be done according to facility policy.
◆ Explain the purpose of the test and how it's done.
◆ Tell the patient who will perform the test and when it will be done.
◆ Make sure the patient has signed an informed consent form.
◆ Document and report the patient's allergies.
◆ Have the patient void before the test.
◆ If local anesthesia is used, inform the patient that he'll feel a burning sensation when the instrument enters the urethra and an urgent need to urinate as the bladder fills with irrigating solution.
◆ Tell the patient that he'll need to lie still.

KEY STEPS
◆ The patient is assisted into the lithotomy position on a cystoscopic table.
◆ The genitalia are cleaned with an antiseptic solution, and the patient is draped.

◆ The urethra is examined with a urethroscope.
◆ The urethroscope is removed and a cystoscope is inserted into the bladder.
◆ The bladder is filled with irrigating solution, and the entire bladder surface wall and ureteral orifices are examined.
◆ The cystoscope is removed and the urethroscope is reinserted.
◆ The bladder neck and various portions of the urethra are examined.
◆ A urine specimen is taken from the bladder for culture and sensitivity testing.
◆ Residual urine volume is measured.
◆ Urine is taken for a cytologic examination if a tumor is suspected.
◆ If a tumor is found, it may be necessary to perform a biopsy or resection.
◆ If a urethral stricture is present, urethral dilatation may be needed before this test.

POSTPROCEDURE CARE
◆ Instruct the patient to abstain from alcohol for 48 hours.
◆ Report flank or abdominal pain, chills, fever, an elevated white blood cell count, a low urine output, lack of voiding within 8 hours after the test, or bright red blood that persists after three voidings.
◆ Apply heat to the lower abdomen to relieve pain and muscle spasm, if ordered.
◆ Monitor the patient's vital signs, intake and output, and bleeding.
◆ Watch for bladder distention.

Interpretation

NORMAL RESULTS
◆ Normal size, shape, and position of the urethra, bladder, and ureteral orifices
◆ Smooth and shiny lower urinary tract mucosal lining

ABNORMAL RESULTS
◆ Structural abnormalities, suggesting an enlarged prostate gland, urethral strictures, calculi, tumors, diverticula, ulcers, and polyps

Diagnostic tests

Echocardiography

Overview

Echocardiography examines the size, shape, and motion of cardiac structures. A transducer directs ultra-high-frequency sound waves toward cardiac structures and converts the echoes to electrical impulses on a screen. With M-mode (motion-mode) echocardiography, a single, pencil-like ultrasound beam strikes the heart and produces a vertical view, recording heart motion and the dimensions of intracardiac structures. Two-dimensional echocardiography is a cross-sectional view of cardiac structures that records lateral motion and spatial relationship between structures. Color Doppler echocardiography detects the pattern of blood flow by changes in color.

PURPOSE
♦ To diagnose and evaluate valvular abnormalities and septal defects
♦ To measure and evaluate the size of the heart's chambers and valves
♦ To evaluate cardiac function or wall motion
♦ To detect pericardial effusion or mural thrombi

Test

PREPARATION
♦ Confirm the patient's identity using two patient identifiers and verify the test to be done according to facility policy.
♦ Explain the purpose of the test and how it's done.
♦ Tell the patient who will perform the test and when it will be done.
♦ Stress the need to remain still during the test to avoid distorting results.
♦ Tell the patient that the test takes 15 to 30 minutes.

KEY STEPS
♦ The patient is placed into a supine position and conductive gel is applied to the chest. The transducer is placed directly over it.

♦ The transducer is systematically angled to direct ultrasonic waves at specific parts of the patient's heart.
♦ During the test, the oscilloscope screen is observed, and findings are recorded.

POSTPROCEDURE CARE
♦ Remove the conductive gel from the patient's skin.

Interpretation

NORMAL RESULTS
♦ Normal heart valve movement
♦ Echo-free space between the interventricular septum and the ventricular wall.

ABNORMAL RESULTS
♦ Narrowing valve due to thickened leaflets and disordered motion and anterior leaflet movement instead of posterior movement during diastole, suggesting mitral stenosis
♦ Ballooning leaflet or leaflets into the left atrium during systole, suggesting mitral valve prolapse
♦ Fluttering aortic valve leaflets during diastole, suggesting aortic insufficiency
♦ Thickening aortic valve, more echoes, suggesting aortic stenosis
♦ Disrupted valve motion and fuzzy echoes, usually on or near the valve, suggesting bacterial endocarditis
♦ Large chamber, suggesting cardiomyopathy, valvular disorders, or heart failure
♦ Small chamber, suggesting restrictive pericarditis
♦ Systolic anterior motion of the mitral valve and asymmetrical septal hypertrophy, suggesting hypertrophic cardiomyopathy
♦ Absent or paradoxical motion in ventricular walls, suggesting myocardial ischemia or infarction
♦ Fluid accumulation in the pericardial space, causing an abnormal echo-free space, or restricted pericardial motion, suggesting pericardial effusion

Electrocardiography

Overview

Electrocardiography measures and records the electrical current generated by the heart. Through electrodes connected to an amplifier and strip chart recorder, the electrical potentials are measured from 12 different leads: the standard limb leads (I, II, III), the augmented limb leads (aV$_F$, aV$_L$, aV$_R$), and the precordial, or chest, leads (V$_1$ through V$_6$). The electrocardiogram displays the P wave, QRS complex, and T wave.

PURPOSE
◆ To identify conduction abnormalities, cardiac arrhythmias, and myocardial ischemia or myocardial infarction (MI)
◆ To document pacemaker performance

PRECAUTIONS
◆ Make sure that the electrodes are firmly attached, and the patient remains still.

Test

PREPARATION
◆ Confirm the patient's identity using two patient identifiers and verify the test to be done according to facility policy.
◆ Explain the purpose of the procedure and how it's done.
◆ Tell the patient who will perform the test and when it will be done.
◆ Note current cardiac drug therapy on the test request form and other pertinent clinical information, such as chest pain or pacemaker placement.
◆ Inform the patient that the test is painless and takes 5 to 10 minutes.

KEY STEPS
◆ Place the patient in a supine or semi-Fowler position and instruct him to remian still.
◆ Expose the chest, ankles, and wrists.
◆ Place the electrodes on the inner aspect of the wrists or upper arms, on the medial aspect of the lower legs, and on the chest, then connect the leadwires.

◆ Press the start button and input any required information.

POSTPROCEDURE CARE
◆ Disconnect the equipment and remove the electrodes.

Interpretation

NORMAL RESULTS
◆ Heart rate 60 to 100 beats/minute
◆ Normal sinus cardiac rhythm
◆ P wave preceding each QRS complex
◆ 0.12 to 0.20 second PR interval
◆ 0.06 to 0.10 second QRS complex
◆ ST segment not more than 0.1 mV
◆ Rounded, smooth, and positive T wave in leads I, II, V$_3$, V$_4$, V$_5$, and V$_6$
◆ Varying QT interval duration but usually 0.36 to 0.44 second

ABNORMAL RESULTS
◆ Heart rate below 60 beats/minute, indicating bradycardia
◆ Heart rate above 100 beats/minute, suggesting tachycardia
◆ Missing P waves, indicating atrioventricular (AV) block, atrial arrhythmia, or junctional rhythm
◆ Short PR interval, indicating a junctional arrhythmia; prolonged PR interval, indicating an AV block
◆ Prolonged QRS complex, indicating intraventricular conduction defects; missing QRS complexes, indicating an AV block or ventricular asystole
◆ ST-segment elevation of 0.2 mV or more above the baseline, indicating myocardial injury; ST-segment depression, indicating myocardial ischemia or injury
◆ T wave inversion in leads I, II, and V$_3$ to V$_6$, indicating myocardial ischemia; peaked T waves, indicating hyperkalemia or myocardial ischemia; variations in T wave amplitude, indicating electrolyte imbalances
◆ Prolonged QT interval, suggesting life-threatening ventricular arrhythmias

Electroencephalography

Overview

Electroencephalography (EEG) is the recording of brain waves by transmitting and magnifying electrical activity through electrodes attached to the scalp. Intracranial electrodes are sometimes surgically implanted to record electroencephalographic changes to locate seizure focus.

PURPOSE
◆ To determine the presence and type of seizures
◆ To help diagnose intracranial lesions
◆ To evaluate brain activity in metabolic disease, head injury, meningitis, encephalitis, psychological disorders and drug intoxication
◆ To help confirm brain death

PRECAUTIONS
◆ Stimulants, such as caffeinated beverages, chocolate, and tobacco, should be avoided for 8 hours before the test.

Test

PREPARATION
◆ Confirm the patient's identity using two patient identifiers and verify the test to be done according to facility policy.
◆ Explain the purpose of the test and how it's done.
◆ Tell the patient who will perform the test and when it will be done.
◆ Withhold medications, such as barbiturates and other sedatives, for 24 to 48 hours before the test per practitioner orders.
◆ If a sleep EEG is ordered, give a sedative to promote sleep during the test.
◆ Instruct the patient to avoid stimulants, such as caffeinated beverages, chocolate, and tobacco, for 8 hours before the test.
◆ Advise the patient to sleep only 4 to 5 hours the night before the test.
◆ Inform the patient that the test takes about 1 hour.

KEY STEPS
◆ The patient is positioned and electrodes are attached to the scalp.
◆ During recording, the patient is carefully observed and movements, such as blinking, swallowing, or talking, are noted; these movements may cause artifacts.
◆ The patient may be tested in various stress situations, such as hyperventilation and photic stimulation, to elicit abnormal patterns not obvious in the resting stage.

POSTPROCEDURE CARE
◆ Monitor the patient for seizures and maintain seizure precautions.
◆ Help the patient remove the electrode paste from his hair.
◆ Have the patient resume drug therapy.
◆ If brain death is confirmed, provide emotional support for the family.

Interpretation

NORMAL RESULTS
◆ Regular alpha waves in waking state when the patient's eyes are closed and he's mentally alert; no alpha waves with visual activity or mental concentration
◆ Decreased alpha waves from apprehension or anxiety
◆ Beta waves when the patient is alert and has his eyes open
◆ Theta waves, indicating drowsiness or emotional stress in adults
◆ Delta waves in deep sleep stages

ABNORMAL RESULTS
◆ Spikes and waves, suggesting seizures
◆ Slow waves, suggesting intracranial lesions
◆ Focal abnormalities in the injured area, suggesting vascular lesions
◆ Generalized, diffuse, and slow brain waves, suggesting metabolic or inflammatory disorders or increased intracranial pressure
◆ Absent EEG pattern or a flat tracing (except for artifacts), indicating brain death

Electromyography

Overview

Electromyography (EMG) is the measurement of nerve conduction time by recording the electrical activity of selected skeletal muscle groups at rest and during voluntary contraction.

PURPOSE

◆ To differentiate between primary muscle disorders and certain metabolic disorders
◆ To identify diseases characterized by central neuronal degeneration
◆ To help diagnose neuromuscular disorders such as myasthenia gravis
◆ To help diagnose radiculomyelopathy
◆ To diagnose peripheral nerve damage

PRECAUTIONS

◆ The procedure is contraindicated in patients with bleeding disorders.

Test

PREPARATION

◆ Confirm the patient's identity using two patient identifiers and verify the test to be done according to facility policy.
◆ Explain the purpose of the test and how it's done.
◆ Tell the patient who will perform the test and when it will be done.
◆ Check for drugs, such as cholinergics, anticholinergics, anticoagulants, and skeletal muscle relaxants that may interfere with test results, and note them on the patient's chart.
◆ Instruct the patient to avoid smoking, coffee, tea, and cola for 2 to 3 hours before the test.
◆ Inform the patient that the test takes at least 1 hour.

KEY STEPS

◆ The patient is positioned in a way that relaxes the muscle to be tested.
◆ Needle electrodes are quickly inserted into the selected muscle by the technician.

◆ A metal plate lies under the patient to serve as a reference electrode.
◆ The resulting electrical signal is recorded during rest and contraction, amplified 1 million times, and displayed on an oscilloscope or computer screen.
◆ Leadwires are usually attached to an audio-amplifier so that voltage fluctuations within the muscle are audible.

POSTPROCEDURE CARE

◆ Apply warm compresses and give analgesics for discomfort.
◆ Monitor the patient for signs and symptoms of infection.
◆ Tell the patient to resume drugs that were withheld.

Interpretation

NORMAL RESULTS

◆ Minimal electrical activity in muscles at rest
◆ Markedly increased electrical activity in muscles during voluntary contraction
◆ A rapid "train" of motor unit potentials during a sustained contraction or one of increasing strength

ABNORMAL RESULTS

◆ Short (low-amplitude) motor unit potentials, with frequent, irregular discharges, suggesting possible primary muscle disease such as muscular dystrophies and multiple sclerosis
◆ Isolated and irregular motor unit potentials with increased amplitude and duration, suggesting possible disorders, such as ALS and peripheral nerve disorders
◆ Normal motor unit potentials progressively diminishing in amplitude with continuing contractions, suggesting possible myasthenia gravis
◆ Other abnormal findings, indicating disorders such as myopathy, hyperaldosteronism, hypothyroidism, and spinal cord disease

Electrophysiology studies

Overview

Electrophysiologic studies (EPS) measure and record the heart's discrete electrical conduction intervals during an electrode catheter's slow withdrawal from the right ventricle through the bundle of His to the sinoatrial node.

PURPOSE
◆ To locate the site of a bundle-branch block and to determine the presence and location of accessory conducting pathways
◆ To identify and obliterate low-threshold sites that induce arrhythmias

PRECAUTIONS
◆ The test is contraindicated in patients with severe uncorrected coagulopathy, recent thrombophlebitis, acute pulmonary embolism, or acute MI.

Test

PREPARATION
◆ Confirm the patient's identity using two patient identifiers and verify the test to be done according to facility policy.
◆ Explain the purpose of the test and how it's done.
◆ Tell the patient who will perform the test and when it will be done.
◆ Make sure that the patient has signed an informed consent form.
◆ Document and report all allergies.
◆ Instruct the patient to fast for at least 6 hours before the test.
◆ Inform the patient that the test usually takes 1 to 3 hours, but may take longer.

KEY STEPS
◆ The patient is placed in the supine position on a special table.
◆ The insertion site (usually the groin or antecubital fossa) is shaved and prepared.
◆ A local anesthetic is injected. A catheter is inserted and advanced into the right ventricle and then slowly withdrawn.

◆ Various parts of the cardiac electroconduction system are stimulated by atrial or ventricular pacing.
◆ Recordings of conduction intervals are taken from each pole of the cathete and arrhythmias are identified.
◆ Drugs may be administered to assess their efficacy in preventing EPS-induced arrhythmias.
◆ After recordings and measurements are complete, the catheter is removed.
◆ The insertion site is cleaned and a sterile dressing is applied.

POSTPROCEDURE CARE
◆ Monitor the patient's cardiac rhythm.
◆ Enforce bed rest for the ordered amount of time.
◆ Monitor the insertion site for bleeding.
◆ Assess for signs and symptoms of embolism.
◆ Monitor for ECG changes.

Interpretation

NORMAL RESULTS
◆ 35 to 55 msec conduction time from the bundle of His to the Purkinje fibers (HV interval)
◆ 45 to 150 msec conduction time from the atrioventricular node to the bundle of His (AH interval)
◆ 20 to 40 msec intra-atrial conduction time (PA interval)

ABNORMAL RESULTS
◆ A prolonged HV interval, suggesting possible acute or chronic disease
◆ AH interval delays, suggesting atrial pacing, chronic conduction system disease, carotid sinus pressure, recent myocardial infarction, and the use of certain drugs
◆ PA interval delays, suggesting possible acquired, surgically induced, or congenital atrial disease and atrial pacing

Endoscopic retrograde cholangiopancreatography

Overview

Endoscopic retrograde cholangiopancreatography is an X-ray of the pancreatic ducts and hepatobiliary tree after a fiberoptic endoscope injects a contrast medium into the duodenal papilla.

PURPOSE
◆ To evaluate obstructive jaundice
◆ To diagnose cancer of the duodenal papilla, pancreas, and biliary ducts
◆ To place stents and drain bile
◆ To aid in gallstone removal

PRECAUTIONS
◆ Inform the practitioner if the patient is hypersensitive to iodine, seafood, or iodinated contrast media.

Test

PREPARATION
◆ Confirm the patient's identity using two patient identifiers and verify the test to be done according to facility policy.
◆ Explain the purpose of the test and how it's done.
◆ Tell the patient who will perform the test and when it will be done.
◆ Make sure that the patient has signed an informed consent form.
◆ Document and report all allergies.
◆ Instruct the patient to fast after midnight before the test.
◆ Give the patient a sedative as ordered.
◆ Inform the patient that the test takes at least 1 hour.

KEY STEPS
◆ The patient is placed in a left lateral position, and the endoscope is inserted into the mouth and advanced, using fluoroscopic guidance, into the stomach and duodenum.
◆ The patient is helped into the prone position.

◆ A cannula is passed through the biopsy channel of the endoscope and contrast medium is injected.
◆ Rapid-sequence X-rays are taken after each contrast injection.
◆ A tissue specimen or fluid may be aspirated for histologic and cytologic examination.
◆ Therapeutic measures (sphincterectomy, stent placement, stone removal, or balloon dilatation) may be performed before endoscope withdrawal as indicated.
◆ After the films are reviewed, the cannula is removed.

POSTPROCEDURE CARE
◆ Have the patient resume his usual diet when the gag reflex returns.
◆ Monitor the patient for abdominal distention, pain, nausea, and vomiting.
◆ Tell the patient to avoid alcohol and driving for 24 hours after the test.

Interpretation

NORMAL RESULTS
◆ A small red or pale duodenal papilla protruding into the lumen
◆ Pancreatic and hepatobiliary ducts joining and emptying through the duodenal papilla and presence of separate orifices
◆ Pancreatic duct, hepatobiliary tree, and gallbladder uniformly filled with contrast medium

ABNORMAL RESULTS
◆ Filling defects in the hepatobiliary tree, strictures, or irregular deviations, suggesting biliary cirrhosis, primary sclerosing cholangitis, calculi, or cancer of the bile ducts
◆ Filling defects, strictures, and irregular pancreatic duct deviations, suggesting pancreatic cysts and pseudocysts, pancreatic tumors, chronic pancreatitis, pancreatic fibrosis, calculi, or papillary stenosis

Endoscopy

Overview

Endoscopy is the visualization of the lining of a hollow viscus with an endoscope, an instrument with a cablelike cluster of glass fibers that transmits light and reflects an image to the scope's optical head or video monitor.

PURPOSE

◆ To diagnose inflammatory, ulcerative, and infectious diseases
◆ To diagnose benign and malignant tumors and other mucosal lesions

PRECAUTIONS

◆ For high-risk procedures, stop warfarin (Coumadin) for 3 to 5 days before the test; low-molecular-weight heparin may be ordered.
◆ Stop nonsteroidal anti-inflammatory drugs or aspirin 3 to 7 days before the study.

Test

PREPARATION

◆ Confirm the patient's identity using two patient identifiers and verify the test to be done according to facility policy.
◆ Explain the purpose of the test and how it's done.
◆ Tell the patient who will perform the test and when it will be done.
◆ Make sure that the patient has signed a consent form.
◆ Document and report all allergies.
◆ Give the patient an I.V. sedative as ordered.
◆ Advise the patient of any dietary and medication restrictions as ordered.
◆ Inform the patient that the test takes about 1 hour.

KEY STEPS

◆ Monitor the patient's vital signs, pulse oximetry, and cardiac rhythm during the procedure.

◆ Follow the procedure for the specific endoscopy to be performed (such as arthroscopy, bronchoscopy, colonoscopy, colposcopy, cystourethroscopy, endoscopic retrograde cholangiopancreatography, esophagogastroduodenoscopy, hysteroscopy, laparoscopy, laryngoscopy, mediastinoscopy, proctosigmoidoscopy, sigmoidoscopy, or thoracoscopy).

POSTPROCEDURE CARE

◆ Provide a safe environment.
◆ Withhold food and fluids until the gag reflex returns.
◆ Monitor the patient's vital signs.
◆ Monitor the patient's respiratory and neurologic status.
◆ Monitor the patient's cardiac rhythm.
◆ Tell the patient to resume his usual medications and diet as ordered.

Interpretation

NORMAL RESULTS

◆ Specific to the endoscopy procedure

ABNORMAL RESULTS

◆ Specific to the endoscopy procedure

Esophagogastroduodenoscopy

Overview

An esophagogastroduodenoscopy (EGD) is the visualization of the lining of the esophagus, stomach, and upper duodenum using a flexible fiber-optic endoscope.

PURPOSE
◆ To detect small or surface lesions or diagnose inflammatory disease, tumors, ulcers, and structural abnormalities
◆ To obtain specimens for laboratory evaluation
◆ To allow for foreign body removal
◆ To evaluate patients with dysphagia, weight loss, upper abdominal pain and dyspepsia
◆ To reestablish patency of upper GI tract with dilation
◆ To place biliary stents

PRECAUTIONS
◆ The procedure is contraindicated in patients with Zenker's diverticulum, a large aortic aneurysm, a recent ulcer perforation, known or suspected viscus perforation, or an unstable cardiac or pulmonary condition.
◆ EGD shouldn't be performed on patients with severe GI bleeding, esophageal diveticula, suspected perforation, or recent GI surgery.

Test

PREPARATION
◆ Confirm the patient's identity using two patient identifiers and verify the test to be done according to facility policy.
◆ Explain the purpose of the test and how it's done.
◆ Tell the patient who will perform the test and when it will be done.
◆ Make sure that the patient has signed an informed consent form.
◆ Document and report all allergies.
◆ Instruct the patient to fast for 6 to 12 hours before the test.
◆ Inform the patient that the test takes about 30 minutes.

KEY STEPS
◆ After assisting the patient into a left lateral position, sedation is administered and the throat is topically anesthetized.
◆ The endoscope is inserted into the mouth and advanced to examine the esophagus and cardiac sphincter, the stomach, and the duodenum.
◆ Air may be instilled to open the bowel lumen and flatten tissue folds.
◆ The endoscope is slowly withdrawn.
◆ Tissue specimens are sent to the laboratory for analysis.

POSTPROCEDURE CARE
◆ Withhold food and fluids until the gag reflex returns.
◆ Provide throat lozenges and warm saline gargles for sore throat.
◆ Instruct the patient not to consume alcohol, operate machinery, or drive for 24 hours after I.V. sedation.
◆ Tell him to report persistent difficult swallowing, pain, fever, black feces, or bloody vomitus.

Interpretation

NORMAL RESULTS
◆ Smooth and yellow-pink esophageal mucosa with fine vascular markings
◆ Orange-red gastric mucosa and rugae in the stomach
◆ Reddish duodenal bulb mucosa marked by a few shallow longitudinal folds
◆ Prominent circular folds in the distal duodenum lined with villi

ABNORMAL RESULTS
◆ Anatomic abnormalities of the stomach and duodenum, suggesting acute or chronic ulcers, benign or malignant tumors, or diverticula
◆ Inflammatory changes, suggesting esophagitis, gastritis, and duodenitis
◆ Anatomic abnormalities of the esophagus, suggesting tumors, varices, Mallory-Weiss syndrome, esophageal hiatal hernia, and stenosis

Evoked potential studies

Overview

Evoked potential (EP) studies measure the brain's electrical response to sensory organs or stimulation of the peripheral nerves to evaluate visual, somatosensory, and auditory nerve pathways. Electrodes attached to the scalp and skin over various peripheral sensory nerves detect and record electronic impulses, and a computer identifies low-amplitude impulses from background brain wave activity, which are averaged from repeated stimuli.

PURPOSE
◆ To help diagnose nervous system lesions and abnormalities
◆ To monitor spinal cord function during spinal surgery and progression or treatment of neurologic disorders
◆ To assess neurologic function
◆ To evaluate neurologic function

Test

PREPARATION
◆ Confirm the patient's identity using two patient identifiers and verify the test to be done according to facility policy.
◆ Explain the purpose of the test and how it's done.
◆ Tell the patient who will perform the test and when it will be done.
◆ Make sure that the patient or responsible family member has signed an informed consent form.
◆ Document and report all allergies.
◆ Inform the patient that the test takes about 45 to 60 minutes.

KEY STEPS
◆ The patient is positioned in a reclining or straight-backed chair or on a bed.
◆ The patient is asked to remain still.
◆ Depending on the specific type of EP study, electrodes may be attached.
◆ Visual EPs are produced by exposing the eye to a rapidly reversing checkerboard pattern.

◆ Somatosensory EPs are produced by electrically stimulating a peripheral sensory nerve.
◆ Auditory brain stem EPs are produced by delivering clicks to the ear.
◆ A computer amplifies and averages the brain's response to each stimulus and plots the results as a waveform.

POSTPROCEDURE CARE
◆ Remove electrode gel.

Interpretation

NORMAL RESULTS
◆ Vary greatly among laboratories and patients
◆ Visual EP test: positive P100 waveform appearing about 100 msec after applying a pattern-shift stimulus
◆ Somatosensory EP test: various waveforms, depending on locations of the stimulating and recording electrodes

ABNORMAL RESULTS
◆ Visual EP test: abnormal (extended) P100 latencies confined to one eye, suggesting a visual pathway lesion anterior to the optic chiasm; bilateral abnormal P100 latencies suggesting multiple sclerosis
◆ Somatosensory EP test: changes in the electrical waveforms, indicating damaged or degenerated nerve pathways to the brain from the eyes, ears, or limbs; absence of activity in a pathway, suggesting complete loss of nerve function in that pathway
◆ Changes suggesting evidence of the type and location of nerve damage
◆ Abnormal upper-limb interwave latencies, suggesting possible cervical spondylosis, intracerebral lesions, or sensorimotor neuropathies
◆ Abnormalities in the lower limb, suggesting peripheral nerve and root lesions such as those in Guillain-Barré syndrome

HIDA scan

Overview

A hepatobiliary (HIDA) scan measures gamma rays emitted from bile after technetium-99m is injected.

PURPOSE
- To diagnose suspected gallbladder disorders
- To help in the differential diagnosis of acute and chronic cholecystitis
- To evaluate the patency of the biliary enteric bypass
- To assess obstructive jaundice when done in conjunction with ultrasound or radiography
- To assess enterogastric reflux

PRECAUTIONS
- Wear gloves while handling the radionuclide.

Test

PREPARATION
- Confirm the patient's identity using two patient identifiers and verify the test to be done according to facility policy.
- Explain the purpose of the test and how it's done.
- Tell the patient who will perform the test and when it will be done.
- Make sure the patient has signed an informed consent form.
- Instruct the patient to fast for at least 4 hours before the test.
- Don't administer meperidine (Demerol) or morphine (Duramorph) for 24 hours before the test.
- Have the patient void before the procedure.
- Make sure the patient has a patent I.V. line.
- Inform the patient that the test takes about 1 to 2 hours.

KEY STEPS
- Place the patient on the table in a supine position.
- Instruct the patient to lie still during the test for the best images.
- The technician administers the radionuclide into the I.V. access device.
- The right upper quadrant of the abdomen will be scanned at various intervals for 1 hour.
- During the test, morphine may be administered to initiate spasms of the sphincter of Oddi.
- If the test is assessing gallbladder function or bile reflux, the patient is given a fatty meal 60 minutes after the radionuclide injection.

POSTPROCEDURE CARE
- Instruct the patient to increase fluid intake for 24 to 48 hours unless contraindicated.

Interpretation

NORMAL RESULTS
- Normal gallbladder shape, size, and function
- Presence of patent cystic and common bile ducts

ABNORMAL RESULTS
- Inability to see the gallbladder 1 or 2 hours after injection, indicating an obstruction of the cystic duct
- Delayed filling of the gallbladder, indicating cholecystitis
- Radionuclide seen in the biliary tree but not in the bowel, indicating obstruction of the common bile duct
- No visualization of the radionuclide within 15 to 30 minutes when morphine is used, indicating acute cholecystitis

Holter monitoring

Overview

A Holtor monitor continuously records heart activity as the patient follows his normal routine, usually for 24 hours. A patient-activated monitor, also known as ambulatory electrocardiography or dynamic monitoring, is worn for 5 to 7 days and allows the patient to manually initiate heart activity recording when symptoms occur.

PURPOSE
◆ To detect cardiac arrhythmias
◆ To evaluate chest pain
◆ To evaluate the effectiveness of antiarrhythmic drug therapy
◆ To monitor pacemaker function
◆ To correlate symptoms and palpitations with actual cardiac events and patient activities
◆ To detect sporadic arrhythmias missed by an exercise or resting electrocardiogram (ECG)

PRECAUTIONS
◆ Avoid placing electrodes over large muscle masses such as the pectorals to limit artifacts.

Test

PREPARATION
◆ Confirm the patient's identity using two patient identifiers and verify the test to be done according to facility policy.
◆ Explain the purpose of the test and how it's done.
◆ Tell the patient who will perform the test and when it will be done.
◆ Provide bathing instructions because some equipment must not get wet.
◆ Instruct the patient to avoid magnets, metal detectors, high-voltage areas, and electric blankets.

◆ Explain the importance of logging activities as well as emotional upsets, physical symptoms, and ingestion of medication in a diary.
◆ Explain how to mark the tape at the onset of symptoms, if applicable.
◆ Explain how to check the recorder to make sure that it's working properly.

KEY STEPS
◆ Electrodes are applied to the chest wall and securely attached to the leadwires and monitor.
◆ A new or fully charged battery is inserted in the recorder.
◆ A tape is inserted and the recorder is turned on.
◆ The electrode attachment circuit is tested by connecting the recorder to a standard ECG machine, noting artifact during normal patient movement.

POSTPROCEDURE CARE
◆ Remove all chest electrodes.
◆ Clean the electrode sites.

Interpretation

NORMAL RESULTS
◆ No significant arrhythmias or ST-segment changes on ECG
◆ Changes in heart rate during various activities

ABNORMAL RESULTS
◆ Abnormalities in cardiac rate or rhythm, suggesting possible serious arrhythmias, which may not be causing symptoms
◆ ST-segment changes coinciding with patient symptoms or increased activity, suggesting possible myocardial ischemia

Hysteroscopy

Overview

Hysteroscopy is the examination of the interior of the uterus through the use of a small-diameter endoscope. It's usually performed in the practitioner's office with a local anesthetic or mild sedative and should be done during the first week after a patient's menstrual cycle ends.

PURPOSE

◆ To investigate abnormal uterine bleeding
◆ To remove polyps
◆ To evaluate infertile patients
◆ To direct the removal of intrauterine devices
◆ To help diagnose and treat intrauterine adhesions
◆ To diagnose uterine fibroids
◆ To remove uterine adhesions or small fibroids
◆ To perform uterine ablation

PRECAUTIONS

◆ Watch for adverse reaction to analgesics.
◆ Watch for signs and symptoms of infection, such as fever and pain.

Test

PREPARATION

◆ Confirm the patient's identity using two patient identifiers and verify the test to be done according to facility policy.
◆ Explain the purpose of the test and how it's done.
◆ Tell the patient who will perform the test and when it will be done.
◆ Make sure that the patient has signed an informed consent form.
◆ Document and report all allergies.
◆ Check the patient's history for hypersensitivity to the anesthetic.
◆ Obtain the results of the patient's last Papanicolaou test.
◆ Assess pregnancy status.
◆ Advise the patient of dietary restrictions as ordered.
◆ Have the patient empty her bladder before the test.

◆ Teach the patient how to collect a 24-hour urine specimen.
◆ Warn the patient that the practitioner may inflate her uterus with carbon dioxide (CO_2); tell her that her body will absorb it but that it may cause upper abdominal or shoulder pain for 24 to 36 hours after the test.
◆ Inform the patient that some vaginal bleeding and mild abdominal cramping may occur after the test.

KEY STEPS

◆ The patient is assisted into a modified dorsal lithotomy position with her legs in stirrups.
◆ A local anesthetic is given by the practitioner.
◆ The vagina is cleaned and the hysteroscope is inserted.
◆ Visualization begins at the level of the internal os.
◆ In contact hysteroscopy, the uterus isn't distended; only the area in direct contact with the hysteroscope is visible.
◆ In panoramic hysteroscopy, an external illumination source and media (such as CO_2) for distention are used; these approaches make the tissue visible from a distance.
◆ Cultures of the vagina and cervix may be taken.

POSTPROCEDURE CARE

◆ Provide the patient with a sanitary pad if needed.
◆ Provide analgesics as needed.
◆ Monitor the patient's vital signs.
◆ Watch the patient for bleeding.

Interpretation

NORMAL RESULTS

◆ Normal size and shape of uterus interior
◆ No adhesions and lesions

ABNORMAL RESULTS

◆ Abnormally shaped uterine interior, suggesting polyps, uterine wall tumors, fibroids, or adhesions

Kidney-ureter-bladder radiography

Overview

Kidney-ureter-bladder radiography, also known as a *flat plate of the abdomen*, is an X-ray of the abdomen used mostly to identify GI conditions.

PURPOSE

♦ To evaluate the size, structure, and position of the kidneys and bladder
♦ To screen for abnormalities, such as calcifications, in the area of the kidneys, ureters, and bladder
♦ To identify bowel obstruction, gallstones, presence of stool in the bowel
♦ To assess positioning of nasogastric tubes or stents

PRECAUTIONS

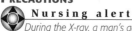 **Nursing alert**

During the X-ray, a man's gonads should be shielded; however, a woman's ovaries can't be shielded because they're too close to the kidneys, ureters, and bladder.

Test

PREPARATION

♦ Confirm the patient's identity using two patient identifiers and verify the test to be done according to facility policy.
♦ Explain the purpose of the study and how it's done.
♦ Explain who will perform the test and when it will be done.
♦ Tell the patient that the test takes only a few minutes.

KEY STEPS

♦ The patient is assisted into a supine position with his arms extended over his head on an X-ray table.
♦ Symmetrical positioning of the iliac crests is noted.
♦ A single X-ray is taken.

POSTPROCEDURE CARE

♦ None is needed.

Interpretation

NORMAL RESULTS

♦ Bilateral kidney shadows, with the right slightly lower than the left
♦ Kidneys about the same size, with the superior poles tilting slightly toward the vertebral column, parallel to the shadows of the psoas muscles
♦ Bladder shadow not as visible as the kidney shadows
♦ Normal amount of intestinal gas

ABNORMAL RESULTS

♦ Bilateral renal enlargement, suggesting polycystic kidney disease, multiple myeloma, lymphoma, amyloidosis, hydronephrosis, or compensatory renal hypertrophy
♦ Unilateral renal enlargement, suggesting a possible tumor, cyst, or hydronephrosis
♦ Abnormally small kidneys, suggesting possible end-stage glomerulonephritis or bilateral atrophic pyelonephritis
♦ An apparent decrease in the size of one kidney, suggesting possible congenital hypoplasia, atrophic pyelonephritis, or ischemia
♦ Renal displacement, suggesting a retroperitoneal tumor
♦ Obliteration or bulging of a portion of the psoas muscle stripe, suggesting possible tumor, abscess, or hematoma
♦ Abnormal location or absence of a kidney, suggesting possible congenital anomalies
♦ A lobulated edge or border, suggesting possible polycystic kidney disease or patchy atrophic pyelonephritis
♦ Opaque bodies, suggesting possible calculi, vascular calcification, cystic tumors, fecaliths, foreign bodies, soft tissue mass or abnormal fluid or gas collection
♦ Excessive stool, suggesting possible bowel obstruction

Laparoscopy, pelvic

Overview

Pelvic laparoscopy is a minimally invasive surgical procedure that allows visualization of the peritoneal cavity using a small fiber-optic telescope (laparoscope) inserted through a small incision in the anterior abdominal wall. This test allows evaluation of the abdominal cavity as well as many types of abdominal surgery, such as tubal ligation and hysterectomy, to be done simultaneously at lower cost and with faster recovery than open surgery.

PURPOSE

◆ To identify the cause of pelvic pain
◆ To detect endometriosis, ectopic pregnancy, or pelvic inflammatory disease (PID)
◆ To evaluate pelvic masses
◆ To evaluate infertility
◆ To stage a carcinoma

PRECAUTIONS

◆ Watch for bleeding and signs and symptoms of infection.

Test

PREPARATION

◆ Confirm the patient's identity using two patient identifiers and verify the test to be done according to facility policy.
◆ Explain the purpose of the test and how it's done.
◆ Tell the patient who will perform the test and when it will be done.
◆ Make sure the patient has signed an informed consent form.
◆ Document and report allergies.
◆ Tell the patient to fast after midnight before the test or for at least 8 hours before surgery.

KEY STEPS

◆ The patient is anesthetized and placed into the lithotomy position.
◆ An incision is made at the inferior rim of the umbilicus.

◆ The peritoneal cavity is insufflated with carbon dioxide or nitrous oxide.
◆ A laparoscope is inserted to examine the pelvis and abdomen.
◆ A second incision may be made just above the pubic hair line for some procedures.
◆ After the examination, minor surgical procedures, such as ovarian biopsy, may be performed.

POSTPROCEDURE CARE

◆ Warn the patient that she may experience pain at the puncture site and in the shoulder, but the pain should disappear within 24 to 36 hours after the procedure.
◆ Provide analgesics.
◆ Monitor the patient's vital signs.
◆ Monitor the patient for adverse reactions to anesthetic.
◆ Tell the patient to resume her usual diet.
◆ Instruct the patient to restrict activity for 2 to 7 days after the procedure.

Interpretation

NORMAL RESULTS

◆ Uterus and fallopian tubes of normal size and shape that are free from adhesions and mobile
◆ Ovaries of normal size and shape
◆ No cysts or endometriosis

ABNORMAL RESULTS

◆ A bubble on the surface of the ovary, suggesting a possible ovarian cyst
◆ Sheets or strands of tissue, suggesting possible adhesions
◆ Small, blue powder burns on the peritoneum or serosa, suggesting endometriosis
◆ Growths on the uterus, suggesting fibroids
◆ An enlarged fallopian tube, suggesting possible hydrosalpinx
◆ An enlarged or ruptured fallopian tube, suggesting a possible ectopic pregnancy
◆ Infection or abscess, suggesting possible PID

Liver-spleen scan

Overview

A liver-spleen scan uses a gamma camera to record the distribution of radioactivity within the liver and spleen after I.V. injection of radioactive colloid, technetium 99m (^{99m}Tc). Focal disease is demonstrated nonspecifically as a cold spot that failed to take up the colloid, although lesions smaller than $^3/_4''$ (2 cm) in diameter or early hepatocellular disease may not be visible. Flow studies may help distinguish metastasis, tumors, cysts, and abscesses.

PURPOSE
◆ To screen for hepatic metastasis and hepatocellular disease
◆ To detect focal disease such as tumors, cysts, or abscesses
◆ To check for hepatomegaly, splenomegaly, and splenic infarcts
◆ To assess the condition of the liver and spleen after abdominal trauma

PRECAUTIONS
◆ A patient shouldn't have more than one radionuclide scan in the same day.

Test

PREPARATION
◆ Confirm the patient's identity using two patient identifiers and verify the test to be done according to facility policy.
◆ Explain the purpose of the test and how it's done.
◆ Explain who will perform the test and when it will be done.
◆ Document and report allergies.
◆ Stress the importance of lying still during the study.
◆ Tell the patient that he need not fast before the test.
◆ Tell him the test takes about 1 hour.

KEY STEPS
◆ ^{99m}Tc is injected I.V by the technician.
◆ After 10 to 15 minutes the abdomen is scanned using various views.
◆ Scintigraphs are reviewed for clarity.
◆ Additional views are obtained as needed.

POSTPROCEDURE CARE
◆ Encourage oral fluid intake to assist elimination of the radioactive material, unless contraindicated.
◆ Monitor the patient's vital signs and respiratory status.
◆ Monitor intake and output.
◆ After the test, instruct the patient to flush the toilet immediately after urinating to reduce exposure to radiation in the urine.

Interpretation

NORMAL RESULTS
◆ Equally bright liver and spleen images
◆ More homogeneous distribution of radioactive colloid in the spleen than in the liver
◆ Various normal indentations and impressions in the liver mimicking focal disease

ABNORMAL RESULTS
◆ Uniformly decreased or patchy appearance, suggesting hepatocellular disease
◆ Uniformly decreased colloid distribution, suggesting hepatitis
◆ Failure to take up the radioactive colloid and the appearance of solitary or multiple focal defects, suggesting cysts, abscesses, hematomas, and tumors
◆ Lentiform defects on the periphery of the liver, suggesting subcapsular hematoma
◆ Linear defects, suggesting hepatic laceration
◆ Focal defects in or next to the spleen, possibly transecting it, suggesting splenic hematoma

Lumbar puncture

Overview

A lumbar puncture, also known as a *spinal tap*, is the insertion of a needle into the spinal column to obtain a cerebral spinal fluid (CSF) sample for qualitative analysis.

PURPOSE
◆ To measure CSF pressure
◆ To help diagnose meningitis, subarachnoid or intracranial hemorrhage, tumors and brain abscesses, neurosyphilis, and chronic central nervous system infections

PRECAUTIONS
◆ The test is contraindicated in patients with increased intracranial pressure.

Test

PREPARATION
◆ Confirm the patient's identity using two patient identifiers and verify the test to be done according to facility policy.
◆ Explain the purpose of the test, how it's done, who will perform the test, and when it will be done.
◆ Make sure the patient has signed an informed consent form.
◆ Note and report allergies.

KEY STEPS
◆ Position the patient on his side with his knees drawn up to his abdomen and his chin tucked against his chest.
◆ The skin site is prepared and draped.
◆ A local anesthetic is injected.
◆ The spinal needle is inserted in the midline between the spinous processes of the vertebrae.
◆ The stylet is removed from the needle; CSF will drip out of the needle if properly positioned.
◆ A stopcock and manometer are attached to the needle to measure the CSF pressure.
◆ Specimens are collected and placed in the appropriate containers.
◆ The needle is removed and a small sterile dressing is applied.

POSTPROCEDURE CARE
◆ Keep the patient lying flat for 4 to 6 hours.
◆ Encourage the patient to drink fluids.
◆ Monitor the patient's neurologic status.
◆ Monitor the puncture site for redness, swelling, and drainage.

Interpretation

NORMAL RESULTS
◆ 50 to 180 mm H_2O pressure
◆ Clear and colorless CSF
◆ Protein level of 15 to 45 mg/dl (SI, 150 to 450 mg/L)
◆ Gamma globulin level 3% to 12% of total protein
◆ Glucose level of 40 to 70 mg/dl (2.2 to 3.9 mmol/L)
◆ 0 to 5 white blood cells; no red blood cells (RBCs)
◆ Chloride level of 118 to 130 mEq/L (118 to 130 mmol/L)
◆ No organisms in Gram stain

ABNORMAL RESULTS
◆ Increased ICP, indicating tumor, hemorrhage, or edema from trauma
◆ Cloudy CSF appearance and decreased chloride level, suggesting infection
◆ Yellow or bloody appearance, suggesting intracranial hemorrhage or spinal cord obstruction
◆ Brown or orange appearance, indicating increased protein levels or RBC breakdown
◆ Increased protein, suggesting tumor, trauma, diabetes mellitus, or blood in CSF
◆ Increased gamma globulin, indicating demyelinating disease or Guillain-Barré syndrome
◆ Increased glucose level, suggesting hyperglycemia
◆ Increased cell count, indicating meningitis, tumor, abscess, or demyelinating disease
◆ RBCs, indicating hemorrhage
◆ Gram-positive or gram-negative organisms, indicating bacterial meningitis

Lung perfusion and ventilation scan

Overview

A lung perfusion and ventilation scan produces a visual image of pulmonary blood flow after a radiopharmaceutical I.V. injection. Air mixed with radioactive gas is inhaled and a nuclear scan differentiates ventilated lung areas from underventilated lung areas.

PURPOSE
- To assess arterial perfusion of the lungs
- To detect pulmonary emboli
- To evaluate pulmonary function
- To identify areas of the lung capable of ventilation, evaluate regional respiratory function, and locate regional hypoventilation

PRECAUTIONS
- This scan is contraindicated in patients hypersensitive to the radiopharmaceutical.

Test

PREPARATION
- Confirm the patient's identity using two patient identifiers and verify the test to be done according to facility policy.
- Explain the purpose of the test and how it's done.
- Explain who will perform the test and when it will be done.
- Document and report allergies.
- Stress the importance of lying still during imaging.
- Make sure the patient has I.V. access.
- Tell him that fasting isn't required before the test.
- Tell the patient that the test takes about 30 minutes.

KEY STEPS
Lung perfusion scan
- With the patient in a supine position and taking moderately deep breaths, the radiopharmaceutical is injected I.V. slowly by the technician over 5 to 10 seconds to allow more even distribution of pulmonary blood flow.
- After the injection, the gamma camera takes a series of single, stationary images in the anterior, posterior, oblique, and both lateral chest views.
- The images are projected onto an oscilloscope screen and show the distribution of radioactive particles.

Lung ventilation scan
- After the patient inhales air mixed with a small amount of radioactive gas through a mask, its distribution in the lungs is monitored on a nuclear scanner.
- The patient's chest is scanned as he exhales.

POSTPROCEDURE CARE
- Monitor the injection site for hematoma and apply warm soaks if one develops.
- Inform the practitioner of abnormal results.

Interpretation

NORMAL RESULTS
- Hot spots (areas of high uptake), indicating normal blood perfusion
- Uniform uptake pattern
- Equal distribution and normal wash-in and wash-out phases in both lungs in the ventilation scan

ABNORMAL RESULTS
- Cold spots (areas of low uptake), indicating poor perfusion, suggesting an embolism
- Decreased regional blood flow, without vessel obstruction, suggesting possible pneumonitis
- Unequal gas distribution in both lungs, indicating poor ventilation or airway obstruction

Magnetic resonance imaging

Overview

Magnetic resonance imaging (MRI) is the use of a powerful magnetic field and radiofrequency waves to produce computerized images of internal organs and tissues, eliminating risks associated with exposure to X-rays.

PURPOSE
◆ To obtain images of internal organs and tissues not readily visible on standard X-rays

PRECAUTIONS
◆ Because MRI works through a powerful magnetic field, it can't be performed on patients with a pacemaker, an aneurysm clip, or other ferrous metal implants.
◆ Metallic or computer-based equipment (such as ventilators and I.V. pumps) can't enter the MRI area because of the magnetic field.

Test

PREPARATION

Nursing alert
Because patients requiring life support equipment, including ventilators, require special preparation, consult with MRI staff in advance of the test.

◆ Confirm the patient's identity using two patient identifiers and verify the test to be done according to facility policy.
◆ Explain the purpose of the test and how it's done.
◆ Tell the patient who will perform the test and when it will be done.
◆ Make sure the patient has signed an informed consent form.
◆ Document and report allergies.
◆ Administer sedation as ordered.
◆ If contrast is to be used, insert an I.V. catheter.

◆ Instruct the patient to remove metal objects he's wearing or carrying.
◆ Advise the patient that he'll be asked to remain still during the procedure.
◆ Warn the patient that the machine makes loud clacking sounds.
◆ Tell the patient the test takes 30 to 60 minutes.

KEY STEPS
◆ Check the patient for metal objects at the scanner room door.
◆ Place the patient in the supine position on a padded scanning table.
◆ The table is positioned in the opening of the scanning gantry.
◆ Use a call bell or intercom to maintain verbal contact.
◆ The patient may wear earplugs if needed.
◆ Varying radiofrequency waves are directed at the area being scanned.
◆ A computer reconstructs information as images on a television screen.

POSTPROCEDURE CARE
◆ Monitor the patient's vital signs.
◆ Inform the practitioner of abnormal results.

Interpretation

NORMAL RESULTS
◆ Normal structures specific to the area tested

ABNORMAL RESULTS
◆ Abnormal tissue or organ structure in the area tested

Multiple-gated acquisition scan

Overview

A multiple-gated acquisition (MUGA) scan shows moving images of the beating heart as well as other features that assess the health of cardiac ventricles in a noninvasive way. It's commonly done when the patient is at rest and then repeated with exercise or after the patient receives certain drugs.

PURPOSE
◆ To assess the function of the heart
◆ To detect certain heart conditions

PRECAUTIONS
◆ Movement during the examination may interfere with the image. Have the patient remain as still as possible.

Test

PREPARATION
◆ Confirm the patient's identity using two patient identifiers and verify the test to be done according to facility policy.
◆ Explain the purpose of the MUGA scan and how it's done.
◆ Tell the patient who will perform the test and when it will be done.
◆ Make sure the patient or a responsible family member has signed an informed consent form.
◆ Tell the patient that he'll receive an I.V. injection of a radioactive tracer and that a detector positioned above his chest will record the circulation of this tracer through the heart.
◆ Inform the patient that he may experience slight discomfort from the needle puncture, but that the imaging itself is painless.
◆ Instruct the patient to remain silent and motionless during imaging, unless otherwise instructed.

KEY STEPS
◆ A radioactive isotope is injected into the patient's vein.
◆ Radioactive isotopes attach to red blood cells and pass through the heart in the circulation.
◆ The isotopes are traced through the heart by a scintillation camera.
◆ For the next minute, the scintillation camera records the first pass of the isotope through the heart so that the aortic and mitral valves can be located.
◆ Using an electrocardiogram, the camera is set to record for selected 60-msec intervals, representing end-systole and end-diastole, and 500 to 1,000 cardiac cycles are recorded on X-ray or other film.

POSTPROCEDURE CARE
◆ None is needed.

Interpretation

NORMAL RESULTS
◆ Symmetrical left ventricle contraction
◆ Even distribution of the isotope

ABNORMAL RESULTS
◆ Asymmetrical blood distribution to the myocardium, producing ventricular wall motion segmental abnormalities, suggesting coronary artery disease or preexisting conditions such as myocarditis
◆ Reduced ejection fractions, indicating cardiomyopathy
◆ Recirculating radioisotope prolonging downslope of scintigraphic data curve, indicating left-to-right shunt
◆ Early arrival of activity in the left ventricle or aorta, signifying a right-to-left shunt

Myelography

Overview

Myelography is a radiologic procedure that combines radiography with fluoroscopy, which shows the flow of injected contrast medium and outlines of structures, to evaluate the spinal subarachnoid space.

PURPOSE
◆ To demonstrate lesions, such as tumors and herniated intervertebral disks, that partially or totally block cerebrospinal fluid (CSF) flow in the subarachnoid space
◆ To detect arachnoiditis, spinal nerve root injury, or tumors in the posterior fossa of the skull

PRECAUTIONS
◆ Notify the radiologist if the patient has a history of epilepsy or of antidepressant or phenothiazine use; phenothiazines given with metrizamide (Amipaque) during myelography increase the risk of toxicity.

Test

PREPARATION
◆ Confirm the patient's identity using two patient identifiers and verify the test to be done according to facility policy.
◆ Explain the purpose of the test and how it's done.
◆ Explain who will perform the test and when it will be done.
◆ Make sure the patient has signed an informed consent form.
◆ Record and report the patient's allergies.
◆ Give the patient a sedative and an anticholinergic.
◆ Instruct the patient to fast for 8 hours before the test.

KEY STEPS
◆ The patient is positioned on his side at the edge of the table with his knees drawn up to his chest.
◆ A lumbar puncture is performed.
◆ Some CSF may be removed for routine laboratory analysis.

◆ The patient is placed in the prone position.
◆ The contrast medium is injected.
◆ If a subarachnoid space obstruction blocks the upward flow of the contrast medium, a cisternal puncture may be performed.
◆ The flow of the contrast medium is studied with fluoroscopy, and X-rays are taken.
◆ The contrast medium is withdrawn, if oil-based, and the needle is removed.
◆ The puncture site is cleaned and a small dressing is applied.

POSTPROCEDURE CARE
◆ If the patient received an oil-based contrast medium, keep him flat in bed for 8 to 12 hours.
◆ If the patient received a water-based contrast medium, elevate the head of the bed 30 to 45 degrees for 6 to 8 hours.
◆ Encourage the patient to drink fluids.
◆ Monitor the patient's vital signs and intake and output.
◆ Monitor the patient's neurologic status.
◆ Observe the puncture site for bleeding and infection.
◆ Monitor the patient for seizure activity.
◆ Instruct the patient to resume his usual diet and activities 1 day after the test.

Interpretation

NORMAL RESULTS
◆ Freely flowing contrast medium through the subarachnoid space
◆ No obstruction or structural abnormality

ABNORMAL RESULTS
◆ Extradural lesions, suggesting herniated intervertebral disks, or metastatic tumors
◆ Lesions within the subarachnoid space, suggesting neurofibromas or meningiomas
◆ Lesions within the spinal cord, suggesting ependymomas or astrocytomas
◆ Fluid-filled cavities in the spinal cord and widening of the cord itself, suggesting possible syringomyelia

Nuclear medicine scan

Overview

A nuclear medicine scan obtains images of specific body organs or systems by a scintillating scanning camera after I.V. injection, inhalation, or oral ingestion of a radioactive tracer compound.

PURPOSE
◆ To produce tissue analysis and images not readily seen on standard X-rays
◆ To detect or rule out malignant lesions when X-ray findings are normal or questionable

PRECAUTIONS
◆ Make sure the patient isn't scheduled for more than one radionuclide scan on the same day.

Test

PREPARATION
◆ Confirm the patient's identity using two patient identifiers and verify the test to be done according to facility policy.
◆ Explain the purpose of the test and how it's done.
◆ Explain who will perform the test and when it will be done.
◆ Document and report allergies.
◆ Check for prior nuclear medicine procedures.
◆ Explain dietary restrictions based on the exact test being done.
◆ Insert an I.V. catheter.
◆ Advise the patient to remain still during the procedure and that he'll be asked to take various positions on a scanner table.
◆ Tell him that the test takes about 1 to 2 hours, but the time may vary based on the exact test.

KEY STEPS
◆ An I.V. tracer isotope is injected by the technician.
◆ The detector of a scintillation camera is directed at the area being scanned and displays the image on a monitor.
◆ Scintigraphs are obtained and reviewed for clarity.
◆ Additional views are obtained, if necessary.

POSTPROCEDURE CARE
◆ Monitor the patient's vital signs.
◆ Assess the injection site.
◆ Watch the patient for infection and orthostatic hypotension.
◆ Inform the practitioner of abnormal results.
◆ Tell the patient to resume his normal diet and activities as ordered.

Interpretation

NORMAL RESULTS
◆ Normal tissues and structures in the area being tested

ABNORMAL RESULTS
◆ Malignant lesions or tissue abnormalities specific to the area being scanned

Persantine thallium imaging

Overview

Persantine thallium imaging is the infusion of dipyridamole (Persantine) to simulate the effects of exercise to assess coronary vessel function for patients who can't tolerate exercise or stress electrocardiography. The infusion increases blood flow to the collateral circulation and away from the coronary arteries, inducing ischemia, and allowing the examiner to evaluate the cardiac vessel response. The heart is scanned immediately after the thallium infusion and again after 2 to 4 hours (diseased vessels can't deliver thallium to the heart, and thallium lingers in diseased areas of the myocardium).

PURPOSE
◆ To identify exercise- or stress-induced arrhythmias
◆ To assess the presence and degree of cardiac ischemia

PRECAUTIONS
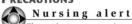 **Nursing alert**
The patient may experience arrhythmias, angina, ST-segment depression, or bronchospasm. Have resuscitation equipment available.

Test

PREPARATION
◆ Confirm the patient's identity using two patient identifiers and verify the test to be done according to facility policy.
◆ Explain the purpose of the test and how it's done.
◆ Explain who will perform the test and when it will be done.
◆ Make sure that the patient has signed the appropriate consent form.
◆ Tell the patient that a painless baseline electrocardiogram (ECG) will precede the test.
◆ Tell the patient to fast before the test and to avoid caffeine and other stimulants.

◆ Instruct the patient to continue taking his regular medications, with the possible exception of beta-adrenergic blockers.
◆ Tell the patient that the test may take up to 4 hours to complete.

KEY STEPS
◆ The patient reclines or sits while a resting ECG is performed. Persantine is either given orally or infused I.V. over 4 minutes. Monitor blood pressure, pulse rate, and cardiac rhythm continuously.
◆ After Persantine administration, the patient is asked to walk. After the Persantine takes effect, thallium is injected.
◆ The patient is placed in a supine position while the scan is performed. The scan is then reviewed. If necessary, a second scan is performed.

POSTPROCEDURE CARE
◆ Report abnormal results.
◆ If the patient must return for further scanning, tell him to rest and to restrict food and fluids in the interim.

Interpretation

NORMAL RESULTS
◆ Distribution of the isotope throughout the left ventricle and no visible defects

ABNORMAL RESULTS
◆ The presence of ST-segment depression, angina, and arrhythmias, strongly suggesting coronary artery disease (CAD)
◆ Persistent ST-segment depression, indicating a myocardial infarction; transient ST-segment depression, indicating ischemia from CAD
◆ Cold spots, indicating CAD or resulting from sarcoidosis, myocardial fibrosis, cardiac contusion, attenuation because of soft tissue (for example, breast or diaphragm), apical cleft, and coronary spasm
◆ Absence of cold spots in the presence of CAD, resulting from insignificant obstruction, single-vessel disease, or collateral circulation

Plethysmography, venous

Overview

A venous plethysmography, also called *occlusive impedance phlebography* measures venous flow in the limbs. Plethysmograph electrodes are applied to the patient's leg to record changes in electrical resistance (impedance) from blood volume variations.

PURPOSE
◆ To detect deep vein thrombosis (DVT)
◆ To screen the patient at high risk for thrombophlebitis
◆ To evaluate the patient with suspected pulmonary embolism

PRECAUTIONS
◆ Decreased peripheral arterial blood flow may interfere with test results.

Test

PREPARATION
◆ Confirm the patient's identity using two patient identifiers and verify the test to be done according to facility policy.
◆ Explain the purpose of the test and how it's done.
◆ Explain who will perform the test and when it will be done.
◆ Keep the room temperature as warm as possible to help prevent the patient's extremities from becoming cold.
◆ Tell the patient the test takes 30 to 45 minutes.

KEY STEPS
◆ Assist the patient into the supine position, elevating the leg to be tested 30 to 35 degrees. To promote venous drainage, place the calf above the patient's heart level.
◆ Ask the patient to flex his knee slightly and to rotate his hips by shifting his weight to the same side as the leg being tested.
◆ After the electrodes (connected to the plethysmograph) have been loosely attached by the technician to the calf about

3″ to 4″ (7.5 to 10 cm) apart, the pressure cuff (connected to the air pressure system) is wrapped snugly around the thigh about 2″ (5 cm) above the knee.
◆ The pressure cuff is inflated to 45 to 60 cm H_2O, allowing full venous distention without interfering with arterial blood flow.
◆ Pressure is maintained for 45 seconds or until the tracing stabilizes.
◆ In a patient with reduced arterial blood flow, pressure is maintained for 2 minutes or longer, after which the pressure cuff is rapidly deflated.
◆ The strip chart tracing, which records the increase in venous volume after cuff inflation and the decrease in venous volume 3 seconds after deflation, is checked.
◆ The test is repeated for the other leg.
◆ If necessary, three to five tracings for each leg are obtained to confirm full venous filling and outflow; the tracing showing the greatest rise and fall in venous volume is used as the test result.
◆ If the result is ambiguous, the position of the patient's leg and placement of the cuff and electrode are checked.

POSTPROCEDURE CARE
◆ Remove the conductive gel from the patient's skin after the test.
◆ Inform the practitioner of abnormal results.

Interpretation

NORMAL RESULTS
◆ A sharp rise in venous volume from temporary venous occlusion; rapid venous outflow from occlusion release

ABNORMAL RESULTS
◆ Increased calf vein pressure and vein distension, suggesting blockage of major deep veins
◆ Reduced filling in the calf vein and venous outflow rates, suggesting significant thrombi in a major deep vein of the lower leg, such as the popliteal, femoral, or iliac vein

Positron emission tomography

Overview

Positron emission tomography (PET) is a nuclear medicine scan that measures metabolic processes, such as glucose metabolism, blood flow, and tissue perfusion, and oxygenation, of the organ being observed. Radioactive chemicals are given to the patient, and sensors placed around the patient detect positrons emitted from the chemicals in organs. Positron counts, along with computed tomography, help record a two- or three-dimensional image of the organ. A PET scan is most commonly used in cardiology, neurology, and oncology.

Purpose
♦ To detect stroke or aneurysm
♦ To diagnose Parkinson's disease and Huntington's disease
♦ To evaluate cranial tumor preoperatively and postoperatively
♦ To assess the size of a myocardial infarction (MI) or detect coronary artery disease
♦ To evaluate the presence or recurrence of cancer or tumors
♦ To evaluate for metastasis of a cancerous tumor

Precautions
♦ Wear gloves while handling the radionuclide.

Test

Preparation
♦ Confirm the patient's identity using two patient identifiers and verify the test to be done according to facility policy.
♦ Explain the purpose of the test and how it's done.
♦ Explain who will perform the test and when it will be done.
♦ Tell the patient to fast for 4 hours before the test and to avoid alcohol, caffeine, and tobacco products for at least 24 hours before the test.
♦ Insert two I.V. catheters.

♦ Tell the patient the test takes 45 to 90 minutes.

Key steps
♦ Position the patient as appropriate for the organs to be scanned.
♦ The radioactive material is injected through an I.V. line.
♦ The gamma rays that are able to penetrate the tissue are recorded outside the body by a series of detectors and are displayed on a computer screen.
♦ If the patient is having a brain scan, he may be asked to perform a series of cognitive activities.
♦ The imaging is done at periodic intervals for up to 1 hour.

Postprocedure care
♦ Inform the practitioner of abnormal results.
♦ Instruct the patient to increase his fluid intake for 24 to 48 hours to help flush the radionuclide from the body, unless otherwise ordered.

Interpretation

Normal results
♦ Normal organ anatomy and physiology, including tissue metabolism, oxygenation, and blood flow

Abnormal results
♦ Various abnormalities depending on the scanned organ
♦ Brain scan abnormalities, indicating strokes, metastasis in the brain, dementia, head trauma, migraines, seizure disorders, and tumors
♦ Cardiac scan abnormalities, indicating necrotic tissue, hypertrophic left ventricle, MI, ischemia, pulmonary edema, and chronic obstructive pulmonary disease
♦ Increased radionuclide uptake, indicating abnormal lymph nodes, tumors, and metastasis

Diagnostic tests

Pulmonary artery catheterization

Overview

Pulmonary artery catheterization, also known as *Swan-Ganz catheterization,* is the insertion of a balloon-tipped, flow-directed catheter for the purpose of obtaining hemodynamic measurements, such as pulmonary artery pressure (PAP) and pulmonary artery wedge pressure (PAWP). It's used for assessment of cardiac, pulmonary, and fluid status to help direct and evaluate treatment.

PURPOSE

◆ To assess right- and left-sided ventricular function
◆ To monitor therapy for complications of acute myocardial infarction, shock, pulmonary edema, systolic murmur, and various cardiac arrhythmias
◆ To monitor fluid status in patients with serious burns, renal disease, noncardiogenic pulmonary edema, or acute respiratory distress syndrome
◆ To establish baseline pressures preoperatively in patients with existing cardiac disease
◆ To differentiate between noncardiac and cardiac pulmonary edema
◆ To monitor the effects of cardiovascular drugs

PRECAUTIONS

◆ Notify the practitioner if there's difficulty in flushing the system.
◆ If a damped waveform occurs, it may be necessary to withdraw the catheter slightly; pulmonary infarction can occur if the catheter remains in a wedged position.
◆ After each PAWP reading, make sure the balloon is completely deflated.
◆ If the patient shows signs of sepsis, treat the catheter as the source of infection and send it to the laboratory for culture when it's removed.

Test

PREPARATION

◆ Confirm the patient's identity using two patient identifiers and verify the test to be done according to facility policy.
◆ Explain the purpose of the study and how it's done.
◆ Explain who will perform the test and where it will be done.
◆ Make sure the patient has signed an informed consent form.
◆ Document and report allergies.
◆ Explain that the catheter will remain in place, causing little or no discomfort, for 48 to 72 hours.
◆ Tell the patient that catheter insertion takes about 30 minutes.

KEY STEPS

◆ The patient is placed in a supine position with his head and shoulders slightly lower than his trunk.
◆ The catheter is introduced into the vein percutaneously.
◆ The catheter is directed into the right atrium.
◆ The catheter balloon is partially inflated.
◆ Venous flow carries the catheter tip through the right atrium and tricuspid valve into the right ventricle and into the pulmonary artery.
◆ The monitor is observed for characteristic pressure waveform changes as the catheter enters each heart chamber.
◆ As the catheter is passed into the chambers on the right side of the heart, the monitor screen is observed for frequent premature ventricular contractions, ventricular tachycardia, and other arrhythmias. If arrhythmias occur, the catheter may be partially withdrawn or medication given to suppress the arrhythmias.
◆ For recording PAWP, the catheter balloon is carefully inflated with the specified

amount of air (no more than 1.5 cc), until a PAWP waveform is obtained.

◆ After PAWP is recorded, the air from the balloon is allowed to return to the syringe.

◆ The monitor screen is observed for a continuous pulmonary artery waveform.

POSTPROCEDURE CARE

◆ Obtain a chest X-ray to verify proper catheter placement and to assess for complications such as pneumothorax.

◆ Monitor the patient's vital signs and cardiac rhythm.

◆ Document PAP, PAWP, and cardiac output per facility policy.

◆ Watch for infection of the insertion site and bleeding.

◆ Watch for signs and symptoms of pulmonary emboli, pulmonary artery perforation, and arrhythmias.

◆ Inform the practitioner of abnormal results.

Interpretation

NORMAL RESULTS

◆ 1 to 6 mm Hg right atrial (RA) pressure
◆ 20 to 30 mm Hg right ventricular (RV) systolic pressure
◆ Less than 5 mm Hg RV end-diastolic pressure
◆ 20 to 30 mm Hg systolic PAP
◆ 10 to 15 mm Hg diastolic PAP
◆ Less than 20 mm Hg mean PAWP
◆ 6 to 12 mm Hg PAWP
◆ 10 mm Hg left atrial pressure

ABNORMAL RESULTS

◆ High RA pressures, suggesting pulmonary disease, right-sided heart failure, fluid overload, or cardiac tamponade
◆ High RV pressures, suggesting pulmonary hypertension, pulmonary valvular stenosis, right-sided heart failure, pericardial effusion, or ventricular septal defects

◆ High PAP, suggesting atrial or ventricular septal defects, pulmonary hypertension, mitral stenosis, chronic obstructive pulmonary disease, pulmonary edema or embolus, or left-sided heart failure

◆ High PAWP, suggesting left-sided heart failure or cardiac tamponade

◆ Low PAWP, suggesting hypovolemia

Pulmonary function tests

Overview

Pulmonary function tests (PFTs) evaluate pulmonary function through a series of spirometric measurements.

PURPOSE
◆ To assess effectiveness of a specific therapeutic regimen
◆ To determine the cause of dyspnea
◆ To determine whether a functional abnormality is obstructive or restrictive
◆ To measure pulmonary dysfunction

PRECAUTIONS

 Nursing alert

PFTs may be contraindicated in patients with acute coronary insufficiency, angina, or recent myocardial infarction. Watch for respiratory distress, changes in pulse rate and blood pressure, coughing, and bronchospasm in these patients.

Test

PREPARATION
◆ Confirm the patient's identity using two patient identifiers and verify the test to be done according to facility policy.
◆ Explain the purpose of the test and how it's done.
◆ Explain who will perform the test and when it will be done.
◆ Withhold bronchodilators for 8 hours as ordered.
◆ Stress the need for the patient to avoid smoking for 12 hours before the tests.
◆ Instruct the patient not to eat a heavy meal before the tests.
◆ Tell the patient the test takes 1 or 2 hours.

KEY STEPS
◆ For tidal volume (V_T), the patient breathes normally into the mouthpiece 10 times.
◆ For expiratory reserve volume (ERV), the patient breathes normally for several breaths and then exhales as completely as possible.
◆ For vital capacity (VC), the patient inhales as deeply as possible and exhales into the mouthpiece as completely as possible. This process is repeated three times, and the largest volume is recorded.
◆ For inspiratory capacity (IC), the patient breathes normally for several breaths and inhales as deeply as possible.
◆ For functional residual capacity (FRC), the patient breathes normally into a spirometer. After a few breaths, the levels of gas in the spirometer and in the lungs reach equilibrium. FRC is calculated by subtracting the spirometer volume from the original volume.
◆ For forced vital capacity (FVC) and forced expiratory volume (FEV), the patient inhales as slowly and deeply as possible and then exhales into the mouthpiece as quickly and completely as possible. This step is repeated three times, and the largest volume is recorded. The volume of air expired at 1 second (FEV_1), at 2 seconds (FEV_2), and at 3 seconds (FEV_3) during all three repetitions is recorded.
◆ For maximal voluntary ventilation, the patient breathes into the mouthpiece as quickly and deeply as possible for 15 seconds.
◆ For diffusing capacity for carbon monoxide, the patient inhales a gas mixture with a low level of carbon monoxide and holds his breath for 10 to 15 seconds before exhaling.

POSTPROCEDURE CARE

◆ Inform the practitioner of abnormal results.

◆ Tell the patient to resume his usual activities, diet, and medications as ordered.

Interpretation

NORMAL RESULTS

◆ Based on age, height, weight, and sex as a percentage
◆ V_T: 5 to 7 mg/kg of body weight
◆ ERV: 25% of VC
◆ IC: 75% of VC
◆ FEV_1: 83% of VC after 1 second
◆ FEV_2: 94% of VC after 2 seconds
◆ FEV_3: 97% of VC after 3 seconds

ABNORMAL RESULTS

◆ FEV_1 less than 80%, suggesting obstructed pulmonary disease
◆ FEV_1-to-FVC ratio greater than 80%, suggesting restrictive pulmonary disease
◆ Low V_T, suggesting possible restrictive disease
◆ Low minute volume (MV), suggesting possible disorders such as pulmonary edema
◆ High MV, suggesting possible acidosis, exercise, or low compliance states
◆ Low carbon dioxide response, suggesting possible emphysema, myxedema, obesity, hypoventilation syndrome, or sleep apnea
◆ Residual volume greater than 35% of total lung capacity after maximal expiratory effort, suggesting obstructive disease
◆ Low IC, suggesting restrictive disease
◆ High FRC, suggesting possible obstructive pulmonary disease
◆ Low total lung capacity (TLC), suggesting restrictive disease
◆ High TLC, suggesting obstructive disease

◆ Low FVC, suggesting flow resistance from obstructive disease or from restrictive disease
◆ Low forced expiratory flow, suggesting obstructive disease of the small and medium-sized airways
◆ Low peak expiratory flow rate, suggesting upper airway obstruction
◆ Low diffusing capacity for carbon monoxide, suggesting possible interstitial pulmonary disease

Sigmoidoscopy

Overview

A sigmoidoscopy is the use of a flexible sigmoidoscope to examine the lining of the descending colon, sigmoid colon, rectum, and anal canal. It's used for colorectal screening and to obtain specimens from suspicious areas of the mucosa via biopsy, cytology brush, or aspirate.

PURPOSE
◆ To help diagnose acute or chronic diarrhea and rectal bleeding
◆ To evaluate changes in bowel habits or stool characteristics
◆ To help assess known ulcerative colitis

PRECAUTIONS
◆ The procedure is contraindicated when the patient has a perforated viscus or acute diverticulitis.

◆ Specimens are obtained from any suspicious area of the intestinal mucosa.
◆ Polyps are biopsied for histologic diagnosis and may be removed with an electrocautery snare.
◆ Aspirate of stools may be obtained for laboratory analysis if indicated.
◆ Before withdrawal of the scope, retroflexion is performed, allowing examination of the internal anal verge and the adjacent rectal mucosa.
◆ The scope is withdrawn, the lining of the colon is thoroughly examined, and air is removed.

POSTPROCEDURE CARE
◆ Monitor the patient's vital signs and observe for rectal bleeding.
◆ Observe for signs of bowel perforation
◆ Tell the patient to resume his previous diet as ordered.

Test

PREPARATION
◆ Confirm the patient's identity using two patient identifiers and verify the test to be done according to facility policy.
◆ Explain the purpose of the test and how it's done.
◆ Explain who will perform the test and when it will be done.
◆ Make sure that the patient has signed an informed consent form.
◆ Document and report allergies.
◆ Withhold food and fluid as ordered.
◆ Tell the patient that he may receive a laxative or enema before the test.
◆ Tell the patient that the test takes 10 to 30 minutes.

KEY STEPS
◆ The patient is placed in the Sims' position on the examination table.
◆ A digital rectal examination is performed.
◆ The flexible sigmoidoscope is slowly advanced to the splenic flexure.

Interpretation

NORMAL RESULTS
◆ Pearly white or pigmented anal canal mucosa, depending on the patient's race
◆ Pink rectal mucosa with a velvety appearance
◆ Less prominent vascular network at the rectosigmoid junction
◆ Three semilunar valves in the proximal half of the rectum
◆ Light pink-orange sigmoid and descending colon mucosa

ABNORMAL RESULTS
◆ Benign, precancerous, or malignant polyps or tumors and various forms of colitis revealed by biopsy
◆ Visible abnormalities of the anus and perineum, indicating external hemorrhoids, anal fissure, anorectal cellulitis or abscess, and perirectal skin tag
◆ Rectal mass, internal hemorrhoids, or anorectal abscess upon digital rectal examination
◆ Inflammatory change, suggesting possible diverticulitis

Slit-lamp examination

Overview

During a slit-lamp examination the ophthalmologist uses an instrument with a special lighting system and a binocular microscope to view the anterior segment of the eye, including eyelids, eyelashes, conjunctiva, sclera, cornea, tear film, anterior chamber, iris, crystalline lens, and vitreous face. This test also allows for evaluation of transparent ocular fluids and tissues.

PURPOSE
◆ To detect and evaluate abnormalities of the anterior segment tissues and structures

PRECAUTIONS
◆ Don't instill mydriatic drops into the eyes of patients with angle-closure glaucoma or in those who have a hypersensitivity reaction to the drops.

Test

PREPARATION
◆ Confirm the patient's identity using two patient identifiers and verify the test to be done according to facility policy.
◆ Explain the purpose of the test and how it's done.
◆ Explain who will perform the test and when it will be done.
◆ Instruct the patient to remove his contact lenses before the test, unless the test is to evaluate the fit of the contact lenses.
◆ Stress the need to remain still during the test.
◆ Tell him that the test takes 5 to 10 minutes.

KEY STEPS
◆ The patient is placed into the examining chair with both feet on the floor.
◆ The patient is asked to place his chin on the rest and his forehead against the bar.
◆ The room lights are dimmed.
◆ The ophthalmologist examines the patient's eyes—starting with the lids and lashes and progressing to the vitreous face—altering light and magnification as needed.
◆ A special camera may be attached to the slit lamp to photograph portions of the eye.
◆ If a corneal abrasion or ulcer is detected, a fluorescein stain allows better visualization.
◆ If a tearing deficiency is suspected, the ophthalmologist may examine the eye after applying a fluorescein or rose bengal stain; he may also perform the Schirmer's tearing test.

POSTPROCEDURE CARE
◆ If dilating drops were instilled, tell the patient that his near vision will be blurred for 40 minutes to 2 hours after the test.

Interpretation

NORMAL RESULTS
◆ Normal anterior segment tissues and structures

ABNORMAL RESULTS
◆ Irregular corneal shape, suggesting possible keratoconus
◆ A parchment-like consistency of the lid skin, with redness, minor swelling, and moderate itching, suggesting a possible hypersensitivity reaction
◆ Early-stage lens opacities, suggesting possible development of cataracts

Tonometry

Overview

Tonometry measures intraocular pressure (IOP). *Indentation tonometry* measures how deeply a known weight depresses the cornea; *applanation tonometry* measures how much force is required to flatten an area of the cornea.

PURPOSE
◆ To measure IOP
◆ To help diagnose and evaluate glaucoma

PRECAUTIONS
◆ Avoid the test in patients with corneal ulcer or infection unless it's performed by a skilled examiner and only in an emergency such as suspected acute angle-closure glaucoma.

Test

PREPARATION
◆ Confirm the patient's identity using two patient identifiers and verify the test to be done according to facility policy.
◆ Explain the purpose of the test and how it's done.
◆ Explain who will perform the test and when it will be done.
◆ Ask the patient to remove his contact lenses, if applicable.
◆ Instruct the patient not to cough or squeeze his eyelids together.
◆ Tell the patient that the test takes only a few minutes and requires his eyes to be anesthetized.
◆ Tell the patient not to rub his eyes for at least 20 minutes after the test to prevent corneal abrasion.

KEY STEPS
◆ The patient is asked to look down. The practitioner raises the patient's superior eyelid with his thumb, places one drop of the topical anesthetic at the top of the sclera, and has the patient blink.
◆ The practitioner checks the tonometer for a zero reading on the steel test block

that comes with the instrument and makes sure the plunger moves freely. The first measurement on each eye is obtained with the 5½-g weight.
◆ The patient is asked to look up and stare at a spot on the ceiling. He is then asked to open his mouth, take a deep breath, and exhale slowly for distraction.
◆ With the thumb and forefinger of one hand, the practitioner holds the lid of his right eye open against the orbital rim.
◆ The tonometer is held vertically with the thumb and forefinger of the other hand, and the footplate is rested on the apex of the cornea.
◆ With the footplate in place, the indicator needle is checked for a rhythmic transmission caused by the ocular pulse, and then the calibrated scale reading that converts to a measurement of IOP is recorded.
◆ If the reading doesn't exceed 4, an additional weight (7½, 10, or 15 g) is added to obtain a reliable result.
◆ The procedure is repeated on the left eye, and the time the test is performed is recorded.

POSTPROCEDURE CARE
◆ Tell the patient that if he feels a scratching sensation on his eye, it should disappear within 4 hours.
◆ The patient may reinsert contact lenses after the anesthetic has worn off or after at least 2 hours.

Interpretation

NORMAL RESULTS
◆ 12 to 20 mm Hg IOP, with diurnal variations (highest point upon waking, lowest point in the evening)

ABNORMAL RESULTS
◆ Increased IOP, requiring further testing for glaucoma
◆ IOP diurnal variations, suggesting supplemental serial measurements at different times on different days

Diagnostic tests

Transcranial Doppler study

Overview

A transcranial Doppler study measures blood flow velocity through the cerebral arteries. This noninvasive test provides information about the presence, quality, and changing nature of circulation to an area of the brain.

PURPOSE
◆ To measure the velocity of blood flow through certain cerebral vessels
◆ To detect and monitor the progression of cerebral vasospasm
◆ To determine the presence of collateral blood flow before surgical ligation or radiologic occlusion of diseased blood vessels

PRECAUTIONS
◆ Accuracy of results may be affected if a dressing is over the test site.

Test

PREPARATION
◆ Confirm the patient's identity using two patient identifiers and verify the test to be done according to facility policy.
◆ Explain the purpose of the test and how it's done.
◆ Explain who will perform the test and when it will be done.
◆ Explain that the test usually takes less than 1 hour, depending on the number of vessels to be examined and any interfering factors.

KEY STEPS
◆ The patient reclines in a chair or on a stretcher or bed.
◆ A small amount of gel is applied to the transcranial "window" (temporal, transorbital, and through the foramen magnum), where bone is thin enough to allow the Doppler signal to enter and be detected.
◆ The technician directs the signal toward the artery being studied and then records the velocities detected.
◆ In a complete study, the middle cerebral arteries, anterior cerebral arteries, ophthalmic arteries, carotid siphon, vertebral arteries, and basilar artery are studied.
◆ The Doppler signal can be transmitted to varying depths.
◆ Waveforms may be printed for later analysis.

POSTPROCEDURE CARE
◆ Remove any remaining gel from the patient's skin.
◆ Inform the practitioner of abnormal results.

Interpretation

NORMAL RESULTS
◆ Normal waveforms and velocities

ABNORMAL RESULTS
◆ High velocities, suggesting that blood flow is too turbulent or the vessel is too narrow; or possible stenosis, vasospasm, or arteriovenous malformation

Diagnostic tests

Transesophageal echocardiography

Overview

Transesophageal echocardiography combines ultrasonography with endoscopy to view the heart's structures. It's performed using a small transducer attached to the end of a gastroscope that's inserted into the esophagus, allowing images to be taken from the posterior aspect of the heart. This test produces high-quality images of the thoracic aorta, except for the superior ascending aorta, which is shadowed by the trachea.

PURPOSE

◆ To visualize and evaluate thoracic and aortic disorders, such as dissection and aneurysm, valvular disease (especially of the mitral valve), endocarditis, and congenital heart disease
◆ To visualize and evaluate intracardiac thrombi, cardiac tumors, cardiac tamponade, and ventricular dysfunction

PRECAUTIONS

◆ Observe closely for a vasovagal response, which may occur with gagging.
◆ Laryngospasm, arrhythmias, or bleeding increases the risk of complications.

Test

PREPARATION

◆ Confirm the patient's identity using two patient identifiers and verify the test to be done according to facility policy.
◆ Explain the purpose of the test and how it's done.
◆ Explain who will perform the test and when it will be done.
◆ Make sure the patient has signed an informed consent form.
◆ Document and report all allergies.
◆ Document and report any loose teeth.
◆ Explain the need for I.V. sedation and continuous monitoring during the study.
◆ Tell the patient to fast for 6 hours before the procedure.
◆ Instruct the patient to remove dentures or oral prostheses.

◆ Tell the patient that the study takes about 2 hours, including preparation and recovery.
◆ If the procedure is done on an outpatient basis, advise the patient to have someone drive him home.

KEY STEPS

◆ Connect the patient to monitors for continual blood pressure, heart rate, and pulse oximetry assessment.
◆ Assist the patient into a supine position on his left side and give him a sedative.
◆ Spray the back of his throat with a topical anesthetic.
◆ Place a bite block in the patient's mouth and instruct him to close his lips around it.
◆ The endoscope is inserted by the cardiologist and is advanced 12″ to 14″ (30 to 36 cm) to the level of the right atrium.
◆ To visualize the left ventricle, the scope is advanced 16″ to 18″ (41 to 46 cm).
◆ Ultrasound images are obtained and reviewed.

POSTPROCEDURE CARE

◆ Ensure the patient's safety and a patent airway until the sedative wears off.
◆ Withhold food and water until his gag reflex returns.
◆ Monitor the patient's level of consciousness and vital signs.
◆ Monitor the patient's respiratory status and cardiac arrhythmias.
◆ Observe for gag reflex.

Interpretation

NORMAL RESULTS

◆ No structural abnormalities
◆ No vegetations or thrombi
◆ No visible tumors

ABNORMAL RESULTS

◆ Structural thoracic and aortic abnormalities, suggesting possible endocarditis, congenital heart disease, intracardiac thrombi, or tumors
◆ Congenital defects, suggesting possible patent ductus arteriosus

Ultrasonography

Overview

Ultrasonography uses high-frequency sound wave echoes that are converted to electrical impulses and amplified by a transducer to display tissue characteristics on a monitor.

PURPOSE
◆ To measure organ size and evaluate structure
◆ To detect foreign bodies and differentiate between a cyst and solid tumor
◆ To monitor tissue response to radiation or chemotherapy

Test

PREPARATION
◆ Confirm the patient's identity using two patient identifiers and verify the test to be done according to facility policy.
◆ Explain the purpose of the test and how it's done.
◆ Explain who will perform the test and when it will be done.
◆ Stress the importance of remaining still during scanning to prevent a distorted image.
◆ Review required dietary restrictions.
◆ Tell the patient the test will take about 30 minutes.

KEY STEPS
◆ Assist the patient into a supine position; use pillows to support the area to be examined.
◆ The technician coats the target area with a water-soluble jelly.
◆ The transducer is used to scan the area, projecting the images on the oscilloscope screen. The image on the screen is photographed for subsequent examination.
◆ The patient may need assistance into right or left lateral positions for subsequent views.

POSTPROCEDURE CARE
◆ Remove the contact jelly from the patient's skin.
◆ Inform the practitioner of abnormal results.

Interpretation

NORMAL RESULTS
◆ Normal structure, movement, and blood flow of internal organs, specific to ultrasonography type (for example, abdominal aorta, gallbladder and biliary system, kidney and perirenal structures, liver, pancreas, pelvic area, spleen, and thyroid)

ABNORMAL RESULTS
◆ Indentification of a solid mass or decreased blood flow in the area tested, specific to ultrasonography type (for example, abdominal aorta, gallbladder and biliary system, kidney and perirenal structures, liver, pancreas, pelvic area, spleen, and thyroid)
◆ Fluid-filled cysts (no further study needed)

Venography, leg

Overview

Leg venography, also known as *ascending contrast phlebography*, assesses deep leg veins after injection of a radiographic contrast medium. This test is done when duplex ultrasound findings are equivocal.

PURPOSE
◆ To confirm a DVT diagnosis
◆ To distinguish clot formation from venous obstruction
◆ To evaluate congenital venous abnormalities
◆ To assess deep vein valvular competence
◆ To locate a suitable vein for arterial bypass grafting
◆ To evaluate chronic venous disease

PRECAUTIONS
◆ Because of the high volume of contrast used, especially if bilateral venography is needed, monitor renal function and hydration status carefully.

Test

PREPARATION
◆ Confirm the patient's identity using two patient identifiers and verify the test to be done according to facility policy.
◆ Explain the purpose of the study and how it's done.
◆ Explain who will perform the study and when it will be done.
◆ Make sure the patient has signed an informed consent form.
◆ Document and report all allergies.
◆ Stop anticoagulant therapy as ordered.
◆ Instruct the patient to restrict food and to drink only clear liquids for 4 hours before the test.
◆ Tell the patient that the test takes 30 to 45 minutes.

KEY STEPS
◆ Position the patient on a tilting X-ray table so that the leg being tested doesn't bear any weight.

◆ Tie a tourniquet around the ankle to expedite venous filling.
◆ Normal saline solution is injected into a superficial vein in the dorsum of the patient's foot, and a contrast medium is injected after placement has been confirmed.
◆ Using a fluoroscope, the distribution of the contrast medium is monitored, and spot films of the thigh and femoroiliac regions are taken from the anteroposterior and oblique views.
◆ Overhead films are taken of the calf, knee, thigh, and femoral area.
◆ After filming, reposition the patient horizontally, quickly elevate the leg being tested, and infuse normal saline solution to flush the contrast medium from the veins.
◆ The fluoroscope is checked to confirm complete emptying.
◆ After the needle is removed, apply a dressing to the injection site.

POSTPROCEDURE CARE
◆ Encourage fluid intake.
◆ If DVT is documented, start appropriate therapy.
◆ Monitor the injection site for bleeding, infection, hematoma, and erythema.

Interpretation

NORMAL RESULTS
◆ Steady opacification of the superficial and deep vasculature with no filling defects

ABNORMAL RESULTS
◆ Consistent filling defects, abrupt termination of a column of contrast material, unfilled major deep veins, or diversion of flow (through collaterals, for example), suggesting DVT
◆ Improper needle placement in a superficial vein, weight-bearing or muscle contraction, or use of tourniquets, producing artifacts of poor filling
◆ Diagnosis errors, usually resulting from incomplete filling

Wound culture and sensitivity

Overview

A wound culture and sensitivity analysis identifies the presence of bacteria in a lesion specimen and their sensitivity to specific antibiotics. The culture may be aerobic (for detection of organisms that require oxygen to grow and typically appear in a superficial wound) or anaerobic (for organisms that need little or no oxygen and exist in areas of poor tissue perfusion, such as postoperative wounds, ulcers, or compound fractures).

PURPOSE
◆ To identify an infectious microbe in a wound
◆ To guide antibiotic therapy

PRECAUTIONS
◆ Because some anaerobes die in the presence of oxygen, place the specimen in the culture tube quickly; make sure no air enters the tube, and check that the double stoppers are secure.
◆ Keep the specimen container upright and send it to the laboratory within 15 minutes to prevent growth or deterioration of microbes.

Test

PREPARATION
◆ Confirm the patient's identity using two patient identifiers and verify the test to be done according to facility policy.
◆ Explain the purpose of the study and how it's done.
◆ Explain who will perform the study and when it will be done.
◆ Tell the patient that the test takes only a few minutes.

KEY STEPS
◆ Maintain sterile technique during the procedure.
◆ Wear personal protective equipment during the procedure.
◆ Prepare a sterile field.

◆ Clean the area around the wound with antiseptic solution.
◆ For an aerobic culture, express the wound and swab as much exudate as possible, or insert the swab deep into the wound and gently rotate it. Immediately place the swab in the aerobic culture tube.
◆ For an anaerobic culture, insert the swab deep into the wound, gently rotate it, and immediately place it in the anaerobic culture tube.
◆ Record recent antimicrobial therapy, the source of the specimen, and the suspected organism on the laboratory request form.
◆ Label the specimen container appropriately with the patient's name, practitioner's name, hospital number, wound site, and time of specimen collection.

POSTPROCEDURE CARE
◆ Clean the area around the wound thoroughly to limit contamination of the culture by normal skin flora.
◆ Make sure no antiseptic solution enters the wound.
◆ Re-dress the wound.
◆ Inform the practitioner of abnormal results.

Interpretation

NORMAL RESULTS
◆ No pathogenic organisms

ABNORMAL RESULTS
◆ Presence of *Staphylococcus aureus*, group A beta-hemolytic streptococci, Proteus species, *Escherichia coli*, and other Enterobacteriaceae, and some Pseudomonas species, suggesting an aerobic wound infection
◆ Presence of *Clostridium, Peptococcus,* and *Streptococcus* species, suggesting an anaerobic wound infection

V Signs and symptoms

Abdominal distention

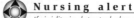

Overview

Abdominal distention (increased abdominal girth resulting from increased intra-abdominal pressure) occurs when fluid and gas can't pass freely through the GI tract. It may also occur as a result of acute bleeding, ascitic fluid accumulation, or air buildup from an abdominal organ perforation. It may be mild or severe, localized or diffuse, and gradual or sudden.

Assessment

HISTORY
◆ Ask about onset and duration.
◆ Obtain a medical history, noting GI or biliary disorders, chronic constipation, abdominal surgery, and recent accidents.

PHYSICAL ASSESSMENT
◆ Observe the recumbent patient for abdominal asymmetry.
◆ Assess abdominal contour.
◆ Check for localized distention, which may cause a sensation of pressure, fullness, or tenderness.
◆ Assess for generalized distention, which may cause perceived bloating, heart pounding, and difficulty breathing when lying flat or breathing deeply.
◆ Inspect for tense, glistening skin and bulging flanks, which may indicate ascites.
◆ Observe for everted or inverted umbilicus.
◆ Inspect the abdomen for signs of inguinal or femoral hernia and for incisions.
◆ Auscultate for bowel sounds, abdominal rubs, and bruits.
◆ Percuss and palpate the abdomen.
◆ Prepare the patient for pelvic or genital examination.
◆ Measure abdominal girth for a baseline value.
◆ Assess for other signs and symptoms, including abdominal pain, fever, nausea, vomiting, anorexia, altered bowel habits, and weight gain or loss.

◆ Nursing alert
If rigidity is detected along with abnormal bowel sounds, and the patient complains of pain, begin emergency interventions. Place the patient in the supine position, administer oxygen, and insert an I.V. line for fluid replacement. Insert a nasogastric (NG) tube to relieve acute intraluminal distention and prepare the patient for surgery.

Causes

MEDICAL
Abdominal cancer
◆ Generalized distention may occur when advanced cancer (ovarian, hepatic, or pancreatic) produces ascites.
◆ Other signs and symptoms include severe abdominal pain, anorexia, jaundice, GI hemorrhage, dyspepsia, weight loss, abdominal mass, and muscle weakness and atrophy.

Abdominal trauma
◆ Acute and dramatic distention may occur with brisk internal bleeding.
◆ Other signs and symptoms include abdominal rigidity with guarding, decreased or absent bowel sounds, vomiting, tenderness, abdominal bruising, pain over the trauma site or scapula, and, if blood loss is significant, hypovolemic shock.

Bladder distention
◆ Distention occurs in the lower abdomen.
◆ If mild, there's slight dullness on percussion above the symphysis pubis; if severe, there's a palpable, smooth, rounded suprapubic mass.

Cirrhosis
◆ Ascites causes generalized distension.
◆ Umbilical eversion and caput medusae (dilated veins around the umbilicus) are common and the patient may have vague

S&S

abdominal pain, hepatomegaly, fever, anorexia, nausea, vomiting, constipation or diarrhea, bleeding tendencies, severe pruritus, palmar erythema, spider angiomas, leg edema, and jaundice (a late sign).

Large-bowel obstruction
◆ Dramatic abdominal distention is preceded by constipation, tympany, high-pitched bowel sounds, and the sudden onset of colicky lower abdominal pain.
◆ Late signs include fecal vomiting and diminished peristaltic waves.

Mesenteric artery occlusion, acute
◆ Abdominal distention usually occurs several hours after the sudden onset of severe, colicky periumbilical pain and rapid or forceful bowel evacuation.
◆ Pain later becomes constant and diffuse.
◆ Late signs and symptoms include fever, tachycardia, tachypnea, hypotension, and cool, clammy skin.

Ovarian cysts
◆ Lower abdominal distention and pain occurs along with umbilical eversion.

Paralytic ileus
◆ Generalized distention occurs with a tympanic percussion note.
◆ Bowel sounds may be absent or hypoactive. Other symptoms include vomiting and severe constipation or flatus with small, frequent stools.

Peritonitis
◆ Localized or generalized abdominal distention occurs with sudden and severe abdominal pain that worsens with movement.
◆ Rebound tenderness and abdominal rigidity may be present.

Small-bowel obstruction
◆ Abdominal distention is most pronounced during late obstruction, especially in the distal small bowel.
◆ Bowel sounds may be hypoactive or hyperactive, with tympany, and the patient may experience colicky periumbilical pain, constipation, nausea, vomiting, drowsiness, malaise, dehydration, and signs of hypovolemic shock.

Toxic megacolon, acute
◆ Dramatic abdominal distention usually develops gradually.
◆ Bowel sounds may be diminished or absent, and the patient may have abdominal pain and rebound tenderness, fever, tachycardia, and dehydration.

Nursing considerations

◆ Withhold food and fluids as ordered.
◆ Assess the patient's pain level, administer analgesics, and evaluate their effects.
◆ Position the patient comfortably, using pillows for support.
◆ If the patient has ascites, elevate the head of the bed to ease breathing.
◆ Insert an NG tube and monitor drainage as ordered.
◆ Prepare the patient for diagnostic tests.

PATIENT TEACHING
◆ Explain the underlying disorder and treatment plan.
◆ Review dietary restrictions.
◆ Explain diagnostic tests.
◆ Teach the patient to use slow breathing to help relieve abdominal discomfort.

S & S

Abdominal pain

Overview

Abdominal pain, which may be acute or chronic and diffuse or localized, arises from the abdominopelvic viscera, the parietal peritoneum, or the capsules of the liver, kidney, or spleen. Visceral pain develops slowly into a deep, dull, aching pain that's poorly localized in the epigastric, periumbilical, or lower midabdominal region. Somatic (parietal, peritoneal) pain produces a sharp, more intense, and well-localized discomfort that rapidly follows the insult and is aggravated by coughing.

Assessment

HISTORY

◆ Obtain a medical history, noting previous abdominal pain; substance abuse; vascular, GI, genitourinary, or reproductive disorders; and menstrual patterns and changes.
◆ Ask the patient to describe the pain, including quality, quantity, frequency, duration, location, radiation, and what aggravates and alleviates the pain. Ask the patient to rate the pain on a scale of 0 to 10.
◆ Ask the patient if he's experienced changes in appetite, increased flatulence, constipation, diarrhea, changes in bowel movements, urinary frequency and urgency, and painful urination.
◆ If the patient complains of constant, steady abdominal pain, it may suggest organ perforation, ischemia, or inflammation or blood in the abdominal cavity.
◆ If the patient complains of intermittent, cramping abdominal pain, it may suggest an obstruction of a hollow organ.

PHYSICAL ASSESSMENT

◆ Take the patient's vital signs.
◆ Assess skin turgor and mucous membranes.
◆ Inspect the patient's abdomen for distention or visible peristaltic waves and measure his abdomen.
◆ Auscultate for bowel sounds and characterize their motility.

◆ Percuss all quadrants, noting the percussion sounds.
◆ Palpate the entire abdomen for masses, rigidity, and tenderness.
◆ Check for costovertebral angle tenderness, abdominal tenderness with guarding, and rebound tenderness.

Causes

MEDICAL
Appendicitis
◆ Pain initially occurs in the epigastric or umbilical region and then localizes at McBurney's point in the right lower quadrant.
◆ Other signs and symptoms include abdominal rigidity, rebound tenderness, nausea, vomiting, constipation (or diarrhea), low-grade fever, and tachycardia.

Cholecystitis
◆ Sudden severe pain occurs in the right upper quadrant, usually after meals. Pain radiates to the right shoulder, chest, or back.
◆ Murphy's sign (inspiratory arrest brought on by palpating the right upper quadrant while the patient takes a deep breath) is common.

Cholelithiasis
◆ Sudden, severe, and paroxysmal pain occurs in the right upper quadrant and radiates to the epigastrium, back, or shoulder blades.
◆ Other signs and symptoms include anorexia, nausea, vomiting (sometimes bilious), abdominal tenderness with guarding, fatty food intolerance, and indigestion.

Diverticulitis
◆ Intermittent, diffuse left-lower-quadrant pain occurs; it may worsen with eating but is relieved by defecation or passage of flatus.
◆ Rupture causes severe left-lower-quadrant pain, abdominal rigidity and, possi-

bly, signs and symptoms of shock and sepsis.

Duodenal ulcer
◆ Localized, steady, gnawing, burning, aching, or hungerlike pain occurs, typically 2 to 4 hours after a meal.
◆ Pain may be high in the midepigastrium and slightly off-center (usually on the right).

Gastritis
◆ Rapid onset of pain occurs, ranging from mild epigastric discomfort to burning in the left upper quadrant.
◆ Other signs and symptoms include belching, fever, malaise, anorexia, nausea, bloody or coffee-ground vomitus, and melena.

Gastroenteritis
◆ Cramping or colicky pain originates in the left upper quadrant and then radiates or migrates to the other quadrants.
◆ Other signs and symptoms include diarrhea, hyperactive bowel sounds, headache, myalgia, nausea, and vomiting.

Intestinal obstruction
◆ Short episodes of intense, colicky, cramping pain occur, alternating with pain-free intervals.
◆ Other signs and symptoms include abdominal distention, nausea and vomiting, and absent bowel sounds (with complete obstruction).

Irritable bowel syndrome
◆ Lower abdominal cramping or pain occurs, aggravated by ingestion of coarse or raw foods and alleviated by defecation or passage of flatus.
◆ Other signs and symptoms include abdominal tenderness, diarrhea alternating with constipation or normal bowel function, small stools with visible mucus, dyspepsia, nausea, and abdominal distention with a feeling of incomplete evacuation. Symptoms increase with stress, anxiety, and emotional lability.

Pancreatitis
◆ With acute pancreatitis, fulminating, continuous upper abdominal pain radiates to both flanks and to the back.
◆ With chronic pancreatitis, severe left-upper-quadrant or epigastric pain radiates to the back.
◆ Other signs and symptoms include nausea, vomiting, tachycardia, abdominal rigidity, rebound tenderness, hypoactive bowel sounds, Turner's sign (ecchymosis of the abdomen or flank) or Cullen's sign (a bluish tinge around the umbilicus) (hemorrhagic pancreatitis), and jaundice.

Ulcerative colitis
◆ Abdominal discomfort leads to lower abdominal cramping pain, increasing with movement and coughing.
◆ Other signs and symptoms include recurrent and possibly severe diarrhea with blood, pus, and mucus; soft, extremely tender abdomen; high-pitched, infrequent bowel sounds; and mild, intermittent fever.

Nursing considerations

◆ Position the patient for comfort.
◆ Monitor the patient's vital signs, pain level and its location, and intake and output.
◆ Withhold food and fluids.
◆ Administer I.V. fluids as ordered.
◆ Insert a nasogastric or other intestinal tube and monitor drainage.
◆ Assist with peritoneal lavage or abdominal paracentesis as needed.

PATIENT TEACHING
◆ Explain the underlying disorder and treatment plan.
◆ Explain diagnostic tests.
◆ Explain which foods and fluids the patient should avoid.
◆ Tell the patient to report changes in bowel habits.
◆ Instruct the patient how to position himself to alleviate symptoms.

Aphasia

Overview

Aphasia, or *dysphasia,* is the impairment of expression or comprehension, impeding communication or making it impossible. It's caused by disease or injury to the written or spoken language centers of the brain. Aphasia may be classified as anomic, Broca's, global, or Wernicke's. Anomic aphasia eventually resolves in more than one-half of patients; global aphasia is usually irreversible. Broca's aphasia, also known as *expressive aphasia,* results from lesions to the medial insular cortex. Wernicke's aphasia, also known as *sensory aphasia,* results from damage to the temporal lobe.

Assessment

HISTORY
◆ Obtain a medical history, noting headaches, hypertension, seizure disorders, or drug use.
◆ Determine the patient's preaphasia ability to communicate and perform routine tasks.

PHYSICAL ASSESSMENT
◆ Perform a complete neurologic examination.
◆ Check for obvious signs of neurologic deficit.
◆ Take the patient's vital signs and assess his level of consciousness (LOC).
◆ Assess the patient's pupillary response, eye movements, and motor function.

Causes

MEDICAL
Alzheimer's disease
◆ Anomic aphasia may begin insidiously and then progress to severe global aphasia.
◆ Other signs and symptoms include behavioral changes, loss of memory, poor judgment, restlessness, myoclonus, incontinence, and muscle rigidity.

Brain abscess
◆ Aphasia, hemiparesis, ataxia, facial weakness, and signs of increased intracranial pressure (ICP) may appear.
◆ Other signs and symptoms include fever, chills, stiff neck, back, or shoulders, nausea, vomiting, and weakness.

Brain tumor
◆ Behavioral changes, memory loss, motor weakness, seizures, auditory hallucinations, visual field deficits, and signs of increased ICP may occur.

Creutzfeldt-Jakob disease
◆ Aphasia with a rapidly progressive dementia may appear.
◆ Other signs and symptoms include myoclonic jerking, ataxia, vision disturbances, and paralysis.

Encephalitis
◆ Transient aphasia with fever, headache, and vomiting may occur.
◆ Other signs and symptoms include seizures, confusion, stupor or coma, hemiparesis, asymmetrical deep tendon reflexes, positive Babinski's reflex, ataxia, myoclonus, nystagmus, oculomotor palsies, and facial weakness.

Head trauma
◆ Sudden aphasia may occur.
◆ Other signs and symptoms include blurred or double vision; headache; pallor; diaphoresis; numbness and paresis; discharge, containing cerebrospinal fluid from the ear or nose; altered respirations; tachycardia; behavioral changes; and increased ICP.

Seizure disorder
◆ Transient aphasia and seizure activity may be observed.

Stroke
◆ Wernicke's, Broca's, or global aphasia may occur.

◆ Other signs and symptoms include decreased LOC, right-sided hemiparesis, homonymous hemianopsia, paresthesia, visual changes, and loss of sensation.

Transient ischemic attack
◆ Sudden aphasia occurs but resolves within 24 hours.
◆ Other signs and symptoms include transient hemiparesis, hemianopsia, paresthesia, dizziness, and confusion.

Nursing considerations

◆ Help the patient communicate by providing a relaxed environment with minimal distracting stimuli.
◆ Monitor neurologic status and vital signs.
◆ Obtain swallowing evaluation and monitor for signs of aspiration pneumonia.

PATIENT TEACHING
◆ Explain the underlying disorder and treatment plan.
◆ Discuss alternate means of communication.
◆ Discuss risk reduction factors for stroke.
◆ Explain the benefits of speech therapy.

Ataxia

Overview

Ataxia, the incoordination and irregularity of voluntary, purposeful movements, may be acute and possibly life-threatening or chronic. It may be classified as cerebellar (resulting from disease of the cerebellum) or sensory (resulting from proprioception).

 Nursing alert

If ataxic movements occur suddenly, examine for signs of increased intracranial pressure and impending herniation. Determine the level of consciousness (LOC) and be alert for pupillary changes, motor weakness or paralysis, neck stiffness or pain, and vomiting. Check vital signs, especially respirations. Elevate the head of the bed. Have emergency resuscitation equipment readily available. Prepare the patient for computed tomography scanning or surgery.

Assessment

HISTORY

- Ask about a history of multiple sclerosis, diabetes, central nervous system infection, neoplastic disease, or stroke.
- Ask about a family history of ataxia.
- Ask about chronic alcohol abuse or prolonged exposure to industrial toxins.
- Find out if the ataxia developed suddenly or gradually.

PHYSICAL ASSESSMENT

- Perform Romberg's test to help distinguish between cerebellar and sensory ataxia.
- Check motor strength.
- Perform a neurologic assessment.

Causes

MEDICAL
Cerebellar abscess
- Limb ataxia occurs on the same side as the lesion, with gait and truncal ataxia.
- Headache is localized behind the ear or in the occipital region.

- Other signs and symptoms include oculomotor palsy, fever, vomiting, altered LOC, and coma.

Cerebellar hemorrhage
- Acute ataxia may affect the trunk, gait, or limbs.
- Other signs and symptoms include repeated vomiting, occipital headache, vertigo, oculomotor palsy, dysphagia, dysarthria, decreased LOC or coma, signal impending herniation.

Creutzfeldt-Jakob disease
- Myoclonic jerking, aphasia, and rapidly progressing dementia may occur.

Diabetic neuropathy
- Sensory ataxia may be observed.
- Other signs and symptoms include arm or leg pain, slight leg weakness, bowel and bladder dysfunction, unsteady gait and, as neuropathy progresses, numbness in the feet.

Diphtheria
- Sensory ataxia may occur within 4 to 8 weeks of symptoms onset.
- Other signs and and symptoms include fever, paresthesia, and paralysis of the limbs and, sometimes, the respiratory muscles.

Hepatocerebral degeneration
- Residual neurologic defects occur, including mild cerebellar ataxia with a wide-based and unsteady gait.
- Other signs and symptoms include altered LOC, dysarthria, rhythmic arm tremors, and choreoathetosis of the face, neck, and shoulders.

Multiple sclerosis
- Cerebellar, speech and sensory ataxia (with spinal cord involvement) may be observed and subside or disappear during remissions.
- Other signs and symptoms include optic neuritis, optic atrophy, numbness and

weakness, diplopia, dizziness, and bladder dysfunction.

Polyneuropathy
◆ Ataxia, severe motor weakness, muscle atrophy, and sensory loss in the limbs occurs.

Spinocerebellar ataxia
◆ Stiff-legged gait ataxia follows fatigue.
◆ Other signs and symptoms eventually include limb ataxia, dysarthria, static tremor, nystagmus, cramps, paresthesia, and sensory deficits.

Stroke
◆ Infarction occurring in the medulla, pons, or cerebellum may lead to ataxia, which may remain as a residual symptom.
◆ Worsening ataxia during the acute phase may indicate extension of stroke or severe swelling of the brain.
◆ Other signs and symptoms include motor weakness, sensory loss, dysphagia and, possibly, altered LOC.

Wernicke's disease
◆ Gait ataxia occurs.
◆ Other signs and symptoms include nystagmus, diplopia, oculomotor palsies, confusion, tachycardia, exertional dyspnea, and orthostatic hypotension.

OTHER
Drugs
◆ Aminoglutethimide (Cytadren) ataxia disappears 4 to 6 weeks after the drug is stopped.
◆ Other drugs causing ataxia include toxic levels of anticonvulsants, anticholinergics, and tricyclic antidepressants.

Toxicity
◆ Chronic arsenic toxicity may cause sensory ataxia along with headache, seizures, altered LOC, motor deficits, and muscle aching.
◆ Chronic mercury toxicity causes gait and limb ataxia, principally of the arms as well

as dysarthria, mood changes, mental confusion, and tremors of the extremities, tongue, and lips.

Nursing considerations
◆ Monitor neurologic status.
◆ Encourage physical therapy to improve function.
◆ If the patient has a brain tumor, prepare him for surgery, chemotherapy, or radiation therapy.
◆ Provide safety measures and initiate fall precautions.

PATIENT TEACHING
◆ Explain the underlying disorder and treatment plan.
◆ Help the patient to identify rehabilitation goals.
◆ Stress safety measures.
◆ Discuss the use of assistive devices.
◆ Refer the patient to counseling as needed.

Babinski's reflex

Overview

Babinski's reflex, also known as *extensor plantar reflex* or *toe sign,* refers to dorsiflexion of the great toe with extension and fanning of the other toes. It's elicited by firmly stroking the side of the sole of the foot with a moderately sharp object. This reflex may be temporary in the postictal stage of a seizure or permanent in cortispinal damage.

Assessment

HISTORY

◆ Ask about recent head trauma, spinal cord injury, or an animal bite.
◆ Ask about personal or family history of neurologic disorders.

PHYSICAL ASSESSMENT

◆ Evaluate other neurologic signs.
◆ Evaluate muscle strength and tone in each extremity.
◆ Observe coordination.
◆ Test deep tendon reflexes (DTRs) in the elbow, antecubital area, wrist, knee, and ankle.
◆ Evaluate pain sensation and proprioception in the feet.

Causes

MEDICAL

Amyotrophic lateral sclerosis

◆ One-sided Babinski's reflex may occur with hyperactive DTRs and spasticity.
◆ Fasciculations are accompanied by muscle atrophy and weakness.
◆ Other signs and symptoms include incoordination; impaired speech; difficulty chewing, swallowing, and breathing; urinary frequency and urgency; and choking and excessive drooling.

Brain tumor

◆ Babinski's reflex may be present if the tumor involves the corticospinal tract.
◆ Other signs and symptoms include hyperactive DTRs, spasticity, seizures, cranial nerve dysfunction, hemiparesis or hemiplegia, decreased pain sensation, unsteady gait, incoordination, headache, emotional lability, and decreased level of consciousness (LOC).

Head trauma

◆ Unilateral or bilateral Babinski's reflex may occur from primary corticospinal damage or secondary injury associated with increased intracranial pressure.
◆ Hyperactive DTRs, spasticity, weakness, and incoordination may occur.
◆ Other signs and symptoms may include headache, vomiting, and decreased LOC, and abnormal pupillary size and response to light.

Meningitis

◆ Babinski's reflex of both feet follows fever, chills, and malaise.
◆ As meningitis progresses, signs and symptoms include decreased LOC, nuchal rigidity, positive Brudzinski's and Kernig's signs, hyperactive DTRs, photophobia, and opisthotonos.

Multiple sclerosis

◆ Babinski's reflex starts in one foot but eventually occurs in both.
◆ Initial signs and symptoms include paresthesia, nystagmus, and blurred or double vision.
◆ Other signs and symptoms include scanning speech (syllables separated by pauses), dysphagia, intention tremor, weakness, incoordination, spasticity, gait ataxia, seizures, paraparesis or paraplegia, bladder incontinence, emotional lability, and loss of pain and temperature sensation and proprioception.

Pernicious anemia

◆ Babinski's reflex occurs in both feet late in the progression of the disorder.
◆ Weakness; sore, burning tongue; and numbness and tingling in the extremities are the classic triad of symptoms in this disorder.
◆ Other signs and symptoms include bleeding gums, positive Romberg's sign, tachycardia, and fatigue.

Spinal cord injury

◆ Babinski's reflex can be elicited as spinal shock resolves. It occurs on one side if the injury affects only one side of the spinal cord (Brown-Séquard's syndrome) and both sides if the injury affects both sides.
◆ Horner's syndrome, which is marked by one-sided ptosis, pupillary constriction, and facial anhidrosis, may occur with lower cervical cord injury.
◆ Other signs and symptoms include variable or total loss of sensation and motor function.

Spinal cord tumor

◆ Babinski's reflex occurs in both feet with paresis and paralysis below the level of the tumor.
◆ Other signs and symptoms include spasticity, hyperactive DTRs, absent abdominal reflexes, incontinence, and diffuse pain at the level of the tumor.

Stroke

◆ Cerebral involvement produces Babinski's reflex in one foot with hemiplegia or hemiparesis, one-sided hyperactive DTRs, hemianopsia, and aphasia.
◆ Brain stem involvement produces Babinski's reflex in both feet with weakness or paralysis, bilateral hyperactive DTRs, cranial nerve dysfunction, incoordination, and unsteady gait.

Nursing considerations

◆ Monitor the patient's neurologic status.
◆ Assist the patient with activity.
◆ Keep his environment free from obstructions.

PATIENT TEACHING

◆ Explain the disorder and treatment plan.
◆ Instruct the patient about the need to call for assistance when getting out of bed.
◆ Discuss ways to maintain a safe environment.
◆ Instruct the patient in the use of adaptive devices.

S & S

Back pain

Overview

Back pain, which may be acute or chronic and constant or intermittent, affects about 80% of the U.S. population. It may be localized or radiate along the spine or legs. Back pain may be referred from abdomen or flank pain, possibly signaling a life-threatening disorder.

Assessment

HISTORY
◆ Obtain a medical, family, and drug history.
◆ Ask about recent injury.
◆ Ask about unusual sensations in the legs.
◆ Ask about diet and alcohol use.

PHYSICAL ASSESSMENT
◆ Observe skin color, especially in the legs.
◆ Observe posture and body alignment.
◆ Palpate skin temperature and femoral, popliteal, posterior tibial, and pedal pulses.
◆ Ask the patient to bend forward, backward, and side to side while you palpate for paravertebral muscle spasms.
◆ Palpate the dorsolumbar spine for point tenderness.
◆ Evaluate patellar tendon (knee), Achilles tendon, and Babinski's reflexes.
◆ Evaluate the strength of the extensor hallucis longus by asking the patient to hold up his big toe against resistance.
◆ Measure leg length and hamstring and quadriceps muscles.
◆ Help the patient into the supine position. Then, grasp his heel and slowly lift his leg. Note the pain's exact location and the angle between the table and his leg when it occurs. Repeat this maneuver with the opposite leg.
◆ Note range of motion of the hip and knee.
◆ Palpate and percuss the flanks to elicit costovertebral angle tenderness.

Causes

MEDICAL
Abdominal aortic aneurysm, dissecting
◆ Lower back pain or dull abdominal pain may initially occur, although upper abdominal pain is more common.
◆ A pulsating epigastrium mass may be palpated; pulsating stops after rupture.
◆ Other signs and symptoms include mottled skin below the waist, absent femoral and pedal pulses, lower blood pressure in the legs than in the arms, abdominal rigidity, mild to moderate tenderness with guarding, and shock, if blood loss is significant.

Ankylosing spondylitis
◆ Sacroiliac pain radiates up the spine and is aggravated by pressure on the side of the pelvis.
◆ Pain is usually most severe in the morning or after a period of inactivity and isn't relieved by rest.
◆ Abnormal rigidity of the lumbar spine with forward flexion is common.

Intervertebral disk rupture
◆ Gradual or sudden lower back pain occurs with or without sciatica.
◆ Pain begins in the back and radiates to the buttocks and legs.
◆ Pain is exacerbated by activity, coughing, and sneezing, and is eased by rest.
◆ The patient walks slowly and rises from sitting to standing with extreme difficulty.
◆ Other signs and symptoms include paresthesia, paravertebral muscle spasm, and decreased reflexes on the affected side.

Lumbosacral sprain
◆ Aching, localized pain and tenderness is associated with muscle spasm upon sideways motion.
◆ Flexion of the spine and movement intensify the pain; rest and lying recumbent with knees and hips flexed relieves it.

Prostate cancer

◆ Chronic, aching back pain may be the only symptom, appearing in the advanced stages.
◆ Late signs and symptoms include hematuria, difficulty initiating a urine stream, dribbling, urine retention, unexplained cystitis, and a decrease in the urine stream.

Pyelonephritis, acute

◆ Progressive flank and lower abdominal pain accompanies back pain or tenderness, especially over the costovertebral angle.
◆ Other signs and symptoms include high fever and chills, nausea, vomiting, flank and abdominal tenderness, and urinary frequency and urgency.

Renal calculi

◆ Colicky pain travels from the costovertebral angle to the flank, suprapubic region, and external genitalia.
◆ If calculi travel down a ureter, the patient may feel excruciating pain.
◆ If calculi are in the renal pelvis and calyces, the patient may feel dull and constant flank pain.
◆ Other signs and symptoms include urinary urgency, hematuria, and agitation.

Sacroiliac strain

◆ Sacroiliac pain may radiate to the buttock, hip, and lateral aspect of the thigh.
◆ Weight bearing on the affected side and abduction with resistance of the leg aggravates the pain.

Spinal stenosis

◆ Back pain occurs with or without sciatica.
◆ Pain may radiate to the toes and may progress to numbness or weakness.

Transverse process fractures and vertebral compression fractures

◆ Severe, localized back pain occurs along with muscle spasm and hematoma in a transverse process fracture.

◆ Pain may not occur for several weeks with a vertebral compression fracture; then, back pain is aggravated by weight bearing, and local tenderness occurs.

Vertebral osteoporosis

◆ Chronic, aching back pain is aggravated by activity and somewhat relieved by rest.
◆ Vertebral collapse, causing a backache with pain that radiates around the trunk, is the most common characteristic.

Nursing considerations

◆ If the cause is life-threatening, monitor the patient closely and provide supportive care.
◆ Look for increasing pain, altered neurovascular condition of the legs, loss of bowel or bladder control, altered vital signs, sweating, and cyanosis.
◆ Withhold food and fluids if surgery is indicated.
◆ Elevate the head of the bed and place a pillow under the knees.
◆ Fit the patient for a corset or lumbosacral support as appropriate.
◆ Apply heat or cold therapy, backboard, foam mattress, or pelvic traction.

PATIENT TEACHING

◆ Explain the cause of back pain and the treatment plan.
◆ Provide information about the use of anti-inflammatory drugs and analgesics.
◆ Discuss lifestyle changes, such as weight loss or correcting posture.
◆ Teach relaxation techniques, such as deep breathing.
◆ Instruct the patient on correct use of corset or lumbosacral support.
◆ Provide information about alternatives to drug therapy, such as biofeedback and transcutaneous electrical nerve stimulation.

Blood pressure decrease

Overview

Decreased blood pressure, also called *hypotension*, is classified as a reading below 90/60 mm Hg or a drop of 30 mm Hg from the baseline. It indicates inadequate intravascular pressure to maintain oxygen requirements that may affect the kidneys, brain, and heart, leading to a change in level of consciousness (LOC) or to myocardial ischemia. It may also reflect an expanded intravascular space or reduced intravascular volume and cardiac output.

Assessment

HISTORY
◆ Ask about such symptoms as weakness, nausea, dizziness, and chest pain.

PHYSICAL ASSESSMENT
◆ Obtain vital signs.

 Nursing alert

If the patient's systolic blood pressure is less than 80 mm Hg, or 30 mm Hg below baseline, suspect shock. Quickly evaluate the patient for decreased LOC. Check the apical pulse for tachycardia; check respirations for tachypnea. Inspect for cool, clammy skin. Elevate the patient's legs above the level of his heart. Start an I.V. line using a large-bore needle to replace fluids and blood or to give drugs. Administer oxygen with mechanical ventilation. Prepare for cardiac or hemodynamic monitoring.

◆ Inspect skin for pallor, sweating, and clamminess.
◆ Palpate peripheral pulses.
◆ Auscultate for abnormal heart, breath, and bowel sounds and abnormal heart and breath rates, and rhythms.
◆ Look for signs of hemorrhage.
◆ Assess for abdominal rigidity, rebound tenderness, and possible sources of infection.
◆ If patient has episodes of dizziness when standing up suddenly, take blood pressure while he's lying down, sitting, and then standing. Compare the readings.

Causes

MEDICAL

Acute adrenal insufficiency
◆ Orthostatic hypotension is a characteristic sign.
◆ Other signs and symptoms include fatigue, weakness, nausea, vomiting, fever, tachycardia, tachypnea, hyperpigmentation, and coma.

Cardiac arrhythmia
◆ Blood pressure fluctuates between normal and low, depending on the type of arrhythmia.
◆ Dizziness, chest pain, difficulty breathing, light-headedness, weakness, fatigue, and palpitations occur.
◆ Pulse rhythm is irregular, and heart rate is greater than 100 beats/minute or less than 60 beats/minute.

Cardiac tamponade
◆ Systolic pressure falls more than 10 mm Hg during inspiration (paradoxical pulse).
◆ Other signs and symptoms include restlessness, cyanosis, tachycardia, jugular vein distention, muffled heart sounds, dyspnea, and Kussmaul's respirations.

Cardiogenic shock
◆ Systolic pressure is less than 80 mm Hg or falls to 30 mm Hg less than baseline.
◆ Tachycardia; narrowed pulse pressure; diminished Korotkoff sounds; peripheral cyanosis; restlessness and anxiety, which may progress to disorientation and confusion; and pale, cool, clammy skin occur.

Diabetic ketoacidosis
◆ Low blood pressure and tachycardia occur.
◆ Other signs and symptoms include polydipsia, polyuria, polyphagia, dehydration, weight loss, breath with fruity odor, Kussmaul's respirations, seizures, confusion, and stupor that may progress to coma.

Heart failure

◆ Blood pressure fluctuates between normal and low.
◆ Auscultation reveals ventricular gallop, tachycardia, crackles, and tachypnea.
◆ Dependent edema, jugular vein distention, and hepatomegaly may occur.
◆ Other signs and symptoms include dyspnea, fatigue, weight gain, sweating, and anxiety.

Hypovolemic shock

◆ Systolic pressure falls to less than 80 mm Hg or 30 mm Hg less than the patient's baseline.
◆ Other signs and symptoms include diminished Korotkoff sounds; narrowed pulse pressure; cyanosis of the extremities; pale, cool, clammy skin; rapid, weak, and irregular pulse; oliguria; confusion; disorientation; restlessness; and anxiety.

Myocardial infarction

◆ Blood pressure may be low or high; a precipitous drop in blood pressure may signal cardiogenic shock.
◆ Other signs and symptoms include chest pain that may radiate to the jaw, shoulder, arm, or epigastrium; dyspnea; anxiety; nausea or vomiting; sweating; and cool, pale, or cyanotic skin.

Neurogenic shock

◆ Low blood pressure and bradycardia occur.
◆ Other signs and symptoms include warm, dry skin and, possibly, motor weakness of the limbs or diaphragm, depending on the cause of shock.

Pulmonary embolism

◆ Low blood pressure with narrowed pulse pressure and diminished Korotkoff sounds occur.
◆ Early signs and symptoms include sharp chest pain, dyspnea, and cough.
◆ Other signs and symptoms include tachycardia, tachypnea, paradoxical pulse, jugular vein distention, and hemoptysis.

Septic shock

◆ Initially, fever and chills occur.
◆ Low blood pressure, tachycardia, and tachypnea may develop early, but the skin remains warm.
◆ Blood pressure continues to decrease, accompanied by a narrowed pulse pressure.

OTHER
Diagnostic tests

◆ A gastric acid stimulation test using histamine and X-ray studies using contrast media may cause low blood pressure.

Drugs

◆ Alpha and beta blockers, anxiolytics, calcium channel blockers, diuretics, general anesthetics, most I.V. antiarrhythmics, monoamine oxidase inhibitors, opioid analgesics, sedatives, and vasodilators can cause low blood pressure.

Nursing considerations

◆ Check vital signs frequently to determine if low blood pressure is constant or intermittent.
◆ Ensure bed rest.
◆ Don't leave a dizzy patient unattended when he's sitting or walking.
◆ Low blood pressure may occur as a result of taking several drugs that have such an adverse effect.

PATIENT TEACHING

◆ Explain the cause of decreased blood pressure and the treatment plan.
◆ Discuss medications and possible adverse effects.
◆ Advise the patient with orthostatic hypotension to stand up slowly from a sitting position and to dangle his feet and rise slowly when getting out of bed.
◆ For patients with vasovagal syncope, discuss how to avoid triggers.
◆ Discuss the need for a cane or walker.

Blood pressure increase

Overview

An increase in blood pressure, known as *hypertension,* is the intermittent or sustained increase in blood pressure exceeding 140/90 mm Hg. Essential hypertension develops insidiously. Blood pressure increases gradually, and the cause is unknown. Secondary hypertension results from an identifiable cause. A sudden and severe increase in blood pressure may indicate a life-threatening condition.

 Nursing alert

If blood pressure is greater than 180/110 mm Hg, suspect hypertensive crisis and treat immediately. Maintain a patent airway in case the patient vomits, and use seizure precautions. Give an I.V. antihypertensive and a diuretic. Insert an indwelling urinary catheter to monitor urine output.

Assessment

HISTORY

◆ Obtain a medical history, noting incidence of diabetes or cardiovascular, cerebrovascular, or renal disease or a family history of high blood pressure.

◆ Ask the patient about the onset of high blood pressure.

◆ Note associated signs and symptoms, including headache, palpitations, blurred vision, sweating, wine-colored urine, and decreased urine output.

◆ Obtain a drug history, including past and present prescriptions, herbal preparations, and over-the-counter (OTC) drugs.

◆ If the patient is taking antihypertensives, determine compliance to the drug regimen.

◆ Explore psychosocial or environmental factors that affect blood pressure control.

◆ Note history of smoking, alcohol use, and dietary habits.

PHYSICAL ASSESSMENT

◆ Perform a funduscopic (ophthalmoscopic) examination.

◆ Perform a cardiovascular assessment; check for carotid bruits and jugular vein distention.

◆ Assess skin color, temperature, and turgor.

◆ Palpate peripheral pulses.

◆ Auscultate for abnormal heart and breath sounds, rates, or rhythms.

◆ Auscultate for abdominal bruits.

◆ Palpate the abdomen for tenderness, masses, and liver or kidney enlargement.

Causes

MEDICAL
Anemia

◆ Elevated systolic pressure may occur.

◆ Other signs and symptoms include pulsations in the capillary beds, bounding pulse, tachycardia, systolic ejection murmur, and pale mucous membranes.

Aortic aneurysm, dissecting

◆ Initially, a sudden rise in systolic pressure occurs, but diastolic pressure remains stable.

◆ Hypotension occurs as the body's ability to compensate fails.

◆ With an abdominal aneurysm, associated signs and symptoms include abdominal and back pain, weakness, sweating, tachycardia, dyspnea, a pulsating abdominal mass, restlessness, confusion, and cool, clammy skin may occur.

◆ With a thoracic aneurysm, associated signs and symptoms include a ripping or tearing sensation in the chest, which may radiate to the neck, shoulders, lower back, or abdomen; pallor; syncope; blindness; loss of consciousness; sweating; dyspnea; tachycardia; cyanosis; leg weakness; murmur; and absent radial and femoral pulses.

Atherosclerosis

◆ Systolic pressure rises, but diastolic pressure remains normal or slightly elevated.

◆ The patient may be asymptomatic.

S & S

◆ Other signs and symptoms may include a weak pulse, flushed skin, tachycardia, angina, and claudication.

Cushing's syndrome
◆ Blood pressure elevates and pulse pressure widens.
◆ Other findings include truncal obesity, moon face, fatigue, muscle weakness, increased facial hair (in women), irregular menstrual cycles, and memory impairment.

Increased intracranial pressure
◆ Respiratory rate increases initially, followed by increased systolic pressure and widened pulse pressure.
◆ Other signs and symptoms include headache, projectile vomiting, decreased level of consciousness, fixed or dilated pupils, and bradycardia (a late sign).

Myocardial infarction
◆ Blood pressure may be high or low.
◆ Crushing chest pain may radiate to the jaw, shoulder, arm, or epigastrium.
◆ Other signs and symptoms include dyspnea, anxiety, nausea, vomiting, fatigue, weakness, diaphoresis, atrial gallop, and murmurs.

Pheochromocytoma
◆ Paroxysmal or sustained elevated blood pressure occurs with possible orthostatic hypotension.
◆ Other findings include anxiety, diaphoresis, palpitations, tremors, pallor, nausea, weight loss, and headache.
◆ Hematuria, life-threatening retroperitoneal bleeding, proteinuria, and colicky abdominal pain may occur in advanced stages.

Renovascular stenosis
◆ Systolic and diastolic pressure rise abruptly.
◆ Other characteristic findings include bruits over the upper abdomen or in the costovertebral angles, hematuria, and acute flank pain.

Thyrotoxicosis
◆ Elevated systolic pressure occurs.
◆ Other findings include widened pulse pressure, tachycardia, bounding pulse, pulsations in the capillary nail beds, palpitations, weight loss, exophthalmos, enlarged thyroid gland, diarrhea, fever, heat intolerance, exertional dyspnea, decreased or absent menses, and warm, moist skin.

OTHER
Drugs
◆ Central nervous system stimulants, corticosteroids, hormonal contraceptives, monoamine oxidase inhibitors, nonsteroidal anti-inflammatory drugs, sympathomimetics, and OTC cold remedies can increase blood pressure.
◆ Cocaine use may increase blood pressure.

Nursing considerations
◆ Monitor the patient's vital signs.
◆ Administer medications to control blood pressure.
◆ Stress the need for follow-up diagnostic tests.

PATIENT TEACHING
◆ Explain the cause of increased blood pressure and the treatment plan.
◆ Emphasize the importance of weight loss, exercise, and smoking and alcohol cessation.
◆ Explain the need for sodium restriction.
◆ Discuss stress management.
◆ Discuss ways of reducing other risk factors for coronary artery disease.
◆ Discuss the importance of regular blood pressure monitoring.
◆ Explain how to take prescribed antihypertensives correctly.
◆ Emphasize the importance of long-term follow-up care.

Bowel sounds, absent

Overview

Absent bowel sounds, or silent bowel sounds, are characterized by the inability to auscultate bowel sounds in any abdominal quadrant with a stethoscope for at least 5 minutes. It happens when mechanical or vascular obstruction or neurogenic inhibition stops peristalsis. Life-threatening complications include bowel perforation, peritonitis, sepsis, and hypovolemic shock.

 Nursing alert

If absent bowel sounds are accompanied by sudden, severe abdominal pain and cramping or severe abdominal distention, insert a nasogastric (NG) or intestinal tube to suction lumen contents and decompress the bowel. Give I.V. fluids and electrolytes. Withhold oral intake if surgery is warranted. Take the patient's vital signs, and watch for signs of shock, such as hypotension, tachycardia, and cool, clammy skin. Measure abdominal girth to establish a baseline.

Assessment

HISTORY
◆ Ask about the onset and description of abdominal pain.
◆ Obtain a description of bowel movements, and ask the patient if he has had diarrhea or has passed pencil-thin stools, a possible sign of a developing luminal obstruction.
◆ Obtain a medical and surgical history, including recent accidents, abdominal tumors, hernias, adhesions from past surgery, acute pancreatitis, diverticulitis, gynecologic infection, uremia, or spinal cord injury.

PHYSICAL ASSESSMENT
◆ Inspect abdominal contour.
◆ Observe for distention.
◆ Auscultate all abdominal quadrants for at least 5 minutes.
◆ Listen for dullness over fluid-filled areas and for tympany over pockets of gas.
◆ Gently percuss and palpate the abdomen.
◆ Palpate for abdominal rigidity and guarding.

Causes

MEDICAL
Abdominal surgery
◆ Bowel sounds are normally temporarily absent after abdominal surgery.

Complete mechanical intestinal obstruction
◆ Absent bowel sounds follow hyperactive sounds.
◆ Colicky abdominal pain, which may radiate, arises in the quadrant with the obstruction.
◆ Other signs and symptoms include abdominal distention, bloating, constipation, nausea, and vomiting.

Mesenteric artery occlusion
◆ Bowel sounds disappear after a brief period of hyperactive sounds.
◆ Midepigastric or periumbilical pain occurs next, followed by abdominal distention, bruits, vomiting, constipation, and signs of shock.
◆ Abdominal rigidity may appear later.

Paralytic ileus

◆ Absent bowel sounds are a hallmark sign.

◆ If paralytic ileus follows acute abdominal infection, fever and abdominal pain may occur.

◆ Other signs and symptoms include abdominal distention, generalized discomfort, and constipation or passage of small, liquid stools.

Nursing considerations

◆ Withhold food and fluids. Give I.V. fluids and electrolytes as prescribed.

◆ Once mechanical obstruction and intra-abdominal sepsis have been ruled out, give drugs to control pain and stimulate peristalsis.

◆ If a bowel obstruction doesn't respond to decompression, early surgical intervention should be considered to avoid the risk of bowel infarct.

After NG or intestinal tube insertion

◆ Elevate the head of the bed at least 30 degrees.

◆ Turn the patient to facilitate passage of the tube through the GI tract.

◆ Ensure tube patency and monitor amount and characteristics of drainage.

PATIENT TEACHING

◆ Explain the cause of absent bowel sounds and the treatment plan.

◆ Explain needed diagnostic tests and therapeutic procedures.

◆ Explain about the need for I.V. fluids while maintaining nothing-by-mouth status.

◆ Explain the need for postoperative ambulation.

Bradycardia

Overview

Bradycardia refers to a heart rate of fewer than 60 beats/minute. It occurs normally in some patients, but can also result from pathologic causes.

 Nursing alert

Bradycardia that occurs along with decreased level of consciousness (LOC), decreased blood pressure, or chest pain requires emergency action. Place the patient on a continuous cardiac monitor, administer atropine sulfate I.V. per advanced cardiac life support protocol, and prepare for pacemaker use.

Assessment

HISTORY
♦ Ask about a family history of slow pulse rate.
♦ Obtain a medical history, including underlying metabolic disorders.
♦ Ask about current drugs and the patient's compliance.
♦ Find out if the patient is an athlete and determine his degree of physical activity.

PHYSICAL ASSESSMENT
♦ Monitor the patient's vital signs, cardiac rhythm, and pulse oximetry.
♦ Note level of LOC and respiratory status.
♦ Perform a complete cardiac assessment.
♦ After detecting bradycardia, look for related signs and symptoms to identify the cause.

Causes

MEDICAL
Cardiac arrhythmia
♦ Bradycardia may be transient, sustained, benign, or life-threatening.
♦ Other signs and symptoms include hypotension, palpitations, dizziness, weakness, dyspnea, chest pain, decreased urine output, altered LOC, syncope, and fatigue.

Cardiomyopathy
♦ Transient or sustained bradycardia may occur.
♦ Other signs and symptoms include dizziness, syncope, edema, fatigue, jugular vein distention, orthopnea, dyspnea, and peripheral cyanosis.

Cervical spinal injury
♦ Bradycardia may be transient or sustained, depending on the severity of the injury.
♦ Other signs and symptoms include hypotension, decreased body temperature, slowed peristalsis, leg paralysis, and partial arm and respiratory muscle paralysis.

Hypothermia
♦ If the patient's core temperature drops below 86° F (30° C), he may not have a palpable pulse or audible heart sounds.
♦ Other signs and symptoms include shivering, peripheral cyanosis, muscle rigidity, bradypnea, and confusion leading to stupor.

Hypothyroidism
♦ Severe bradycardia is accompanied by fatigue, constipation, unexplained weight gain, and sensitivity to cold.
♦ Related signs and symptoms include cool, dry, thick skin; sparse, dry hair; facial swelling; periorbital edema; thick, brittle nails; and confusion leading to stupor.

Myocardial infarction
♦ Sinus bradycardia is common and may not be symptomatic.
♦ Abnormal heart sounds may be heard on auscultation.
♦ Other signs and symptoms include an aching, burning, or viselike pressure in the chest, which may radiate to the jaw, shoulder, arm, back, or epigastric area; nausea and vomiting; cool, clammy, and pale or cyanotic skin; anxiety; and dyspnea.

S&S

OTHER

Diagnostic tests

◆ Cardiac catheterization and electrophysiologic studies can induce temporary bradycardia.

Drugs

◆ Protamines and some antiarrhythmics, beta-adrenergic blockers, cardiac glycosides, calcium channel blockers, sympatholytics, and topical miotics may cause transient bradycardia.

◆ Not taking a thyroid replacement may cause bradycardia.

Invasive treatments

◆ Cardiac surgery can result in edema or damage to the conduction tissue, causing bradycardia.

◆ Suctioning can induce hypoxia and vagal stimulation, causing bradycardia.

Nursing considerations

◆ Monitor cardiac rhythm, respiratory rate, and LOC.

◆ Prepare the patient for 24-hour Holter monitoring.

 Age considerations

Fetal bradycardia, characterized by a heart rate less than 120 beats/minute, may occur during prolonged labor or complications of delivery. Sinus node dysfunction is the most common bradyarrhythmia in elderly patients.

PATIENT TEACHING

◆ Explain the cause of bradycardia and the treatment plan.

◆ Teach the patient about signs and symptoms he should report.

◆ Give instructions for pulse measurement, and explain the parameters for calling the practitioner and seeking emergency care.

◆ If a patient is getting a pacemaker, explain its use.

S & S

Breast pain

Overview

Breast pain, also called *mastalgia,* commonly results from benign breast disease. It may occur in one or both breasts during rest or movement, and may be aggravated by manipulation or palpation. The pain may be dull or sharp and cyclic, intermittent, or constant. Breast pain may occur before menstruation from increased mammary blood flow from hormonal changes or during pregnancy from hormonal changes. Breast pain from benign breast disease is rare in postmenopausal women. Trauma from falls or physical abuse is another cause.

Assessment

HISTORY

◆ Ask the patient when the pain started and to describe it.
◆ Ask the patient to point to the exact location of pain, if possible.
◆ Ask about duration of pain (constant or intermittent).
◆ Find out if the patient is nursing, pregnant, menopausal, or postmenopausal.
◆ Question the patient about injury or changes to breast.

PHYSICAL ASSESSMENT

◆ With the patient standing or sitting with arms at the sides, note breast size, symmetry, and contour, and the appearance of the skin.
◆ Note the size, shape, and symmetry of the nipples and areolae.
◆ Repeat your inspection with the patient's arms raised over her head and then with her hands pressed against her hips.
◆ Palpate the breasts with the patient seated and then lying down with a pillow placed under the shoulder on the side being examined.
◆ Palpate the nipple, noting tenderness and nodules; check for discharge.
◆ Palpate axillary lymph nodes, noting any enlargement.

Causes

MEDICAL

Areolar gland abscess

◆ Inflamed Montgomery glands cause pain.
◆ The abscess is tender and palpable and is located on the periphery of the areola.
◆ Other signs and symptoms include fever, local swelling, drainage, and malaise.

Breast abscess, acute

◆ Local pain, tenderness, erythema, peau d'orange, and warmth are associated with a breast abscess.
◆ Other signs and symptoms include malaise, fever, chills, and enlarged axillary nodes.

Fat necrosis

◆ Local pain and tenderness may develop along with ecchymosis; erythema; a firm, irregular, fixed mass; skin dimpling; and nipple retraction.

Fibrocystic breast disease

◆ Cysts may cause pain before menstruation and produce no symptoms afterward.
◆ Later, pain may persist throughout the cycle.
◆ Cysts feel firm, mobile, and well-defined.
◆ A clear, serous nipple discharge may come from one or both breasts.
◆ The patient may experience signs and symptoms of premenstrual syndrome.

Intraductal papilloma

◆ Breast pain or tenderness may occur in one breast.
◆ Serous or bloody nipple discharge is the primary sign.

Mammary duct ectasia

◆ Burning pain and itching around the areola may occur.
◆ Inflammation with pain, tenderness, erythema, and acute fever, or with pain and tenderness alone, may develop and subside in 7 to 10 days.

◆ Other signs and symptoms include a rubbery, subareolar breast nodule; swelling and erythema around the nipple; nipple retraction; a bluish green discoloration or peau d'orange of the skin overlying the nodule; a thick, sticky, multicolored nipple discharge from multiple ducts; axillary lymphadenopathy; and breast ulcer (late sign).

Mastitis
◆ Pain in one breast may be severe.
◆ Skin is typically red and warm at the inflammation site.
◆ High fever, chills, malaise, and fatigue are systemic findings.
◆ Other signs and symptoms include peau d'orange, breast dimpling, a firm area of induration, and nipple deviation, inversion, or flattening.

Sebaceous cyst, infected
◆ Pain may be reported with this cutaneous cyst.
◆ Other signs and symptoms include a small, well-delineated nodule, localized erythema, and induration.

Nursing considerations

◆ Provide comfort measures, such as warm or cold compresses.
◆ Provide emotional support for the patient.
◆ Emphasize the importance of monthly breast self-examinations.

PATIENT TEACHING
◆ Explain the diagnostic tests to be performed.
◆ Explain the cause of breast pain and the treatment plan.
◆ Instruct the patient on wearing the correct type of brassiere.
◆ Explain the use of warm or cold compresses.
◆ Teach the techniques of breast self-examination, and stress the importance of monthly self-examinations.

Breath with fruity odor

Overview

Fruity breath odor results from respiratory elimination of excess acetone. It characteristically occurs with ketoacidosis, a potentially life-threatening condition.

Assessment

HISTORY

◆ Ask about the onset and duration of odor.
◆ Find out about changes in breathing patterns.
◆ Ask about other signs and symptoms, including increased thirst, frequent urination, weight loss, fatigue, and abdominal pain.
◆ Ask the female patient if she has had candidal vaginitis or vaginal secretions with itching.
◆ If the patient has a history of diabetes mellitus, ask about stress, infections, and noncompliance to the treatment regimen.
◆ If anorexia nervosa is suspected, obtain a dietary and weight history.
◆ Note current medications.

PHYSICAL ASSESSMENT

◆ Take the patient's vital signs and obtain weight.
◆ Assess skin turgor and the condition of mucous membranes.
◆ Check serum blood glucose and urine ketone levels.

Causes

MEDICAL

Anorexia nervosa

◆ Severe weight loss may produce fruity breath odor.
◆ Nausea, constipation, and cold intolerance may be present.
◆ Dental enamel erosion and scars or calluses in the dorsum of the hand may indicate induced vomiting.

Ketoacidosis

◆ With alcoholic ketoacidosis, fruity breath odor occurs with vomiting, abdominal pain, abrupt onset of Kussmaul's respirations, signs of dehydration, minimal food intake over several days, and normal or slightly decreased blood glucose levels.
◆ With starvation ketoacidosis, fruity breath odor occurs with signs of cachexia and dehydration, decreased level of consciousness, bradycardia, and a history of severely limited food intake.
◆ With diabetic ketoacidosis, fruity breath odor occurs along with polydipsia, polyuria, nocturia, weak and rapid pulse, hunger, weight loss, weakness, fatigue, nausea, vomiting, abdominal pain, and, eventually, Kussmaul's respirations, orthostatic hypotension, dehydration, tachycardia, confusion, stupor, and coma.

OTHER

Drugs

◆ Drugs that cause metabolic acidosis, such as nitroprusside (Nitropress) and salicylates, can result in fruity breath odor.
◆ Low-carbohydrate diets may cause ketoacidosis and a fruity breath odor.

S & S

Nursing considerations

◆ Administer I.V. fluids as ordered.
◆ Monitor the patient's vital signs and intake and output.
◆ Monitor the patient's serum blood glucose level.
◆ Maintain an appropriate diet.

Age considerations

Consider factors such as poor oral hygiene, increased dental caries, decreased salivary function, poor dietary intake, and use of multiple drugs when evaluating the condition of an elderly patient with mouth odor.

PATIENT TEACHING

◆ Explain the cause of fruity breath odor and the treatment plan.
◆ Explain the signs of hyperglycemia.
◆ Emphasize the importance of wearing medical identification.
◆ Refer the patient to psychologist or support group as needed.

Brudzinski's sign

Overview

Brudzinski's sign is the flexion of the hips and knees in response to passive flexion of the neck. It signals meningeal irritation and may be an early indicator of life-threatening meningitis and subarachnoid hemorrhage.

Assessment

HISTORY

◆ Ask the patient about signs of increased intracranial pressure (ICP), such as headache, neck pain, nausea, and vision disturbances.

◆ Ask about a history of hypertension, spinal arthritis, recent head trauma, open-head injury, dental work or abscessed teeth, endocarditis, or I.V. drug abuse.

PHYSICAL ASSESSMENT

◆ Observe for altered level of consciousness (LOC), pupillary changes, bradycardia, widened pulse pressure, Cheyne-Stokes or Kussmaul's respirations, and vomiting.

◆ Evaluate cranial nerve function, noting any motor or sensory deficits.

◆ Look for Kernig's sign (resistance to knee extension after flexion of the hip), which is a further indication of meningeal irritation.

◆ Look for signs of central nervous system infection, such as fever and nuchal rigidity.

Causes

MEDICAL
Meningitis

◆ A positive Brudzinski's sign can usually be elicited 24 hours after onset.

◆ As ICP increases, arterial hypertension, bradycardia, widened pulse pressure, Cheyne-Stokes or Kussmaul's respirations, and coma may develop.

◆ Other signs and symptoms include headache, a positive Kernig's sign, nuchal rigidity, irritability or restlessness, deep stupor or coma, vertigo, fever, chills, malaise, hyperalgesia, muscular hypotonia, opisthotonos, symmetrical deep tendon reflexes, papilledema, ocular and facial palsies, nausea, vomiting, photophobia, diplopia, and unequal, sluggish pupils.

Age considerations

In infants with meningeal irritation, bulging fontanels, a weak cry, fretfulness, vomiting, and poor feeding appear earlier than does Brudzinski's sign.

Subarachnoid hemorrhage

◆ Brudzinski's sign may be elicited within minutes after initial bleeding.

◆ Focal signs, such as hemiparesis, vision disturbances, or aphasia, may occur.

◆ As ICP increases, arterial hypertension, bradycardia, widened pulse pressure, Cheyne-Stokes or Kussmaul's respirations, and coma may develop.

◆ Other signs and symptoms include sudden onset of severe headache, nuchal rigidity, altered LOC, dizziness, photophobia, cranial nerve palsies, nausea, vomiting, fever, and a positive Kernig's sign.

S & S

Nursing considerations

◆ Elevate the patient's head 30 to 60 degrees to promote venous return and administer an osmotic diuretic as ordered.
◆ Provide constant ICP monitoring and perform frequent neurologic checks.
◆ Monitor vital signs, fluid intake and urine output, and cardiorespiratory status.

PATIENT TEACHING
◆ Explain the cause of Brudzinski's sign and the treatment plan.
◆ Discuss the signs and symptoms of meningitis and subdural hematoma.
◆ Tell the patient when to seek immediate medical attention.

S & S

Chest expansion, asymmetrical

Overview

Asymmetrical chest expansion, which may be a sign of a life-threatening disorder, is an uneven extension of portions of the chest wall during inspiration. It may develop suddenly or gradually and may affect one or both sides of the chest wall.

 Nursing alert

If asymmetrical chest expansion is present, always suspect flail chest and treat it as a life-threatening emergency. Take the patient's vital signs, and assess for signs of acute respiratory distress. Administer oxygen by nasal cannula, mask, or mechanical ventilation, depending on the severity of respiratory distress. Insert an I.V. catheter to allow fluid replacement and administration of drugs for pain. Draw a blood sample for arterial blood gas analysis, and connect the patient to a cardiac monitor. Continue to watch for signs of respiratory distress.

Assessment

HISTORY
◆ Ask about the onset, duration, and extent of dyspnea or pain during breathing.
◆ Obtain a history of pulmonary or systemic illness, thoracic surgery, or blunt or penetrating chest trauma.

PHYSICAL ASSESSMENT
◆ Note any respiratory distress and provide supportive measures as appropriate.
◆ Palpate the trachea for midline positioning.
◆ Examine the posterior chest wall for tenderness or deformity.
◆ Evaluate the extent of asymmetrical chest expansion.
◆ Palpate for vocal or tactile fremitus on both sides of the chest. Note asymmetrical vibrations and areas of enhanced, diminished, or absent fremitus.
◆ Percuss and auscultate to detect air and fluid in the lungs and pleural spaces.

◆ Auscultate all lung fields for abnormal breath sounds.
◆ Examine the patient's anterior chest wall.

Causes

MEDICAL
Bronchial obstruction
◆ Lack of chest movement indicates complete obstruction; lagging chest signals partial obstruction.
◆ Intercostal bulging during expiration and hyperresonance on percussion suggests air trapped in the chest.
◆ Other signs and symptoms may include dyspnea, accessory muscle use, decreased or absent breath sounds, and suprasternal, substernal, or intercostal retractions.

Flail chest
◆ The unstable portion of the chest wall collapses inward during inspiration and balloons outward during expiration.
◆ Ecchymoses and severe localized pain occur with traumatic injury to the chest wall.
◆ Rapid and shallow respirations, tachycardia, and cyanosis may also occur.

Hemothorax
◆ Bleeding into the pleural space causes the chest to lag during inspiration. Other signs and symptoms include signs of traumatic chest injury, stabbing pain at the injury site, anxiety, dullness on percussion, tachypnea, tachycardia, hypoxemia, and signs of shock.

Myasthenia gravis
◆ Progressive loss of ventilatory muscle function produces asynchrony of the chest and abdomen during inspiration.
◆ Shallow respirations and increased muscle weakness cause severe dyspnea, tachypnea, and possible apnea.

Phrenic nerve dysfunction

◆ The paralyzed hemidiaphragm fails to contract downward; onset may be gradual or sudden.

◆ Asynchrony of the thorax and upper abdomen during inspiration develops on the affected side.

Pneumonia

◆ Inspiratory lagging chest or chest-abdomen asynchrony occurs.

◆ Other signs and symptoms include fever, chills, tachycardia, fatigue, productive cough with rust-colored sputum, tachypnea, dyspnea, crackles, rhonchi, and chest pain that worsens with deep breathing.

Pneumothorax

◆ Lagging chest occurs on the affected side at end inspiration.

◆ Sudden, stabbing chest pain occurs that may radiate to the arms, face, back, or abdomen.

◆ Other signs and symptoms include tachypnea, tympany on percussion, decreased or absent breath sounds on the affected side, tachycardia, restlessness, and anxiety, subcutaneous crepitation, and mediastinal and tracheal deviation from the affected side.

OTHER
Treatments

◆ Pneumonectomy and surgical removal of several ribs can cause asymmetrical chest expansion.

◆ Mainstem bronchi intubation may also cause chest lag or the absence of chest movement.

Nursing considerations

◆ Give supplemental oxygen as needed.
◆ Monitor respiratory status and pulse oximetry.
◆ Prepare the patient for pulmonary studies.
◆ Maintain chest tube and monitor function and drainage.

PATIENT TEACHING

◆ Explain the cause of asymmetrical chest expansion and the treatment plan.
◆ Explain to the patient or caregiver how to recognize early signs and symptoms of respiratory distress and what to do if they occur.
◆ Teach the patient coughing and deep-breathing exercises.
◆ Teach the patient techniques that can help reduce his anxiety.
◆ Teach the patient about all hospital procedures, tests, and interventions, such as chest tube insertion and oxygen administration.

S & S

Chest pain

Overview

Chest pain results from disorders that affect thoracic or abdominal organs and may indicate acute and life-threatening disorders. It may be sudden or gradual in onset, steady or intermittent, mild or acute and may radiate to the arms, neck, jaw, or back.

 Nursing alert

Consider chest pain a life-threatening condition that needs immediate attention. If chest pain is present, administer oxygen, obtain an electrocardiogram (ECG), place the patient on a cardiac monitor, and obtain serum cardiac markers. Administer medication for pain relief, such a nitrates or opioids.

Assessment

HISTORY

◆ Ask about the onset and radiation of pain and its duration, quality, quantity, and what aggravates or alleviates it.
◆ Obtain a history of cardiac or pulmonary disease, chest trauma, GI disease, or sickle cell anemia.
◆ Obtain a drug history, including tobacco use.

PHYSICAL ASSESSMENT

◆ Take vital signs; note tachypnea, fever, tachycardia, oxygen saturation, paradoxical pulse, and hypertension or hypotension.
◆ Look for jugular vein distention and peripheral edema.
◆ Observe breathing pattern; inspect the chest for asymmetrical expansion.
◆ Auscultate for pleural rub, crackles, rhonchi, wheezing, diminished or absent breath, murmurs, clicks, gallops, and pericardial rub sounds.
◆ Palpate for lifts, heaves, thrills, gallops, tactile fremitus, and abdominal masses or tenderness.

Causes

MEDICAL
Angina pectoris

◆ Chest discomfort may be described as pain or a sensation of indigestion or expansion.
◆ Pain usually occurs in the retrosternal region behind the sternum and typically lasts 2 to 10 minutes; it may radiate to the neck, jaw, and arms.
◆ Other signs and symptoms include dyspnea, nausea, vomiting, tachycardia, and diaphoresis.
◆ With Prinzmetal's angina, pain occurs at rest and with shortness of breath, nausea, vomiting, dizziness, and palpitations.

Anxiety

◆ Intermittent, sharp, stabbing pain occurs behind the left breast.
◆ Other signs and symptoms include precordial tenderness, palpitations, fatigue, headache, insomnia, breathlessness, nausea, vomiting, diarrhea, and tremors.

Aortic aneurysm, dissecting

◆ Excruciating tearing, ripping, stabbing chest and neck pain begins suddenly and radiates to the upper and lower back and abdomen.
◆ Other signs and symptoms include abdominal tenderness; tachycardia; hypotension; pale, cool, diaphoretic, and mottled skin below the waist; weak or absent femoral or pedal pulses; a palpable abdominal mass; and systolic bruit.

Asthma

◆ Diffuse and painful chest tightness, dry cough, and mild wheezing arise suddenly.
◆ Signs may progress to a productive cough, audible wheezing, severe dyspnea, rhonchi, crackles, prolonged expirations, intercostal and supraclavicular retractions on inspiration, accessory muscle use, flaring nostrils, and tachypnea.

Bronchitis

◆ Burning chest pain or a sensation of substernal tightness occurs in the acute form.
◆ Other findings include a cough that's initially dry but later productive, low-grade fever, chills, sore throat, tachycardia, muscle and back pain, rhonchi, crackles, and wheezing.

Cardiomyopathy

◆ Hypertrophic cardiomyopathy may cause angina-like chest pain, dyspnea, cough, dizziness, syncope, gallops, murmurs, and bradycardia associated with tachycardia.
◆ A medium-pitched systolic ejection murmur may be heard along the left sternal border and top of the heart.
◆ Palpation of peripheral pulses reveals a characteristic double impulse (pulsus bisferiens).

Cholecystitis

◆ Epigastric or right-upper-quadrant pain occurs abruptly because of gallbladder inflammation.
◆ Pain may be sharp or intensely aching, steady or intermittent, and may radiate to the back or right shoulder.
◆ An abdominal mass, rigidity, distention, or tenderness may be palpable in the right-upper abdomen.
◆ Other signs and symptoms include Murphy's sign, nausea, and vomiting.

Esophageal spasm

◆ Substernal chest pain mimics angina and may last up to 1 hour. Pain may radiate to the neck, jaw, arms, or back.
◆ Other findings include dysphagia for solid foods, bradycardia, and nodal rhythm.

Hiatal hernia

◆ Heartburn and sternal ache or pressure occur and may radiate to left shoulder and arm.
◆ Pain occurs after a meal and with bending or lying down.

Mitral valve prolapse

◆ Sharp, stabbing precordial chest pain or precordial aching may occur.
◆ A systolic murmur at the apex follows a midsystolic click.
◆ Other signs and symptoms include cardiac awareness, migraine headache, dizziness, weakness, episodic severe fatigue, dyspnea, tachycardia, mood swings, and palpitations.

Muscle strain

◆ Strain may cause a superficial and continuous ache or pulling sensation in the chest that may be aggravated by lifting, pulling, or pushing heavy objects.
◆ Fatigue, weakness, and rapid swelling of the affected area occur with acute strain.

Myocardial infarction

◆ Crushing substernal pain occurs that isn't relieved by nitroglycerin (Nitrostat).
◆ Pain lasts 15 minutes to hours and may radiate to the left arm, jaw, neck, or shoulder blades.
◆ Other signs and symptoms include pallor, clammy skin, dyspnea, diaphoresis, nausea, vomiting, anxiety, restlessness, murmurs, crackles, hypotension or hypertension, a feeling of impending doom, and an atrial gallop.

Pancreatitis

◆ Acute form causes intense pain in the epigastric area that radiates to the back and worsens in a supine position.
◆ Extreme restlessness, mottled skin, tachycardia, and cold, sweaty extremities may occur with severe pancreatitis.
◆ Massive hemorrhage, with resultant shock and coma, occurs with sudden, severe pancreatitis.

Peptic ulcer

◆ Sharp and burning pain arises in the epigastric region hours after food intake, commonly during the night, and is relieved by food or antacids.

◆ Other signs and symptoms include nausea, vomiting, melena, and epigastric tenderness.

Pericarditis
◆ Sharp or cutting precordial or retrosternal pain is aggravated by deep breathing, coughing, and position changes and radiates to the shoulder and neck.
◆ Other findings include pericardial rub, fever, tachycardia, and dyspnea.

Pleurisy
◆ Sharp, usually one-sided, pain in the lower aspects of the chest arises abruptly, reaching maximum intensity within a few hours.
◆ Deep breathing, coughing, or thoracic movement aggravates pain.
◆ Decreased breath sounds, inspiratory crackles, and a pleural rub may be heard on auscultation.

Pneumonia
◆ Pleuritic chest pain increases with deep inspiration.
◆ Other findings include shaking chills; fever; a dry, hacking cough that later becomes productive; crackles; rhonchi; tachycardia; tachypnea; myalgia; dyspnea, abdominal pain; anorexia; cyanosis; decreased breath sounds; and diaphoresis.

Pneumothorax
◆ Sudden, severe, sharp chest pain typically presents on one side and increases with chest movement.
◆ Dyspnea and cyanosis progressively worsen.
◆ Breath sounds are decreased or absent on the affected side, with hyperresonance or tympany, subcutaneous crepitation, and decreased vocal fremitus.
◆ Other signs and symptoms include asymmetrical chest expansion, tachypnea, tachycardia, anxiety, and restlessness.

Pulmonary embolism
◆ Sudden dyspnea occurs with intense angina-like or pleuritic pain that's aggravated by deep breathing and thoracic movement.
◆ Cyanosis and distended jugular veins occur with a large embolus.
◆ Other findings include tachypnea, diaphoresis, crackles, and signs of hypoxia.

Pulmonary hypertension, primary
◆ Angina-like pain develops late and typically occurs on exertion.
◆ Pain may radiate to the neck.
◆ Other signs and symptoms include exertional dyspnea, fatigue, syncope, weakness, cough, and hemoptysis.

Sickle cell crisis
◆ Pain may be vague at first and located in the back, hands, or feet.
◆ As pain worsens, it becomes generalized or localized to the abdomen or chest, causing severe pleuritic pain.

Tuberculosis
◆ Pleuritic chest pain and fine crackles occur after coughing.
◆ Other signs and symptoms include night sweats, anorexia, weight loss, fever, malaise, dyspnea, fatigue, mild to severe productive cough, hemoptysis, dullness on percussion, increased tactile fremitus, and amphoric breath sounds.

OTHER
Chinese restaurant syndrome
◆ A reaction to excessive ingestion of monosodium glutamate mimics the signs of an acute myocardial infarction.

Drugs
◆ Abrupt withdrawal from beta-adrenergic blockers can cause rebound angina in patients with coronary heart disease.

Nursing considerations

◆ Monitor the patient's vital signs and pulse oximetry.
◆ Assess the patient's pain level, administer nitrates or analgesics as ordered, and evaluate their effects.
◆ Prepare the patient for cardiopulmonary studies.
◆ Obtain cardiac markers, ECGs, and arterial blood gas values as ordered.

PATIENT TEACHING

◆ Teach the patient about the underlying diagnosis and ways to prevent future chest pain.
◆ Alert the patient or caregiver to signs and symptoms that require immediate medical attention.
◆ Explain the diagnostic tests the patient needs.
◆ Teach about the administration, dosage, and possible adverse effects of prescribed medications.

Cheyne-Stokes respirations

Overview

Cheyne-Stokes respirations, a waxing and waning period of hyperpnea that alternates with a shorter period of apnea, may occur normally in patients with heart or lung disease or those who live at high altitudes. They usually indicate increased intracranial pressure (ICP) from a deep cerebral or brain stem lesion or a metabolic disturbance in the brain. Cheyne-Stokes respirations may also occur normally in elderly people during sleep.

Assessment

HISTORY
◆ Obtain a medical and surgical history.
◆ Ask about any recent head injury or change in neurologic status.
◆ Ask about drug use.

PHYSICAL ASSESSMENT
◆ Perform a complete physical examination, focusing on the neurologic and cardiorespiratory systems.

 Nursing alert

Quickly take vital signs in a patient with a history of head trauma, recent brain surgery, or another brain insult. Elevate the head of the bed 30 degrees, and perform a rapid neurologic examination. Watch for signs of rising ICP, and anticipate ICP monitoring. Time the hyperpnea and apnea periods, being alert for prolonged apnea periods. Assess vital signs and neurologic status frequently to detect changes. Maintain airway patency, and administer oxygen as needed. Mechanical ventilation may be necessary if the patient's condition worsens.

Causes

MEDICAL
Adams-Stokes syndrome
◆ Adams-Stokes attacks may precede Cheyne-Stokes respirations.
◆ A syncopal episode associated with atrioventricular block occurs.

◆ Other signs and symptoms include hypotension, a heart rate between 20 and 50 beats/minute, confusion, shaking, and paleness.

Heart failure
◆ Cheyne-Stokes respirations may occur along with exertional dyspnea and orthopnea in left-sided heart failure.
◆ Other signs and symptoms include fatigue, weakness, tachycardia, tachypnea, and crackles.

Hypertensive encephalopathy
◆ Severe hypertension precedes Cheyne-Stokes respirations.
◆ Other signs and symptoms include decreased level of consciousness (LOC), vomiting, seizures, severe headaches, vision disturbances, and transient paralysis.

Increased ICP
◆ Cheyne-Stokes respirations are the first irregular respiratory pattern to occur as ICP rises.
◆ Late signs of increased ICP include bradycardia and widened pulse pressure.
◆ Accompanying signs and symptoms include decreased LOC, hypertension, headache, vomiting, impaired motor movement, and vision disturbances.

Renal failure
◆ Cheyne-Stokes respirations occur with end-stage chronic renal failure.
◆ Other signs and symptoms include bleeding gums, oral lesions, ammonia breath odor, and marked changes in every body system.

OTHER
Drugs
◆ Large doses of an opioid, hypnotic, or barbiturate drugs can precipitate a Cheyne-Stokes respiratory pattern.

Nursing considerations

◆ Monitor the patient's vital signs and pulse oximetry. Note periods of apnea.
◆ Monitor neurologic status.

PATIENT TEACHING

◆ Explain the causes and treatments of conditions leading to Cheyne-Stokes respirations.
◆ Teach the patient and a responsible person to recognize the difference between sleep apnea and Cheyne-Stokes respirations.

Costovertebral angle tenderness

Overview

Costovertebral angle (CVA) tenderness is pain elicited by percussing the CVA just to the side of the spine and the 12th rib. The pain then travels forward, below the ribs toward the umbilicus. It accompanies un-elicited, dull, constant flank pain and indicates sudden distention of the renal capsule.

Assessment

HISTORY
◆ Find out about other signs and symptoms of renal or urologic dysfunction.
◆ Ask about voiding habits and the onset and description of any recent changes.
◆ Obtain a personal or family history of urinary tract infections, congenital anomalies, calculi, other obstructive nephropathies or uropathies, or renovascular disorders.

PHYSICAL ASSESSMENT
◆ Obtain the patient's vital signs.
◆ If the patient has hypertension and bradycardia, look for other autonomic effects of renal pain.
◆ Inspect, auscultate, and gently palpate and percuss the abdomen for clues to the underlying cause of CVA tenderness.
◆ Look for abdominal distention, hypoactive bowel sounds, and palpable masses.

Age considerations
Advanced age and cognitive impairment reduce an older patient's ability to perceive pain or describe its intensity.

Causes

MEDICAL
Perirenal abscess
◆ Exquisite CVA tenderness occurs with flank pain that may radiate to the groin or down the leg.
◆ Other signs and symptoms include dysuria, persistent high fever, chills, erythema of the skin, and a palpable abdominal mass.

Pyelonephritis, acute
◆ CVA tenderness occurs with persistent high fever, chills, flank pain, anorexia, nausea and vomiting, weakness, dysuria, hematuria, nocturia, urinary urgency and frequency, and tenesmus.
◆ Bacterial infection of the renal pelvis occurs.

Renal artery occlusion
◆ CVA tenderness and flank pain occur.
◆ Other signs and symptoms include severe, continuous upper abdominal pain; nausea; vomiting; hematuria; decreased bowel sounds; and high fever.

Renal calculi
◆ CVA tenderness occurs with waves of waxing and waning flank pain that may radiate to the groin, testicles, suprapubic area, or labia, caused by calculi of the urinary tract system.
◆ Other signs and symptoms include nausea, vomiting, severe abdominal pain, abdominal distention, and decreased bowel sounds.

Renal vein occlusion
◆ CVA tenderness and flank pain occur.
◆ Other signs and symptoms include sudden, severe back pain; fever; oliguria; edema; and hematuria.

S & S

Nursing considerations

◆ Give prescribed drugs for pain.
◆ Monitor the patient's vital signs.
◆ Monitor fluid intake and urine output.
◆ Collect blood samples and urine specimens as ordered.

PATIENT TEACHING

◆ Explain the cause of CVA tenderness and the treatment plan.
◆ Explain dietary restrictions the patient needs to follow.
◆ Tell the patient to drink at least 2 qt (2 L) of fluids daily unless he's instructed otherwise.
◆ Explain which signs and symptoms of kidney infection he should report.
◆ Emphasize the importance of taking the full course of prescribed antibiotics.

S & S

Crackles

Overview

Crackles, also known as *rales* or *crepitations*, are nonmusical clicking or rattling noises heard during auscultation of breath sounds. They may be on one or both sides, moist- or dry-sounding. Crackles usually occur during inspiration and recur constantly from one respiratory cycle to the next. They indicate abnormal movement of air through fluid-filled airways.

Assessment

HISTORY

◆ Ask about the onset, duration, and description of cough and pain.
◆ Note the sputum's consistency, amount, odor, and color.
◆ Obtain a medical history, including incidence of cancer, respiratory or cardiovascular problems, surgery, or trauma.
◆ Find out about smoking and alcohol use.
◆ Obtain a drug and occupational history.
◆ Ask about recent weight loss, anorexia, nausea, vomiting, fatigue, weakness, vertigo, hoarseness, difficulty swallowing, and syncope.
◆ Determine exposure to respiratory irritants.

PHYSICAL ASSESSMENT

◆ Take vital signs, and examine the patient for signs of respiratory distress or airway obstruction. Check the depth and rhythm of respirations. Check for increased accessory muscle use and chest-wall motion, retractions, stridor, or nasal flaring.
◆ Examine the nose and mouth for signs of infection.
◆ Assess breath odor.
◆ Check the neck for masses, tenderness, lymphadenopathy, swelling, or vein distention.
◆ Inspect the chest for abnormal configuration or uneven expansion.
◆ Percuss the chest for dullness, tympany, or flatness.

◆ Auscultate the lungs for other abnormal, diminished, or absent breath sounds.
◆ Auscultate for abnormal heart sounds.
◆ Check the hands and feet for edema or clubbing.

Causes

MEDICAL

Acute respiratory distress syndrome

◆ Diffuse, fine to coarse crackles are usually heard in the dependent portions of the lungs.
◆ Other signs and symptoms include cyanosis, nasal flaring, tachypnea, tachycardia, grunting respirations, rhonchi, dyspnea, anxiety, and decreased level of consciousness.

Bronchiectasis

◆ Persistent, coarse crackles are heard over the affected area of the lung.
◆ Chronic cough that produces copious amounts of mucopurulent sputum accompanies crackles.
◆ Other signs and symptoms include exertional dyspnea, rhonchi, weight loss, fatigue, and late clubbing.

Bronchitis, chronic

◆ Coarse crackles are usually heard at the lung base.
◆ Other signs and symptoms include prolonged expirations, wheezing, rhonchi, exertional dyspnea, tachypnea, cyanosis, clubbing, and persistent, productive cough.

Interstitial fibrosis of the lungs

◆ Cellophane-like crackles can be heard over all lobes.
◆ Other signs and symptoms as the disease progresses include nonproductive cough, dyspnea, fatigue, weight loss, cyanosis, pleuritic chest pain, nasal flaring, and cyanosis.

Legionnaires' disease

◆ Diffuse, moist crackles are heard.

◆ Early signs and symptoms include malaise, fatigue, weakness, anorexia, myalgia, and diarrhea.

◆ Within 12 to 48 hours, a dry cough develops, with accompanying sudden high fever and chills.

◆ Other signs and symptoms include pleuritic chest pain, tachypnea, and dyspnea.

Lung abscess

◆ Fine to medium and moist inspiratory crackles occur.

◆ Other signs and symptoms include sweats, anorexia, weight loss, fever, fatigue, weakness, dyspnea, clubbing, pleuritic chest pain, pleural rub, and a cough that produces large amounts of foul-smelling, purulent, bloody sputum.

Pneumonia

◆ Bacterial pneumonia produces diffuse, fine crackles.

◆ Mycoplasmal pneumonia produces medium to fine crackles.

◆ Viral pneumonia causes gradually developing, diffuse crackles.

◆ Other signs and symptoms include fever, tachypnea, pleuritic chest pain, dyspnea, rhonchi, and a dry cough that becomes productive.

Pulmonary edema

◆ Moist, bubbling crackles on inspiration are one of the first signs.

◆ Other signs and symptoms include exertional dyspnea; paroxysmal nocturnal dyspnea, then orthopnea; tachycardia; tachypnea; ventricular gallop; and a cough that's initially nonproductive, but later produces frothy, bloody sputum.

Pulmonary embolism

◆ Fine to coarse crackles and severe dyspnea are early signs and may be accompanied by angina or pleuritic chest pain.

◆ Cough may be nonproductive or produce blood-tinged sputum.

◆ Other signs and symptoms include pleural rub, wheezing, chest dullness on percussion, decreased breath sounds, and signs of circulatory collapse.

Pulmonary tuberculosis

◆ Fine crackles occur after coughing.

◆ Sputum may be scant, mucoid or copious, and purulent.

◆ Other signs and symptoms include hemoptysis, malaise, dyspnea, pleuritic chest pain, fatigue, night sweats, weakness, weight loss, and amphoric breath sounds.

Sarcoidosis

◆ Fine, basilar, end-inspiratory crackles occur.

◆ Other signs and symptoms include malaise, fatigue, weakness, weight loss, cough, dyspnea, and tachypnea.

Nursing considerations

◆ Administer oxygen and monitor pulse oximetry.

◆ Elevate the head of the bed to ease the patient's breathing.

◆ Administer fluids to liquefy secretions and relieve mucous membrane inflammation.

◆ If crackles result from cardiogenic pulmonary edema, give a diuretic, as prescribed.

◆ Turn the patient every 1 to 2 hours, and encourage deep breathing and coughing exercises.

◆ Monitor respiratory status.

PATIENT TEACHING

◆ Explain the cause of crackles and the treatment plan.

◆ Teach the patient effective coughing techniques.

◆ Teach him to avoid respiratory irritants.

◆ Provide information on smoking cessation.

◆ Teach the patient energy conservation techniques, particularly with chronic disorders.

Crepitation, subcutaneous

Overview

Subcutaneous crepitation, a crackling sound on palpation of the skin that's accompanied by bubbles that feel like small, unstable nodules, results from trapping of air or gas bubbles in the subcutaneous tissue. Edema develops in the affected area, and if edema occurs in the neck or upper chest, it may cause life-threatening airway occlusion.

Assessment

HISTORY

◆ Ask the patient if he is having difficulty breathing.
◆ Ask about the onset, location, and severity of any associated pain.
◆ Obtain a medical and surgical history, including recent thoracic surgery, diagnostic tests, and respiratory therapy as well as trauma or chronic pulmonary disease.

PHYSICAL ASSESSMENT

◆ Palpate the affected skin frquently to evaluate the location and extent of crepitus and whether crepitation is increasing.
◆ Perform abbreviated cardiac, pulmonary, and GI assessments as the patient's condition allows. Note if tracheal deviation is present.
◆ When the patient is stabilized, perform a complete physical examination.

Causes

MEDICAL
Esophageal rupture

◆ Subcutaneous crepitation may be palpable in the neck, chest wall, or supraclavicular fossa.
◆ With cervical esophagus rupture, excruciating pain in the neck or supraclavicular area, resistance to passive neck movement, local tenderness, soft-tissue swelling, dysphagia, odynophagia, and orthostatic vertigo may occur.
◆ With intrathoracic esophagus rupture, findings include a positive Hamman's sign; severe retrosternal, epigastric, neck, or scapular pain; dyspnea; tachypnea; asymmetrical chest movement; tachycardia; and hypotension.

Orbital fracture

◆ Subcutaneous crepitation of the eyelid and orbit develops when fracture allows air from the nasal sinus to escape into subcutaneous tissue.
◆ Periorbital ecchymosis is the most common sign.
◆ Other signs and symptoms include facial and eyelid edema, diplopia, and impaired extraocular movements.

Pneumothorax

◆ Subcutaneous crepitation occurs in the upper chest and neck in severe cases.
◆ One-sided chest pain increases on inspiration.
◆ Other signs and symptoms include dyspnea, anxiety, restlessness, tachypnea, cyanosis, tachycardia, accessory muscle use, asymmetrical chest expansion, decreased or absent breath sounds on the affected side, and a nonproductive cough.

Tracheal rupture

◆ Abrupt subcutaneous crepitation of the neck and anterior chest wall occurs.
◆ Other signs and symptoms include severe dyspnea with nasal flaring, tachycardia, accessory muscle use, tracheal deviation, hypotension, cyanosis, extreme anxiety, hemoptysis, and mediastinal emphysema with a positive Hamman's sign.

OTHER

Diagnostic tests
◆ Endoscopic tests can rupture or perforate respiratory or GI organs, producing subcutaneous crepitation.

Respiratory treatments
◆ Intermittent positive-pressure breathing and mechanical ventilation can rupture alveoli, producing subcutaneous crepitation.

Thoracic surgery
◆ If air escapes into the tissue in the area of the incision, subcutaneous crepitation can occur.

Nursing considerations

◆ Monitor vital signs and pulse oximetry.
◆ Monitor respiratory status and provide supportive measures as needed.
◆ Obtain a chest X-ray as indicated.
◆ Assess the extent of crepitation; note an increase or a decrease.

PATIENT TEACHING
◆ Explain the cause of subcutaneous crepitation and the treatment plan.
◆ Explain diagnostic tests and procedures the patient needs.
◆ Explain the signs and symptoms of subcutaneous crepitation to report.

Cyanosis

Overview

Cyanosis is a bluish or bluish-black discoloration of the skin and mucous membranes from excessive concentration of unoxygenated hemoglobin in the blood. It's classified as central (inadequate oxygenation of systemic arterial blood) or peripheral (sluggish peripheral circulation). Cyanosis isn't always an accurate gauge of oxygenation.

Nursing alert

If sudden, localized cyanosis occurs with other signs of arterial occlusion, protect the affected limb from injury, but don't massage it. If central cyanosis stems from a pulmonary disorder or shock, perform a rapid evaluation. Take immediate steps to maintain an airway, assist breathing, and monitor circulation.

Assessment

HISTORY

◆ Obtain a medical history, including cardiac, pulmonary, and hematologic disorders, and previous surgery.
◆ Evaluate the patient's mental status while obtaining his history.
◆ Ask about the onset, aggravating and alleviating factors, and characteristics of the cyanosis.

PHYSICAL ASSESSMENT

◆ Obtain vital signs and pulse oximetry, and evaluate respiratory rate and rhythm.
◆ Check for nasal flaring and accessory muscle use.
◆ Inspect the skin, lips, and nail bed color and mucous membranes.
◆ Inspect for asymmetrical chest expansion or barrel chest.
◆ Inspect the abdomen for ascites.
◆ Palpate peripheral pulses, test capillary refill, and note edema.
◆ Percuss and palpate for liver enlargement and tenderness.
◆ Percuss the lungs for dullness or hyperresonance.

◆ Auscultate for decreased or adventitious breath sounds, heart rate and rhythm, and the abdominal aorta and femoral arteries for bruits.

Causes

MEDICAL

Arteriosclerotic occlusive disease, chronic

◆ Peripheral cyanosis occurs in the legs whenever they're in a dependent position.
◆ Other findings include intermittent claudication and burning pain at rest, paresthesia, pallor, muscle atrophy, weak leg pulses, impotence, and leg ulcers and gangrene (late signs).

Bronchiectasis

◆ Chronic central cyanosis develops.
◆ The classic sign is chronic productive cough with copious, foul-smelling, mucopurulent sputum, or hemoptysis.
◆ Other signs and symptoms include dyspnea, recurrent fever and chills, weight loss, and clubbing.

Chronic obstructive pulmonary disease

◆ Chronic central cyanosis that's aggravated by exertion occurs in advanced stages.
◆ Barrel chest and clubbing are late signs.
◆ Other signs and symptoms include exertional dyspnea, productive cough with thick sputum, anorexia, weight loss, pursed-lip breathing, tachypnea, accessory muscle use, and wheezing.

Heart failure

◆ With left-sided heart failure, central cyanosis occurs with tachycardia, fatigue, dyspnea, cold intolerance, orthopnea, cough, ventricular or atrial gallop, and crackles.
◆ With right-sided heart failure, peripheral cyanosis occurs with fatigue, peripheral edema, ascites, jugular vein distention, and hepatomegaly.

◆ Acute or chronic cyanosis may occur as a late sign.

Peripheral arterial occlusion, acute
◆ Acute cyanosis of the arm or leg is accompanied by sharp or aching pain that worsens with movement.
◆ Paresthesia, weakness, decreased or absent pulse, and pale, cool skin occur in the affected extremity.

Pneumonia
◆ Acute central cyanosis is usually preceded by fever, shaking chills, cough with purulent sputum, crackles, rhonchi, and pleuritic chest pain that's exacerbated by deep inspiration.
◆ Other signs and symptoms include tachycardia, dyspnea, tachypnea, diminished breath sounds, diaphoresis, myalgia, fatigue, headache, and anorexia.

Pneumothorax
◆ Acute central cyanosis is a cardinal sign.
◆ Rapid, shallow respirations; weak, rapid pulse; pallor; jugular vein distention; anxiety; and absence of breath sounds over the affected lobe may also occur.
◆ Other signs and symptoms include asymmetrical chest movement and shortness of breath.

Pulmonary edema
◆ Acute central cyanosis occurs.
◆ Other signs and symptoms include dyspnea; orthopnea; frothy, blood-tinged sputum; tachycardia; tachypnea; crackles; ventricular gallop; cold, clammy skin; hypotension; weak, thready pulse; and confusion.

Pulmonary embolism
◆ Acute central cyanosis occurs.
◆ Other signs and symptoms include syncope, jugular vein distention, dyspnea, chest pain, tachycardia, paradoxical pulse, dry cough or productive cough with blood-tinged sputum, fever, restlessness, and diaphoresis.

Raynaud's disease
◆ Exposure to cold or stress causes the fingers or hands to blanch, turn cold, then become cyanotic, and finally to redden with return of normal temperature.
◆ Numbness and tingling may also develop.

Shock
◆ Acute peripheral cyanosis develops in the hands and feet.
◆ Feet may be cold, clammy, and pale.
◆ Central cyanosis develops with progression of shock and organ system failures.
◆ Other signs and symptoms include confusion, hypotension, and a rapid, weak pulse.

Nursing considerations

◆ Provide supplemental oxygen and monitor pulse oximetry and arterial blood gas values.
◆ Assist with endotracheal intubation when necessary.
◆ Position the patient comfortably to ease breathing.
◆ Give a diuretic, bronchodilator, antibiotic, or cardiac drug as prescribed.
◆ Provide rest periods to prevent dyspnea; encourage energy conservation.

PATIENT TEACHING
◆ Explain the cause of cyanosis and the treatment plan.
◆ Instruct the patient to seek medical attention if cyanosis occurs.
◆ Discuss the safe use of oxygen in the home.
◆ Explain medication use and possible adverse effects.
◆ Discuss the importance of frequent rest periods and follow-up care.

S & S

Decerebrate posture

Overview

Decerebrate posture, also known as *decerebrate rigidity* or *abnormal extensor reflex,* indicates upper brain stem damage. It may occur spontaneously or be elicited by noxious stimuli and is characterized by internally rotated and extended arms, pronated wrists, flexed fingers, stiffly extended legs, and forced plantar flexion of the feet.

Assessment

HISTORY
◆ Determine when the patient's level of consciousness (LOC) began to deteriorate.
◆ Ask if onset was abrupt or gradual and occurred with other signs or symptoms.
◆ Obtain a medical history, asking about diabetes, liver disease, cancer, blood clots, and aneurysm.
◆ Ask about recent trauma or accidents.

PHYSICAL ASSESSMENT
◆ Take vital signs.
◆ Determine LOC using the Glasgow Coma Scale.
◆ Evaluate pupils for size, equality, and response to light.
◆ Test deep tendon reflexes and cranial nerve reflexes.
◆ Check for doll's eye sign.
◆ Check if the patient's airway is patent.

Causes

MEDICAL
Brain stem infarction
◆ Coma may occur with decerebrate posture.
◆ Absence of doll's eye sign, a positive Babinski's reflex, and flaccidity occur with deep coma.

Brain stem tumor
◆ Hemiparesis or quadriparesis, cranial nerve palsies, vertigo, dizziness, ataxia, and vomiting may occur.
◆ Decerebrate posture is a late sign that occurs with coma.

Cerebral lesion
◆ Increased intracranial pressure (ICP) may produce decerebrate posture, a late sign.
◆ Other signs and symptoms include coma, abnormal pupil size and response to light, and the classic triad of increased ICP: bradycardia, increasing systolic blood pressure, and widening pulse pressure.

Hepatic encephalopathy
◆ Decerebrate posture occurs as a late sign with coma resulting from increased ICP and ammonia toxicity.
◆ Other signs and symptoms include fetor hepaticus, a positive Babinski's reflex, and hyperactive deep tendon reflexes.

Hypoglycemic encephalopathy
◆ Decerebrate posture and coma may occur.
◆ Low glucose levels are characteristic.
◆ Muscle spasms, twitching, and seizures progress to flaccidity.

Hypoxic encephalopathy
◆ Decerebrate posture occurs along with coma, positive Babinski's reflex, absence of doll's eye sign, hypoactive deep tendon reflexes, fixed pupils, and respiratory arrest.

Pontine hemorrhage
◆ Decerebrate posture occurs rapidly along with coma.
◆ Other signs and symptoms include paralysis, absence of doll's eye sign, a positive Babinski's reflex, and small, reactive pupils.

Posterior fossa hemorrhage

◆ Decerebrate posture occurs with vomiting, headache, vertigo, ataxia, stiff neck, drowsiness, papilledema, and cranial nerve palsies.

◆ Coma and respiratory arrest eventually may occur.

OTHER

Diagnostic tests

◆ Removing spinal fluid during a lumbar puncture may cause the brain stem to compress, causing decerebrate posture and coma.

Nursing considerations

◆ Insert an artificial airway, if needed, to prevent aspiration. (If you suspect spinal cord injury, don't disrupt spinal alignment.)

◆ Suction as needed.

◆ Give supplemental oxygen; intubation and mechanical ventilation may be required.

◆ Keep emergency resuscitation equipment readily available.

◆ Monitor the patient's neurologic status and vital signs.

◆ Look for symptoms of increased ICP and neurologic deterioration.

◆ Provide supportive care as indicated.

PATIENT TEACHING

◆ Teach the patient and family about the medical diagnosis, prognosis, and treatment plan.

◆ Provide emotional support to the patient and his family.

Decorticate posture

Overview

Decorticate posture, which may occur spontaneously or be elicited by noxious stimuli, signals corticospinal damage, usually from stroke or head injury. It's characterized by adducted arms, flexion of the elbows, flexed wrists and fingers on the chest, and extended and internally rotated legs with plantar flexion of the feet. The stimulus intensity, the duration of the posture, and the spontaneous episode frequency depend on the cerebral injury severity and location. The prognosis for decorticate posture is more favorable than for decerebrate posture.

Assessment

HISTORY

◆ Check for symptoms, such as headache, dizziness, nausea, changes in vision, numbness or tingling, and behavioral changes. If a symptom is present, ask when it began.

◆ Obtain a medical history, asking about cerebrovascular disease, cancer, meningitis, encephalitis, upper respiratory tract infection, bleeding or clotting disorders, or recent trauma.

PHYSICAL ASSESSMENT

◆ Obtain vital signs and evaluate level of consciousness (LOC).

◆ Test motor and sensory functions.

◆ Evaluate pupil size, equality, and response to light.

◆ Test cranial nerve function and deep tendon reflexes.

Causes

MEDICAL
Brain abscess

◆ Decorticate posture may occur along with aphasia, behavioral changes, altered vital signs, decreased LOC, hemiparesis, headache, dizziness, seizures, nausea, and vomiting.

Brain tumor

◆ Decorticate posture results from increased intracranial pressure (ICP).

◆ Other signs and symptoms include headache, behavioral changes, memory loss, diplopia, blurred vision or vision loss, seizures, ataxia, apraxia, aphasia, sensory loss, paresthesia, vomiting, papilledema, and signs of hormonal imbalance.

Head injury

◆ Decorticate posture may result, depending on the injury.

◆ Other signs and symptoms include headache, nausea, vomiting, dizziness, irritability, decreased LOC, aphasia, hemiparesis, seizures, and pupillary dilation.

Stroke

◆ A stroke involving the cerebral cortex produces decorticate posture on one side of the body.

◆ Other signs and symptoms include hemiplegia, dysarthria, dysphagia, sensory loss, apraxia, agnosia, aphasia, memory loss, decreased LOC, homonymous hemianopia, and blurred vision.

Nursing considerations

◆ Monitor the patient's neurologic status and vital signs frequently to detect signs of deterioration.
◆ Look for other signs of increased ICP.
◆ Maintain a patent airway and prevent aspiration.
◆ If you suspect spinal cord injury, don't disrupt spinal alignment. Intubation and mechanical ventilation may be required.

PATIENT TEACHING
◆ Explain the signs and symptoms of decreased LOC and seizures.
◆ Discuss the patient's or caregiver's concerns about quality-of-life.
◆ Provide referrals as appropriate.
◆ Explain to the caregiver how to keep the patient safe, especially during a seizure.

Dizziness

Overview

Dizziness, the sensation of imbalance or faintness, commonly results from inadequate blood flow and oxygen supply to the cerebrum and spinal cord. It may be associated with giddiness, weakness, confusion, and blurred or double vision. It's commonly confused with vertigo, a sensation of revolving in space or of surroundings revolving about oneself, and its associated symptoms of nausea, vomiting, nystagmus, staggering gait, and tinnitus or hearing loss.

Assessment

HISTORY

◆ Obtain a medical history, noting diabetes mellitus, head injury, anxiety disorders, and cardiovascular, pulmonary, and kidney disease.
◆ Take a drug history and determine whether the patient is taking antihypertensives.
◆ Determine the onset and characteristics of dizziness.
◆ Ask about emotional stress.
◆ Ask about other signs and symptoms, such as palpitations, chest pain, diaphoresis, shortness of breath, and chronic cough.

PHYSICAL ASSESSMENT

◆ Check neurologic status, including level of consciousness (LOC), motor and sensory functions, and reflexes.
◆ Inspect for poor skin turgor and dry mucous membranes.
◆ Auscultate heart rate and rhythm and breath and heart sounds.
◆ Inspect for barrel chest, clubbing, cyanosis, and accessory muscle use.
◆ Check for orthostatic hypotension.
◆ Palpate for edema and capillary refill time.

Causes

MEDICAL
Anemia
◆ Dizziness is aggravated by postural changes or exertion.
◆ Other signs and symptoms include pallor, dyspnea, fatigue, tachycardia, and bounding pulse.

Cardiac arrhythmias
◆ Dizziness lasts for several seconds or longer and may precede fainting.
◆ Other signs and symptoms include palpitations; irregular, rapid, or thready pulse; hypotension; weakness; blurred vision; paresthesia, and confusion.

Carotid sinus hypersensitivity
◆ Brief episodes of dizziness after stimulation of one or both carotid arteries usually result in fainting.
◆ Other signs and symptoms include sweating, nausea, and pallor.

Generalized anxiety disorder
◆ Continuous dizziness may intensify as the disorder worsens.
◆ Other signs and symptoms include persistent anxiety, insomnia, difficulty concentrating, fidgeting, cold and clammy hands, dry mouth, frequent urination, tachycardia, tachypnea, diaphoresis, palpitations, and irritability.

Hypertension
◆ Dizziness may precede fainting or may be relieved by rest.
◆ Other signs and symptoms include headache, blurred vision, and retinal changes.

Hyperventilation syndrome
◆ Dizziness lasts a few minutes.
◆ With frequent hyperventilation, dizziness occurs between episodes.
◆ Other signs and symptoms include apprehension, diaphoresis, pallor, dyspnea,

chest tightness, palpitations, trembling, fatigue, and peripheral and circumoral paresthesia.

Hypoglycemia

◆ Dizziness, headache, clouding of vision, restlessness, and mental status changes can result from fasting hypoglycemia.
◆ Other signs and symptoms include trembling, cold sweats, and tachycardia.

Hypovolemia

◆ Dizziness results from lack of circulating volume.
◆ Other signs and symptoms include orthostatic hypotension, thirst, poor skin turgor, and flattened jugular veins.

Orthostatic hypotension

◆ Dizziness may end in fainting or disappear with rest after position change.
◆ Other findings include dim vision, spots before the eyes, pallor, diaphoresis, hypotension, tachycardia, and signs of dehydration.

Panic disorder

◆ Dizziness may accompany acute attacks of panic.
◆ Other signs and symptoms include anxiety, dyspnea, palpitations, chest pain, a choking or smothering sensation, vertigo, paresthesia, hot and cold flashes, diaphoresis, and trembling or shaking.

Postconcussion syndrome

◆ Dizziness, headache, emotional lability, alcohol intolerance, fatigue, anxiety and, possibly, vertigo occur 1 to 3 weeks after a head injury.
◆ Dizziness or other symptoms are intensified by physical or mental stress.

Transient ischemic attack

◆ Dizziness of varying severity, diplopia, blindness or visual field deficits, ptosis, tinnitus, hearing loss, paresis, and numbness occur.

OTHER
Drugs
◆ Antihistamines, antihypertensives, anxiolytics, central nervous system depressants, decongestants, opioids, and vasodilators commonly cause dizziness.
◆ Herbal remedies such as St. John's wort can produce dizziness.

Nursing considerations

◆ If the patient is dizzy, provide for his safety.
◆ Determine the severity and onset of the dizziness, and ask if he has a headache or blurred vision.
◆ Take the patient's blood pressure, and check for orthostatic hypotension.
◆ Determine if the patient is at risk for hypoglycemia.
◆ Have the patient lie down, and recheck vital signs every 15 minutes.
◆ Monitor the patient's neurologic status and intake and output.
◆ Assess cardiac rhythm and pulse oximetry. Obtain a capillary blood glucose level, if indicated.

PATIENT TEACHING
◆ Teach the patient about the underlying disease process and treatment.
◆ Teach the patient how to control dizziness.
◆ Teach the patient safety measures for when dizziness happens in the future.

S & S

Dyspepsia

Overview

Dyspepsia, the feeling of uncomfortable fullness after meals, occurs from altered gastric secretions that lead to excess stomach acidity. It results in belching, heartburn and, possibly, cramping and abdominal distention.

Assessment

HISTORY

◆ Ask about the onset, duration, and description of symptoms.
◆ Ask about alleviating and aggravating factors.
◆ Ask the patient about nausea, vomiting, melena, hematemesis, cough, chest pain, or urine changes.
◆ Obtain a drug and surgical history.
◆ Obtain a medical history, including renal, cardiovascular, or pulmonary disorders.
◆ Ask whether the patient has an unusual or overwhelming amount of emotional stress.

PHYSICAL ASSESSMENT

◆ Inspect the abdomen for distention, ascites, scars, obvious hernias, jaundice, uremic frost, and bruising.
◆ Auscultate for bowel sounds and characterize their motility.
◆ Percuss then palpate the abdomen, noting any tenderness, pain, organ enlargement, or tympany.
◆ Auscultate for gallops and crackles.
◆ Percuss the lungs to detect consolidation.
◆ Note peripheral edema and swelling of lymph nodes.

Causes

MEDICAL

Cholelithiasis

◆ Dyspepsia may occur, typically after intake of fatty foods.

◆ Other signs and symptoms include diaphoresis, tachycardia, jaundice with pruritus, dark urine, clay-colored stools, and biliary colic.

Cirrhosis

◆ Dyspepsia occurs and is relieved by ingestion of an antacid.
◆ Other signs and symptoms include jaundice, hepatomegaly, ascites, abdominal distention, and epigastric or right-upper-quadrant pain.

Duodenal ulcer

◆ Dyspepsia ranges from a vague fullness or pressure to a boring or aching sensation.
◆ Symptom occurs $1\frac{1}{2}$ to 3 hours after eating and is relieved by ingestion of food or antacids.
◆ Pain may awaken the patient at night with heartburn and fluid regurgitation.

Gastric dilation, acute

◆ Dyspepsia is an early symptom.
◆ Nausea, vomiting, upper abdominal distention, succussion splash, and apathy occur.
◆ Dehydration and gastric bleeding may also occur.

Gastric ulcer

◆ Dyspepsia and heartburn occur after eating.
◆ Epigastric pain may occur with vomiting, fullness, weight loss, GI bleeding, and abdominal distention and may not be relieved by food.

Gastritis, chronic

◆ Dyspepsia is relieved by antacids; lessened by smaller, more frequent meals; and aggravated by spicy foods or excessive caffeine.
◆ Other findings include anorexia, a feeling of fullness, vague epigastric pain, belching, nausea, and vomiting.

GI cancer

◆ Chronic dyspepsia occurs along with anorexia, fatigue, jaundice, melena, hematemesis, constipation, weight loss, weakness, syncope, and abdominal pain.

Heart failure

◆ With right-sided heart failure, transient dyspepsia may occur with chest tightness and pain or ache in the right upper quadrant because of vascular congestion.
◆ Other signs and symptoms include hepatomegaly, anorexia, bloating, ascites, tachycardia, jugular vein distention, tachypnea, dyspnea, orthopnea, edema, and fatigue.

Hepatitis

◆ Before an attack, moderate to severe dyspepsia along with fever, malaise, arthralgia, coryza, myalgia, nausea, vomiting, an altered sense of taste or smell, and hepatomegaly occur.
◆ Jaundice marks the onset of an attack; as jaundice clears, dyspepsia and other GI effects also diminish.

Hiatal hernia

◆ Dyspepsia occurs when gastric reflux through the hernia causes esophagitis, esophageal ulceration, or stricture.
◆ Dyspepsia is accompanied by heartburn and retrosternal or substernal chest pain.

Pancreatitis, chronic

◆ A feeling of fullness or dyspepsia may occur with epigastric pain that radiates to the back or through the abdomen.
◆ Other signs and symptoms include anorexia, nausea, vomiting, jaundice, dramatic weight loss, Turner's sign or Cullen's sign, hyperglycemia, and steatorrhea.

Uremia

◆ Dyspepsia may be the earliest and most important GI complaint.
◆ As the disease progresses, edema, pruritus, pallor, hyperpigmentation, uremic frost, ecchymoses, irritability, drowsiness, muscle twitching, seizures, weight gain, and oliguria may occur.

OTHER
Drugs

◆ Antibiotics, antihypertensives, corticosteroids, diuretics, and nonsteroidal anti-inflammatory drugs may cause dyspepsia.

Pregnancy

◆ Hormone changes slow the digestive process and relax the cardiac sphincter, allowing gastric reflux.
◆ This problem may increase in later pregnancy because of the pressure of the fetus on the mother's internal organs.

Surgery

◆ After GI surgery, postoperative gastritis can cause dyspepsia.

Nursing considerations

◆ Monitor the patient's GI status.
◆ Give an antacid 30 minutes before or 1 hour after a meal.
◆ Provide food to relieve dyspepsia.
◆ If drugs cause dyspepsia, give them after meals.

PATIENT TEACHING

◆ Explain the cause of dyspepsia and the treatment plan.
◆ Discuss the importance of small, frequent meals.
◆ Describe foods or liquids the patient should avoid.
◆ Discuss stress reduction techniques the patient can use.
◆ Instruct the patient to avoid lying down for 2 to 3 hours after eating and to avoid tight or constrictive clothing.

S & S

Dyspnea

Overview

Dyspnea (shortness of breath indicating cardiopulmonary dysfunction) may arise suddenly or slowly and subside rapidly or persist for years.

Assessment

HISTORY

◆ Ask about the symptom's onset and progression.
◆ Determine aggravating and alleviating factors.
◆ Ask the patient if he has a cough.
◆ Obtain a history, including trauma, upper respiratory tract infection, deep vein phlebitis, orthopnea, paroxysmal nocturnal dyspnea, fatigue, smoking, or exposure to occupational hazards.
◆ Ask about current orthopnea, paroxysmal nocturnal dyspnea, or progressive fatigue.

PHYSICAL ASSESSMENT

◆ Look for pursed-lip exhalation, clubbing, peripheral edema, barrel chest, diaphoresis, jugular vein distention, and edema.
◆ Obtain the patient's vital signs and a pulse oximetry reading.
◆ Auscultate for crackles, egophony, bronchophony, abnormal heart sounds or rhythms, and whispered pectoriloquy.
◆ Palpate the abdomen for hepatomegaly.

Causes

MEDICAL

Acute respiratory distress syndrome

◆ Acute dyspnea is usually the first complaint.
◆ Progressive respiratory distress occurs with restlessness, anxiety, decreased mental acuity, tachycardia, tachypnea, and crackles and rhonchi.

Asthma

◆ Dyspneic attacks occur with audible wheezing, dry cough, accessory muscle use, nasal flaring, intercostal and supra-clavicular retractions, tachypnea, tachycardia, diaphoresis, prolonged expiration, flush or cyanosis, and anxiety.

Cor pulmonale

◆ Chronic dyspnea begins gradually with exertion and progressively worsens until it occurs even at rest.
◆ Other signs and symptoms include chronic productive cough, wheezing, tachypnea, jugular vein distention, edema, fatigue, weakness, and hepatomegaly.

Emphysema

◆ Progressive exertional dyspnea occurs.
◆ Other signs and symptoms include barrel chest, accessory muscle use, diminished breath sounds, anorexia, weight loss, malaise, peripheral cyanosis, tachypnea, pursed-lip breathing, prolonged expiration, a chronic and productive cough, and late clubbing.

Flail chest

◆ Sudden dyspnea is accompanied by paradoxical chest movement, severe chest pain, hypotension, tachypnea, tachycardia, and cyanosis.
◆ Bruising and decreased or absent breath sounds occur over the affected side.

Heart failure

◆ Dyspnea occurs gradually with orthopnea, tachypnea, tachycardia, palpitations, ventricular gallop, fatigue, dependent edema, jugular vein distention, paroxysmal nocturnal dyspnea, hepatosplenomegaly, cough, and weight gain.

Myocardial infarction

◆ Dyspnea occurs suddenly with crushing substernal chest pain that may radiate to the back, neck, jaw, and arms.
◆ Other signs and symptoms include nausea, vomiting, diaphoresis, vertigo, tachycardia, anxiety, and pale, cool, clammy skin.

Pleural effusion

◆ Dyspnea develops slowly and progressively worsens over time.
◆ Initial signs and symptoms include pleural friction rub and pleuritic pain that worsens with cough and deep breathing.
◆ Other signs and symptoms include dullness on percussion, tachypnea, and decreased breath sounds.

Pneumonia

◆ Dyspnea occurs suddenly with fever, shaking chills, pleuritic chest pain, and a productive cough.
◆ Other signs and symptoms include fatigue, headache, myalgia, anorexia, abdominal pain, crackles, rhonchi, tachycardia, tachypnea, cyanosis, decreased breath sounds, and diaphoresis.

Pneumothorax

◆ Acute dyspnea occurs that's unrelated to the severity of pain.
◆ Sudden, stabbing chest pain radiates to the arms, face, back, or abdomen.
◆ Other signs and symptoms include anxiety, restlessness, dry cough, cyanosis, tachypnea, decreased or absent breath sounds on the affected side, splinting, and accessory muscle use.

Pulmonary edema

◆ Acute dyspnea is preceded by signs of heart failure.
◆ Other signs and symptoms include tachycardia, tachypnea, crackles, ventricular gallop, thready pulse, hypotension, diaphoresis, cyanosis, marked anxiety, and a cough that's dry or produces copious amounts of pink, frothy sputum.

Pulmonary embolism

◆ Acute dyspnea usually occurs with sudden pleuritic chest pain.
◆ Other signs and symptoms include tachycardia, tachypnea, productive cough with blood-tinged sputum, decreased breath sounds, diaphoresis, anxiety, and, with a massive embolism, signs of shock.

Shock

◆ Sudden dyspnea occurs, progressively worsening over time.
◆ Other signs and symptoms include severe hypotension, tachypnea, tachycardia, decreased peripheral pulses, decreased mental acuity, restlessness, anxiety, and cool, clammy skin.

Tuberculosis

◆ Dyspnea occurs with chest pain, crackles, and productive cough.
◆ Other signs and symptoms include night sweats, fever, anorexia, weight loss, palpitations on mild exertion, and dullness on percussion.

Nursing considerations

◆ Monitor the patient's vital signs and pulse oximetry.
◆ Position the patient comfortably, usually in a high Fowler or forward-leaning position.
◆ Give a bronchodilator, an antiarrhythmic, a diuretic, and an analgesic, as prescribed.
◆ Monitor the patient's respiratory status.

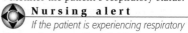 **Nursing alert**

If the patient is experiencing respiratory distress, give oxygen if needed. Ensure patent I.V. access and begin cardiac and oxygen saturation monitoring. A chest tube may need to be inserted for severe pneumothorax, continuous positive airway pressure, endotracheal intubation, and mechanical ventilation.

PATIENT TEACHING

◆ Teach the patient about the underlying condition, diagnostic tests, and treatment.
◆ Teach the patient about pursed-lip, diaphragmatic breathing and chest splinting.
◆ Instruct the patient to avoid chemical irritants, pollutants, and people with respiratory infections.
◆ Teach the patient with chronic dyspnea about oxygen use, if prescribed, and energy conservation.

Edema, generalized

Overview

Generalized edema, the excessive accumulation of interstitial fluid throughout the body, may be chronic or progressive.

Assessment

HISTORY

◆ Note the onset, location, and description of edema.
◆ Ask about shortness of breath or pain.
◆ Obtain a medical history, including incidence of previous burns and cardiac, renal, hepatic, endocrine, and GI disorders.
◆ Find out about recent weight gain and urine output changes.
◆ Ask the patient to describe his diet.
◆ Obtain a drug history.

PHYSICAL ASSESSMENT

◆ Compare the patient's arms and legs for symmetrical edema.
◆ Note ecchymoses and cyanosis.
◆ Assess the back, sacrum, and hips of a bedridden patient for dependent edema.
◆ Palpate peripheral pulses, noting any coolness in hands and feet.
◆ Perform complete cardiac and respiratory assessments.

> **Nursing alert**
> *If the patient has severe edema, take his vital signs and determine the degree of pitting. Check for jugular vein distention and cyanotic lips. Auscultate the lungs and heart. Look for signs of heart failure or pulmonary congestion. Place the patient in Fowler's position and prepare to administer oxygen and an I.V. diuretic as prescribed. Have emergency resuscitation equipment readily available.*

Causes

MEDICAL
Angioneurotic edema or angioedema
◆ Recurrent attacks of acute, painless, nonpitting edema involving the skin and mucous membranes may result from food or drug allergy, heredity, or emotional stress.

◆ Abdominal pain, nausea, vomiting, and diarrhea accompany visceral edema.
◆ Dyspnea and stridor accompany life-threatening laryngeal edema.

Burns
◆ Severe generalized edema may occur within 2 days of a major burn.
◆ Depending on the degree of edema, signs and symptoms of reduced or absent circulation and airway obstruction may occur.

Cirrhosis
◆ Edema is a late sign.
◆ Other signs and symptoms include abdominal pain, anorexia, nausea, vomiting, hepatomegaly, ascites, jaundice, pruritus, bleeding tendencies, musty breath, lethargy, mental changes, and asterixis.

Heart failure
◆ Severe, generalized pitting edema may follow leg edema.
◆ Edema may improve with exercise or elevation of limbs and is worst at the end of day.
◆ Other classic, late signs and symptoms include hemoptysis, cyanosis, clubbing, crackles, marked hepatosplenomegaly, and a ventricular gallop.

Myxedema
◆ Generalized nonpitting edema occurs with dry, flaky, inelastic, waxy, pale skin; puffy face; and upper eyelid droop.
◆ Other signs and symptoms include masklike facies, hair loss or coarsening, hoarseness, weight gain, fatigue, cold intolerance, bradycardia, constipation, abdominal distention, menorrhagia, impotence, and infertility.

Nephrotic syndrome
◆ Edema is initially localized around the eyes, and then becomes generalized and pitting.

♦ Other signs and symptoms include ascites, anorexia, fatigue, malaise, depression, and pallor.

Pericardial effusion
♦ Generalized pitting edema may be most prominent in arms and legs.
♦ Other signs and symptoms include chest pain, dyspnea, orthopnea, nonproductive cough, pericardial friction rub, jugular vein distention, dysphagia, and fever.

Renal failure
♦ Generalized pitting edema occurs as a late sign.
♦ With chronic renal failure, edema is less likely to become generalized; its severity depends on the degree of fluid overload.
♦ Other signs and symptoms include oliguria, hypertension, dyspnea, and crackles.

Septic shock
♦ A late sign, generalized edema typically develops rapidly. Edema becomes pitting and moderately severe.
♦ Other signs and symptoms include cool skin, hypotension, oliguria, anxiety, and signs of respiratory failure.

OTHER
Drugs
♦ Drugs that cause sodium retention, such as antihypertensives, corticosteroids, androgenic and anabolic steroids, estrogens, and nonsteroidal anti-inflammatory drugs, may aggravate or cause generalized edema.
♦ In patients with cardiac or renal disease, I.V. saline solution infusions and enteral feedings may cause sodium and fluid overload, resulting in generalized edema.

Treatments
♦ Enteral feedings and I.V. saline solution infusions may cause sodium and fluid overload.

Nursing considerations

♦ Position the patient with his limbs above heart level to promote drainage.
♦ Reposition the patient frequently.
♦ If the dyspnea develops, lower the patient's limbs, elevate the head of the bed, and administer oxygen.
♦ Prevent skin breakdown by placing a pressure mattress on the patient's bed.
♦ Restrict fluids and sodium, and administer a diuretic or I.V. albumin as prescribed.
♦ Monitor intake and output and daily weight.
♦ Monitor electrolyte levels.

PATIENT TEACHING
♦ Explain the cause of edema and the treatment plan.
♦ Describe signs and symptoms of edema that the patient should report.
♦ Discuss foods and fluids the patient should avoid.

Epistaxis

Overview

Epistaxis (nosebleed) occurs in the anteriorinferior nasal septum or at the point where the inferior turbinates meet the nasopharynx. Bleeding may be mild to severe or even life-threatening and usually involves only one nostril.

Assessment

HISTORY

◆ Ask about recent trauma or surgery.
◆ Obtain a description of past epistaxis.
◆ Take a medical history, including incidence of hypertension, bleeding or liver disorders, and other recent illnesses.
◆ Find out what drugs the patient is taking, especially anti-inflammatory drugs, anticoagulants, or recreational drugs.

PHYSICAL ASSESSMENT

◆ Inspect for other signs of bleeding.
◆ Look for trauma injuries.
◆ If the patient has severe epistaxis, quickly take vital signs and look for signs of hypovolemic shock.

Causes

MEDICAL
Aplastic anemia

◆ Epistaxis is accompanied by ecchymoses, retinal hemorrhages, menorrhagia, petechiae, and signs of GI bleeding.
◆ Other signs and symptoms may include fatigue, dyspnea, headache, tachycardia, and pallor.

Coagulation disorders

◆ Epistaxis, ecchymoses, petechiae, menorrhagia, GI bleeding, and bleeding from the gums, mouth, and I.V. puncture sites may occur.

Hypertension

◆ Severe hypertension can produce extreme epistaxis with accompanying dizziness, a throbbing headache, anxiety, peripheral edema, nocturia, nausea, vomiting, drowsiness, and mental impairment.

Leukemia

◆ With acute leukemia, sudden epistaxis is accompanied by high fever and other types of abnormal bleeding tendencies.
◆ With chronic leukemia, epistaxis is a late sign that may be accompanied by other bleeding tendencies, extreme fatigue, weight loss, hepatosplenomegaly, bone tenderness, macular or nodular skin lesions, pallor, weakness, dyspnea, tachycardia, palpitations, and headache.

Maxillofacial injury

◆ Severe epistaxis may occur with accompanying facial pain; swelling; open-bite malocclusion or inability to open the mouth; diplopia; conjunctival hemorrhage; lip edema; and buccal, mucosal, and soft palatal ecchymoses.

Nasal fracture

◆ One or both nostrils may bleed.
◆ Nasal swelling, periorbital ecchymoses and edema, pain, nasal deformity, and crepitation of the nasal bones may occur.

Polycythemia vera

◆ Spontaneous epistaxis is a common sign.
◆ Other signs and symptoms include bleeding gums; ecchymoses; ruddy cyanosis of the face, nose, ears, and lips; headache; dizziness; vision disturbances; hypertension; chest pain; splenomegaly; epigastric pain; pruritus; dyspnea; and congestion of the conjunctiva, retina, and oral mucous membranes.

Sarcoidosis

◆ Oozing epistaxis may occur along with extensive nasal mucosal lesions, a nonproductive cough, substernal pain, malaise, and weight loss.
◆ Other signs and symptoms include tachycardia; arrhythmias; parotid enlargement; cervical lymphadenopathy; skin le-

sions; hepatosplenomegaly; and arthritis in the ankles, knees, and wrists.

Sinusitis, acute
◆ Bloody or blood-tinged nasal discharge may become purulent and copious 48 hours after onset.
◆ Other signs and symptoms include nasal congestion, pain, and tenderness; malaise; headache; low-grade fever; and red, edematous nasal mucosa.

Skull fracture
◆ Epistaxis is direct or indirect, depending on the type of fracture.
◆ With a severe skull fracture, signs and symptoms include severe headache, decreased level of consciousness, hemiparesis, dizziness, seizures, projectile vomiting, and decreased pulse and respirations.
◆ With a basilar fracture, signs and symptoms include raccoon eyes; Battle's sign; bleeding from the pharynx, ears, and conjunctiva; and leakage of cerebrospinal fluid or brain tissue from the nose or ears.
◆ With a sphenoid fracture, blindness may also occur.
◆ With a temporal fracture, deafness in one ear or facial paralysis may also occur.

Systemic lupus erythematosus
◆ Oozing epistaxis occurs.
◆ Other signs and symptoms include butterfly rash, lymphadenopathy, joint pain and stiffness, anorexia, nausea, vomiting, myalgia, and weight loss.

OTHER
Chemical irritants
◆ Some chemicals, such as phosphorus, sulfuric acid, ammonia, printer's ink, and chromates, irritate the nasal mucosa, producing epistaxis.

Drugs
◆ Anticoagulants or anti-inflammatories can cause or worsen epistaxis.
◆ Frequent cocaine use may cause epistaxis.

Vigorous nose blowing
◆ Vigorous nose blowing may rupture superficial blood vessels and cause epistaxis.

Nursing considerations

◆ Unless you suspect a nasal fracture, control bleeding by pinching the nares closed, and then place gauze under the nose.
◆ Monitor for signs of hypovolemic shock.
◆ Have a hypovolemic patient lie down and turn his head to the side to prevent aspiration.
◆ If the patient isn't hypovolemic, have him sit upright and tilt his head forward, and check airway patency.
◆ If the patient is unstable, begin cardiac monitoring and give oxygen.
◆ If external pressure doesn't control the bleeding, insert cotton saturated with a vasoconstrictor and local anesthetic into the nose as prescribed.
◆ For severe epistaxis, insert a large-gauge I.V. catheter for fluid and blood replacement.
◆ If bleeding persists, insert anterior or posterior nasal packing.
◆ Administer humidified oxygen by face mask to a patient with posterior packing.

PATIENT TEACHING
◆ Explain the cause of epistaxis and the treatment plan.
◆ Teach the patient or caregiver pinching pressure techniques.
◆ Discuss ways to prevent epistaxis.

S & S

Fatigue

Overview

Fatigue, the feeling of excessive tiredness, lack of energy, or exhaustion with a strong desire to rest or sleep, reflects hypermetabolic and hypometabolic states in which nutrients needed for cellular energy and growth are lacking.

Assessment

HISTORY
◆ Review the pattern, onset, and duration of fatigue.
◆ Ask if the patient has other symptoms.
◆ Ask about viral or bacterial illness or stress.
◆ Ask about nutrition and appetite or weight changes.
◆ Review the medical and psychiatric history for disorders that produce fatigue.
◆ Ask about a family history of chronic disorders.
◆ Obtain a drug and alcohol history.
◆ Ask about carbon monoxide exposure.

PHYSICAL ASSESSMENT
◆ Observe the patient's general appearance for overt signs of depression or organic illness.
◆ Evaluate mental status.
◆ Take the patient's vital signs and obtain pulse oximetry reading.
◆ Perform a complete physical examination.

Causes

MEDICAL
Acquired immunodeficiency syndrome
◆ Fatigue, fever, night sweats, weight loss, diarrhea, and a cough may develop.
◆ Signs of opportunistic infection and malnutrition may be apparent.

Anemia
◆ Fatigue after mild activity is a common initial symptom.

◆ Other signs and symptoms include listlessness, irritability, inability to concentrate, pallor, tachycardia, and dyspnea.

Anxiety
◆ Chronic anxiety invariably produces fatigue characterized as nervous exhaustion.
◆ Other signs and symptoms include apprehension, indecisiveness, restlessness, insomnia, trembling, and increased muscle tension.

Cancer
◆ Unexplained fatigue is typically the earliest sign.
◆ Other signs and symptoms vary with the type of cancer but may include pain, nausea, vomiting, anorexia, weight loss, abnormal bleeding, and a palpable mass.

Chronic fatigue syndrome
◆ Fatigue is incapacitating.
◆ Other signs and symptoms include sore throat, myalgia, low-grade fever, painful lymph nodes, sleep disturbances, and cognitive dysfunction.

Chronic obstructive pulmonary disease
◆ Progressive fatigue and dyspnea are the earliest symptoms.
◆ Other signs and symptoms include a chronic and productive cough, weight loss, barrel chest, cyanosis, slight dependent edema, and poor exercise tolerance.

Depression
◆ Persistent fatigue unrelated to exertion accompanies chronic depression.
◆ Other signs and symptoms include insomnia, slowed speech, agitation or bradykinesia, irritability, loss of concentration, feelings of worthlessness, and persistent thoughts of death.

Diabetes mellitus
◆ Insidious or abrupt fatigue is the most common symptom of this disorder.

◆ Other signs and symptoms include weight loss, blurred vision, polyuria, polydipsia, and polyphagia.

Heart failure
◆ Persistent fatigue and lethargy are characteristic.
◆ Left-sided heart failure produces exertional and paroxysmal nocturnal dyspnea, orthopnea, and tachycardia.
◆ Right-sided heart failure produces jugular vein distention and, possibly, a slight but persistent nonproductive cough.

Hypothyroidism
◆ Fatigue occurs early, along with forgetfulness, cold intolerance, weight gain, metrorrhagia, and constipation.
◆ Other signs and symptoms include coarse hair and alopecia; anorexia; edema; dry, flaky skin; and thinning nails.

Myasthenia gravis
◆ Easy fatigability and muscle weakness, which worsen as the day progresses, are classic symptoms.
◆ Symptoms worsen with exertion and subside with rest.

Myocardial infarction
◆ Fatigue can be severe, and occurs more often in women.
◆ Other signs and symptoms include chest, neck, arm, or back pain, dyspnea, anxiety, pallor, cold sweat, increased or decreased blood pressure, and abnormal heart sounds.

Renal failure
◆ Sudden fatigue occurs with drowsiness and lethargy.
◆ Chronic renal failure causes insidious fatigue and lethargy with marked changes in all body systems.
◆ Other signs and symptoms include oliguria, increased blood pressure, and weight gain.

Systemic lupus erythematosus
◆ Fatigue occurs with generalized aching, malaise, low-grade fever, headache, and irritability.
◆ Other signs and symptoms include joint pain and stiffness, butterfly rash, photosensitivity, Raynaud's phenomenon, patchy alopecia, and mucous membrane ulcers.

Thyrotoxicosis
◆ Fatigue may occur with enlarged thyroid gland, tachycardia, palpitations, tremors, weight loss despite increased appetite, diarrhea, dyspnea, nervousness, diaphoresis, heat intolerance, amenorrhea, and exophthalmos.

OTHER
Drugs
◆ Antihypertensives and sedatives may cause fatigue.
◆ In the patient taking digoxin (Lanoxin), fatigue may signal toxicity.

Nursing considerations
◆ Help the patient determine and pace activities.
◆ Encourage rest periods.
◆ Take measures to reduce pain and nausea.
◆ If fatigue results from a psychogenic cause, refer the patient for psychological counseling.

PATIENT TEACHING
◆ Teach the patient about the underlying disease and treatment plan.
◆ Educate the patient about lifestyle modifications, including diet and exercise.
◆ Stress the importance of pacing his activities and planning rest periods.
◆ Discuss stress management techniques.

S & S

Flank pain

Overview

Flank pain in one or both flanks indicates renal and upper urinary tract disease or trauma. It may range from a dull ache to a severe stabbing or throbbing pain, and may be constant or intermittent. Flank pain may be unaffected by position changes and typically responds to analgesics or treatment of underlying disorder.

Assessment

HISTORY
◆ Ask about the onset, location, intensity, pattern, and duration of pain.
◆ Ask what alleviates or aggravates the pain.
◆ Explore precipitating events to pain.
◆ Ask about the patient's normal fluid intake and urine output and recent changes.
◆ Obtain a medical history, including incidence of urinary tract infection (UTI), obstruction, renal disease, or recent streptococcal infection.

PHYSICAL ASSESSMENT
◆ Obtain the patient's vital signs.
◆ Palpate the flank area and percuss the costovertebral angle (CVA).
◆ Inspect, auscultate, percuss and palpate the abdomen.
◆ Obtain a urine sample.

 Nursing alert
If the patient has suffered trauma, quickly look for a visible or palpable flank mass, other injuries, CVA tenderness, hematuria, Turner's sign, and signs of shock. If one or more signs of shock are present, insert an I.V. catheter to allow fluid or drug infusion. Insert an indwelling urinary catheter to monitor urine output and evaluate hematuria.

Causes

MEDICAL
Bladder cancer
◆ Dull, constant flank pain radiates to the legs, back, and perineum.

◆ Initial signs include gross, painless, intermittent hematuria, usually with clots.
◆ Other signs and symptoms include urinary frequency and urgency, nocturia, dysuria, or pyuria; bladder distention; and pain in the bladder, rectum, pelvis, back, or legs.

Cystitis, bacterial
◆ Flank pain occurs along with perineal, lower back, and suprapubic pain.
◆ Other signs and symptoms include dysuria, nocturia, hematuria, urinary frequency and urgency, tenesmus, fatigue, and low-grade fever.

Glomerulonephritis, acute
◆ Constant and moderately intense flank pain occurs.
◆ Classic signs and symptoms include moderate facial and generalized edema, hematuria, oliguria or anuria, and fatigue.

Obstructive uropathy
◆ With acute obstruction, flank pain may be excruciating.
◆ With gradual obstruction, pain is typically a dull ache.
◆ A palpable abdominal mass, CVA tenderness, and bladder distention vary with the site and cause of the obstruction.
◆ Other signs and symptoms include nausea, vomiting, abdominal distention, anuria alternating with periods of oliguria and polyuria, and hypoactive bowel sounds.

Pancreatitis, acute
◆ Flank pain may develop as severe epigastric or left-upper-quadrant pain that radiates to the back.
◆ A severe attack causes extreme pain, nausea, persistent vomiting, abdominal tenderness and rigidity, hypoactive bowel sounds, restlessness, low-grade fever, tachycardia, hypotension, and positive Turner's and Cullen's signs.

Perirenal abscess

◆ Intense pain in one flank and CVA tenderness accompany dysuria, persistent high fever, and chills.

Polycystic kidney disease

◆ Dull, aching, pain in both flanks is an early symptom; pain may become severe and colicky if cysts rupture and clots migrate or cause obstruction.
◆ Early signs and symptoms include polyuria, increased blood pressure, and signs of UTI.

Pyelonephritis, acute

◆ Intense, constant flank pain develops.
◆ Typical signs and symptoms include dysuria, nocturia, hematuria, urgency, frequency, and tenesmus.
◆ Other signs and symptoms include persistent high fever, chills, anorexia, weakness, fatigue, and CVA tenderness.

Renal calculi

◆ Flank pain may be dull or severe. Other signs and symptoms include intense nausea, vomiting, CVA tenderness, hematuria, hypoactive bowel sounds, and UTI signs and symptoms.

Renal cancer

◆ Classic signs and symptoms include pain in one flank that's dull and vague, gross hematuria, and a palpable flank mass.
◆ Signs of advanced disease include weight loss, leg edema, nausea, and vomiting. Other signs and symptoms include fever, increased blood pressure, and urine retention.

Renal infarction

◆ Constant, severe pain in one flank and tenderness typically accompany persistent, severe upper abdominal pain.
◆ Other signs and symptoms include CVA tenderness, anorexia, nausea, vomiting, fever, hypoactive bowel sounds, hematuria, and oliguria or anuria.

Renal trauma

◆ Variable flank pain is common.
◆ A visible or palpable flank mass and CVA or abdominal pain, which may be severe and radiate to the groin, may also develop.
◆ Other signs and symptoms include hematuria, oliguria, abdominal distention, Turner's sign, hypoactive bowel sounds, nausea, vomiting and, with severe injury, signs of shock.

Renal vein thrombosis

◆ Severe pain in one flank and lower back pain with CVA and epigastric tenderness are typical.
◆ Other signs and symptoms include fever, hematuria, and leg edema.

Nursing considerations

◆ Give drugs for pain as prescribed.
◆ Monitor the patient's vital signs and intake and output.

PATIENT TEACHING

◆ Explain the patient's underlying condition, treatment plan, and signs and symptoms to report.
◆ Explain the importance of increased fluid intake, unless contraindicated.
◆ Stress the importance of taking drugs as prescribed.
◆ Stress the importance of keeping follow-up appointments.

S & S

Gag reflex abnormalities

Overview

Normal gag reflex, the protective mechanism that prevents aspiration of food, fluid, and vomitus, is elicited by touching the posterior wall of the oropharynx with a tongue blade or by suctioning the throat. It's characterized by prompt elevation of the palate, constriction of the pharyngeal musculature, and a sensation of retching. An abnormal gag reflex (either decreased or absent) interferes with the ability to swallow and, more importantly, increases susceptibility to life-threatening aspiration.

Nursing alert

If you detect an abnormal gag reflex, immediately stop the patient's oral intake to prevent aspiration. Quickly evaluate his level of consciousness (LOC). If it's decreased, place him in a side-lying position to prevent aspiration; if not, place him in Fowler's position. Have suction equipment readily available.

Assessment

HISTORY

◆ Ask the patient, or a family member if the patient can't communicate, about the onset and duration of swallowing difficulties and if it's more difficult to swallow liquids than solids.

◆ If the patient also has trouble chewing, suspect more widespread neurologic involvement because chewing involves different cranial nerves.

◆ Explore the patient's medical history for vascular and degenerative disorders.

PHYSICAL ASSESSMENT

◆ Assess the patient's respiratory status for evidence of aspiration.

◆ Perform a neurologic examination.

Causes

MEDICAL
Basilar artery occlusion

◆ This disorder may suddenly diminish or obliterate the gag reflex.

◆ Other signs and symptoms include sensory loss, dysarthria, facial weakness, extraocular muscle palsies, quadriplegia, and decreased LOC.

Brain stem glioma

◆ This lesion causes gradual loss of the gag reflex.

◆ Involvement of the corticospinal pathways causes spasticity and paresis of the arms and legs as well as gait disturbances.

◆ Other signs and symptoms reflect bilateral brain stem involvement and include diplopia and facial weakness.

Bulbar palsy

◆ Loss of the gag reflex reflects temporary or permanent paralysis of muscles supplied by cranial nerves IX and X.

◆ Other signs and symptoms include jaw and facial muscle weakness, dysphagia, loss of sensation at the base of the tongue, increased salivation, fasciculations and, possibly, difficulty articulating and breathing.

Wallenberg's syndrome

◆ Paresis of the palate and an impaired gag reflex usually develop within hours to days of stroke of the brain stem.

◆ Other signs and symptoms may include analgesia and thermanesthesia occurring ipsilaterally on the face and contralaterally on the body as well as vertigo, nystagmus, ipsilateral ataxia of the arm and leg, signs of Horner's syndrome (unilateral ptosis and miosis, hemifacial anhidrosis), and uncontrollable hiccups.

OTHER

Anesthesia

◆ General and local throat anesthesia can produce temporary loss of the gag reflex.

Nursing considerations

◆ Continually assess the patient's ability to swallow.

◆ If his gag reflex is absent, provide tube feedings as ordered; if it's merely diminished, try pureed foods.

◆ Stay with him while he eats and observe for choking.

◆ Remember to keep suction equipment handy in case of aspiration.

◆ Keep accurate intake and output records, and assess the patient's nutritional status daily.

◆ Refer the patient to a speech therapist to determine his aspiration risk, and develop an exercise program to strengthen specific muscles.

PATIENT TEACHING

◆ Teach the patient about the underlying diagnosis and treatment plan.

◆ Advise the patient to take small amounts and eat slowly while sitting or in high Fowler's position.

◆ Teach the patient about scheduled diagnostic studies, such as swallow studies, computed tomography scan, magnetic resonance imaging, EEG, lumbar puncture, and arteriography.

Gallop, atrial

Overview

An atrial gallop, also known as *presystolic gallop,* refers to a fourth heart sound (S_4) heard or palpated before the first heart sound (S_1). It's a low-pitched sound that originates from left atrial contraction and is best heard with the bell of the stethoscope pressed lightly against the cardiac apex.

 Age considerations

Atrial gallop may occur normally in older patients.

Assessment

HISTORY

◆ Obtain a medical history, including incidence of hypertension, angina, cardiomyopathy, or valvular stenosis.
◆ Ask about the frequency and severity of anginal attacks.

PHYSICAL ASSESSMENT

◆ Obtain the patient's vital signs.
◆ Perform a complete cardiopulmonary examination.

Causes

MEDICAL
Anemia

◆ An atrial gallop may accompany compensatory increased cardiac output.
◆ Other signs and symptoms may include fatigue, pallor, dyspnea, tachycardia, a bounding pulse, crackles, and a systolic bruit over the carotid arteries.

Angina

◆ An intermittent atrial gallop typically occurs during an attack.
◆ The gallop may be accompanied by paradoxical second heart sound (S_2) or a new murmur.

◆ Other signs and symptoms include chest tightness, pressure, aching, or burning that radiates to the neck, jaw, left shoulder, and arm; dyspnea; tachycardia; increased blood pressure; diaphoresis; dizziness; nausea; and vomiting.

Aortic insufficiency, acute

◆ Atrial gallop is accompanied by a soft, short diastolic murmur along the left sternal border.
◆ S_2 may be soft or absent and a soft, short midsystolic murmur may be heard over the second right intercostal space.
◆ Other signs and symptoms include tachycardia, dyspnea, jugular vein distention, crackles, cool extremities, and angina.

Aortic stenosis

◆ Atrial gallop occurs with severe valvular obstruction.
◆ Auscultation reveals a harsh, crescendo-decrescendo (louder-then-softer), systolic-ejection murmur.
◆ Angina and syncope are principal symptoms.

Atrioventricular block

◆ First-degree atrioventricular (AV) block may cause an atrial gallop accompanied by a faint S_1, but the patient remains asymptomatic.
◆ Second-degree AV block produces an atrial gallop.
◆ Third-degree AV block produces an atrial gallop that varies in intensity with S_1.
◆ Other signs and symptoms include hypotension, light-headedness, dizziness, angina, and syncope.

Cardiomyopathy

◆ Atrial gallop is accompanied by such signs and symptoms as dyspnea, orthopnea, crackles, fatigue, syncope, chest pain, palpitations, edema, jugular vein distention, third heart sound (S_3), and tachycardia-bradycardia syndrome.

Hypertension

◆ Atrial gallop is an early symptom.
◆ Other signs and symptoms include headache, weakness, epistaxis, tinnitus, dizziness, and fatigue.

Mitral insufficiency

◆ Atrial gallop occurs with an S_3.
◆ Other signs and symptoms include a harsh holosystolic murmur, fatigue, dyspnea, tachypnea, orthopnea, tachycardia, crackles, and jugular vein distention.

Myocardial infarction

◆ Atrial gallop signifies a myocardial infarction and may persist after the infarction heals.
◆ Crushing substernal chest pain may radiate to the back, neck, jaw, shoulder, and left arm.
◆ Other signs and symptoms include dyspnea, restlessness, anxiety, a feeling of impending doom, diaphoresis, fatigue, pallor, clammy skin, nausea, vomiting, and increased or decreased blood pressure.

Pulmonary embolism

◆ Right-sided atrial gallop is heard along the lower left sternal border with a loud pulmonic closure sound.
◆ Other signs and symptoms include tachycardia, tachypnea, fever, chest pain, diaphoresis, syncope, cyanosis, and a nonproductive or productive cough with blood-tinged sputum.

Thyrotoxicosis

◆ Atrial gallop occurs with an S_3.
◆ Other signs and symptoms include tachycardia, bounding pulse, widened pulse pressure, palpitations, weight loss despite increased appetite, enlarged thyroid gland, dyspnea, nervousness, heat intolerance, and fatigue.

Nursing considerations

◆ Monitor the patient's vital signs and cardiovascular status.
◆ Monitor for signs and symptoms of heart failure.
◆ Give drugs and oxygen as prescribed.

PATIENT TEACHING

◆ Discuss with the patient ways to reduce his cardiac risk.
◆ Teach the patient the correct way to measure his pulse rate.
◆ Emphasize conditions that require medical attention.
◆ Stress the importance of follow-up appointments.

S & S

Gallop, ventricular

Overview

A ventricular gallop refers to a third heart sound (S_3) auscultated after the second heart sound (S_2). It may be physiologic or pathologic. It's associated with rapid ventricular filling in early diastole. A venetricular gallop is best heard along the lower left sternal border or over the xiphoid region on inspiration (right-sided) or at the apex on expiration (left-sided).

Age considerations

A ventricular gallop may occur normally in children and adults up to age 40 and during the third trimester of pregnancy.

Assessment

HISTORY
◆ Ask about location, frequency, and duration of chest pain if present, and what aggravates and alleviates it.
◆ Ask about palpitations, dizziness, syncope, difficulty breathing, or cough.
◆ Obtain a medical history, including incidence of cardiac disorders.
◆ Obtain a drug history.

PHYSICAL ASSESSMENT
◆ Auscultate for murmurs or abnormalities in the first heart sound (S_1) and S_2.
◆ Listen for pulmonary crackles.
◆ Assess peripheral pulses.
◆ Palpate the liver.
◆ Assess for jugular vein distention and peripheral edema.

Causes

MEDICAL
Aortic insufficiency
◆ In acute cases, ventricular and atrial gallops may occur with a soft, short diastolic murmur. Other signs and symptoms include tachycardia, dyspnea, jugular vein distention, and crackles.

◆ In chronic cases, a ventricular gallop and a high-pitched, blowing, decrescendo diastolic murmur occur. Other signs and symptoms include tachycardia, palpitations, angina, fatigue, dyspnea, orthopnea, and crackles.

Cardiomyopathy
◆ Ventricular gallop is a common symptom.
◆ When associated with fluctuating pulse and altered S_1 and S_2, it signals advanced heart disease.
◆ Other signs and symptoms include fatigue, dyspnea, orthopnea, chest pain, palpitations, syncope, crackles, peripheral edema, jugular vein distention, and an atrial gallop.

Heart failure
◆ Ventricular gallop is a classic symptom.
◆ Other signs and symptoms of left-sided heart failure include sinus tachycardia, fatigue, exertional dyspnea, paroxysmal nocturnal dyspnea, orthopnea, and a dry cough.
◆ Other signs and symptoms of right-sided heart failure include jugular vein distention, tachypnea, chest tightness, palpitations, anorexia, nausea, dependent edema, weight gain, slowed mental response, hepatomegaly, and pallor.

Mitral insufficiency
◆ In acute cases, ventricular gallop may be accompanied by an early or holosystolic decrescendo murmur at the apex, an atrial gallop, and a widely split S_2.
◆ Other signs and symptoms of acute valvular disease include tachycardia, tachypnea, orthopnea, dyspnea, crackles, jugular vein distention, peripheral edema, hepatomegaly, and fatigue.
◆ In chronic cases, ventricular gallop is progressively severe and accompanied by fatigue, exertional dyspnea, and palpitations.

Thyrotoxicosis
◆ Ventricular and atrial gallops may occur.
◆ Other signs and symptoms include an enlarged thyroid gland, weight loss despite increased appetite, heat intolerance, diaphoresis, nervousness, tremors, tachycardia, palpitations, diarrhea, and dyspnea.

Nursing considerations

◆ Assess for tachycardia, dyspnea, crackles, and jugular vein distention.
◆ To prevent pulmonary edema, give oxygen, diuretics, and other drugs, such as digoxin (Lanoxin) and angiotensin-converting enzyme inhibitors as prescribed.

PATIENT TEACHING
◆ Teach the patient about the underlying condition and treatment plan.
◆ Explain dietary and fluid restrictions the patient needs to follow.
◆ Stress the importance of scheduled rest periods.
◆ Explain signs and symptoms of fluid overload that the patient should report.
◆ Teach the patient how to measure and monitor his daily weight.

Headache

Overview

Headache, the most common neurologic symptom, is pain in an area of the head. A headache may be vascular, caused by a muscle contraction, or a combination of both. Benign in 90% of cases, it may be localized or generalized, producing mild to severe pain.

Assessment

HISTORY

◆ Ask about the characteristics and location of the headache.
◆ Find out about precipitating or alleviating factors.
◆ Obtain a drug and alcohol history.
◆ Find out about recent head trauma, nausea, vomiting, photophobia, or vision changes.
◆ Ask about associated drowsiness, confusion, dizziness, or seizures.

PHYSICAL ASSESSMENT

◆ Evaluate level of consciousness (LOC).
◆ Check the patient's vital signs.
◆ Be alert for signs of increased intracranial pressure (ICP).
◆ Check pupil size and response to light.
◆ Note any neck stiffness.

Causes

MEDICAL
Brain abscess
◆ Headache is localized to the abscess site and intensifies over a few days and is aggravated by strain.
◆ Other signs and symptoms include nausea, vomiting, focal or generalized seizures, changes in LOC and, depending on the location of the abscess, aphasia, impaired visual acuity, hemiparesis, ataxia, tremors, and personality changes.

Brain tumor
◆ Headache is localized near the tumor site but becomes generalized as the tumor grows.
◆ Pain is usually intermittent, deep-seated, dull, and most intense in the morning; aggravating factors include coughing, stooping, Valsalva's maneuver, and changes in head position; and alleviating factors include sitting and rest.
◆ Other signs and symptoms include personality changes, altered LOC, motor and sensory dysfunction, and signs of increased ICP.

Encephalitis
◆ A severe, generalized headache is characteristic.
◆ Within 48 hours, the patient's LOC typically deteriorates.
◆ Other signs and symptoms include fever, nuchal rigidity, irritability, seizures, nausea, vomiting, photophobia, cranial nerve palsies, and focal neurologic deficits.

Glaucoma, acute angle-closure
◆ Excruciating headache as well as acute eye pain, blurred vision, halo vision, nausea, and vomiting may occur in this ophthalmic emergency.
◆ Other signs and symptoms include conjunctival injection, a cloudy cornea, and a moderately dilated, fixed pupil.

Hypertension
◆ A slightly throbbing occipital headache on awakening may occur; severity decreases during the day (if diastolic pressure remains greater than 120 mm Hg, the headache is constant).
◆ Other signs and symptoms include atrial gallop, restlessness, confusion, nausea, vomiting, blurred vision, seizures, and altered LOC.

Intracerebral hemorrhage
◆ A severe generalized headache may develop.
◆ Signs and symptoms vary with the size and location of the hemorrhage but may include altered LOC, hemiplegia, hemiparesis, abnormal pupil size and response, aphasia, seizures, irregular respirations, positive Babinski's reflex, and decorticate or decerebrate posture.

Meningitis
◆ Onset of a severe, constant, generalized headache is sudden and worsens with movement.
◆ Other signs and symptoms include altered LOC, seizures, fever, chills, nuchal rigidity, ocular palsies, facial weakness, hearing loss, positive Kernig's sign and Brudzinski's sign, hyperreflexia, opisthotonos, and signs of increased ICP.

Postconcussion syndrome
◆ A generalized or localized headache may develop 1 to 30 days after head trauma and last for 2 to 3 weeks. Pain may be aching, pounding, pressing, stabbing, or throbbing.
◆ Other signs and symptoms include giddiness or dizziness, blurred vision, fatigue, insomnia, inability to concentrate, noise and alcohol intolerance, fever, chills, malaise, chest pain, nausea, vomiting, and diarrhea.

Sinusitis, acute
◆ A dull periorbital headache is usually aggravated by bending over or touching the face and is relieved by sinus drainage.
◆ Other signs and symptoms may include fever, sinus tenderness, nasal turbinate edema, sore throat, malaise, cough, and nasal discharge.

Subdural hematoma
◆ Headache develops and LOC decreases.
◆ In acute cases, early signs and symptoms include drowsiness, confusion, and agitation that may progress to coma; late signs include signs of increased ICP and focal neurologic deficits.
◆ In chronic cases, pounding headache fluctuates in severity and is located over the hematoma.

Temporal arteritis
◆ A throbbing unilateral headache in the temporal or frontotemporal region may be accompanied by vision loss, hearing loss, confusion, and fever.
◆ The temporal arteries are tender, swollen, nodular and, possibly, erythematous.

OTHER
Diagnostic tests
◆ Lumbar puncture or myelogram may produce a throbbing frontal headache that worsens on standing.

Drugs
◆ Indomethacin (Indocin), vasodilators, and drugs with a vasodilating effect may produce headaches.
◆ Withdrawal from vasopressors may also result in headaches.

Nursing considerations

◆ Monitor the patient's vital signs and LOC.
◆ Watch for a change in the headache's severity or location.
◆ Administer an analgesic, darken the room, and minimize stimuli to ease the headache.

PATIENT TEACHING
◆ Discuss the underlying disorder, diagnostic testing, and treatment options.
◆ Explain the signs of reduced LOC and seizures that the patient or his caregivers should report.
◆ Explain ways to maintain a safe, quiet environment and reduce environmental stress.
◆ Discuss the use of analgesics.

Hearing loss

Overview

Hearing loss is classified as conductive (resulting from external or middle ear disorders), sensorineural (resulting from disorders of the inner ear or of the eighth cranial nerve), mixed (resulting from a combination of conductive and sensorineural factors), or functional (resulting from psychological factors). It may be temporary or permanent and partial or complete.

Assessment

HISTORY

◆ Ask for a description of the hearing loss and when it started.
◆ Obtain a medical history, including incidence of chronic ear infections, ear surgery, ear or head trauma, and recent upper respiratory tract infection.
◆ Obtain a drug history.
◆ Ask for a description of the occupational environment.
◆ Ask about other signs and symptoms, such as pain; discharge; ringing, buzzing, hissing, or other noises; and dizziness.

PHYSICAL ASSESSMENT

◆ Inspect the external ear for inflammation, boils, foreign bodies, and discharge.
◆ Apply pressure to the tragus and mastoid to elicit tenderness.
◆ During otoscopic examination, note color change, perforation, bulging, or retraction of tympanic membrane.
◆ Evaluate hearing acuity.
◆ Perform the Weber's and Rinne tests.

Causes

MEDICAL
Acoustic neuroma

◆ Unilateral, progressive, sensorineural hearing loss occurs; tinnitus, vertigo, and facial paralysis may also develop.

External ear canal tumor, malignant

◆ Progressive conductive hearing loss occurs with deep, boring ear pain; purulent discharge; and facial paralysis.

Furuncle

◆ Reversible conductive hearing loss may occur.
◆ Other signs and symptoms include a sense of fullness in the ear, pain on palpation of the tragus or auricle and, with boil rupture, pain relief and a purulent, necrotic discharge.

Head trauma

◆ Conductive or sensorineural hearing loss is sudden in onset.
◆ Headache and bleeding from the ear occur.

Hypothyroidism

◆ Reversible sensorineural hearing loss may occur.
◆ Other signs and symptoms include bradycardia, weight gain despite anorexia, mental dullness, cold intolerance, facial edema, brittle hair, and dry, pale, cool and doughy skin.

Ménière's disease

◆ Intermittent, unilateral sensorineural hearing loss that involves only low tones progresses to constant hearing loss that involves other tones.
◆ Other signs and symptoms include intermittent severe vertigo, nausea, vomiting, a sensation of fullness in the ear, a roaring or hollow-seashell tinnitus, diaphoresis, and nystagmus.

Otitis externa

◆ Conductive hearing loss occurs.
◆ Acute form produces pain, headache on the affected side, low-grade fever, lymphadenopathy, itching, and a foul-smelling sticky yellow discharge.
◆ Malignant form involves visible debris in the ear canal, pruritus, tinnitus, and severe ear pain.

Otitis media

◆ In the acute and chronic forms, hearing loss develops gradually.

◆ Other signs and symptoms of the acute form include upper respiratory tract infection with sore throat, cough, nasal discharge, and intermittent or constant ear pain.

◆ Other signs and symptoms of the chronic form include purulent ear drainage, earache, nausea, and vertigo.

◆ In the serous form, a stuffy feeling in the ear occurs with pain that worsens at night.

Otosclerosis

◆ Unilateral conductive hearing loss usually begins in the early 20s and may gradually progress to bilateral mixed loss.

◆ Tinnitus and the ability to hear better in a noisy environment may occur.

Skull fracture

◆ Sudden, unilateral, sensorineural hearing loss may occur if the auditory nerve is damaged. Other signs and symptoms include ringing tinnitus, blood behind the tympanic membrane, and scalp wounds.

Temporal arteritis

◆ Unilateral, sensorineural hearing loss may occur along with throbbing unilateral facial pain, pain behind the eye, temporal or frontotemporal headache and, occasionally, vision loss.

◆ Other signs and symptoms include malaise, weakness, myalgia, and a nodular, swollen artery.

Temporal bone fracture

◆ Sudden, unilateral, sensorineural hearing loss is accompanied by hissing tinnitus.

◆ Other signs and symptoms may include a perforated tympanic membrane, loss of consciousness, Battle's sign, and facial paralysis.

Tympanic membrane perforation

◆ Abrupt hearing loss occurs with ear pain, tinnitus, vertigo, and sensation of fullness in the ear.

OTHER

Drugs

◆ Chloroquine (Aralen), cisplatin (Platinol-AQ), vancomycin (Vancocin) , and aminoglycosides may cause irreversible hearing loss.

◆ Loop diuretics, quinine (Quinamm), quinidine (Cardioquin), and high doses of erythromycin (ERYC) or salicylates may cause reversible hearing loss.

Radiation therapy

◆ Radiation of the middle ear, thyroid, face, skull, or nasopharynx may cause eustachian tube dysfunction, resulting in hearing loss.

Surgery

◆ Myringotomy, myringoplasty, simple or radical mastoidectomy, or fenestrations may cause scarring that result in hearing loss.

Nursing considerations

◆ When talking to the patient, face him and speak slowly and clearly.

◆ Treat the underlying disorder appropriately, and assess if the patient's level of hearing loss changes.

◆ Provide an alternate method of communication as appropriate.

PATIENT TEACHING

◆ Teach the patient about underlying diagnosis and treatment options.

◆ Explain the importance of ear protection and avoidance of loud noise.

◆ Stress the importance of following instructions for taking prescribed antibiotics.

Hematemesis

Overview

Hematemesis is bright red or blood-streaked vomitus from fresh or recent bleeding and usually indicates GI bleeding above the jejunum. Hematemesis may be life-threatening if massive (500 to 1,000 ml of blood). Dark red, brown, or black vomitus indicates blood retained in the stomach or partially digested.

Assessment

HISTORY

◆ Ask about the onset, amount, color, and consistency of vomitus.
◆ Ask for a description of stools.
◆ Ask about associated nausea, flatulence, diarrhea, or weakness.
◆ Obtain a medical history, including incidence of ulcers or liver or coagulation disorders.
◆ Find out about alcohol use.
◆ Obtain a drug history, including aspirin and other nonsteroidal anti-inflammatory drugs.

PHYSICAL ASSESSMENT

◆ Check for orthostatic hypotension.
◆ Obtain other vital signs.
◆ Inspect the mucous membranes, nasopharynx, and skin for signs of bleeding.
◆ Palpate the abdomen for tenderness, pain, or masses.
◆ Note lymphadenopathy.

 Nursing alert

If the patient has massive hematemesis, check vital signs. If you detect signs of shock, place the patient in a supine position and elevate his feet. Start a large-bore I.V. line for emergency fluid replacement. Send a blood sample for typing and crossmatching, hemoglobin level, and hematocrit; administer oxygen. Emergency endoscopy may be necessary to locate and treat the source of bleeding. Prepare to insert a nasogastric (NG) tube for suction or iced lavage.

Causes

MEDICAL
Anthrax, GI

◆ Initial findings include loss of appetite, nausea, vomiting, and fever.
◆ Signs and symptoms may progress to hematemesis, abdominal pain, and severe bloody diarrhea.

Coagulation disorders

◆ GI bleeding and moderate to severe hematemesis may occur.
◆ Other signs and symptoms vary with the specific coagulation disorder and may include epistaxis and ecchymoses.

Esophageal cancer

◆ Hematemesis is a late sign and occurs with steady chest pain that radiates to the back.
◆ Other signs and symptoms include substernal fullness, severe dysphagia, nausea, vomiting with nocturnal regurgitation and aspiration, hemoptysis, fever, hiccups, sore throat, melena, and halitosis.

Esophageal rupture

◆ Severity of hematemesis depends on the cause of the rupture.
◆ Severe retrosternal, epigastric, neck, or scapular pain accompanied by chest and neck edema may occur.
◆ Other signs and symptoms include subcutaneous crepitation in the chest wall, supraclavicular fossa, and neck, and signs of respiratory distress.

Esophageal varices, ruptured

◆ Coffee-ground or massive, bright red vomitus may occur.
◆ Other signs and symptoms include signs of shock, abdominal distention, and melena or painless hematochezia, ranging from slight oozing to massive rectal hemorrhage.

Gastric cancer

◆ Painless, bright red or dark brown vomitus is a late sign.
◆ Other signs and symptoms include upper-abdominal discomfort, anorexia, mild nausea, and chronic dyspepsia unrelieved by antacids and exacerbated by food.

Gastritis, acute

◆ Hematemesis and melena are the most common signs.
◆ Other signs and symptoms include mild epigastric discomfort, nausea, fever, malaise, and, with massive blood loss, signs of shock.

GI leiomyoma

◆ Hematemesis occurs, possibly with dysphagia and weight loss.

Mallory-Weiss syndrome

◆ Hematemesis and melena may occur preceded by severe vomiting, retching, or straining.
◆ Signs of shock may accompany severe bleeding.

Peptic ulcer

◆ Hematemesis may occur.
◆ Other signs and symptoms include melena or hematochezia, chills, fever, and signs of shock.

OTHER

Esophageal injury by caustic substances

◆ Hematemesis occurs with epigastric and anterior or retrosternal chest pain that's intensified by swallowing.

Treatments

◆ Nose or throat surgery and traumatic NG or endotracheal intubation may cause hematemesis.

Nursing considerations

◆ Monitor vital signs; watch for signs of shock.
◆ Administer blood products and fluids as needed.
◆ Monitor hemoglobin and hematocrit levels.
◆ Check stools for occult blood.
◆ Keep accurate intake and output records.
◆ Place the patient on bed rest in a low or semi-Fowler position.
◆ Keep suctioning equipment nearby and use as needed.
◆ Provide frequent oral hygiene.
◆ Give a histamine-2 blocker and antacids as prescribed.
◆ Prepare the patient for endoscopic evaluation as needed.

PATIENT TEACHING

◆ Discuss the underlying condition and treatment options.
◆ Explain foods or fluids the patient should avoid as appropriate.
◆ Stress the importance of avoiding alcohol, if applicable.
◆ Teach the patient and family about all hospital procedures and testing.

S & S

Hematuria

Overview

Hematuria, the abnormal presence of blood in urine, is a cardinal sign of renal and urinary tract disorders. It results from rupture or perforation of vessels in the renal system or urinary tract or from impaired glomerular filtration, which allows red blood cells (RBCs) to seep into the urine. Blood cells may be microscopic (confirmed by occult blood) or macroscopic (immediately visible). Hematuria is classified as initial (occurring at the start of urination), terminal (occurring at the end of urination), or total (occurring throughout urination).

Assessment

HISTORY

◆ Ask about the onset, description, and severity of hematuria.
◆ Ask whether the patient has associated pain or burning.
◆ Obtain a medical history, including incidence of renal, urinary, prostatic, or coagulation disorders, and recent abdominal or flank trauma.
◆ Find out about recent strenuous exercise.
◆ Take a drug history, noting use of anticoagulants or aspirin.

PHYSICAL ASSESSMENT

◆ Percuss and palpate the abdomen and flanks.
◆ Percuss the costovertebral angle (CVA) to elicit tenderness.
◆ Check the urinary meatus for bleeding or other abnormalities.
◆ Obtain a urine specimen for testing.
◆ Perform a vaginal or digital rectal examination.

Causes

MEDICAL
Bladder cancer

◆ Gross hematuria occurs with pain in bladder, rectum, pelvis, flank, back, or leg.

◆ Other signs and symptoms include nocturia, dysuria, urinary frequency and urgency, vomiting, diarrhea, and insomnia.

Bladder trauma

◆ Hematuria occurs with lower abdominal pain.
◆ Other signs and symptoms include anuria despite a strong urge to void; swelling of the scrotum, buttocks, or perineum; and signs of shock.

Calculi

◆ Bladder calculi causes gross hematuria, pain that's referred to the lower back or penile or vulvar area, and bladder distention.
◆ Renal calculi causes microscopic or gross hematuria, colicky pain (cardinal sign) that travels from the CVA to the flank, suprapubic region, and external genitalia when a calculus is passed; nausea; vomiting; restlessness; fever; chills; and abdominal distention.

Coagulation disorders

◆ Macroscopic hematuria is the first sign of hemorrhage.
◆ Other signs and symptoms include epistaxis, purpura, and signs of GI bleeding.

Cystitis

◆ Bacterial cystitis usually produces macroscopic hematuria with urinary urgency and frequency, dysuria, perineal and lumbar pain, suprapubic discomfort, and nocturia.
◆ Chronic interstitial cystitis occasionally causes grossly bloody hematuria with urinary frequency, dysuria, nocturia, and tenesmus.
◆ Viral cystitis usually produces hematuria, urinary urgency and frequency, dysuria, nocturia, tenesmus, and fever.

Glomerulonephritis

◆ The acute form causes gross hematuria that tapers off to microscopic hematuria and RBC casts.

◆ Other acute signs and symptoms include oliguria or anuria, flank and abdominal pain, edema, and increased blood pressure.

◆ The chronic form causes hematuria that's accompanied by proteinuria, generalized edema, and increased blood pressure.

Prostatitis

◆ Macroscopic hematuria occurs at the end of urination.

◆ Urinary frequency and urgency and dysuria occur followed by visible bladder distention.

◆ Acute form causes fatigue, malaise, myalgia, arthralgia, fever, chills, nausea, vomiting, perineal and lower back pain, decreased libido, and a tender, swollen, firm prostate on palpation.

◆ Chronic form causes persistent urethral discharge, dull perineal pain, ejaculatory pain, and decreased libido.

Pyelonephritis, acute

◆ Microscopic or macroscopic hematuria progresses to grossly bloody hematuria.

◆ After the infection resolves, microscopic hematuria may persist for a few months.

◆ Other signs and symptoms include persistent high fever, flank pain, CVA tenderness, dysuria, urinary frequency and urgency, nocturia, and tenesmus.

Renal cancer

◆ Grossly bloody hematuria; dull, aching flank pain; and a smooth, firm, palpable flank mass are the classic triad of signs and symptoms.

◆ Colicky pain occurs accompanied by the passage of clots, CVA tenderness, fever, and increased blood pressure.

Renal infarction

◆ Gross hematuria occurs.

◆ Constant, severe flank and upper abdominal pain occurs with CVA tenderness, anorexia, nausea, and vomiting.

Renal trauma

◆ Microscopic or gross hematuria occurs.

◆ Other signs and symptoms include flank pain, a palpable flank mass, oliguria, hematoma or ecchymoses over the upper abdomen or flank, nausea, vomiting, hypoactive bowel sounds and, in severe trauma, signs of shock.

Sickle cell anemia

◆ Gross hematuria occurs.

◆ Other signs and symptoms include tachycardia, heart murmurs, polyarthralgia, dyspnea, chest pain, impaired growth and development, hepatomegaly, and jaundice.

Urethral trauma

◆ Initial hematuria occurs with blood at the urinary meatus, local pain, and penile or vulvar ecchymoses.

Drugs

◆ Drugs that may cause hematuria include anticoagulants, aspirin, analgesics, cyclophosphamide (Cytoxan), metyrosine (Demser), penicillin (Pen-Vee K), rifampin (Rifadin), and thiabendazole (Mintezol).

Nursing considerations

◆ Monitor intake and output, including the hematuria amount and pattern.

◆ If the patient has an indwelling urinary catheter in place, ensure its patency; irrigate if necessary.

◆ Irrigate the bladder as ordered.

PATIENT TEACHING

◆ Discuss the underlying condition, diagnostic testing, and treatment options.

◆ Encourage the patient to increase fluid intake.

◆ Tell the patient signs and symptoms to report to the practitioner.

Hemoptysis

Overview

Hemoptysis is the expectoration of blood or bloody sputum from the lungs or tracheobronchial tree. It usually results from chronic bronchitis, lung cancer, or bronchiectasis.

 Nursing alert
Massive hemoptysis can cause airway obstruction and asphyxiation.

Assessment

HISTORY

◆ Ask about the onset and extent of hemoptysis.
◆ Obtain a medical history of cardiac, pulmonary, or bleeding disorders; recent infection; and exposure to tuberculosis.
◆ Ask about the date and results of the last tuberculin tine test.
◆ Obtain a drug history, including use of anticoagulants and herbal supplements.
◆ Obtain a smoking history.

PHYSICAL ASSESSMENT

◆ Obtain vital signs.
◆ Examine the nose, mouth, and pharynx for sources of bleeding.
◆ Inspect the chest; look for abnormal movement during breathing and use of accessory muscles.
◆ Observe respiratory rate, depth, and rhythm.
◆ Examine the skin for lesions.
◆ Palpate the chest to assess the diaphragm level and check for tenderness, respiratory excursion, fremitus, and abnormal pulsations.
◆ Percuss the chest for flatness, dullness, resonance, hyperresonance, and tympany.
◆ Auscultate for breath sounds, heart murmurs, bruits, and pleural rubs.
◆ Obtain sputum sample, and examine it for quantity, amount of blood, and color, odor, and consistency.

Causes

MEDICAL
Bronchial adenoma
◆ Recurring hemoptysis occurs along with a chronic cough and local wheezing.
◆ Recurrent infection, dyspnea, and wheezing may also occur.

Bronchiectasis
◆ Hemoptysis appearance varies from blood-tinged sputum to frank blood, depending on extent of bronchial blood vessel erosion.
◆ Other signs and symptoms include chronic cough, coarse crackles, late clubbing, fever, weight loss, fatigue, weakness, malaise, dyspnea on exertion, and copious, foul-smelling, and purulent sputum.

Coagulation disorders
◆ Hemoptysis occurs with multisystem hemorrhaging and purpuric lesions.

Laryngeal cancer
◆ Hemoptysis occurs, but hoarseness is the usual early sign.
◆ Other signs and symptoms include dysphagia, dyspnea, stridor, cervical lymphadenopathy, and neck pain.

Lung cancer
◆ Recurring hemoptysis is an early sign. Other signs and symptoms include a productive cough, dyspnea, fever, anorexia, weight loss, wheezing, and chest pain (a late sign).

Pneumonia
◆ *Klebsiella* pneumonia produces dark brown or red tenacious sputum that the patient has difficulty expelling from his mouth.
◆ Pneumococcal pneumonia causes pinkish or rust-colored mucoid sputum; onset is marked by sudden shaking chills, a rap-

idly rising temperature, tachycardia, and tachypnea.

Pulmonary edema
◆ Frothy, blood-tinged pink sputum accompanies severe dyspnea, orthopnea, gasping, anxiety, cyanosis, diffuse crackles, a ventricular gallop, and cold, clammy skin.
◆ Other signs and symptoms include tachycardia, lethargy, arrhythmias, tachypnea, hypotension, and a thready pulse.

Pulmonary embolism with infarction
◆ Hemoptysis is a common sign.
◆ Other symptoms include dyspnea and anginal or pleuritic chest pain.

Pulmonary tuberculosis
◆ Hemoptysis is a common sign.
◆ Other signs and symptoms include chronic productive cough, fine crackles after coughing, dyspnea, dullness to percussion, increased tactile fremitus, night sweats, and pleuritic chest pain.

OTHER
Diagnostic tests
◆ Lung or airway injury from bronchoscopy, laryngoscopy, mediastinoscopy, or lung biopsy may cause bleeding and hemoptysis.

Treatments
◆ Traumatic or prolonged intubation may produce hemoptysis.
◆ Surgery to the lungs, throat, or upper airways may cause hemoptysis.

Nursing considerations

◆ To protect the nonbleeding lung, place the patient in the lateral decubitus position, with the suspected bleeding lung facing down.

◆ Monitor the patient's respiratory status, vital signs, and blood test results closely.
◆ Administer oxygen as needed. Monitor pulse oximetry.
◆ If the patient is receiving anticoagulants, determine any changes that need to be made in diet or medications because these factors may affect clotting.

If the patient coughs up a copious amount of blood
◆ Endotracheal intubation may be required.
◆ Suction frequently to remove blood.
◆ Lavage may be necessary to loosen tenacious secretions or clots.
◆ Insert an I.V. line for fluid replacement, drug administration, and blood transfusion, if needed.
◆ Bronchoscopy should be performed to identify the bleeding site.
◆ Monitor vital signs to detect shock.

PATIENT TEACHING
◆ Teach the patient about the cause of hemoptysis and the treatment plan.
◆ Teach the patient and family about all hospital procedures and tests.
◆ Explain the importance of reporting recurrent episodes.
◆ Give the patient instructions for providing sputum samples.

Hepatomegaly

Overview

Hepatomegaly refers to enlargement of the liver and indicates potentially reversible primary or secondary liver disease. It may be confirmed by palpation, percussion, or radiologic tests.

Assessment

HISTORY
◆ Ask about alcohol use.
◆ Determine exposure to hepatitis.
◆ Obtain a drug history.
◆ Ask about the location and description of any associated abdominal pain.

PHYSICAL ASSESSMENT
◆ Inspect the skin and sclerae for jaundice, dilated veins, scars from previous surgery, and spider angiomas.
◆ Inspect the contour of the abdomen and measure abdominal girth.
◆ Percuss the liver.
◆ During deep inspiration, palpate the liver's edge.
◆ Take vital signs.
◆ Assess nutritional status.
◆ Evaluate level of consciousness.
◆ Watch for personality changes, irritability, agitation, memory loss, inability to concentrate, poor mentation, and in a severely ill patient, coma.

Causes

MEDICAL
Cirrhosis
◆ In the late stage of this disease, the liver becomes enlarged, nodular, and hard.
◆ Other late signs and symptoms affect all body systems and include jaundice, ascites, hypoxia, encephalopathy, bleeding disorders, and portal hypertension.

Diabetes mellitus
◆ Hepatomegaly, and right-upper-quadrant tenderness along with polydipsia, polyphagia, and polyuria may occur in overweight patients with poorly controlled diabetes.

Heart failure
◆ Hepatomegaly occurs along with jugular vein distention, cyanosis, nocturia, dependent edema of the legs and sacrum, steady weight gain, confusion and, possibly, nausea, vomiting, abdominal discomfort, and anorexia.
◆ Massive right-sided failure may cause anasarca, oliguria, severe weakness, and anxiety.
◆ If left-sided failure precedes right-sided failure, signs and symptoms include dyspnea, orthopnea, paroxysmal nocturnal dyspnea, tachypnea, arrhythmias, tachycardia, and fatigue.

Hepatitis
◆ Hepatomegaly occurs in the icteric phase and continues during the recovery phase.
◆ Early signs and symptoms include nausea, vomiting, fatigue, malaise, photophobia, sore throat, cough, and headache.
◆ Other signs and symptoms of the icteric phase include liver tenderness, slight weight loss, dark urine, clay-colored stools, jaundice, pruritus, right-upper-quadrant pain, and splenomegaly.

Leukemia and lymphomas
◆ Moderate to massive hepatomegaly, splenomegaly, and abdominal discomfort are common.
◆ Other signs and symptoms include malaise, low-grade fever, fatigue, weakness, tachycardia, weight loss, bleeding disorders, and anorexia.

Liver cancer
◆ Primary liver tumors cause irregular, nodular, firm hepatomegaly, with pain or tenderness in the right upper quadrant and a friction rub or bruit over the liver.
◆ Metastatic liver tumors cause hepatomegaly, but accompanying signs and symptoms reflect the primary cancer.
◆ Other signs and symptoms include ascites, jaundice, and a palpable right-upper-quadrant mass.

Mononucleosis, infectious
◆ Hepatomegaly may occur.
◆ Prodromal symptoms include headache, malaise, and extreme fatigue.
◆ After 3 to 5 days, signs and symptoms include sore throat, cervical lymphadenopathy, temperature fluctuations, stomatitis, palatal petechiae, periorbital edema, splenomegaly, exudative tonsillitis, pharyngitis, and a maculopapular rash.

Obesity
◆ Hepatomegaly may occur along with respiratory difficulties, cardiovascular disease, diabetes, renal disease, gallbladder disease, and psychological difficulties.

Pancreatic cancer
◆ Hepatomegaly accompanies anorexia, weight loss, abdominal or back pain, and jaundice.
◆ Other signs and symptoms include nausea, vomiting, fever, fatigue, weakness, pruritus, and skin lesions.

Nursing considerations
◆ Provide bed rest, relief from stress, and adequate nutrition.
◆ Monitor and restrict dietary protein as needed.
◆ Give hepatotoxic drugs or drugs metabolized by the liver in very small doses, if at all.
◆ Treat the underlying condition as indicated.

PATIENT TEACHING
◆ Explain the treatment plan for the underlying disorder and diagnostic tests.
◆ Stress avoiding alcohol and people with infections.
◆ Emphasize the importance of personal hygiene.
◆ Discuss the importance of pacing activities and rest periods.

Jaundice

Overview

Jaundice, also known as *icterus*, is a yellow discoloration of skin, mucous membranes, or sclerae of the eyes caused by excessive bilirubin levels in the blood. The discoloration is easier to detect in natural light. In people with dark skin, jaundice is usually detected by the sclerae.

Assessment

HISTORY
◆ Ask about the onset of jaundice.
◆ Ask about associated pruritus, clay-colored stools, dark urine, fatigue, fever, chills, GI signs or symptoms, and cardiopulmonary symptoms.
◆ Obtain a medical history, including incidence of cancer; liver, pancreatic or gallbladder disease; hepatitis; or gallstones.
◆ Ask about drug and alcohol use.
◆ Find out about recent weight loss.

PHYSICAL ASSESSMENT
◆ If possible, perform the physical examination in a room with natural light.
◆ Rule out hypercarotenemia, which is more prominent on the palms and soles and doesn't affect the sclera.
◆ Inspect the skin for texture, dryness, hyperpigmentation, spider angiomas, petechiae, and xanthomas.
◆ Note clubbed fingers and gynecomastia.
◆ Palpate the abdomen for tenderness, pain, and swelling.
◆ Palpate and percuss the liver and spleen for enlargement.
◆ Test for ascites.
◆ Auscultate for arrhythmias, murmurs, or gallops.
◆ Palpate lymph nodes for swelling.
◆ Obtain baseline data on the patient's mental status.

Causes

MEDICAL
Carcinoma
◆ Cancer of the hepatopancreatic ampulla produces fluctuating jaundice, occult bleeding, mild abdominal pain, recurrent fever, weight loss, pruritus, back pain, and chills.
◆ Hepatic cancer produces jaundice, right-upper-quadrant discomfort and tenderness, nausea, weight loss, slight fever, ascites, edema, and an irregular, nodular, firm, enlarged liver.
◆ With pancreatic cancer, progressive jaundice may be the only sign. Other signs and symptoms include weight loss, back or abdominal pain, anorexia, nausea, vomiting, fever, steatorrhea, fatigue, weakness, diarrhea, pruritus, and skin lesions.

Cholangitis
◆ Jaundice along with right-upper-quadrant pain and high fever with chills indicates Charcot's triad, a hallmark sign.
◆ Other signs and symptoms include pruritus and clay-colored stools.

Cholecystitis
◆ Nonobstructive jaundice occurs.
◆ Biliary colic typically peaks abruptly, persists for 2 to 4 hours, then localizes to the right upper quadrant and becomes constant.

Cholelithiasis
◆ Jaundice and biliary colic are common.
◆ Pain is severe and steady in the right upper quadrant or epigastrium, radiates to the right scapula or shoulder, and intensifies over several hours.

Cirrhosis
◆ With Laënnec's cirrhosis, mild to moderate jaundice occurs with pruritus; common early signs and symptoms include ascites, weakness, leg edema, nausea, vomiting, diarrhea or constipation, anorexia, mas-

sive hematemesis, weight loss, and right-upper-quadrant pain.

◆ With primary biliary cirrhosis, fluctuating jaundice may appear years after the onset of other signs and symptoms, such as pruritus that worsens at bedtime (commonly the first sign), weakness, fatigue, weight loss, and vague abdominal pain.

Heart failure
◆ Jaundice occurs with severe right-sided heart failure.

◆ Other signs and symptoms include jugular vein distention, cyanosis, dependent edema, weight gain, weakness, confusion, hepatomegaly, nausea, vomiting, abdominal discomfort, anorexia, and ascites (a late sign).

Hemolytic anemia, acquired
◆ Prominent jaundice appears with dyspnea, fatigue, pallor, tachycardia, and palpitations.

◆ With rapid hemolysis, chills, fever, irritability, headache, abdominal pain, and signs of shock may appear.

Hepatitis
◆ Jaundice occurs late and is preceded by dark urine and clay-colored stools.

◆ During the icteric phase, weight loss, anorexia, right-upper-quadrant pain and tenderness, and an enlarged liver occur.

◆ Other signs and symptoms include nausea, vomiting, malaise, arthralgias, myalgias, pharyngitis, cough, diarrhea or constipation, and low-grade fever.

Pancreatitis, acute
◆ Jaundice may occur.

◆ Severe epigastric pain may radiate to the back and is relieved by lying with the knees flexed on the chest or sitting up and leaning forward.

◆ Other signs and symptoms include nausea, persistent vomiting, Turner's or Cullen's sign, fever, and abdominal distention, rigidity, and tenderness.

Sickle cell anemia
◆ Jaundice occurs with impaired growth and development, increased susceptibility to infection, thrombotic complications, leg ulcers, swollen and painful joints, fever, chills, bone aches, and chest pain.

OTHER
Drugs
◆ Jaundice may occur with drugs that cause hepatic injury, such as acetaminophen (Tylenol), isoniazid (Nydrazid), hormonal contraceptives, sulfonamides, mercaptopurine (Purinethol), erythromycin estolate (Ilosone), niacin (Niacor), troleandomycin (TAO), androgenic steroids, 3-hydroxy-3-methylglutaryl coenzyme A (HMG-CoA) reductase inhibitors, phenothiazines, ethanol, methyldopa (Aldoril), rifampin (Rifadin), phenytoin (Dilantin), phenylbutazone (Butazolodine), and I.V. tetracycline (Sumycin).

Nursing considerations

◆ To decrease pruritus, frequently bathe the patient, apply an antipruritic lotion such as calamine, and administer diphenhydramine (Benadryl) or hydroxyzine (Vistaril).

◆ Monitor the patient's neurologic status.

◆ Assess GI status and monitor the appearance of stools.

PATIENT TEACHING
◆ Discuss the underlying condition, diagnostic tests, and treatment options.

◆ Teach the patient appropriate dietary changes.

◆ Discuss ways to reduce pruritus.

Jaw pain

Overview

Jaw pain, which may develop gradually or abruptly and may signal a life-threatening disorder, may arise from the maxilla, mandible, or temporomandibular joint (TMJ). It's usually caused by disorders of the teeth, soft tissue, or glands of the mouth or throat or from local trauma or infection.

 Nursing alert

Sudden severe jaw pain, especially when associated with chest pain, shortness of breath, or arm pain, may signal acute coronary syndrome or myocardial infarction. If these symptoms occur, obtain an electrocardiogram and blood samples for cardiac enzyme levels. Administer oxygen, morphine sulfate, and a vasodilator as indicated.

Assessment

HISTORY

- Determine the onset, character, intensity, and frequency of jaw pain.
- Ask whether the jaw pain radiates to other areas.
- Ask about recent trauma, surgery, or procedures.
- Ask about associated signs and symptoms, such as joint or chest pain, dyspnea, palpitations, fatigue, headache, malaise, anorexia, weight loss, intermittent claudication, diplopia, and hearing loss.
- Ask about aggravating or alleviating factors.

PHYSICAL ASSESSMENT

- Inspect the painful area for redness; palpate for edema or warmth.
- Look for facial asymmetry.
- Check the TMJs, noting crepitus and ability to open the mouth.
- Palpate the parotid area for pain and swelling.
- Inspect and palpate the oral cavity for lesions, elevation of the tongue, or masses.

Causes

MEDICAL
Angina pectoris
- Jaw and left arm pain may radiate from the substernal area.
- Other signs and symptoms include shortness of breath, nausea, vomiting, tachycardia, dizziness, diaphoresis, and palpitations.

Hypocalcemic tetany
- Painful muscle contractions of the jaw and mouth occur with paresthesia and carpopedal spasms.
- Other signs and symptoms include weakness, fatigue, palpitations, hyperreflexia, positive Chvostek's and Trousseau's signs, muscle twitching, choreiform movements, muscle cramps and, with severe hypocalcemia, laryngospasm with stridor, cyanosis, seizures, and arrhythmias.

Ludwig's angina
- Severe jaw pain in the mandibular area occurs with tongue elevation, sublingual edema, fever, and drooling caused by cellulitis.
- Progressive disease produces dysphagia, dysphonia, stridor, and dyspnea.

Myocardial infarction
- Crushing substernal pain may radiate to the lower jaw, left arm, neck, back, or shoulder blades.
- Other signs and symptoms include pallor, clammy skin, dyspnea, excessive diaphoresis, nausea, vomiting, anxiety, restlessness, a feeling of impending doom, low-grade fever, decreased or increased blood pressure, arrhythmias, an atrial gallop, new murmurs, and crackles.

Osteomyelitis
- Aching jaw pain may occur along with warmth, swelling, tenderness, erythema, and restricted jaw movement.

Tachycardia, sudden fever, nausea, and malaise may occur with acute osteomyelitis.

Sinusitis
◆ Maxillary sinusitis produces intense boring pain in the maxilla and cheek that may radiate to the eye along with a feeling of fullness, increased pain on percussion of the first and second molars and, in those with nasal obstruction, the loss of the sense of smell.
◆ Sphenoid sinusitis produces chronic pain at the mandibular ramus and vertex of the head and in the temporal area.

Suppurative parotitis
◆ Onset of jaw pain, high fever, and chills is abrupt.
◆ Other signs and symptoms include erythema and edema of the overlying skin; a tender, swollen gland; and pus at the second molar.

Temporal arteritis
◆ Sharp jaw pain occurs after chewing or talking.
◆ Other signs and symptoms include low-grade fever; generalized muscle pain; malaise; fatigue; anorexia; weight loss; throbbing, unilateral headache in the frontotemporal regions; swollen, nodular, tender and, possibly, pulseless temporal arteries; and erythema of the overlying skin.

TMJ disorders
◆ Jaw pain at the TMJ; spasm and pain of the masticating muscle; clicking, popping, or crepitus of the TMJ; and restricted jaw movement may occur.
◆ Other signs and symptoms include localized pain that may radiate to other head and neck areas, teeth clenching, bruxism, ear pain, headache, deviation of the jaw to the affected side upon opening the mouth, and jaw subluxation or dislocation, especially after yawning.

Trauma
◆ Jaw pain may occur with swelling and decreased jaw mobility.
◆ Other signs and symptoms include hypotension, tachycardia, lacerations, ecchymoses, hematomas, blurred vision, and rhinorrhea or otorrhea.

Trigeminal neuralgia
◆ Paroxysmal attacks of intense unilateral jaw pain stopping at the facial midline or rapid-fire shooting sensations in one division of the trigeminal nerve, usually the mandibular or maxillary division, occur.
◆ Pain is felt mainly over the lips and chin and in the teeth; mouth and nose areas may be hypersensitive; and corneal reflexes are diminished or absent, if the ophthalmic branch is involved.

OTHER
Drugs
◆ Some drugs, such as phenothiazines, affect the extrapyramidal tract, causing dyskinesias; others cause tetany of the jaw from hypocalcemia.

Nursing considerations

◆ Assess the patient's vital signs and level of consciousness. Initiate emergency supportive measures, if appropriate.
◆ If pain is severe, withhold food, liquids, and oral medications until a diagnosis is confirmed.
◆ Administer an analgesic.
◆ Apply an ice pack if the jaw is swollen.
◆ Discourage the patient from talking or moving the jaw.

PATIENT TEACHING
◆ Explain the disorder and the treatments needed.
◆ Teach the patient the proper way to insert mouth splints, if indicated.
◆ Discuss ways to reduce stress.
◆ Review possible triggers and ways to avoid them.

S & S

Jugular vein distention

Overview

Jugular vein distention (JVD), the abnormal fullness and height of pulse waves in internal or external jugular veins, reflects increased venous pressure in the right side of the heart and indicates increased central venous pressure. It's characterized by a pulse wave height greater than 1¼″ to 1½″ (3 to 4 cm) above the angle of Louis with the patient in a supine position and his head elevated 45 degrees.

Assessment

HISTORY

♦ Find out about recent weight gain or swelling.
♦ Ask about associated chest pain, shortness of breath, paroxysmal nocturnal dyspnea, anorexia, nausea, or vomiting.
♦ Obtain a medical history, including incidence of cancer or cardiac, pulmonary, hepatic, or renal disease, recent trauma or surgery.
♦ Obtain a drug history, noting use of diuretics.
♦ Ask about diet history, especially sodium intake.

PHYSICAL ASSESSMENT

♦ Check vital signs.

 Nursing alert

Suspect cardiac tamponade if a patient with jugular vein distention also has hypotension; a paradoxical pulse; pale, clammy skin; and sudden anxiety and dyspnea. Elevate the foot of the bed 20 to 30 degrees, give supplemental oxygen, and monitor cardiac status and rhythm, oxygen saturation, and mental status. Start an I.V. line for medication administration, and keep cardiopulmonary resuscitation equipment readily available. Assemble equipment for emergency pericardiocentesis.

♦ Inspect and palpate for edema.
♦ Weigh the patient and compare weight to his baseline.

♦ Auscultate lungs for crackles and heart for gallops, pericardial friction rub, and muffled heart sounds.
♦ Inspect for abdominal distention.
♦ Palpate and percuss for an enlarged liver.

Causes

MEDICAL
Cardiac tamponade
♦ JVD occurs along with anxiety, restlessness, cyanosis, chest pain, dyspnea, hypotension, and clammy skin.
♦ Other signs and symptoms include tachycardia, tachypnea, muffled heart sounds, a pericardial friction rub, weak or absent peripheral pulses that decrease during inspiration (pulsus paradoxus), and hepatomegaly.

Heart failure
♦ Right-sided heart failure commonly causes JVD, weakness, cyanosis, dependent edema, steady weight gain, confusion, and hepatomegaly. Other signs and symptoms of right-sided failure include nausea, vomiting, abdominal discomfort, anorexia, and ascites (a late sign).
♦ JVD is a late sign in left-sided heart failure. Other signs and symptoms of left-sided failure include fatigue, dyspnea, orthopnea, paroxysmal nocturnal dyspnea, tachypnea, tachycardia, crackles, a ventricular gallop, and arrhythmias.

Hypervolemia
♦ JVD occurs along with rapid weight gain, elevated blood pressure, bounding pulse, peripheral edema, dyspnea, and crackles.

Pericarditis, chronic constrictive
♦ JVD is a progressive sign and more prominent on inspiration (known as Kussmaul's sign).
♦ Other signs and symptoms include chest pain, dependent edema, hepatomegaly, ascites, and pericardial friction rub.

S & S

Superior vena cava obstruction

◆ JVD may occur along with facial, neck, and upper arm edema.

Nursing considerations

◆ Monitor the patient's vital signs and cardiopulmonary status.
◆ If the patient has cardiac tamponade, prepare him for pericardiocentesis.
◆ Restrict fluids and monitor intake and output.
◆ Insert an indwelling urinary catheter, if necessary.
◆ If the patient has heart failure, administer a diuretic as ordered.
◆ Routinely change the patient's position to avoid skin breakdown from peripheral edema.
◆ Prepare the patient for central venous or pulmonary artery catheter insertion.

PATIENT TEACHING

◆ Discuss the underlying condition, diagnostic tests, and treatment options.
◆ Explain foods or fluids the patient should avoid.
◆ Teach the patient to perform daily weight monitoring.
◆ Explain signs and symptoms the patient should report to the practitioner.
◆ Explain the importance of and help plan scheduled rest periods.

Level of consciousness, decreased

Overview

Decreased level of consciousness (LOC) nvolves a cerebral disturbance of communications within the reticular activating system and may signal a life-threatening disorder. Decreased LOC ranges from lethargy to stupor to coma. It may deteriorate suddenly or gradually, and can remain altered temporarily or permanently. The most easily identified indicator of decreased LOC is change in mental status.

Assessment

HISTORY

◆ Ask family about headaches, dizziness, nausea, vision or hearing disturbances, weakness, and fatigue.
◆ Determine whether the family has noticed any changes in behavior, personality, memory, or temperament.
◆ Obtain a medical history, including incidence of neurologic disease or cancer and recent trauma or infection.
◆ Obtain a history of drug and alcohol use.

PHYSICAL ASSESSMENT

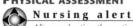
Nursing alert
After evaluating the patient's airway, breathing, and circulation, use the Glasgow Coma Scale to determine LOC and to obtain baseline data.

◆ Perform a complete neurologic examination.
◆ Perform a physical assessment.

Causes

MEDICAL
Brain abscess
◆ Decreased LOC varies from drowsiness to deep stupor.
◆ Early signs and symptoms include constant intractable headache, nausea, vomiting, and seizures.
◆ Other signs and symptoms include personality changes, confusion, abnormal behavior, dizziness, facial weakness, aphasia, ataxia, tremor, and hemiparesis.

Brain tumor
◆ LOC decreases slowly from lethargy to coma.
◆ Apathy, behavior changes, memory loss, decreased attention span, morning headache, dizziness, aphasia, seizures, vision loss, ataxia, and sensorimotor disturbances may occur.
◆ In the final stages, signs include decorticate or decerebrate posture.

Cerebral contusion
◆ Unconscious patients may have dilated, nonreactive pupils and decorticate or decerebrate posture.
◆ Conscious patients may be drowsy, confused, disoriented, agitated, or violent.
◆ Other signs and symptoms include blurred or double vision, fever, headache, pallor, diaphoresis, seizures, impaired mental status, tachycardia, altered respirations, aphasia, and hemiparesis.

Diabetic ketoacidosis
◆ Decrease in LOC is rapid and ranges from lethargy to coma.
◆ Polydipsia, polyphagia, and polyuria precede decreased LOC secondary to fluid shift from elevated glucose level.
◆ Other signs and symptoms include weakness, anorexia, abdominal pain, nausea, vomiting, orthostatic hypotension, fruity breath odor, Kussmaul's respirations, warm and dry skin, and a rapid, thready pulse.

Encephalopathy
◆ Hepatic encephalopathy involves decreased LOC that ranges from slight personality changes to coma depending on the stage.
◆ Hypertensive encephalopathy involves LOC that progressively decreases from lethargy to stupor to coma.

◆ Hypoglycemic encephalopathy involves LOC that rapidly deteriorates from lethargy to coma.

◆ Hypoxic encephalopathy involves a sudden or gradual decrease in LOC, leading to coma and brain death.

◆ Uremic encephalopathy involves LOC that decreases gradually from lethargy to coma.

Hyperosmolar hyperglycemic nonketotic syndrome
◆ LOC decreases rapidly from lethargy to coma.

◆ Early signs and symptoms include polyuria, polydipsia, weight loss, and weakness.

◆ Later signs and symptoms include hypotension, poor skin turgor, dry skin and mucous membranes, tachycardia, tachypnea, oliguria, and seizures.

Intracerebral hemorrhage
◆ Steady loss of consciousness occurs within hours and is accompanied by severe headache, dizziness, nausea, and vomiting.

◆ Other signs and symptoms include increased blood pressure, irregular respirations, Babinski's reflex, seizures, aphasia, decreased sensations, hemiplegia, decorticate or decerebrate posture, and dilated pupils.

Stroke
◆ With thrombotic stroke, LOC changes may be abrupt or take several minutes, hours, or days to evolve.

◆ With embolic stroke, LOC changes occur suddenly and peak immediately.

◆ With hemorrhagic stroke, LOC changes develop over minutes or hours, depending on the extent of the bleeding.

◆ Other signs and symptoms of stroke include disorientation, intellectual deficits, personality changes, emotional lability, dysarthria, dysphagia, ataxia, aphasia, agnosia, unilateral sensorimotor loss, vision disturbances, incontinence, and seizures.

Subdural hemorrhage, acute
◆ Agitation and confusion are followed by progressively decreasing LOC from somnolence to coma.

◆ Other signs and symptoms include headache, fever, unilateral pupil dilation, decreased pulse and respiratory rates, widening pulse pressure, seizures, hemiparesis, and Babinski's reflex.

OTHER
Alcohol
◆ Alcohol causes varying degrees of sedation, irritability, and incoordination; intoxication causes stupor.

Drugs
◆ Overdose of barbiturates, other central nervous system depressants, or aspirin can cause sedation and other degrees of decreased LOC.

Nursing considerations

◆ Reassess LOC and neurologic status at least hourly.

◆ Monitor intracranial pressure and intake and output.

◆ Ensure airway patency.

◆ Keep the patient on bed rest with the head of the bed elevated to at least 30 degrees.

◆ Maintain seizure precautions.

PATIENT TEACHING
◆ Discuss the underlying condition, diagnostic tests, and treatment options with the patient and his family as appropriate for the patient's mental status or LOC.

◆ Teach safety and seizure precautions.

◆ Provide referrals to sources of support.

◆ Discuss quality-of-life issues.

S & S

Lymphadenopathy

Overview

Lymphadenopathy, which may be generalized or localized, is the enlargement of one or more lymph nodes. A node more than ³⁄₈″ (1 cm) in diameter, or persistent enlargement, is cause for concern.

Assessment

HISTORY
◆ Ask about the onset, location, and description of swelling.
◆ Find out about recent infections or health problems.
◆ Ask about previous biopsies and personal or family history of cancer.

PHYSICAL ASSESSMENT
◆ Note the size of palpable lymph nodes and whether they're fixed or mobile, tender or nontender, and erythematous.
◆ Note the texture of palpable nodes.
◆ If lymph nodes are erythematous, check the area drained by that part of the lymph system for signs of infection.
◆ Palpate and percuss the spleen.

Causes

MEDICAL
Acquired immunodeficiency syndrome
◆ Lymphadenopathy occurs with fatigue, night sweats, afternoon fevers, diarrhea, weight loss, and cough with several concurrent infections.

Anthrax, cutaneous
◆ Lymphadenopathy, malaise, headache, and fever may develop.
◆ A small, elevated itchy lesion resembling an insect bite may progress into a painless, necrotic-centered ulcer.

Chronic fatigue syndrome
◆ Lymphadenopathy may occur with incapacitating fatigue, sore throat, low-grade fevers, myalgia, cognitive dysfunction, and sleep disturbances.

◆ Other signs and symptoms include arthralgia with arthritis, headache, and memory deficits.

Cytomegalovirus infection
◆ Generalized lymphadenopathy is accompanied by fever, malaise, and hepatosplenomegaly.
◆ Other signs and symptoms include a pruritic rash of small, erythematous macules that progresses to papules and then to vesicles.

Hodgkin's disease
◆ The extent of lymphadenopathy reflects the stage of malignancy.
◆ Early signs and symptoms include pruritus, fatigue, weakness, night sweats, malaise, weight loss, and fever.

Leukemia
◆ In acute lymphocytic leukemia, generalized lymphadenopathy is accompanied by fatigue, malaise, pallor, prolonged bleeding time, swollen gums, weight loss, bone or joint pain, hepatosplenomegaly, and low fever.
◆ In chronic lymphocytic leukemia, generalized lymphadenopathy appears early along with fatigue, malaise, and fever.
◆ Late signs and symptoms of the chronic form include hepatosplenomegaly, severe fatigue, weight loss, bone tenderness, edema, pallor, dyspnea, tachycardia, palpitations, bleeding, anemia, and macular or nodular lesions.

Lyme disease
◆ As disease progresses, lymphadenopathy, constant malaise and fatigue, and intermittent headache, fever, chills, and aches develop.
◆ Arthralgia and, eventually, neurologic and cardiac abnormalities may develop.

Mononucleosis, infectious
◆ Painful lymphadenopathy involves cervical, axillary, and inguinal nodes.
◆ Prodromal symptoms of headache, malaise, and fatigue appear 3 to 5 days be-

fore the appearance of the classic triad of lymphadenopathy, sore throat, and temperature fluctuations with an evening peak.

Non-Hodgkin's lymphoma
◆ Painless enlargement of one or more peripheral lymph nodes is the most common sign.
◆ Generalized lymphadenopathy characterizes stage IV.
◆ Other signs and symptoms include dyspnea, cough, hepatosplenomegaly, fever, night sweats, fatigue, malaise, and weight loss.

Rheumatoid arthritis
◆ Lymphadenopathy is an early, nonspecific finding.
◆ Later signs and symptoms include joint tenderness, swelling, and warmth; joint stiffness after inactivity; subcutaneous nodules on the elbows; joint deformity; muscle weakness; and muscle atrophy.

Sarcoidosis
◆ Generalized hilar and right paratracheal forms of lymphadenopathy with splenomegaly are common.
◆ Initial signs and symptoms include arthralgia, fatigue, malaise, weight loss, and pulmonary symptoms.

Syphilis
◆ Localized lymphadenopathy occurs with a painless canker that develops at site of sexual exposure.
◆ In the second stage, generalized lymphadenopathy occurs along with a macular, papular, pustular, or nodular rash on the arms, trunk, palms (a diagnostic sign), soles, face, and scalp.
◆ Other signs and symptoms include headache, malaise, anorexia, weight loss, nausea, vomiting, sore throat, and low fever.

Systemic lupus erythematosus
◆ Generalized lymphadenopathy accompanies butterfly rash (hallmark sign), photosensitivity, Raynaud's phenomenon, and joint pain and stiffness.
◆ Other signs and symptoms include pleuritic chest pain, cough, fever, anorexia, and weight loss.

Tuberculous lymphadenitis
◆ Lymphadenopathy may be generalized or restricted to superficial lymph nodes.
◆ Lymph nodes may become fluctuant and drain to surrounding tissue.
◆ Other signs and symptoms include fever, chills, weakness, and fatigue.

OTHER
Drugs
◆ Phenytoin (Dilantin) may cause generalized lymphadenopathy.

Immunizations
◆ Typhoid vaccination may cause generalized lymphadenopathy.

Nursing considerations
◆ If the patient has a temperature, provide an antipyretic, a tepid sponge bath, or a hypothermia blanket.
◆ If diagnostic tests reveal infection, check your facility's policy regarding infection control.

PATIENT TEACHING
◆ Teach the patient about the underlying condition, diagnostic tests, and treatment options.
◆ Teach the patient ways to prevent infection.
◆ Explain signs and symptoms of infection the patient should report to the practitioner.
◆ Explain the reasons for isolation as needed.
◆ Stress the importance of a healthy diet and rest.

Melena

Overview

Melena (black, tarry stools containing digested blood) commonly indicates upper GI bleeding. When severe, it can signal acute GI bleeding and life-threatening hypovolemic shock.

Assessment

HISTORY

◆ Ask about the onset of melena.
◆ Determine the frequency and quantity of bowel movements.
◆ Ask about hematemesis or hematochezia.
◆ Find out about the use of anti-inflammatory drugs, alcohol, other GI irritants, or iron supplements.
◆ Obtain a drug history, noting the use of warfarin (Coumadin) and other anticoagulants.

PHYSICAL ASSESSMENT

◆ Inspect the mouth and nasopharynx for bleeding.
◆ Auscultate, percuss, and palpate the abdomen.
◆ Perform a cardiovascular assessment to detect signs and symptoms of shock.

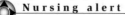 **Nursing alert**

If the patient has severe melena, take orthostatic vital signs and look for other signs of hypovolemic shock. Insert a large-bore I.V. line to administer replacement fluids and allow blood transfusion. Obtain hematocrit, prothrombin time, International Normalized Ratio, and partial thromboplastin time. Place the patient flat with his head turned to the side and his feet elevated. Administer supplemental oxygen as needed.

Causes

MEDICAL

Colon cancer

◆ Early right-sided tumor growth may cause melena and abdominal aching, pressure, or cramps. As it progresses, signs and symptoms include weakness, fatigue, anemia, diarrhea or obstipation, anorexia, weight loss, vomiting, and signs and symptoms of obstruction.
◆ Early left-sided tumor growth may cause rectal bleeding with intermittent abdominal fullness or cramping and rectal pressure. As the tumor progresses, signs and symptoms include melena (usually develops late in the disease), obstipation, diarrhea, and pencil-shaped stools.

Esophageal cancer

◆ Melena is a late sign along with painful dysphagia, anorexia, and regurgitation.
◆ Earlier signs and symptoms include painless dysphagia, rapid weight loss, steady chest pain with substernal fullness, nausea, vomiting, and hematemesis.

Esophageal varices, ruptured

◆ Melena, hematochezia, and hematemesis may occur.
◆ Melena is preceded by signs of shock.
◆ Agitation or confusion signal developing hepatic encephalopathy.

Gastric cancer

◆ Melena and altered bowel habits may occur late.
◆ Other signs and symptoms include insidious onset of upper abdominal or retrosternal discomfort and chronic dyspepsia unrelieved by antacids and exacerbated by food, anorexia, nausea, hematemesis, pallor, fatigue, weight loss, and a feeling of abdominal fullness.

Gastritis
◆ Melena and hematemesis are common signs.
◆ Other signs and symptoms include mild epigastric or abdominal discomfort that's made worse by eating, belching, nausea, vomiting, and malaise.

Mallory-Weiss syndrome
◆ Melena and hematemesis follow vomiting of large amounts of bright red blood.
◆ Epigastric or back pain, and signs and symptoms of shock may occur.

Mesenteric vascular occlusion
◆ Slight melena occurs along with 2 to 3 days of persistent, mild abdominal pain.
◆ Later, abdominal pain becomes severe and may be accompanied by tenderness, distention, guarding, and rigidity.
◆ Anorexia, vomiting, fever, and profound shock may also develop.

Peptic ulcer
◆ Melena may signal life-threatening hemorrhage.
◆ Other signs and symptoms include decreased appetite; nausea; vomiting; hematemesis; hematochezia; left epigastric pain that's gnawing, burning, or sharp; and signs and symptoms of shock.

Small-bowel tumors
◆ Tumors may bleed and produce melena.
◆ Other signs and symptoms include abdominal pain, distention, and increasing frequency and rising pitch of bowel sounds.

Thrombocytopenia
◆ Melena or hematochezia may accompany other manifestations of bleeding tendency.
◆ Malaise, fatigue, weakness, and lethargy are typical.

OTHER
Drugs
◆ Aspirin, nonsteroidal anti-inflammatory drugs (NSAIDs), or alcohol may cause melena.

Nursing considerations

◆ Monitor the patient's vital signs, and assess for signs of hypovolemic shock.
◆ Encourage bed rest.
◆ Provide perianal care.
◆ Insert a nasogastric tube and assess amount and characteristics of drainage if ordered.
◆ Monitor hemoglobin and hematocrit and administer blood transfusions as ordered.

PATIENT TEACHING
◆ Explain the underlying disorder and treatment plan.
◆ Explain the changes in bowel elimination that the patient needs to report.
◆ Stress the importance of undergoing colorectal cancer screening.
◆ Explain the need to avoid aspirin, other NSAIDs, and alcohol.

S & S

Menorrhagia

Overview

Menorrhagia, abnormally heavy or long menstrual bleeding of 80 ml or more per monthly period, may occur as a single episode or chronically.

Assessment

HISTORY

◆ Obtain a menstural history including age at menarche, average duration of menstrual periods, interval between them, date of the last menses, and recent changes in her normal menstrual pattern. Have the patient describe the character and amount of bleeding.

◆ Obtain information about method of birth control, the number of pregnancies and outcome of each, dates of her most recent pelvic examination and Papanicolaou smear, and the details of any previous gynecologic infections or neoplasms.

◆ If possible, obtain a pregnancy history of the patient's mother, and determine if the patient was exposed in utero to diethylstilbestrol (DES), a drug linked to vaginal and cervical diseases.

◆ Ask about general health and medical history, including a history of thyroid, adrenal, or hepatic disease; blood dyscrasias; or tuberculosis, because these may predispose the patient to menorrhagia; and about past surgical procedures; and any recent emotional stress.

◆ Find out if the patient has undergone X-ray or other radiation therapy.

◆ Obtain a thorough drug and alcohol history, noting the use of anticoagulants or aspirin.

PHYSICAL ASSESSMENT

◆ Obtain vital signs.

◆ Use menstrual pads to examine the quality and quantity of bleeding. Then prepare the patient for a pelvic examination to help determine the cause of bleeding.

◆ Obtain a blood sample and urine specimen for pregnancy testing.

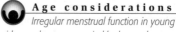 **Age considerations**

Irregular menstrual function in young girls may be accompanied by hemorrhage and resulting anemia. In such patients, evaluate hemodynamic status by taking orthostatic vital signs. Insert a large-gauge I.V. line to begin fluid replacement if the patient shows signs of hypovolemic shock, such as pallor, tachycardia, tachypnea, and cool, clammy skin. Place the patient in a supine position with her feet elevated, and administer supplemental oxygen as needed.

Causes

MEDICAL
Blood dyscrasias

◆ Menorrhagia is one of several possible signs of a bleeding disorder.

◆ Other associated signs and symptoms include epistaxis, bleeding gums, purpura, hematemesis, hematuria, and melena.

Endometriosis

◆ Menorrhagia may occur, however, the classic symptom is dysmenorrhea.

◆ A tender fixed adnexal mass is commonly palpable on bimanual examination.

◆ Other signs and symptoms depend on the location of the ectopic tissue outside the uterus but may include dyspareunia, suprapubic pain, dysuria, nausea, vomiting, abdominal cramps, cyclic pelvic pain, and infertility.

S & S

Hypothyroidism

◆ Menorrhagia is a common early sign and is accompanied by such nonspecific findings as fatigue, cold intolerance, constipation, and weight gain despite anorexia.

◆ As hypothyroidism progresses, intellectual and motor activity decrease; the skin becomes dry, pale, cool, and doughy; the hair becomes dry and sparse; and the nails become thick and brittle.

◆ Deep tendon reflexes are delayed, and bradycardia and abdominal distention may occur.

Uterine fibroids

◆ Menorrhagia is the most common sign, but other forms of abnormal uterine bleeding as well as dysmenorrhea or leukorrhea may occur.

◆ Other related signs and symptoms include abdominal pain, a feeling of abdominal heaviness, backache, constipation, urinary urgency or frequency, and an enlarged uterus, which is usually nontender.

OTHER
Drugs

◆ Use of hormonal contraceptives may cause sudden onset of profuse, prolonged menorrhagia.

◆ Anticoagulants have been associated with excessive menstrual flow.

Intrauterine devices

◆ Menorrhagia may result from the use of intrauterine contraceptive devices.

Nursing considerations

◆ Monitor the patient's vital signs and observe for signs of hypovolemia.

◆ Infuse I.V. fluids as ordered and encourage the patient to maintain adequate fluid intake.

◆ Monitor intake and output, and estimate uterine blood loss by recording the number of sanitary napkins or tampons used during menstruation.

◆ Obtain blood samples for hematocrit, prothrombin time, partial thromboplastin time, and International Normalized Ratio levels.

PATIENT TEACHING

◆ Teach the patient about the cause of menorrhagia and treatment options.

◆ Teach her how to monitor blood loss and maintain fluid volume by adequate fluid intake.

S & S

Muscle flaccidity

Overview

Muscle flaccidity involves weak, soft muscles that have decreased resistance to movement, increased mobility, and greater than normal range of motion (ROM). It results from disrupted muscle innervation. Flaccid muscles may be localized to a limb or muscle group or generalized over the entire body, and onset may be acute from trauma or chronic from neurologic disease.

 Nursing alert

If the patient's muscle flaccidity results from trauma, make sure his cervical spine has been stabilized. Quickly determine his respiratory status. If you note signs and symptoms of respiratory insufficiency (dyspnea, shallow respirations, nasal flaring, cyanosis, and decreased oxygen saturation), administer oxygen by nasal cannula or mask. Intubation and mechanical ventilation may be necessary.

Assessment

HISTORY
◆ Ask about the onset and duration of muscle flaccidity and any precipitating factors.
◆ Ask about associated signs and symptoms, notably weakness, other muscle changes, and sensory loss or paresthesia.

PHYSICAL ASSESSMENT
◆ Examine the affected muscles for atrophy, which indicates a chronic problem.
◆ Test muscle strength, and check deep tendon reflexes in all limbs.
◆ Perform a neurologic assessment.

Causes

MEDICAL
Amyotrophic lateral sclerosis
◆ Progressive muscle weakness and paralysis are accompanied by generalized flaccidity.
◆ Effects typically begin in one hand, spread to the arm, and then develop in the other hand and arm. Eventually, they spread to the trunk, neck, tongue, larynx, pharynx, and legs; progressive respiratory muscle weakness leads to respiratory insufficiency.
◆ Other signs and symptoms include muscle cramps and coarse fasciculations, hyperactive deep tendon reflexes (DTRs), slight leg muscle spasticity, dysphagia, dysarthria, excessive drooling, and depression.

Brain lesions
◆ Frontal and parietal lobe lesions may cause contralateral flaccidity, weakness or paralysis, and eventually, spasticity and possibly contractures.
◆ Other signs and symptoms include hyperactive DTRs, positive Babinski's reflex, loss of proprioception, stereognosis, graphesthesia, anesthesia, and thermanesthesia.

Cerebellar disease
◆ Generalized muscle flaccidity or hypotonia is accompanied by ataxia, dysmetria, intention tremor, slight muscle weakness, fatigue, and dysarthria.

Guillain-Barré syndrome
◆ Progression of muscle flaccidity is typically symmetrical and ascending, moving from the feet to the arms and facial nerves within 24 to 72 hours of the syndrome's onset.
◆ Associated signs and symptoms include sensory loss or paresthesia, absent DTRs, tachycardia (or, less often, bradycardia), fluctuating hypertension and orthostatic hypotension, diaphoresis, incontinence, dysphagia, dysarthria, hypernasality, and facial diplegia.
◆ Weakness may progress to total motor paralysis and respiratory failure.

Huntington's disease
◆ Besides flaccidity, progressive mental status changes and choreiform movements are major symptoms.
◆ Other signs and symptoms include poor balance, hesitant or explosive speech, dys-

S&S

phagia, impaired respirations, and incontinence.

Muscle disease
◆ Muscle weakness and flaccidity are features of myopathies and muscular dystrophies.

Peripheral nerve trauma
◆ Flaccidity, paralysis, and loss of sensation and reflexes in the innervated area may occur.

Peripheral neuropathy
◆ Flaccidity usually occurs in the legs as a result of chronic progressive muscle weakness and paralysis, which may also cause mild to sharp burning pain, glossy red skin, anhidrosis, and loss of vibration sensation.
◆ Paresthesia, hyperesthesia, or anesthesia may affect the hands and feet.
◆ DTRs may be hypoactive or absent.

Poliomyelitis
◆ Damage to the anterior horn cells in the spinal cord and brain stem causes flaccid weakness and loss of reflexes.
◆ The large proximal muscles of the limbs are most commonly affected.

Seizure disorder
◆ Brief periods of syncope and generalized flaccidity commonly follow a generalized tonic-clonic seizure.

Spinal cord injury
◆ Spinal shock may result in acute muscle flaccidity or spasticity below the level of injury.
◆ Other signs and symptoms that occur below the level of injury may include paralysis; absent DTRs; analgesia; thermanesthesia; loss of proprioception and vibration, touch, and pressure sensation; anhidrosis (usually unilateral); hypotension; bowel and bladder dysfunction; and impotence or priapism.

◆ Injury in the C1 to C5 region can produce respiratory paralysis and bradycardia.

Nursing considerations

◆ Monitor the patient's musculoskeletal and neurologic status.
◆ Initiate fall prevention measures and ensure patient safety.
◆ Provide regular, systematic, passive ROM exercises to preserve joint mobility and to increase circulation.
◆ Reposition and assess a patient with generalized flaccidity every 2 hours to protect him from skin breakdown.
◆ Pad bony prominences and other pressure points.
◆ Prevent thermal injury by testing bath water before the patient bathes.
◆ Treat isolated flaccidity by supporting the affected limb in a sling or with a splint.
◆ Provide assistive devices as apporpriate.
◆ Consult physical and occupational therapy to formulate a personalized therapy regimen and foster independence.
◆ Prepare the patient for diagnostic tests, such as cranial and spinal X-rays, computed tomography scans, and electromyography.

PATIENT TEACHING
◆ Teach the patient and his family about the underlying diagnosis and treatment plan.
◆ Teach the patient and his family how to do ROM exercises at home and why it's important that they be done.
◆ Teach the patient and his family the importance of frequent position changes and other pressure ulcer prevention techniques.
◆ Teach the patient and his family about prescribed medications and possible adverse effects.
◆ Encourage the patient to use assistive devices as instructed.

Muscle weakness

Overview

Muscle weakness, the inability of a muscle to function at an appropriate level, is detected by observing and measuring the strength of an individual muscle or muscle group.

 Age considerations
Some decreased muscle strength occurs with aging.

Assessment

HISTORY

◆ Determine the onset and location of weakness.
◆ Ask what aggravates or alleviates the weakness.
◆ Find out about other symptoms, including muscle or joint pain, altered sensory function, and fatigue.
◆ Obtain a medical history, including incidence of hyperthyroidism, musculoskeletal or neurologic problems, recent trauma, and family history of chronic muscle weakness.
◆ Obtain an alcohol and drug history.

PHYSICAL ASSESSMENT

◆ Test major muscles on both sides.
◆ Test for range of motion (ROM) at all major joints.
◆ Test sensory function in the involved areas.
◆ Test deep tendon reflexes (DTRs) on both sides.

Causes

MEDICAL
Amyotrophic lateral sclerosis

◆ Muscle weakness and atrophy in one hand rapidly spread to the arm and then to the other hand and arm.
◆ Eventually, weakness and atrophy spread to the trunk, neck, tongue, larynx, pharynx, and legs; respiratory insufficiency results from progressive respiratory muscle weakness.

Guillain-Barré syndrome

◆ Rapidly progressive, symmetrical weakness and pain ascend from the feet to the arms and facial nerves, and may progress to motor paralysis and respiratory failure.
◆ Other signs and symptoms include sensory loss or paresthesia, muscle flaccidity, absent DTRs, tachycardia or bradycardia, fluctuating hypertension and orthostatic hypotension, diaphoresis, bowel and bladder incontinence, facial diplegia, dysphagia, dysarthria, and hypernasality.

Hypothyroidism

◆ Reversible weakness and atrophy of proximal limb muscles may occur.
◆ Other signs and symptoms include muscle cramps; cold intolerance; weight gain despite anorexia; mental dullness; dry, pale, doughy skin; puffy face, hands, and feet; impaired hearing and balance; and bradycardia.

Multiple sclerosis

◆ Muscle weakness in one or more limbs may progress to atrophy, spasticity, and contractures.
◆ Other signs and symptoms include diplopia, blurred vision, vision loss, nystagmus, hyperactive DTRs, sensory loss or paresthesia, dysarthria, dysphagia, incoordination, ataxic gait, intention tremors, emotional lability, and urinary dysfunction.

Myasthenia gravis

◆ Gradually progressive skeletal muscle weakness and fatigue are the principal symptoms.
◆ Other early signs include weak eye closure, ptosis, diplopia, a masklike facies, difficulty chewing and swallowing, nasal regurgitation of fluid with hypernasality, and a hanging jaw and bobbing head.

Parkinson's disease

◆ Muscle weakness accompanies rigidity.
◆ Other signs and symptoms include a pill-rolling tremor in one hand, propulsive

gait, dysarthria, bradykinesia, drooling, dysphagia, a masklike facies, and a high-pitched, monotonous voice.

Peripheral neuropathy
◆ Muscle weakness progresses slowly to flaccid paralysis.
◆ Other signs and symptoms include loss of vibration sense; paresthesia, hyperesthesia, or anesthesia in the hands and feet; hypoactive or absent DTRs; mild to sharp burning pain; anhidrosis; and glossy, red skin.

Potassium imbalance
◆ With hypokalemia, temporary muscle weakness occurs and may be accompanied by nausea, vomiting, diarrhea, decreased mentation, leg cramps, diminished reflexes, malaise, polyuria, dizziness, hypotension, and arrhythmias.
◆ With hyperkalemia, weakness progresses to flaccid paralysis and may be accompanied by irritability, confusion, hyperreflexia, paresthesia or anesthesia, oliguria, anorexia, nausea, diarrhea, abdominal cramps, tachycardia or bradycardia, and arrhythmias.

Rhabdomyolysis
◆ Muscle weakness or pain occurs with fever, nausea, vomiting, malaise, dark urine, and signs of acute renal failure.

Rheumatoid arthritis
◆ Symmetric muscle weakness may accompany increased warmth, swelling, and tenderness in involved joints; pain; and stiffness.

Spinal trauma and disease
◆ Severe muscle weakness leading to flaccidity or spasticity and, eventually, paralysis, occurs.

Stroke
◆ Weakness may progress to hemiplegia and atrophy.

◆ Other signs and symptoms include dysarthria, aphasia, ataxia, apraxia, agnosia, ipsilateral paresthesia or sensory loss, visual disturbance, altered level of consciousness, personality changes, bowel and bladder dysfunction, headache, and seizures.

OTHER
Drugs
◆ Aminoglycoside antibiotics may worsen weakness in patients with myasthenia gravis.
◆ Generalized muscle weakness can result from prolonged corticosteroid use, digoxin (Lanoxin), and excessive doses of dantrolene (Dantrium).

Immobility
◆ Immobilization, prolonged bed rest, or inactivity can lead to overall muscle weakness.

Nursing considerations
◆ Monitor musculoskeletal status.
◆ Provide assistive devices as needed.
◆ Protect the patient from injury.
◆ If sensory loss occurs, guard against pressure ulcer formation and thermal injury.
◆ With chronic weakness, provide ROM exercises or splint the limbs as needed.
◆ Encourage participation in physical therapy program, but allow for adequate rest periods.
◆ Give drugs for pain as needed.

PATIENT TEACHING
◆ Teach the patient and family about the underlying disorder and treatment plan.
◆ Teach the patient how to use assistive devices as needed.
◆ Explain the importance of frequent position changes and rest periods.
◆ Teach the patient about prescribed medications and possible adverse effects.

S & S

Nausea

Overview

Nausea is the sensation of impending vomiting or the profound revulsion to food.

Assessment

HISTORY

◆ Ask about the onset and description of nausea.
◆ Determine aggravating or alleviating factors.
◆ Obtain a medical history, including incidence of GI, endocrine, and metabolic disorders; cancer; and infections.
◆ Ask about vomiting, abdominal pain, and changes in bowel habits.
◆ Ask about recent exposure to illness.
◆ Ask about the possibility of pregnancy.

PHYSICAL ASSESSMENT

◆ Obtain the patient's vital signs.
◆ Inspect the skin for jaundice, bruises, and spider angiomas; assess skin turgor.
◆ Inspect for abdominal distention.
◆ Auscultate for bowel sounds and bruits.
◆ Palpate for abdominal rigidity and tenderness and test for rebound tenderness.
◆ Palpate and percuss the liver.

Causes

MEDICAL
Cholecystitis, acute
◆ Nausea typically follows severe right-upper-quadrant pain that may radiate to the back or shoulders, commonly after meals.
◆ Other signs and symptoms include vomiting, flatulence, abdominal tenderness, rigidity and distention, fever with chills, diaphoresis, and a positive Murphy's sign.

Cholelithiasis
◆ Nausea accompanies severe right-upper-quadrant or epigastric pain.
◆ Other signs and symptoms include vomiting, abdominal tenderness and guarding, flatulence, belching, epigastric burning,

tachycardia, restlessness and, with occlusion of the common bile duct, jaundice, clay-colored stools, fever, and chills.

Diverticulitis
◆ Nausea, intermittent crampy abdominal pain, constipation or diarrhea, low-grade fever and, in many cases, a palpable, fixed mass occur.
◆ Other signs and symptoms include anorexia, bloody stools, and flatulence.

Electrolyte imbalances
◆ Nausea and vomiting occur along with cardiac arrhythmias, tremors or seizures, anorexia, malaise, and weakness.

Gastritis
◆ Nausea is common, especially after ingestion of alcohol, aspirin, spicy foods, or caffeine.
◆ Vomiting, epigastric pain, belching, and malaise may also occur.

Gastroenteritis
◆ Nausea, vomiting, diarrhea, and abdominal cramping occur.
◆ Other signs and symptoms include fever, malaise, hyperactive bowel sounds, abdominal pain and tenderness, and signs of dehydration and electrolyte imbalance.

Hepatitis
◆ Nausea is an early symptom.
◆ Vomiting, fatigue, myalgia, arthralgia, headache, anorexia, photophobia, pharyngitis, cough, and fever also occur early in the preicteric phase.

Hyperemesis gravidarum
◆ Unremitting nausea and vomiting persist beyond the first trimester of pregnancy.
◆ Other signs and symptoms include weight loss, signs of dehydration, headache, and delirium.

Intestinal obstruction
◆ Nausea, vomiting, constipation, and abdominal pain occur.

◆ Other signs and symptoms include abdominal distention and tenderness, visible peristaltic waves, and hyperactive (in partial obstruction) or hypoactive or absent bowel sounds (in complete obstruction).

Irritable bowel syndrome
◆ Nausea, dyspepsia, and abdominal distention may occur.
◆ Other signs and symptoms include lower abdominal pain and tenderness relieved by defecation, diurnal diarrhea alternating with constipation or normal bowel function, small stools with visible mucus, and a feeling of incomplete evacuation.

Labyrinthitis
◆ Nausea and vomiting occur with vertigo, progressive hearing loss, nystagmus, and tinnitus.

Ménière's disease
◆ Sudden, brief, recurrent attacks of nausea, vomiting, vertigo, tinnitus, nystagmus and, eventually, hearing loss occur.

Migraine headache
◆ Nausea and vomiting may occur along with photophobia, light flashes, increased sensitivity to noise, light-headedness, partial vision loss, and paresthesia of the lips, face, and hands.

Myocardial infarction
◆ Nausea and vomiting may occur, but the cardinal symptom is severe substernal chest pain that may radiate to the left arm, jaw, or neck.
◆ Other signs and symptoms include dyspnea, pallor, clammy skin, diaphoresis, altered blood pressure, and arrhythmias.

Pancreatitis, acute
◆ Nausea, usually followed by vomiting, is an early symptom.
◆ Other signs and symptoms include severe upper abdominal pain that may radiate to the back, abdominal tenderness and rigidity, anorexia, diminished bowel sounds, and fever.

Peptic ulcer
◆ Nausea and vomiting follow attacks of sharp or gnawing, burning epigastric pain when the stomach is empty or after ingesting alcohol, caffeine, or aspirin.

Peritonitis
◆ Nausea and vomiting accompany acute abdominal pain.
◆ Other signs and symptoms include fever, chills, tachycardia, hypoactive or absent bowel sounds, abdominal rigidity and tenderness, diaphoresis, hypotension, and shallow respirations.

OTHER
Drugs
◆ Antineoplastics, opiates, ferrous sulfate (Feosol), levodopa (Dopar), oral potassium chloride replacements, estrogens, sulfasalazine (Azulfadine), antibiotics, quinidine (Quinaglute), anesthetics, digoxin (Lanoxin), theophylline (Slo-Phyllin) overdose, and nonsteroidal anti-inflammatory drugs can cause nausea.

Nursing considerations

◆ Evaluate fluid, electrolyte, and acid-base balance.
◆ Elevate the patient's head or position him on his side.
◆ Be prepared to insert a nasogastric tube, if needed.
◆ Administer I.V. fluids as ordered.
◆ Monitor serum electrolytes if extensive vomiting occurs.

PATIENT TEACHING
◆ Teach the patient about the underlying diagnosis and treatment plan.
◆ Discuss what aggravates nausea and how to avoid it.

S & S

Nuchal rigidity

Overview

Nuchal rigidity is neck stiffness that prevents forward flexion of the head. With meningeal irritation, pain and muscle spasms also occur.

Assessment

HISTORY

◆ Obtain a patient history, relying on family members if an altered level of consciousness (LOC) prevents the patient from responding. Ask about the onset and duration of neck stiffness; precipitating factors; associated signs and symptoms, such as a headache, a fever, nausea and vomiting; and motor and sensory changes.
◆ Check for a history of hypertension, head trauma, cerebral aneurysm or arteriovenous malformation, endocarditis, recent infection (such as sinusitis or pneumonia), or recent dental work.
◆ Obtain a complete drug history.
◆ If the patient has no other signs of meningeal irritation, ask about a history of arthritis or neck trauma.

PHYSICAL ASSESSMENT

◆ To prevent severe spinal cord damage, make sure that there's no cervical spine misalignment, such as a fracture or dislocation, before testing for nuchal rigidity.
◆ Attempt to passively flex the patient's neck and touch his chin to his chest. If meningeal irritation is present, this maneuver triggers pain and muscle spasms.

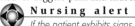 **Nursing alert**

If the patient exhibits signs and symptoms of meningeal irritation, attempt to elicit Kernig's and Brudzinski's signs. Quickly evaluate the patient's LOC. Take his vital signs. If you note signs of increased intracranial pressure (ICP), such as increased systolic pressure, bradycardia, and a widened pulse pressure, start an I.V. line for drug administration and deliver oxygen, as necessary. Keep the head of the bed elevated. Draw a sample for blood studies, such as a complete blood count and electrolytes.

◆ Inspect the patient's hands for swollen, tender joints, and palpate the neck for pain or tenderness.
◆ Assess the neurologic system.

Causes

MEDICAL
Cervical arthritis
◆ Nuchal rigidity develops gradually. Initially, neck stiffness occurs in the early morning or after a period of inactivity. Stiffness then becomes increasingly severe and frequent, and may even affect other joints, especially those in the hands.
◆ Pain on movement, especially with lateral motion or head turning, is common.

Encephalitis
◆ Nuchal rigidity is accompanied by signs of meningeal irritation, such as positive Kernig's and Brudzinski's signs.
◆ Usually, nuchal rigidity appears abruptly and is preceded by a headache, vomiting, and fever.
◆ Other signs and symptoms include a rapidly decreasing LOC, progressing from lethargy to coma within 24 to 48 hours of onset, seizures, ataxia, hemiparesis, nystagmus, and cranial nerve palsies, such as dysphagia and ptosis.

Listeriosis
◆ Nuchal rigidity occurs with fever, headache, and a change in the LOC.
◆ Initial signs and symptoms include myalgia, abdominal pain, nausea, vomiting, and diarrhea.
◆ If listeriosis spreads to the nervous system, meningitis may develop.
◆ Listeriosis infection during pregnancy may lead to premature delivery, infection of the neonate, or stillbirth.

Meningitis
◆ Nuchal rigidity, an early sign, is accompanied by other signs of meningeal irritation, including positive Kernig's and Brudzinski's signs, hyperreflexia, fever

with chills, confusion, headache, photophobia, irritability, vomiting and, possibly, opisthotonos.

♦ Cranial nerve involvement may cause ocular palsies, facial weakness, and hearing loss.

♦ An erythematous papular rash occurs in some forms of viral meningitis; a purpuric rash may occur in meningococcal meningitis.

Subarachnoid hemorrhage

♦ Nuchal rigidity develops immediately after bleeding into the subarachnoid space.

♦ Related signs and symptoms include positive Kernig's and Brudzinski's signs, an abrupt onset of a severe headache, photophobia, fever, nausea and vomiting, dizziness, cranial nerve palsies, focal neurologic signs (such as hemiparesis or hemiplegia), and signs of increased ICP (such as bradycardia and altered respirations).

♦ LOC may deteriorate rapidly, possibly progressing to coma.

Nursing considerations

♦ Prepare the patient for diagnostic tests, such as computed tomography scans, magnetic resonance imaging, and cervical spinal X-rays.

♦ Monitor the patient's vital signs, intake and output, and neurologic status closely.

♦ Avoid routine administration of opioid analgesics because these may mask signs of increasing ICP.

♦ Enforce strict bed rest; keep the head of the bed elevated at least 30 degrees to help minimize ICP.

♦ Assist the patient in finding a comfortable position to obtain adequate rest.

PATIENT TEACHING

♦ Teach the patient about the underlying diagnosis and treatment plan.

♦ Teach family members how they can participate in the patient's care.

Oliguria

Overview

Oliguria, urine output of less than 400 ml per 24 hours, is a major sign of renal and urinary tract disorders and typically occurs abruptly. It may signal serious, possibly life-threatening hemodynamic instability.

Assessment

HISTORY

◆ Ask about usual voiding patterns and the onset and description of oliguria.
◆ Ask about pain or burning on urination, fever, loss of appetite, thirst, dyspnea, chest pain, or recent weight gain or loss.
◆ Record the patient's daily fluid intake.
◆ Obtain a medical history, including incidence of renal, urinary tract, or cardiovascular disorders; recent traumatic injury or surgery with significant blood loss; and recent transfusions.
◆ Ask about alcohol use.
◆ Obtain a drug history.
◆ Ask about exposure to nephrotoxic agents, such as heavy metals, organic solvents, anesthetics, or radiographic contrast media.

PHYSICAL ASSESSMENT

◆ Take vital signs and weigh the patient.
◆ Palpate the kidneys for tenderness and enlargement.
◆ Percuss for costovertebral angle (CVA) tenderness.
◆ Inspect the flanks for edema or erythema.
◆ Auscultate the heart and lungs for abnormal sounds and the flank area for bruits.
◆ Assess for edema or signs of dehydration.
◆ Obtain a urine specimen, and inspect it for abnormal color, odor, or sediment; measure its specific gravity.

Causes

MEDICAL

Acute tubular necrosis

◆ Oliguria, an early sign, may occur abruptly (in shock) or gradually (in nephrotoxicity) and persist for about 2 weeks, followed by polyuria.
◆ Other signs and symptoms include signs of hyperkalemia, uremia, and heart failure.

Calculi

◆ Oliguria or anuria may occur.
◆ Excruciating pain radiates from the CVA to the flank, the suprapubic region, and the external genitalia.
◆ Other signs and symptoms include urinary frequency and urgency, dysuria, hematuria or pyuria, nausea, vomiting, hypoactive bowel sounds, abdominal distention and, possibly, fever and chills.

Glomerulonephritis, acute

◆ Oliguria or anuria occurs.
◆ Other signs and symptoms include mild fever, fatigue, gross hematuria, proteinuria, generalized edema, elevated blood pressure, headache, nausea, vomiting, flank and abdominal pain, and signs of pulmonary congestion.

Heart failure

◆ With left-sided heart failure, oliguria occurs due to decreased renal perfusion.
◆ With advanced failure, orthopnea, cyanosis, clubbing, ventricular gallop, diastolic hypertension, cardiomegaly, and hemoptysis occur.
◆ Other signs and symptoms include dyspnea, fatigue, weakness, peripheral edema, distended neck veins, tachycardia, tachypnea, crackles, and a dry or productive cough.

Hypovolemia

◆ Oliguria may occur along with orthostatic hypotension, apathy, lethargy, fatigue, muscle weakness, anorexia, nausea, thirst, dizziness, sunken eyeballs, poor skin turgor, and dry mucous membranes.

Pyelonephritis, acute
◆ Oliguria, high fever with chills, fatigue, flank pain, CVA tenderness, weakness, nocturia, dysuria, hematuria, urinary frequency and urgency, and tenesmus occur.

Renal artery occlusion, bilateral
◆ Oliguria or, more commonly, anuria may accompany severe, constant upper abdominal and flank pain, nausea and vomiting, hypoactive bowel sounds, fever, and diastolic hypertension.

Renal failure, chronic
◆ Oliguria is a major sign of end-stage chronic renal failure.
◆ Eventually, seizures, coma, and uremic frost develop.
◆ Other signs and symptoms include uremic fetor, peripheral edema, elevated blood pressure, emotional lability, coarse muscle twitching, muscle cramps, peripheral neuropathies, anorexia, metallic taste in the mouth, pruritus, pallor, and yellow- or bronze-tinged skin.

Renal vein occlusion, bilateral
◆ Occasionally, oliguria occurs with acute low back and flank pain, CVA tenderness, fever, pallor, hematuria, enlarged and palpable kidneys, edema and, possibly, signs of uremia.

Sepsis
◆ Oliguria, fever, chills, restlessness, confusion, diaphoresis, anorexia, vomiting, diarrhea, pallor, hypotension, and tachycardia occur.
◆ Signs of local infection may develop.

Toxemia of pregnancy
◆ Oliguria may be accompanied by elevated blood pressure, dizziness, diplopia, blurred vision, nausea and vomiting, irritability, and frontal headache.

◆ Oliguria is preceded by generalized edema and sudden weight gain of more than 3 lb (1.4 kg) per week during the second trimester or more than 1 lb (0.5 kg) per week during the third trimester.
◆ If the condition progresses to eclampsia, seizures and coma may occur.

Urethral stricture
◆ Oliguria is accompanied by chronic urethral discharge, urinary frequency and urgency, dysuria, pyuria, and diminished urine stream.

OTHER
Diagnostic tests
◆ Radiographic studies that use contrast media may cause nephrotoxicity and oliguria.

Drugs
◆ Oliguria may result from drugs that cause decreased renal perfusion (diuretics), nephrotoxicity (most notably aminoglycosides and chemotherapeutics), urine retention (adrenergics and anticholinergics), or urinary obstruction associated with precipitation of urinary crystals (sulfonamides and acyclovir [Zovirax]).

Nursing considerations

◆ Monitor the patient's vital signs, intake and output, and daily weight.
◆ Restrict fluids to 20 to 34 oz (600 ml to 1,000 ml) more than the urinary output for the previous day, if indicated.
◆ Provide diet low in sodium, potassium, and protein.
◆ Monitor serum electrolyte levels, blood urea nitrogen level, and creatinine.

PATIENT TEACHING
◆ Teach about the underlying diagnosis and treatment plan.
◆ Explain fluid and dietary restrictions.
◆ Teach about the administration, dosage, and possible adverse effects of prescribed medications.

Orthopnea

Overview

Orthopnea, difficulty breathing in a supine position, is a common symptom of cardiopulmonary disorders that produce dyspnea. It results from increased hydrostatic pressure in the pulmonary vasculature related to being in the supine position. It may be described as two- or three-pillow orthopnea, which refers to how many pillows a patient uses to help him breathe better during sleep.

Assessment

HISTORY

◆ Ask about the onset and description of orthopnea.
◆ Note how many pillows are used for sleeping.
◆ Obtain a medical history, including incidence of cardiopulmonary disorders, such as myocardial infarction, rheumatic heart disease, heart failure, valvular disease, asthma, emphysema, or chronic bronchitis.
◆ Find out about tobacco and alcohol use.
◆ Ask about associated cough, dyspnea, fatigue, weakness, loss of appetite, or chest pain.
◆ Obtain a drug history.

PHYSICAL ASSESSMENT

◆ Take vital signs.
◆ Check for other signs of increased respiratory effort, such as accessory muscle use, shallow respirations, and tachypnea.
◆ Inspect for a barrel chest.
◆ Inspect skin for pallor or cyanosis, and inspect the fingers for clubbing.
◆ Observe and palpate for edema.
◆ Check for jugular vein distention.
◆ Auscultate the lungs and heart.
◆ Monitor oxygen saturation.

Causes

MEDICAL

Chronic obstructive pulmonary disease

◆ Orthopnea and other dyspneic complaints are accompanied by accessory muscle use, tachypnea, tachycardia, and paradoxical pulse.
◆ Related signs and symptoms include diminished breath sounds, rhonchi, crackles, and wheezing on auscultation; dry or productive cough with copious sputum; anorexia; weight loss; and edema.
◆ Barrel chest, cyanosis, and clubbing are late signs.

Left-sided heart failure

◆ If heart failure is acute, orthopnea may begin suddenly; if chronic, it may be constant.
◆ Early signs and symptoms include progressively severe dyspnea, Cheyne-Stokes respirations, paroxysmal nocturnal dyspnea, fatigue, weakness, a cough that may occasionally produce clear or blood-tinged sputum, tachycardia, tachypnea, and crackles.
◆ Late signs and symptoms include cyanosis, clubbing, ventricular gallop, and hemoptysis.

Mediastinal tumor

◆ Orthopnea is an early sign.
◆ As the tumor enlarges, signs and symptoms include retrosternal chest pain; dry cough; hoarseness; dysphagia; stertorous respirations; palpitations; cyanosis; suprasternal retractions on inspiration; tracheal deviation; dilated jugular and superficial chest veins; and edema of the face, neck, and arms.

Valvular heart disease

◆ Orthopnea may occur.

◆ Other signs and symptoms of aortic insufficiency include fatigue, dyspnea, palpitations, dizziness, and angina. With heart failure, orthopnea, paroxysmal nocturnal dyspnea, and cough may also occur.

◆ Other signs and symptoms of aortic stenosis include syncope, angina, and dyspnea on exertion.

◆ Other signs and symptoms of mitral insufficiency include fatigue, dyspnea, palpitations, and angina.

◆ Other signs and symptoms of mitral stenosis include fatigue, weakness, dyspnea on exertion, nocturnal dyspnea, and palpitations.

Nursing considerations

◆ Monitor the patient's vital signs and pulse oximetry.

◆ Place the patient in semi-Fowler's or high Fowler's position. Alternatively, have the patient lean over a bedside table with his chest forward.

◆ Administer oxygen as indicated.

◆ Administer diuretics, as ordered, and monitor intake and output.

PATIENT TEACHING

◆ Discuss the underlying condition, diagnostic tests, and treatment options.

◆ Explain the signs and symptoms the patient should report.

◆ Explain dietary and fluid restrictions the patient needs to follow.

◆ Discuss daily weight measurement.

◆ Explain energy conservation measures as appropriate.

S & S

Palpitations

Overview

Palpitations, the conscious awareness of one's own heartbeat, feels like a pounding, jumping, turning, fluttering, flopping, or skipping beat. It's usually felt over the precordium or in the throat or neck, may be regular or irregular, fast or slow, paroxysmal or sustained.

Assessment

History

◆ Ask about the onset and description of palpitations.

◆ Inquire about aggravating and alleviating factors.

◆ Note associated signs and symptoms, such as dizziness, syncope, weakness, fatigue, angina, and pale, cool skin.

◆ Obtain a medical history, including cardiovascular or pulmonary disorder, or hypoglycemia.

◆ Obtain a drug history, including recently prescribed digoxin (Lanoxin).

◆ Ask about caffeine, tobacco, and alcohol use.

Physical assessment

◆ Obtain vital signs.

 Nursing alert

Suspect cardiac arrhythmia if hypotension and an irregular or abnormal pulse occur along with dizziness or shortness of breath and pale, cool, clammy skin. Begin cardiac monitoring and, if needed, prepare the patient for electrical cardioversion. Insert an I.V. catheter to administer an antiarrhythmic, if needed.

◆ Perform a complete cardiac and pulmonary assessment, which includes auscultating for gallops and murmurs and abnormal breath sounds.

Causes

Medical

Anemia

◆ Palpitations occur, especially on exertion, with pallor, fatigue, and dyspnea.

◆ Other findings include systolic ejection murmur, bounding pulse, tachycardia, crackles, an atrial gallop, and a systolic bruit over the carotid arteries.

Anxiety attack, acute

◆ Palpitations may be accompanied by diaphoresis, facial flushing, trembling, and an impending sense of doom.

◆ Hyperventilation may lead to dizziness, weakness, and syncope.

◆ Other findings include tachycardia, precordial pain, shortness of breath, restlessness, and insomnia.

Cardiac arrhythmias

◆ Paroxysmal or sustained palpitations may be accompanied by dizziness, weakness, and fatigue.

◆ Other findings include an irregular, rapid, or slow pulse rate; decreased blood pressure; confusion; pallor; chest pain; syncope; oliguria; and diaphoresis.

Hypertension

◆ Sustained palpitations may occur alone or with headache, dizziness, tinnitus, and fatigue.

◆ Blood pressure typically exceeds 140/90 mm Hg.

Hypocalcemia

◆ Palpitations occur with weakness, fatigue, muscle twitching, hyperactive deep tendon reflexes, chorea, and positive Chvostek's and Trousseau's signs.

◆ Paresthesia progresses to muscle tension and carpopedal spasms.

S & S

Hypoglycemia

◆ Sustained palpitations occur with fatigue, irritability, hunger, cold sweats, tremors, tachycardia, anxiety, and headache.

◆ Eventually, blurred or double vision, muscle weakness, hemiplegia, and altered level of consciousness develop.

Mitral prolapse

◆ Paroxysmal palpitations accompany sharp, stabbing, or aching precordial pain and midsystolic click, followed by an apical systolic murmur.

◆ Other findings include dyspnea, dizziness, severe fatigue, migraine headache, anxiety, paroxysmal tachycardia, crackles, and peripheral edema.

Mitral stenosis

◆ Early on, sustained palpitations accompany exertional dyspnea and fatigue.

◆ Loud first heart sound or opening snap and a rumbling diastolic murmur at the apex are heard on auscultation.

◆ Other findings include an atrial gallop and, with advanced disease, orthopnea, dyspnea at rest, paroxysmal nocturnal dyspnea, peripheral edema, jugular vein distention, ascites, hepatomegaly, and atrial fibrillation.

Pheochromocytoma

◆ Paroxysmal palpitations occur with dramatically elevated blood pressure (the main sign).

◆ Other findings include tachycardia, headache, chest or abdominal pain, diaphoresis, warm and pale or flushed skin, paresthesia, tremors, insomnia, nausea, vomiting, and anxiety.

Thyrotoxicosis

◆ Sustained palpitations may be accompanied by tachycardia, dyspnea, diarrhea, nervousness, tremors, diaphoresis, heat intolerance, weight loss despite increased appetite, atrial or ventricular gallop and, possibly, exophthalmos.

OTHER

Drugs

◆ Drugs, such as atropine, beta-adrenergic blockers, calcium channel blockers, digoxin (Lanoxin), ganglionic blockers, minoxidil (Loniten), and sympathomimetics, that precipitate cardiac arrhythmias or increase cardiac output may cause palpitations.

Exercise

◆ Exercise can cause palpitations.

Herbal remedies

◆ Herbal dietary supplements such as ginseng may cause adverse reactions including palpitations and an irregular heartbeat.

Nursing considerations

◆ Monitor the patient's vital signs and cardiac rhythm.

◆ Monitor for signs of reduced cardiac output.

◆ Prepare for procedures such as cardioversion.

◆ Provide supplemental oxygen.

◆ Administer antiarrhythmics as ordered.

◆ Provide for rest periods.

PATIENT TEACHING

◆ Teach about the underlying disorder and treatment options.

◆ Teach about the administration, dosage, and possible adverse effects of prescribed medications.

◆ Explain diagnostic tests.

◆ Teach the patient how to reduce anxiety.

S & S

Paralysis

Overview

Paralysis, the total loss of voluntary motor function from severe cortical or pyramidal tract damage, can be local or widespread, symmetrical or asymmetrical, transient or permanent, and spastic or flaccid. It's classified as paraplegia, quadriplegia, or hemiplegia.

 Nursing alert

If paralysis develops suddenly, suspect trauma or acute vascular insult. Immobilize the patient's spine, determine level of consciousness (LOC), take vital signs, and assess for signs of increasing intracranial pressure (ICP). Elevate the patient's head 30 degrees, if possible, to reduce ICP. Evaluate respiratory status, administer oxygen, and prepare the patient for intubation and mechanical ventilation as needed.

Assessment

HISTORY
◆ Determine the onset, duration, intensity, and progression of paralysis.
◆ Ask about events preceding the paralysis.
◆ Obtain a medical history, including history of neurologic or neuromuscular disease, recent infectious illness, sexually transmitted disease, cancer, recent injury, or recent immunizations.
◆ Find out about fever, headache, vision disturbances, dysphagia, nausea and vomiting, bowel or bladder dysfunction, muscle pain or weakness, and fatigue.

PHYSICAL ASSESSMENT
◆ Perform a complete neurologic examination.
◆ Test cranial nerve, motor, and sensory function, and deep tendon reflexes (DTRs).
◆ Assess strength in all major muscle groups, noting any muscle atrophy.

Causes

MEDICAL
Amyotrophic lateral sclerosis
◆ Spastic or flaccid paralysis occurs in the major muscle groups and progresses to total paralysis.
◆ Early findings include progressive muscle weakness, fasciculations, hyperreflexia, and muscle atrophy. Later, respiratory distress, dysarthria, drooling, choking, and difficulty chewing occur.

Bell's palsy
◆ Transient paralysis in muscles occurs on one side of the face.
◆ Increased tearing and drooling, inability to close the eyelid, and a diminished or absent corneal reflex occur.

Guillain-Barré syndrome
◆ A rapidly developing, reversible paralysis begins as leg muscle weakness and ascends symmetrically; respiratory muscle paralysis may be life-threatening.

Head trauma
◆ Sudden paralysis may occur; location and extent vary, depending on the injury.
◆ Other findings include decreased LOC, sensory disturbances, headache, blurred or double vision, nausea, vomiting, and focal neurologic disturbances.

Multiple sclerosis
◆ Paralysis waxes and wanes until the later stages, when it may become permanent; it ranges from monoplegia to quadriplegia.
◆ Late findings vary and may include muscle weakness and spasticity; hyperreflexia; intention tremor; gait ataxia; dysphagia; dysarthria; impotence; constipation; and urinary frequency, urgency, and incontinence.

Myasthenia gravis
◆ Muscle weakness and fatigue produce paralysis of certain muscle groups.

◆ Paralysis is usually transient in early stages but becomes more persistent as the disease progresses.
◆ Other findings include ptosis, diplopia, lack of facial mobility, dysphagia, dyspnea, and shallow respirations.

Neurosyphilis
◆ Irreversible hemiplegia may occur in the late stages, accompanied by dementia, cranial nerve palsies, meningitis, personality changes, tremors, and abnormal reflexes.

Peripheral nerve trauma
◆ Loss of motor and sensory function in the innervated area may occur.
◆ Muscles become flaccid and atrophied, and reflexes are lost.

Rabies
◆ Progressive flaccid paralysis, vascular collapse, coma, and death may occur within 2 weeks of contact with an infected animal.
◆ Early symptoms include fever; headache; hyperesthesia; photophobia; and excessive salivation, lacrimation, and perspiration.

Spinal cord injury
◆ Complete spinal cord transection results in permanent spastic paralysis below the level of the injury; reflexes may return after spinal shock resolves.
◆ Partial transection causes variable paralysis and paresthesia.

Spinal cord tumor
◆ Paresis, pain, paresthesia, and variable sensory loss may occur.
◆ Condition may progress to spastic paralysis with hyperactive DTRs, and bladder and bowel incontinence.

Stroke
◆ Contralateral paresis or paralysis may result if the motor cortex is involved.
◆ Other findings include headache, vomiting, seizures, decreased LOC, dysphagia,

ataxia, contralateral paresthesia or sensory loss, apraxia, aphasia, vision disturbances, and bowel and bladder dysfunction.

Subarachnoid hemorrhage
◆ Sudden paralysis (temporary or permanent) may occur.
◆ Other findings include severe headache, mydriasis, photophobia, aphasia, decreased LOC, nuchal rigidity, vomiting, and seizures.

Transient ischemic attack
◆ Transient paresis or paralysis may occur on one side along with paresthesia, blurred or double vision, dizziness, aphasia, dysarthria, and decreased LOC.

OTHER
Drugs
◆ Neuromuscular blockers produce paralysis.

Nursing considerations

◆ Monitor the patient's neurologic status.
◆ Reposition the patient every 2 hours, assess skin integrity, and provide skin care.
◆ Administer frequent chest physiotherapy.
◆ Perform passive range-of-motion (ROM) exercises.
◆ Apply splints as ordered.
◆ Arrange for physical, speech, and occupational therapy as appropriate.

PATIENT TEACHING
◆ Explain the underlying disorder and treatment plan.
◆ Provide referrals to social and psychological services.
◆ Teach the patient and his family how to provide care at home, including measures such as passive ROM exercises, frequent turning, and chest physiotherapy.

S & S

Paresthesia

Overview

Paresthesia describes abnormal sensations, such as numbness, prickling, or tingling, along peripheral nerve pathways. It may develop suddenly or gradually and may be transient or permanent.

Assessment

HISTORY

◆ Ask about the onset and nature of abnormal sensations.
◆ Ask about other findings, such as sensory loss and paresis.
◆ Find out about recent traumatic injury, surgery, or invasive procedures.
◆ Take a medical history, including neurologic, cardiovascular, metabolic, renal, and chronic inflammatory disorders.

PHYSICAL ASSESSMENT

◆ Assess level of consciousness (LOC) and cranial nerve function.
◆ Test muscle strength and deep tendon reflexes (DTRs) in affected limbs.
◆ Evaluate light touch, pain, temperature, vibration, and position sensation.
◆ Note skin color and temperature, and palpate pulses.

Causes

MEDICAL
Arterial occlusion, acute
◆ Sudden paresthesia and coldness occurs in the affected extremity; it may occur in one or both legs with a saddle embolus.
◆ Paresis, intermittent claudication, aching pain at rest, mottling, and absent pulses occur below the occlusion.

Guillain-Barré syndrome
◆ Transient paresthesia may precede muscle weakness, which usually begins in the legs and ascends to the arms and facial nerves.

◆ Other findings include dysarthria, dysphagia, nasal speech, orthostatic hypotension, bladder and bowel incontinence, diaphoresis, tachycardia and, possibly, life-threatening respiratory muscle paralysis.

Head trauma
◆ Paresthesia may occur with a concussion or contusion.
◆ Other findings include variable paresis or paralysis, decreased LOC, headache, blurred or double vision, nausea, vomiting, dizziness, and seizures.

Herniated disk
◆ Paresthesia may occur along with severe pain, muscle spasms, and weakness.

Migraine headache
◆ Paresthesia in hands, face, and perioral area may signal an impending migraine headache.
◆ Other early findings include scotomas, hemiparesis, confusion, dizziness, and photophobia.

Multiple sclerosis
◆ An early symptom, paresthesia commonly waxes and wanes until the later stages when it becomes permanent.
◆ Other findings include muscle weakness, spasticity, and hyperreflexia.

Peripheral neuropathy
◆ Progressive paresthesia may occur in all extremities.
◆ Other findings include muscle weakness that may progress to flaccid paralysis and atrophy, loss of vibration sensation, diminished or absent DTRs, and cutaneous changes.

Raynaud's disease
◆ Exposure to cold or stress turns fingers pale, cold, and cyanotic; with rewarming, they become red, throbbing, aching, swollen, and paresthetic.

Seizure disorder

♦ Paresthesia of the lips, fingers, and toes results from seizures originating in the parietal lobe.

♦ Paresthesia may act as auras that precede tonic-clonic seizures.

Spinal cord injury

♦ Paresthesia may occur in partial spinal cord transection, after spinal shock resolves, at or below the level of the lesion.

♦ Sensory and motor loss varies.

Spinal cord tumor

♦ Paresthesia, paresis, pain, and sensory loss occur.

♦ Eventually, paresis may cause spastic paralysis with hyperactive DTRs and, possibly, bladder and bowel incontinence.

Stroke

♦ Although contralateral paresthesia may occur, sensory loss is more common.

♦ Associated findings vary and may include contralateral hemiplegia, decreased LOC, and homonymous hemianopsia.

Thoracic outlet syndrome

♦ Paresthesia occurs suddenly when the affected arm is raised and abducted.

♦ The arm becomes pale and cool, with diminished pulses.

Transient ischemic attack

♦ Abrupt paresthesia is limited to an isolated body part.

♦ Other findings include decreased LOC, dizziness, unilateral vision loss, nystagmus, aphasia, dysarthria, tinnitus, facial weakness, dysphagia, and ataxic gait.

OTHER
Drugs

♦ Chemotherapeutics, chloroquine (Aralen), D-penicillamine (Depen), isoniazid (Nydrazid), nitrofurantoin (Macrobid), parenteral gold therapy, and phenytoin

(Dilantin) may produce transient paresthesia.

Radiation therapy

♦ Long-term radiation therapy may cause peripheral nerve damage, resulting in paresthesia.

Nursing considerations

♦ Monitor the patient's neurologic status.

♦ Help the patient perform daily activities as needed.

♦ If sensory deficits are present, protect the patient from injury.

PATIENT TEACHING

♦ Teach about the underlying diagnosis and treatment plan.

♦ Discuss safety measures.

♦ Tell the patient signs and symptoms to report to the practitioner.

Pericardial friction rub

Overview

A pericardial friction rub occurs when two inflamed layers of the pericardium slide over each other causing a scratching, grating, or crunching sound that ranges from faint to loud. A pericardial friction rub may be presystolic, systolic, and diastolic. The rub is best heard along the lower left sternal border during deep inspiration.

Assessment

HISTORY

◆ Take a medical history, noting instances of cancer, cardiac dysfunction, myocardial infarction, cardiac surgery, pericarditis, rheumatoid arthritis, chronic renal failure, infection, systemic lupus erythematosus, or trauma.
◆ Obtain a description of any chest pain, including its character, location, and aggravating and alleviating factors.

PHYSICAL ASSESSMENT

◆ Take the patient's vital signs, noting hypotension, tachycardia, irregular pulse, tachypnea, and fever.
◆ Inspect for jugular vein distention, edema, ascites, and hepatomegaly.
◆ Auscultate heart sounds; to listen for a pericardial friction rub, have the patient sit upright, lean forward and exhale.
◆ Auscultate the lungs for crackles.

Causes

MEDICAL
Pericarditis

◆ Pericardial rub, the classic sign of acute pericarditis, is accompanied by sharp precordial or retrosternal pain that radiates to the left shoulder, neck, and back.
◆ Pain worsens with deep breathing, coughing, and lying flat.
◆ Pain lessens when the patient sits up and leans forward.
◆ Other acute condition findings include fever, dyspnea, tachycardia, and arrhythmias.
◆ With the chronic condition, a pericardial rub develops gradually and may be accompanied by peripheral edema, ascites, Kussmaul's sign, hepatomegaly, dyspnea, orthopnea, paradoxical pulse, and chest pain.

OTHER
Drugs

◆ Chemotherapeutics and procainamide (Pronestyl) may cause pericarditis.

Treatments

◆ Cardiac surgery and high-dose radiation therapy may cause pericardial friction rub.

Nursing considerations

◆ Monitor the patient's cardiovascular status.

◆ If the pericardial friction rub disappears, look for signs of cardiac tamponade; if the signs develop, prepare the patient for pericardiocentesis.

◆ Ensure that the patient gets adequate rest.

◆ Give an anti-inflammatory, antiarrhythmic, diuretic, or antimicrobial, as ordered, to treat the underlying cause.

◆ Anticipate pericardiectomy to promote cardiac filling and contraction.

PATIENT TEACHING

◆ Teach about the underlying disorder and treatments.

◆ Explain what the patient can do to minimize symptoms.

Polyuria

Overview

Polyuria is the daily production and excretion of more than 3 L of urine. Urine is nearly colorless and has a low specific gravity.

Assessment

HISTORY

◆ Explore the frequency and pattern of polyuria.
◆ Ask for a description of patterns and amounts of daily fluid intake.
◆ Ask about fatigue, increased thirst, or weight loss.
◆ Obtain a medical history of vision deficits, headaches, head trauma, urinary tract obstruction, diabetes mellitus, renal disorder, chronic hypokalemia or hypercalcemia, or psychiatric disorder.
◆ Obtain a drug history.

PHYSICAL ASSESSMENT

◆ Obtain vital signs, noting increased body temperature, tachycardia, and orthostatic hypotension.
◆ Inspect for signs of dehydration.
◆ Perform a neurologic assessment, noting changes in level of consciousness.
◆ Palpate the bladder and inspect the urethral meatus.
◆ Obtain a urine specimen and check its specific gravity.

Causes

MEDICAL
Acute tubular necrosis

◆ During the diuretic phase, urine output of more than 8 L/day gradually subsides after about 1 week.
◆ Urine specific gravity (1.101 or less) increases as polyuria subsides.
◆ Related findings include weight loss, decreasing edema, and nocturia.

Diabetes insipidus

◆ Polyuria of about 5 L/day occurs along with a urine specific gravity of 1.005 or less.
◆ Other findings include polydipsia, nocturia, fatigue, and signs of dehydration.

Diabetes mellitus

◆ Polyuria is seldom more than 5 L/day, and urine specific gravity is typically more than 1.020.
◆ Other findings include polydipsia, polyphagia, weight loss, frequent urinary tract infections and yeast vaginitis, fatigue, signs of dehydration, and nocturia.

Glomerulonephritis, chronic

◆ Polyuria gradually progresses to oliguria.
◆ Usually, urine output is less than 4 L/day; specific gravity is about 1.010.
◆ Other findings include anorexia, nausea, vomiting, drowsiness, fatigue, edema, headache, elevated blood pressure, dyspnea, nocturia, hematuria, frothy or malodorous urine, and proteinuria.

Hypercalcemia

◆ Polyuria of more than 5 L/day occurs with a urine specific gravity of about 1.010.
◆ Other findings include polydipsia, nocturia, constipation, paresthesia and, occasionally, hematuria, and pyuria.
◆ With severe hypercalcemia, anorexia, vomiting, stupor progressing to coma, and renal failure occur.

Hypokalemia

◆ Prolonged potassium depletion causes polyuria of less than 5 L/day with a urine specific gravity of about 1.010.
◆ Other findings include polydipsia, circumoral and foot paresthesia, hypoactive deep tendon reflexes, fatigue, hypoactive bowel sounds, nocturia, arrhythmias, and muscle cramping, weakness, or paralysis.

Postobstructive uropathy
◆ After resolution of a urinary tract obstruction, polyuria with usually more than 5 L/day and a urine specific gravity of less than 1.010 occurs for several days before gradually subsiding.
◆ Other findings include bladder distention, edema, nocturia, and weight loss.

Pyelonephritis
◆ Polyuria of less than 5 L/day with a low but variable urine specific gravity occurs in acute disease along with persistent high fever, flank pain, hematuria, costovertebral angle tenderness, chills, weakness, dysuria, urinary frequency and urgency, tenesmus, and nocturia.
◆ Chronic pyelonephritis produces polyuria of less than 5 L/day that declines as renal function worsens; urine specific gravity is usually about 1.010 but may be higher if proteinuria is present. Other findings include irritability, paresthesia, fatigue, nausea, vomiting, diarrhea, drowsiness, anorexia, pyuria and, in late stages, elevated blood pressure.

Sickle cell anemia
◆ Polyuria occurs with a urinary output of less than 5 L/day with a specific gravity of about 1.020.
◆ Additional findings include polydipsia, fatigue, abdominal cramps, arthralgia, priapism, and, occasionally, leg ulcers and bony deformities.

OTHER
Diagnostic tests
◆ Radiographic tests that use contrast media may cause transient polyuria.

Drugs
◆ Diuretics, cardiotonics, vitamin D, demeclocycline (Declomycin), phenytoin (Dilantin), and lithium (Eskalith) may produce polyuria.

Nursing considerations
◆ Record intake and output, and weigh the patient daily.
◆ Monitor the patient's vital signs.
◆ Encourage fluid intake to maintain adequate fluid balance.

PATIENT TEACHING
◆ Teach the patient about the underlying disorder and treatment plan.
◆ Explain fluid replacement.
◆ Teach the patient to monitor his weight.
◆ Discuss signs and symptoms of dehydration that the patient needs to report to the practitioner.

S & S

Pupils, nonreactive

Overview

A nonreactive pupil fails to constrict in response to light or dilate when light is removed. It may signal a life-threatening emergency or brain death, but it may also occur with optic drug use.

Assessment

HISTORY

◆ Obtain medical history including recent infection.
◆ Ask about the use of eyedrops and when they were last instilled.
◆ Find out about pain and its location, intensity, and duration.
◆ Ask about recent trauma.
◆ Obtain information from family members if the patient is unable to respond.

PHYSICAL ASSESSMENT

◆ Assess the patient's neurologic status.

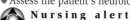 **Nursing alert**

If the patient is unconscious and has nonreactive pupils, quickly take his vital signs. Look for decerebrate or decorticate posture, bradycardia, elevated systolic blood pressure, and widened pulse pressure. One dilated, nonreactive pupil may be an early sign of uncal brain herniation. Emergency surgery to decrease intracranial pressure (ICP) may be necessary. Insert an I.V. line to administer a diuretic, an osmotic agent, or a corticosteroid to treat increased ICP as ordered. The patient may need controlled hyperventilation.

◆ Check visual acuity in both eyes.
◆ Test the pupillary reaction to accommodation.
◆ Examine the cornea and iris for abnormalities.
◆ Cover the affected eye with a protective metal shield.

Causes

MEDICAL

Botulism
◆ Nonreactive pupils and mydriasis in both eyes usually appear 12 to 36 hours after ingestion of tainted food.
◆ Other early findings include blurred vision, diplopia, ptosis, strabismus, extraocular muscle palsies, anorexia, nausea, vomiting, diarrhea, and dry mouth.
◆ Vertigo, deafness, hoarseness, nasal voice, dysarthria, and dysphagia follow.
◆ Progressive muscle weakness and absent deep tendon reflexes evolve over 2 to 4 days, resulting in severe constipation and paralysis of respiratory muscles with respiratory distress.

Encephalitis
◆ Initially sluggish pupils become dilated and nonreactive.
◆ Decreased accommodation and other symptoms of cranial nerve palsies develop.
◆ A decreased level of consciousness (LOC), high fever, headache, vomiting, and nuchal rigidity occur within 48 hours.
◆ Aphasia, ataxia, nystagmus, hemiparesis, and photophobia may occur with seizures.

Glaucoma, acute angle-closure
◆ A moderately dilated, nonreactive pupil occurs in the affected eye.
◆ Sudden blurred vision is followed by excruciating pain in and around the affected eye.
◆ Other findings include seeing halos around white lights at night, conjunctival injection, corneal clouding, and decreased visual acuity.
◆ Nausea and vomiting occur with severely elevated intraocular pressure (IOP).

Ocular trauma
◆ A transient or permanent nonreactive, dilated pupil may result from severe damage to the iris or optic nerve.
◆ Eye pain, eye edema, and ecchymoses may occur.
◆ A V-shaped notch in the pupillary rim, indicating a tear in the iris sphincter muscle, may be seen on slit-lamp examination.

Uveitis
◆ In anterior uveitis, a small, nonreactive pupil appears suddenly and is accompanied by severe eye pain, conjunctival injection, and photophobia.
◆ With posterior uveitis, similar features develop insidiously, along with blurred vision and distorted pupil shape.

Wernicke's disease
◆ Nonreactive pupils occur late in this disease related to thiamine deficiency.
◆ Initial findings include an intention tremor accompanied by a sluggish pupillary reaction.
◆ Other ocular findings include diplopia, gaze paralysis, nystagmus, ptosis, decreased visual acuity, and conjunctival injection.
◆ Orthostatic hypotension, tachycardia, ataxia, apathy, and confusion may also occur.

OTHER
Drugs
◆ Instillation of a topical mydriatic or cycloplegic may induce a temporarily nonreactive pupil in the affected eye.
◆ Opiates cause pinpoint pupils with a minimal light response that can be seen only with a magnifying glass.
◆ Atropine (AtroPen) poisoning produces widely dilated, nonreactive pupils.

Nursing considerations
◆ Monitor the patient's vital signs and LOC.
◆ If the patient is conscious, monitor his pupillary light reflex.
◆ If the patient is unconscious, close his eyes to prevent corneal exposure.

PATIENT TEACHING
◆ Explain to the patient and his family the underlying condition, diagnostic tests, and treatment options.
◆ Teach proper methods for instilling eye drops.
◆ Explain methods of reducing photophobia.
◆ Stress the importance of follow-up care to check IOP.

S & S

Respirations, shallow

Overview

Shallow respirations, a diminished volume of inspired air during ventilation, may lead to an accelerated respiratory rate as the patient attempts to obtain enough oxygen. Inadequate gas exchange may result as muscles tire and increased respiration diminishes. Shallow respirations may develop suddenly or gradually and may last briefly or become chronic, and are a key sign of respiratory distress and neurologic deterioration.

Assessment

HISTORY

♦ If possible, obtain a complete medical history, including chronic respiratory disorders or respiratory tract infection, neurologic or neuromuscular disease, surgery, and trauma.
♦ Ask if the patient has had a tetanus booster within the past 10 years.
♦ Obtain a smoking history.
♦ Obtain a drug history and explore the possibility of drug abuse.
♦ Determine the onset and duration of shallow respirations.
♦ Ask about factors that exacerbate or relieve shallow respirations.
♦ Ask about changes in appetite, weight, activity level, and behavior.

PHYSICAL ASSESSMENT

♦ Obtain vital signs and pulse oximetry.
♦ Evaluate the patient's level of consciousness (LOC) and his orientation to time, person, and place.
♦ Test muscle strength and deep tendon reflexes.
♦ Inspect the chest for deformities or abnormal movements.
♦ Inspect the extremities for cyanosis, edema, and digital clubbing.
♦ Palpate for expansion and diaphragmatic tactile fremitus.
♦ Percuss for hyperresonance or dullness.

♦ Auscultate for diminished, absent, or adventitious breath sounds, and for abnormal or distant heart sounds.
♦ Examine the abdomen for distention, tenderness, or masses.

Causes

MEDICAL
Acute respiratory distress syndrome
♦ Rapid, shallow respirations and dyspnea appear initially, sometimes after the patient appears stable.
♦ Other findings include intercostal and suprasternal retractions, diaphoresis, rhonchi, crackles, restlessness, apprehension, decreased LOC, cyanosis, and tachycardia.

Asthma
♦ Rapid, shallow respirations occur along with wheezing, rhonchi, a dry cough, dyspnea, prolonged expirations, intercostal and supraclavicular retractions on inspiration, nasal flaring, chest tightness, tachycardia, diaphoresis, and the use of accessory muscles.

Chronic bronchitis
♦ Shallow respirations result from chronic airway inflammation.
♦ Other findings include a nonproductive, hacking cough that later becomes productive; prolonged expirations; wheezing; dyspnea; accessory muscle use; barrel chest; cyanosis; tachypnea; scattered rhonchi; coarse crackles; and late-stage clubbing.

Emphysema
♦ Increased breathing effort causes muscle fatigue, leading to chronic shallow respirations.
♦ Other findings include dyspnea, anorexia, malaise, tachypnea, diminished breath sounds, cyanosis, pursed-lip breathing, accessory muscle use, barrel chest, chronic and productive cough, and late-stage clubbing.

Flail chest

◆ Decreased air movement results in rapid, shallow respirations and paradoxical chest wall motion.

◆ Other findings include tachycardia, hypotension, ecchymoses, cyanosis, and pain over the affected area.

Fractured ribs

◆ Sharp, severe pain on inspiration may cause shallow respirations.

◆ Other findings include dyspnea, cough, splinting, and tenderness and edema at the fracture site.

Guillain-Barré syndrome

◆ Progressive ascending paralysis causes rapid or progressive onset of shallow respirations.

◆ Other findings include paresthesia, dysarthria, diminished or absent corneal reflex, nasal speech, dysphagia, ipsilateral loss of facial muscle control, and flaccid paralysis.

Myasthenia gravis

◆ Progressive respiratory muscle weakness leads to shallow respirations, dyspnea, and cyanosis.

◆ Other findings include fatigue, weak eye closure, ptosis, diplopia, and difficulty chewing and swallowing.

Pneumonia

◆ Pulmonary consolidation results in rapid, shallow respirations.

◆ Accompanying findings include dyspnea, fever, shaking chills, chest pain, cough, tachycardia, decreased breath sounds, crackles, rhonchi, myalgia, fatigue, anorexia, headache, and cyanosis.

Pneumothorax

◆ Shallow respirations and dyspnea begin suddenly.

◆ Related findings include tachycardia, tachypnea, nonproductive cough, cyanosis, accessory muscle use, asymmetrical chest expansion, anxiety, restlessness, subcutaneous crepitation, diminished or absent breath sounds on the affected side, and sudden, sharp, severe chest pain that worsens with movement.

Spinal cord injury

◆ Diaphragmatic breathing and shallow respirations may occur in injury to the C5 to C8 cervical vertebrae.

◆ Other findings include quadriplegia with flaccidity followed by spastic paralysis, areflexia, hypotension, sensory loss below the level of injury, and bowel and bladder incontinence.

OTHER

Drugs

◆ Anesthetics, hypnotics and sedatives, magnesium sulfate, neuromuscular blockers, and opioids may produce slow, shallow respirations.

Surgery

◆ After abdominal or chest surgery, pain from chest splinting and decreased chest wall motion may cause shallow respirations.

Nursing considerations

◆ Monitor the patient's vital signs and pulse oximetry.

◆ Give oxygen, a bronchodilator, a mucolytic, an expectorant, or an antibiotic.

◆ Position the patient upright to ease his breathing.

◆ Monitor the patient for increasing lethargy, which may indicate rising carbon dioxide levels.

◆ Monitor respiratory and neurologic status.

PATIENT TEACHING

◆ Teach about the underlying diagnosis and treatment plan.

◆ Explain the importance of coughing and deep breathing.

◆ Teach about the administration, dosage, and possible adverse effects of prescribed medications.

Rhonchi

Overview

Rhonchi, continuous adventitious breath sounds detected by auscultation, are louder and lower-pitched than crackles, and may be described as rattling, sonorous, bubbling, rumbling, or musical. Rhonchi are commonly heard over large airways such as the trachea and can occur when air flows through passages that have been narrowed by secretions, a tumor or foreign body, bronchospasm, or mucosal thickening.

Assessment

HISTORY

◆ Obtain a smoking history.
◆ Ask about a history of asthma or other pulmonary disorder.
◆ Obtain a drug history.

PHYSICAL ASSESSMENT

◆ Obtain vital signs, including oxygen saturation.
◆ Characterize the patient's respirations as rapid or slow, shallow or deep, and regular or irregular.
◆ Inspect the chest, noting the use of accessory muscles.
◆ Listen for audible wheezing or gurgling.
◆ Auscultate for other abnormal breath sounds and note their location.
◆ Percuss the chest, and note the frequency and productivity of cough.

Causes

MEDICAL

Acute respiratory distress syndrome

◆ Initial features include dyspnea, rhonchi, crackles, and rapid shallow respirations.
◆ Intercostal and suprasternal retractions, diaphoresis, and fluid accumulation occur with developing hypoxemia.
◆ As hypoxemia worsens, findings include difficulty breathing, restlessness, apprehension, decreased level of consciousness, cyanosis, motor dysfunction, and tachycardia.

Aspiration of foreign body

◆ Inspiratory and expiratory rhonchi and wheezing occur.
◆ Other findings include diminished breath sounds over the obstructed area, fever, pain, and cough.

Asthma

◆ Rhonchi, crackles and, commonly, wheezing occur.
◆ Other findings include apprehension, a dry cough that later becomes productive, prolonged expirations, accessory muscle use, nasal flaring, tachypnea, tachycardia, diaphoresis, flushing or cyanosis, and intercostal and supraclavicular retractions on inspiration.

Bronchiectasis

◆ Lower-lobe rhonchi and crackles occur along with a cough that produces mucopurulent, foul-smelling sputum (classic sign).
◆ Other findings include fever, weight loss, exertional dyspnea, fatigue, malaise, halitosis, weakness, and late-stage clubbing.

Bronchitis

◆ Sonorous rhonchi and wheezing occur in acute tracheobronchitis along with chills, sore throat, fever, muscle and back pain, substernal tightness, and a cough that becomes productive as secretions increase.

◆ Scattered rhonchi, coarse crackles, wheezing, high-pitched piping sounds, and prolonged expirations occur with chronic bronchitis along with exertional dyspnea, increased accessory muscle use, barrel chest, cyanosis, tachypnea, and late-stage clubbing.

Emphysema

◆ Sonorous rhonchi may occur, but faint, high-pitched wheezing is more typical.

◆ Other findings include weight loss; anorexia; malaise; barrel chest; peripheral cyanosis; exertional dyspnea; accessory muscle use on inspiration; tachypnea; grunting expirations; late-stage clubbing; and a mild, chronic cough with scant sputum.

Pneumonia

◆ Bacterial pneumonias can cause rhonchi and a dry cough that later becomes productive.

◆ Related findings include shaking chills, high fever, myalgia, headache, pleuritic chest pain, tachypnea, tachycardia, dyspnea, cyanosis, diaphoresis, decreased breath sounds, and fine crackles.

OTHER
Diagnostic tests

◆ Pulmonary function tests or bronchoscopy can loosen secretions and mucus, causing rhonchi.

Respiratory therapy

◆ Respiratory therapy may produce rhonchi from loosened secretions and mucus.

Nursing considerations

◆ Monitor the patient's vital signs and pulse oximetry.

◆ Place the patient in semi-Fowler's position, and administer oxygen as indicated.

◆ Give an antibiotic, a bronchodilator, and an expectorant as ordered.

◆ Promote coughing, deep breathing, and use of incentive spirometry.

◆ Provide pulmonary physiotherapy with postural drainage and percussion.

◆ Use tracheal suctioning, if necessary.

PATIENT TEACHING

◆ Explain the underlying cause and treament plan.

◆ Teach deep-breathing and coughing techniques.

◆ Stress the need for increasing fluid intake.

◆ Discuss increasing activity levels.

S & S

Seizures, absence

Overview

Absence seizures, also known as *petit mal seizures*, are benign, generalized seizures of unknown cause that are thought to originate subcortically. They occur as brief episodes of unconsciousness without warning, usually lasting 3 to 20 seconds and possibly occurring 100 or more times per day. They cause periods of inattention, with amnesia occurring after the seizure.

Patients tend not to experience warning signs before an absence seizure. In fact, the patient may not even be aware of the seizure's occurrence.

Simple absence seizures involve staring. Complex absence seizures involve staring as well as muscle activity, such as eye blinking or chewing movements of the mouth.

 Age considerations
Absence seizures usually begin between ages 4 and 12.

Assessment

HISTORY
◆ Obtain a history of the seizures from the parents and the child, including:
  ● how long they have been occurring
  ● how long each one lasts
  ● how far apart they are.
◆ Find out if the patient has been treated for seizures in the past.
◆ Ask family members whether they have noticed a change in behavior or deteriorating schoolwork.
◆ Ask about triggering events, such as flashing lights or hyperventilation.

PHYSICAL ASSESSMENT
◆ Evaluate absence seizure occurrence and duration by reciting a series of numbers and then asking the patient to repeat them after the attack ends. If the patient has had an absence seizure, he'll be unable to do this. Alternatively, if the seizures are occurring within minutes of each other, ask the patient to count for about 5 minutes. He'll stop counting during a seizure and resume when it's over.
◆ Look for accompanying automatisms (automatic repetitive behavior).

Causes

MEDICAL
Idiopathic epilepsy
◆ Absence seizure may be accompanied by learning disabilities.
◆ Absence seizures may produce automatisms, such as repetitive lip smacking, or mild clonic or myoclonic movements, including mild jerking of the eyelids.
◆ The patient may drop an object that he's holding, and muscle relaxation may cause him to drop his head or arms or to slump.

Nursing considerations

◆ Prepare the patient for diagnostic tests, such as computed tomography scan, magnetic resonance imaging, and EEG.
◆ Provide emotional support to the patient and his family.
◆ Ensure a safe environment for the patient.

PATIENT TEACHING

◆ Teach the patient and his family about these seizures and how to recognize their onset, pattern, and duration.
◆ Teach the family how to care for the patient during a seizure.
◆ Include the child's teacher and school nurse in the teaching process, if possible.
◆ If the seizures are being controlled with drug therapy, emphasize the importance of strict compliance.
◆ Teach about the administration, dosage, and possible adverse effects of prescribed medications.

S & S

Seizures, complex partial

Overview

Complex partial seizures occur when focal seizures begin in the temporal lobe and cause partial alterations of consciousness. They're usually preceded by an aura—a complex hallucination, illusion, or sensation—and may cause audiovisual, auditory, or olfactory hallucinations. Other types of auras include sensations of déjà vu, unfamiliarity with surroundings, or depersonalization, and they may cause confusion, drowsiness, and amnesia after the seizure occurs. Repeated complex partial seizures commonly lead to generalized seizures.

Assessment

HISTORY
◆ Ask about the occurrence of an aura.
◆ Ask witnesses for a description of the seizure.
◆ Find out about previous seizures or therapies.
◆ Ask about a history of head trauma.

PHYSICAL ASSESSMENT
◆ Examine the patient for injury after the seizure.
◆ Ensure a patent airway.
◆ Perform a complete neurologic assessment.

Causes

MEDICAL
Brain abscess
◆ If the temporal lobe is affected, complex partial seizures commonly occur after the abscess resolves.
◆ Headache, nausea, vomiting, generalized seizures, a decreased level of consciousness (LOC), central facial weakness, auditory receptive aphasia, hemiparesis, and ocular disturbances may occur.

Head trauma
◆ Trauma to the temporal lobe may produce complex partial seizures months or years later.
◆ Seizures may decrease in frequency and eventually stop.
◆ Generalized seizures and behavior and personality changes may occur.

Temporal lobe tumor
◆ Complex partial seizures may be the first sign.
◆ Other findings include headache, pupillary changes, and mental dullness.
◆ Increased intracranial pressure may cause a decreased LOC, vomiting, and papilledema.

Nursing considerations

◆ After the seizure, reorient the patient to his surroundings and protect him from injury.
◆ Keep the patient in bed until he's fully alert.
◆ Remove harmful objects from the area.
◆ Provide emotional support to the patient and his family.
◆ Monitor for therapeutic drug levels.

PATIENT TEACHING
◆ Discuss methods for coping with seizures.
◆ Instruct the patient and his family in safety measures to take during a seizure.
◆ Teach about the administration, dosage, and possible adverse effects of prescribed medications.
◆ Emphasize compliance with drug therapy.
◆ Tell the patient to carry medical identification.

Seizures, generalized tonic-clonic

Overview

Generalized tonic-clonic seizures, also known as *grand mal seizures,* are caused by paroxysmal, uncontrolled discharge of central nervous system neurons, leading to neurologic dysfunction. They extend to the entire brain and result in uncontrolled muscle rigidity, violent muscle contractions, and loss of consciousness. An aura may precede the seizure, with a postictal period following the seizure in which the patient experiences sleepiness and confusion.

Assessment

HISTORY

◆ Obtain a description of the seizure, including onset, duration, body area affected, characteristics, and progression.
◆ Ask about unusual sensations before the seizure.
◆ Find out about a personal and family history of seizures.
◆ Obtain a drug history.
◆ Ask about head trauma, sleep deprivation, or emotional or physical stress at the time of seizure.
◆ Obtain a medical history.

PHYSICAL ASSESSMENT

◆ If a head injury is suspected, observe the patient closely for loss of consciousness, unequal or nonreactive pupils, and focal neurologic signs.
◆ Examine the arms, legs, face, and tongue for injury, residual paralysis, or limb weakness.
◆ Obtain vital signs.
◆ Complete a neurologic assessment.
◆ Observe for adequate oxygenation.

Causes

MEDICAL
Alcohol withdrawal syndrome
◆ Seizures as well as status epilepticus may occur 7 to 48 hours after sudden alcohol withdrawal.

◆ Other findings include restlessness, hallucinations, profuse diaphoresis, and tachycardia.

Brain abscess
◆ Generalized seizures may occur in the acute stage of abscess formation or after the abscess disappears.
◆ Constant headache, nausea, vomiting, and focal seizures are early signs and symptoms.
◆ Other findings include decreased level of consciousness (LOC), ocular disturbances, aphasia, hemiparesis, abnormal behavior, and personality changes.

Brain tumor
◆ Generalized seizures may occur, depending on the tumor's location and type.
◆ Other findings include a slowly decreasing LOC, morning headache, dizziness, confusion, focal seizures, vision loss, motor and sensory disturbances, aphasia, and ataxia.

Eclampsia
◆ Generalized seizures are a hallmark sign.
◆ Other findings include severe frontal headache, nausea, vomiting, vision disturbances, increased blood pressure, fever, peripheral edema, oliguria, irritability, hyperactive deep tendon reflexes (DTRs), decreased LOC, and sudden weight gain.

Encephalitis
◆ Seizures are an early sign, indicating a poor prognosis. Seizures may also occur after recovery as a result of residual damage.
◆ Other findings include fever, headache, photophobia, nuchal rigidity, neck pain, vomiting, aphasia, ataxia, hemiparesis, nystagmus, irritability, cranial nerve palsies, and myoclonic jerks.

Head trauma
◆ Generalized seizures may occur at the time of injury; focal seizures may occur months later.

◆ Other findings include decreased LOC; soft-tissue injury of the face, head, or neck; clear or bloody drainage from the mouth, nose, or ears; facial edema; bony deformity of the face, head, or neck; Battle's sign; and lack of response to oculocephalic and oculovestibular stimulation; motor and sensory deficits; altered respirations; and signs of increasing intracranial pressure.

Hypertensive encephalopathy
◆ Seizures with increased blood pressure, decreased LOC, intense headache, vomiting, transient blindness, paralysis, and Cheyne-Stokes respirations occur with this life-threatening disorder.

Hyponatremia
◆ Seizure develops when sodium level falls below 125 mEq/L, especially if the decrease is rapid.
◆ Other findings include orthostatic hypotension, headache, muscle twitching and weakness, fatigue, oliguria or anuria, cold and clammy skin, decreased skin turgor, irritability, lethargy, confusion, and stupor or coma.

Hypoparathyroidism
◆ Generalized seizures occur as a result of worsening tetany.
◆ Chronic condition produces neuromuscular irritability, Chvostek's sign, dysphagia, tetany, and hyperactive DTRs.

Renal failure, chronic
◆ Onset of twitching, trembling, myoclonic jerks, and generalized seizures is rapid.
◆ Other signs and symptoms include anuria or oliguria, fatigue, malaise, irritability, decreased mental acuity, muscle cramps, peripheral neuropathies, pruritus, uremic frost, anorexia, constipation or diarrhea, ammonia breath odor, nausea and vomiting, ecchymoses, petechiae, GI bleeding, mouth and gum ulcers, hypertension, and Kussmaul's respirations.

Stroke
◆ Seizures (focal more often than generalized) may occur within 6 months of an ischemic stroke.
◆ Other findings vary but may include decreased LOC, contralateral hemiplegia, dysarthria, dysphagia, ataxia, sensory loss on one side, apraxia, agnosia, aphasia, visual deficits, memory loss, personality changes, emotional lability, and incontinence.

OTHER
Drugs
◆ Amphetamines, isoniazid (Nydrazid), phenothiazines, tricyclic antidepressants, and vincristine (Oncovin) may cause seizures in patients with preexisting epilepsy.
◆ Toxic levels of some drugs, such as cimetidine (Tagamet), lidocaine (Xylocaine), meperidine (Demerol), penicillins, and theophylline (Theo-Dur), may cause generalized seizures.

Nursing considerations

◆ Support the patient's respiratory status, if indicated.
◆ Protect the patient from injury.
◆ Monitor the patient after the seizure for recurring seizure activity.
◆ Monitor for therapeutic drug levels.
◆ Monitor vital signs and neurologic status.

PATIENT TEACHING
◆ Explain the underlying disorder, if appropriate, and treatment plan.
◆ Teach about the administration, dosage, and possible adverse effects of prescribed medications. Stress compliance with drug therapy.
◆ Teach the patient's family how to provide safety during a seizure, and what to report to the practitioner about the seizure.
◆ Tell the patient to carry medical identification.

Seizures, simple partial

Overview

Simple partial seizures, also known as *focal seizures*, result from an irritable focus in the cerebral cortex and vary in type and pattern. They last about 30 seconds and don't alter level of consciousness (LOC). Motor simple partial seizures include jacksonian seizures and epilepsia partialis continua. Somatosensory simple partial seizures include visual, olfactory, and auditory seizures.

Assessment

HISTORY
◆ Obtain a description of the seizure activity.
◆ Ask about events leading up to the seizure.
◆ Ask if the patient can describe an aura or recognize its onset.
◆ Ask about LOC, tonicity and clonicity, cyanosis, tongue biting, and urinary incontinence.
◆ Ask about a history of head trauma, stroke, or infection with fever, headache, or stiff neck.

PHYSICAL ASSESSMENT
◆ Perform a complete physical assessment, focusing on the neurologic assessment.
◆ Check LOC.
◆ Test for residual deficits and sensory disturbances.

Causes

MEDICAL
Brain abscess
◆ Seizures may occur in the acute stage of abscess formation or after resolution of the abscess.
◆ Decreased LOC varies from drowsiness to deep stupor.
◆ Early findings reflect increased intracranial pressure, such as a constant, intractable headache, nausea, and vomiting.
◆ Later findings include ocular disturbances, such as nystagmus, decreased visual acuity, and unequal pupils.
◆ Other findings vary with the abscess site and may include aphasia, hemiparesis, and personality changes.

Brain tumor
◆ Simple partial seizures are commonly the earliest indicators.
◆ Morning headache, dizziness, confusion, vision loss, and motor and sensory disturbances may occur.
◆ Other findings include aphasia, generalized seizures, ataxia, decreased LOC, papilledema, vomiting, increased systolic blood pressure, widening pulse pressure and, eventually, decorticate posture.

Head trauma
◆ Penetrating wounds are associated with simple partial seizures.
◆ Seizures usually begin 3 to 15 months after injury, decrease in frequency after several years, and eventually stop.
◆ Generalized seizures and a decreased LOC may progress to coma.

Multiple sclerosis

◆ Simple partial or generalized seizures may occur in the late stages.

◆ Other findings include visual deficits, paresthesia, constipation, muscle weakness, spasticity, paralysis, hyperreflexia, intention tremor, gait ataxia, dysphagia, dysarthria, emotional lability, impotence, and urinary frequency, urgency, and incontinence.

Neurofibromatosis

◆ Multiple brain lesions cause focal seizures and, at times, generalized seizures.

◆ Other findings include café-au-lait spots, multiple skin tumors, scoliosis, kyphoscoliosis, dizziness, ataxia, progressive monocular blindness, nystagmus, and endocrine abnormalities.

Stroke

◆ Simple partial seizures may occur up to 6 months after a stroke's onset; generalized seizures may also occur.

◆ Accompanying effects vary and may include decreased LOC, contralateral hemiplegia, dysarthria, dysphagia, ataxia, unilateral sensory loss, apraxia, agnosia, and aphasia.

◆ Other findings include vision deficits, memory loss, poor judgment, personality changes, emotional lability, headache, urinary incontinence or retention, and vomiting.

Nursing considerations

◆ Remain with the patient during the seizure, maintain his safety, and provide reassurance.

◆ Monitor the patient's neurologic status.

◆ Give anticonvulsants as prescribed.

◆ Provide emotional support.

◆ Monitor for therapeutic drug levels.

PATIENT TEACHING

◆ Explain the underlying disorder, if applicable, and the treatment plan.

◆ Teach the patient's family how to document seizures.

◆ Teach about the administration, dosage, and possible adverse effects of prescribed medications. Stress the importance of complying with the prescribed drug regimen.

◆ Provide information on maintaining a safe environment.

◆ Tell the patient to carry medical identification.

S & S

Skin, mottled

Overview

Mottled skin refers to patchy skin discolorations that signify changes in deep, middle, or superficial dermal blood vessels. This sign may indicate an emergency condition, such as a ruptured abdominal aortic aneurysm.

Assessment

HISTORY

◆ Ask about the onset of mottled skin (sudden or gradual).
◆ Determine precipitating, aggravating, and alleviating factors.
◆ Ask about associated pain, numbness, or tingling in the extremity.
◆ Obtain a medical history, including history of cardiovascular disease, respiratory illness or abdominal aneurysm.

PHYSICAL ASSESSMENT

◆ Obtain vital signs and pulse oximetry.
◆ Observe the patient's skin color.
◆ Palpate the arms and legs for skin texture, swelling, and temperature differences.
◆ Check capillary refill time.
◆ Palpate for pulses and note their quality.
◆ Note breaks in the skin, muscle appearance, and hair distribution.
◆ Assess motor and sensory function.

Causes

MEDICAL
Abdominal aortic aneurysm, ruptured
◆ Mottling of lower extremites may extend to the abdomen.
◆ Other findings include retroperitoneal pain, hypotension, altered level of consciousness (LOC) and signs of hypovolemia.

Arterial occlusion, acute
◆ Temperature and color changes that develop at the level of obstruction are initial signs of this disorder.
◆ Pallor may change to blotchy cyanosis and mottling.
◆ Other findings include sudden onset of pain in the extremity, diminished or absent pulses, cool extremity, increased capillary refill time, pallor, diminished reflexes and, possibly, paresthesia, paresis, and a sensation of cold in the affected area.

Arteriosclerosis obliterans
◆ Leg pallor, cyanosis, blotchy erythema, and mottled skin develop.
◆ Other findings include intermittent claudication, diminished or absent pedal pulses, paresthesia, increased capillary refill time, and leg coolness.

Buerger's disease
◆ Color changes and mottling, particularly livedo networking in the lower extremities, occur.
◆ Intermittent claudication and erythema along extremity blood vessels can occur.
◆ During cold exposure, feet become cold, cyanotic, and numb; later, they become hot, red, and tingling.
◆ Other possible findings include impaired peripheral pulses and peripheral neuropathy.

Hypovolemic shock
◆ Vasoconstriction commonly produces skin mottling, initially in the knees and elbows.
◆ As shock worsens, mottling becomes generalized.
◆ Early signs include sudden onset of pallor, cool skin, restlessness, thirst, tachypnea, and slight tachycardia.
◆ As shock progresses, other findings include cool, clammy skin; rapid, thready pulse; hypotension; narrowed pulse pres-

S & S

sure; decreased urine output; subnormal temperature; confusion; and decreased LOC.

Livedo reticularis, idiopathic or primary
◆ Symmetrical, diffuse mottling may involve the hands, feet, arms, legs, buttocks, and trunk.
◆ Initially, networking is intermittent and most pronounced on exposure to cold or stress; eventually, mottling persists even with warming.

Polycythemia vera
◆ Mottling, hemangiomas, purpura, rubor, ulcerative nodules, and scleroderma-like lesions develop.
◆ Other symptoms include headache, a vague feeling of fullness in the head, dizziness, vertigo, vision disturbances, dyspnea, and aquagenic pruritus.

Rheumatoid arthritis
◆ Skin mottling may occur.
◆ Early findings include joint pain and stiffness with subcutaneous nodules on the elbows.

Systemic lupus erythematosus
◆ Mottling occurs most commonly on the outer arms.
◆ Other findings include a butterfly rash, nondeforming joint pain and stiffness, photosensitivity, Raynaud's phenomenon, patchy alopecia, seizures, fever, anorexia, weight loss, lymphadenopathy, and emotional lability.

OTHER
Thermal exposure
◆ Prolonged thermal exposure, such as from a heating pad or hot water bottle, may cause localized, reticulated, brown-to-red mottling.

Nursing considerations
◆ Monitor the patient's vital signs, intake and output, and peripheral pulses.
◆ Treat the underlying condition as ordered.

PATIENT TEACHING
◆ Teach about the underlying condition and treatment plan.
◆ Encourage the patient to avoid tight clothing and overexposure to cold or heating devices.
◆ Teach about the administration, dosage, and possible adverse effects of prescribed medications.

S & S

Splenomegaly

Overview

Splenomegaly, the enlargement of the spleen, results from any process that triggers lymphadenopathy, such as infection or inflammation, cancer, increased blood cell destruction, or vascular congestion from portal hypertension. It's detected by light palpation under the left costal margin.

HISTORY

◆ Ask about fatigue; frequent colds, sore throats, or other infections; bruising; left-upper-quadrant pain; abdominal fullness; and early satiety.
◆ Obtain a complete medical history.
◆ Ask about recent trauma or surgery.

PHYSICAL ASSESSMENT

◆ Complete an abdominal assessment.

⬥ Nursing alert

If the patient has a history of abdominal or thoracic trauma, don't palpate the abdomen because this may aggravate internal bleeding. Instead, examine for left-upper-quadrant pain and signs of shock. If these signs are present, suspect splenic rupture. Insert an I.V. catheter for emergency fluid and blood replacement, and administer oxygen. Catheterize the patient to evaluate urine output and begin cardiac monitoring. Prepare the patient for possible surgery.
◆ Examine the skin for pallor and ecchymoses.
◆ Palpate the axillae, groin, and neck for lymphadenopathy.

Causes

MEDICAL
Cirrhosis
◆ Moderate to severe splenomegaly occurs with advanced cirrhosis.
◆ Late findings also include jaundice, hepatomegaly, leg edema, hematemesis, and ascites.
◆ Signs of hepatic encephalopathy may also occur, such as asterixis, fetor hepaticus, slurred speech, and decreased level of consciousness that may progress to coma.

Endocarditis, subacute infective
◆ The spleen is enlarged but nontender.
◆ A suddenly changing murmur or the discovery of a new murmur in the presence of a fever is a classic sign.
◆ Other findings include anorexia, pallor, weakness, fever, night sweats, fatigue, tachycardia, weight loss, arthralgia, petechiae, hematuria, Osler's nodes, and Janeway lesions.

Hepatitis
◆ Splenomegaly may occur. Characteristic findings include dark urine, clay-colored stools, anorexia, malaise, pruritus, hepatomegaly, vomiting, jaundice, and fatigue.

Histoplasmosis
◆ Splenomegaly and hepatomegaly occur.
◆ Other findings include lymphadenopathy, jaundice, fever, anorexia, and signs and symptoms of anemia.

Hypersplenism, primary
◆ Splenomegaly accompanies anemia, neutropenia, or thrombocytopenia.
◆ Left-sided abdominal pain may occur.

Leukemia

♦ Moderate to severe splenomegaly is an early sign.

♦ With chronic granulocytic leukemia, findings include hepatomegaly, lymphadenopathy, fatigue, malaise, pallor, fever, gum swelling, bleeding tendencies, weight loss, anorexia, and abdominal, bone, and joint pain.

♦ Acute leukemia may produce dyspnea, tachycardia, and palpitations.

Lymphoma

♦ Moderate to massive splenomegaly is a late sign.

♦ Other late findings include hepatomegaly, painless lymphadenopathy, night sweats, fever, fatigue, weight loss, malaise, and scaly dermatitis with pruritus.

Mononucleosis, infectious

♦ Splenomegaly, a common sign, is most pronounced during second and third weeks of illness.

♦ The classic triad includes sore throat, cervical lymphadenopathy, and fluctuating temperature with an evening peak.

♦ Hepatomegaly, jaundice, and a maculopapular rash may develop.

Pancreatic cancer

♦ Moderate to severe splenomegaly may occur if a tumor compresses the splenic vein.

♦ Other characteristic findings include abdominal or back pain, anorexia, nausea, vomiting, weight loss, GI bleeding, jaundice, pruritus, skin lesions, emotional lability, weakness, and fatigue.

Polycythemia vera

♦ Splenomegaly results in easy satiety, abdominal fullness, and left-upper-quadrant

pain or pleuritic chest pain late in the disease.

♦ Finger and toe paresthesia, impaired mentation, tinnitus, blurred or double vision, scotoma, increased blood pressure, pruritus, epigastric distress, weight loss, hepatomegaly, bleeding tendencies, and intermittent claudication occur.

♦ Other possible findings include deep purplish red oral mucous membranes, headache, dyspnea, dizziness, vertigo, weakness, and fatigue.

Splenic rupture

♦ Splenomegaly may result from massive abdominal or thoracic hemorrhage that predisposes the spleen to rupture.

♦ Other findings include abdominal rigidity, left-upper-quadrant pain, Kehr's sign, and signs of shock.

Nursing considerations

♦ Monitor the patient's vital signs and blood count.

♦ Prepare the patient for diagnostic tests.

♦ Provide measures to treat the underlying disorder.

PATIENT TEACHING

♦ Teach about underlying diagnosis and treatment plan.

♦ Instruct the patient to avoid infection.

♦ Emphasize the importance of complying with drug therapy.

S & S

Stridor

Overview

Stridor, a loud, harsh, musical respiratory sound that results from an obstruction in the trachea or larynx, is usually heard during inspiration, but may also occur during expiration in severe upper airway obstruction. It may begin as a low-pitched croaking and progress to high-pitched crowing as respirations become more vigorous.

HISTORY
◆ Ask about the onset of stridor.
◆ Ask about previous instances of stridor.
◆ Note whether the patient has a current respiratory tract infection.
◆ Ask about a history of allergies, tumors, or respiratory and vascular disorders.
◆ Note recent exposure to smoke or noxious fumes or gases.
◆ Ask about associated pain or cough.

PHYSICAL ASSESSMENT
◆ Check vital signs, including oxygen saturation.
◆ Examine the mouth for excessive secretions, foreign matter, inflammation, and swelling.
◆ Assess the neck for swelling, masses, subcutaneous crepitation, and scars.
◆ Observe the chest for decreased or asymmetrical expansion.
◆ Auscultate for wheezes, rhonchi, crackles, rubs, and other abnormal breath sounds.
◆ Percuss for dullness, tympany, or flatness.
◆ Inspect for burns or signs of trauma.

◈ Nursing alert
Abrupt end of stridor signals complete airway obstruction. If you detect complete airway obstruction, clear the airway with back blows or abdominal thrusts. Give oxygen or prepare to assist with emergency endotracheal intubation or tracheostomy and mechanical ventilation. Suction aspirated vomitus or blood.

Causes

MEDICAL
Airway trauma
◆ Acute airway obstruction results in the sudden onset of stridor.
◆ Other findings include dysphonia, dysphagia, hemoptysis, cyanosis, accessory muscle use, intercostal retractions, nasal flaring, tachypnea, progressive dyspnea, and shallow respirations.

Anaphylaxis
◆ Upper airway edema and laryngospasm cause stridor and other signs of respiratory distress.
◆ Typically, respiratory effects are preceded by a feeling of impending doom or fear, weakness, diaphoresis, sneezing, nasal pruritus, urticaria, erythema, and angioedema.
◆ Other common findings include chest or throat tightness, dysphagia and, possibly, signs of shock.

Anthrax, inhalation
◆ Initial findings include fever, chills, weakness, cough, and chest pain.
◆ The second stage develops abruptly with rapid deterioration marked by stridor, fever, dyspnea, and hypotension generally leading to death within 24 hours.

Aspiration of a foreign body
◆ Sudden stridor is characteristic in this life-threatening situation.
◆ Other findings include abrupt onset of dry, paroxysmal coughing, gagging, or choking; hoarseness; tachycardia; wheezing; dyspnea; tachypnea; intercostal muscle retractions; diminished breath sounds; cyanosis; anxiety; and shallow respirations.

S & S

Epiglottiditis

◆ Stridor occurs along with fever, sore throat, and a croupy cough in this life-threatening situation.

◆ Other findings include cough that may progress to severe respiratory distress with sternal and intercostal retractions, nasal flaring, cyanosis, and tachycardia.

Hypocalcemia

◆ Stridor results from laryngospasm. Other findings include paresthesia, carpopedal spasm, hyperactive deep tendon reflexes, muscle twitching and cramping, and positive Chvostek's and Trousseau's signs.

Inhalation injury

◆ Laryngeal edema and bronchospasms, resulting in stridor, may develop within 48 hours after inhalation of smoke or noxious fumes.

◆ Other findings include singed nasal hairs, orofacial burns, coughing, hoarseness, sooty sputum, crackles, rhonchi, wheezes, dyspnea, accessory muscle use, intercostal retractions, and nasal flaring.

Laryngitis, acute

◆ Mild to severe hoarseness is the chief sign.

◆ Severe laryngeal edema, resulting in stridor and dyspnea, may occur.

◆ Other findings include sore throat, dysphagia, dry cough, malaise, and fever.

Mediastinal tumor

◆ Compression of the trachea and bronchi results in stridor.

◆ Other findings include hoarseness, brassy cough, tracheal shift or tug, dilated neck veins, swelling of the face and neck, stertorous respirations, dyspnea, dysphagia, suprasternal retractions on inspiration, and pain in the chest, shoulder, or arm.

Thoracic aortic aneurysm

◆ If the trachea is compressed, stridor, dyspnea, wheezing, and a brassy cough may result.

◆ Other findings include hoarseness or complete voice loss, dysphagia, jugular vein distention, prominent chest veins, tracheal tug, paresthesia or neuralgia, and edema of the face, neck, and arms.

OTHER

Diagnostic tests

◆ Bronchoscopy or laryngoscopy may precipitate laryngospasm and stridor as a result of airway irritation.

Treatments

◆ Neck surgery, such as thyroidectomy, may cause laryngeal paralysis and stridor.

◆ After prolonged intubation, the patient may exhibit laryngeal edema and stridor when the tube is removed.

Nursing considerations

◆ Provide supportive emergency measures as indicated.

◆ Monitor the patient's vital signs, pulse oximetry, and respiratory status.

◆ Prepare the patient for diagnostic tests.

◆ Offer reassurance and calm the patient.

◆ Administer antibiotics and respiratory treatments as ordered.

PATIENT TEACHING

◆ Teach about the underlying diagnosis and the treatment plan.

◆ Explain all procedures and treatments.

◆ Teach about the administration, dosage, and possible adverse effects of prescribed medications.

◆ Review safety measures if stridor resulted from foreign body aspiration.

Syncope

Overview

Syncope, a transient loss of consciousness, may be associated with impaired cerebral blood supply or cerebral hypoxia, and may be abrupt and last for seconds to minutes.

HISTORY
◆ Obtain a description of the syncopal episode and its duration.
◆ Ask about precipitating factors.
◆ Ask about preceding symptoms, including weakness, light-headedness, nausea, or diaphoresis.
◆ Ask about associated headache.
◆ Obtain a history of previous syncopal episodes, cardiac arrhythmias, and medication use.

PHYSICAL ASSESSMENT
◆ Obtain the patient's vital signs.
◆ Examine the patient for any injuries from falling during syncope.
◆ Perform a complete cardiac and neurologic assessment.

Causes

MEDICAL
Aortic arch syndrome
◆ Syncope may be accompanied by weak or abruptly absent carotid pulses and unequal or absent radial pulses.
◆ Early findings include night sweats, pallor, nausea, anorexia, weight loss, arthralgia, and Raynaud's phenomenon.
◆ Other findings include hypotension in the arms; neck, shoulder, and chest pain; paresthesia; intermittent claudication; bruits; vision disturbances; and dizziness.

Aortic stenosis
◆ A classic late sign, syncope is accompanied by exertional dyspnea and angina.
◆ Fatigue, orthopnea, paroxysmal nocturnal dyspnea, palpitations, atrial and ventricular gallops, and diminished carotid pulses occur.
◆ A harsh, crescendo-decrescendo systolic ejection murmur that's loudest at the right sternal border of the second intercostal space may be heard.

Cardiac arrhythmias
◆ Decreased cardiac output and impaired cerebral circulation may cause syncope.
◆ Other findings may include chest pain, diaphoresis, confusion, anxiety, signs of stroke, or cardiac arrest.
◆ Syncope may develop without warning in Stokes-Adams syndrome; asystole during syncope may precipitate spasm and myoclonic jerks, if prolonged.

Carotid sinus hypersensitivity
◆ Syncope is triggered by compression of the carotid sinus.
◆ Preceding findings include palpitations, pallor, confusion, diaphoresis, dyspnea, and hypotension.

Hypoxemia
◆ Syncope, confusion, tachycardia, restlessness, tachypnea, dyspnea, cyanosis, and incoordination may occur.

Orthostatic hypotension
◆ Syncope occurs when the patient rises quickly from a recumbent position.
◆ Other findings include tachycardia, pallor, dizziness, blurred vision, nausea, and diaphoresis.

Transient ischemic attack
◆ Syncope and decreased level of consciousness may result.
◆ Other findings vary with the affected artery but may include vision loss, nystagmus, aphasia, dysarthria, unilateral numbness, hemiparesis or hemiplegia, tinnitus, facial weakness, dysphagia, and staggering or uncoordinated gait.

Vagal glossopharyngeal neuralgia
◆ Localized pressure may trigger pain in the base of the tongue, pharynx, larynx, tonsils, and ear, resulting in syncope.

OTHER
Diagnostic tests
◆ Tilt-table tests cause syncope to help identify a cardiogenic source of the symptom.

Drugs
◆ Occasionally, griseofulvin (Grifulvin), indomethacin (Indocin), and levodopa (Dopar) may produce syncope.
◆ Prazosin hydrochloride (Minipress) may cause severe orthostatic hypotension and syncope, usually after the first dose. Other medications that cause orthostatic hypotension include antihypertensives, diuretics, monamine oxidase inhibitors, morphine (MS Contin), nitrates, phenothiazines, spinal anesthesia, and tricyclic antidepressants.
◆ Quinidine (Quinaglute) may cause syncope, and possibly death, associated with ventricular fibrillation.

Nursing considerations

 Nursing alert
If you see the patient faint, provide supportive emergency measures as indicated. Ensure a patent airway and patient safety. Take vital signs. Place the patient in a supine position, elevate his legs, and loosen any tight clothing. Be alert for tachycardia, bradycardia, or an irregular pulse. Place the patient on a cardiac monitor to detect arrhythmias. If an arrhythmia appears, give oxygen and insert an I.V. catheter for drug or fluid administration. Be prepared to begin cardiopulmonary resuscitation. Cardioversion, defibrillation, or insertion of a temporary pacemaker may also be required.

◆ Monitor the patient's vital signs, pulse oximetry, cardiac rhythm, and neurologic status.
◆ Prepare the patient for diagnostic studies.

PATIENT TEACHING
◆ Discuss the underlying condition and the treatment plan.
◆ Teach about the administration, dosage, and possible adverse effects of prescribed medications.
◆ Tell the patient to avoid standing for prolonged periods of time and to make position changes slowly.
◆ Teach the patient what measures to take if he's feeling faint.

Tachycardia

Overview

Tachycardia, a heart rate greater than 100 beats/minute, is detected by counting the apical, carotid, or radial pulse, or by observing it on a cardiac monitor or electrocardiogram (ECG). It can be a normal response to physical exertion or psychological stress, or it may indicate a more serious disorder.

Assessment

HISTORY

◆ Ask about palpitations, dizziness, shortness of breath, weakness, fatigue, syncope, and chest pain.
◆ Ask about a history of trauma, diabetes, and cardiac, pulmonary, or thyroid disorders.
◆ Obtain an alcohol and drug history.

PHYSICAL ASSESSMENT

◆ Inspect for pallor or cyanosis.
◆ Assess pulses and blood pressure and note peripheral edema.
◆ Auscultate the heart and lungs for abnormal sounds and rhythms.

Causes

MEDICAL

Acute respiratory distress syndrome

◆ Tachycardia, crackles, rhonchi, dyspnea, tachypnea, nasal flaring, and grunting respirations occur with this disorder.
◆ Other findings include cyanosis, anxiety, and decreased level of consciousness (LOC).

Adrenocortical insufficiency

◆ A rapid, weak pulse with progressive weakness and fatigue occur.
◆ Other findings include abdominal pain, nausea, vomiting, altered bowel habits, weight loss, orthostatic hypotension, irritability, bronze skin, decreased libido, and syncope.

Anemia

◆ Tachycardia and bounding pulse occur with severe anemia.
◆ Related findings include fatigue, pallor, dyspnea, bleeding tendencies, atrial gallop, crackles, and a systolic bruit over the carotid arteries.

Anxiety

◆ The patient may experience tachycardia, tachypnea, chest pain, cold and clammy skin, light-headedness, dry mouth, and nausea.

Aortic insufficiency

◆ Tachycardia with a bounding pulse and a large, diffuse apical heave occurs with a high-pitched, blowing diastolic murmur starting with the second heart sound.
◆ Other findings include angina, dyspnea, palpitations, strong and abrupt carotid pulsations, pallor, syncope, and signs of heart failure.

Cardiac tamponade

◆ Tachycardia commonly occurs with paradoxical pulse, dyspnea, and tachypnea.
◆ Other findings include anxiety, cyanosis, clammy skin, hypotension, jugular vein distention, narrowed pulse pressure, pericardial rub, muffled heart sounds, chest pain, and hepatomegaly.

Diabetic ketoacidosis

◆ A rapid, thready pulse with Kussmaul's respirations is the cardinal sign.
◆ Other findings include decreased LOC, dehydration, and oliguria with ketosis.

Heart failure

◆ Tachycardia with a ventricular gallop, fatigue, dyspnea, orthopnea, and leg edema occur.

Hypovolemia

◆ Tachycardia and hypotension occur, along with decreased urine output, fatigue, muscle weakness, decreased skin turgor, sunken eyeballs, thirst, syncope, and dry skin and tongue.

S & S

Hypoxemia

◆ Tachycardia with dyspnea, tachypnea, and cyanosis occur.
◆ Other findings include confusion, restlessness, and disorientation, progressing to coma.

Myocardial infarction

◆ Tachycardia or bradycardia may occur with crushing substernal chest pain that may radiate to the left arm, jaw, neck, or shoulder.
◆ Related findings include pallor, clammy skin, fatigue, dyspnea, diaphoresis, atrial gallop, a new murmur, crackles, nausea, vomiting, anxiety, restlessness, and increased or decreased blood pressure.

Pneumothorax

◆ Tachycardia occurs along with dyspnea, chest pain, tachypnea, and cyanosis.
◆ Other findings include dry cough, subcutaneous crepitation, absent or decreased breath sounds, reduced or absent chest movement on the affected side, and decreased vocal fremitus.

Pulmonary embolism

◆ Tachycardia is preceded by sudden dyspnea, angina, or pleuritic chest pain.
◆ Other findings may include weak peripheral pulse, tachypnea, low-grade fever, restlessness, diaphoresis, and a dry cough or a cough with blood-tinged sputum.

Shock

◆ Tachycardia, tachypnea, skin temperature changes, hypotension, apprehension, and decreased LOC occur before cardiac collapse.

Thyrotoxicosis

◆ Tachycardia, an enlarged thyroid, nervousness, heat intolerance, weight loss despite increased appetite, diaphoresis, tremors, palpitations and, possibly, exophthalmos are classic findings.

OTHER
Diagnostic tests

◆ Cardiac catheterization and electrophysiologic studies may induce transient tachycardia.

Drugs and alcohol

◆ Acetylcholinesterase inhibitors, alpha blockers, anticholinergics, beta-adrenergic bronchodilators, nitrates, phenothiazines, sympathomimetics, and vasodilators may cause tachycardia.
◆ Excessive caffeine intake and alcohol intoxication may cause tachycardia.

Surgery and pacemakers

◆ Cardiac surgery and pacemaker malfunction or wire irritation may cause tachycardia.

Nursing considerations

◆ Monitor the patient's vital signs, cardiac rhythm, and pulse oximetry.

◆ Nursing alert

If the patient has symptomatic tachycardia, increased or decreased blood pressure, drowsiness, and confusion, obtain an ECG. Give oxygen, and begin cardiac monitoring. Insert an I.V. catheter for fluid, blood, and drug administration, and keep resuscitation equipment nearby.
◆ Obtain a resting 12-lead ECG if tachycardia worsens, the cardiac rhythm changes, or the patient complains of chest pain.
◆ Administer oxygen, I.V. fluids, or medications as ordered.

PATIENT TEACHING

◆ Teach about underlying diagnosis and the treatment plan.
◆ Explain the possibility of tachycardia recurrence and signs and symptoms to report.
◆ Discuss the use of antiarrhythmics, pacemaker, internal defibrillator, or ablation therapy.
◆ Teach the patient how to take his pulse and when to notify the practitioner.

Tachypnea

Overview

Tachypnea, an abnormally fast respiratory rate of 20 or more breaths/minute, may indicate an impending pulmonary event or be a normal response to increased physical activity or emotion.

Assessment

HISTORY

◆ Ask about the onset, precipitating factors, and characteristics of tachypnea.
◆ Ask about a history of pulmonary or cardiac conditions or anxiety attacks.
◆ Find out about other signs and symptoms, such as diaphoresis, chest pain, or recent weight loss.
◆ Obtain a drug history.

PHYSICAL ASSESSMENT

◆ Take the patient's vital signs, including oxygen saturation.
◆ Auscultate the chest for abnormal heart and breath sounds.
◆ Record the color, amount, and consistency of sputum.
◆ Check for jugular vein distention.
◆ Examine the skin for pallor, cyanosis, edema, and warmth or coolness.

Causes

MEDICAL

Acute respiratory distress syndrome

◆ Tachypnea, an early finding, gradually worsens as fluid accumulates in the lungs.
◆ Other findings include accessory muscle use, grunting expirations, suprasternal and intercostal retractions, crackles, and rhonchi.

Anxiety

◆ Tachypnea may occur with tachycardia, restlessness, chest pain, nausea, and light-headedness.

Aspiration of a foreign body

◆ With partial obstruction, a dry, paroxysmal cough with rapid, shallow respirations develops abruptly.
◆ Other findings include dyspnea, gagging or choking, intercostal retraction, nasal flaring, cyanosis, decreased or absent breath sounds, hoarseness, and stridor or coarse wheezing.

Asthma

◆ Tachypnea is common along with mild wheezing and a dry cough in initial stages.
◆ If left untreated, asthma progresses to a productive cough, prolonged expirations, intercostal and supraclavicular retractions on inspiration, severe wheezing, rhonchi, flaring nostrils, tachycardia, diaphoresis, and flushing or cyanosis.

Cardiac arrhythmias

◆ Tachypnea may occur along with hypotension, dizziness, palpitations, weakness, fatigue and, possibly, decreased level of consciousness (LOC).

Cardiac tamponade

◆ Tachypnea is accompanied by tachycardia, dyspnea, and paradoxical pulse.
◆ Related findings include muffled heart sounds, pericardial rub, chest pain, hypotension, narrowed pulse pressure, hepatomegaly, anxiety, cyanosis, clammy skin, and jugular vein distention.

Emphysema

◆ Tachypnea is accompanied by exertional dyspnea, anorexia, malaise, peripheral cyanosis, pursed-lip breathing, accessory muscle use, chronic productive cough, and late-stage clubbing and barrel chest.

Flail chest
◆ Tachypnea usually appears early.
◆ Other findings include paradoxical chest wall movement, rib bruises and palpable fractures, localized chest pain, hypotension, diminished breath sounds, dyspnea, and accessory muscle use.

Hyperosmolar hyperglycemic nonketotic syndrome
◆ Rapidly deteriorating LOC occurs with tachypnea, tachycardia, hypotension, seizures, oliguria, and signs of dehydration.

Hypoxia
◆ Tachypnea occurs, possibly with restlessness, impaired judgment, tachycardia, dyspnea, and cyanosis.

Pneumonia, bacterial
◆ Tachypnea is usually preceded by a painful, hacking, dry cough that rapidly becomes productive.
◆ Other findings include high fever, shaking chills, headache, dyspnea, pleuritic chest pain, tachycardia, grunting respirations, nasal flaring, and cyanosis.

Pneumothorax
◆ Tachypnea occurs and is typically accompanied by severe, sharp, one-sided chest pain.
◆ Other findings include dyspnea, tachycardia, accessory muscle use, asymmetrical chest expansion, dry cough, cyanosis, anxiety, and restlessness.
◆ Deviated trachea occurs with tension pneumothorax.

Pulmonary edema
◆ Tachypnea, an early sign, is accompanied by exertional dyspnea, paroxysmal nocturnal dyspnea and, later, orthopnea.
◆ Other findings include productive cough with pink frothy sputum, crackles, tachycardia, and a ventricular gallop.

Pulmonary embolism, acute
◆ Sudden tachypnea occurs with dyspnea, angina or pleuritic pain, tachycardia, a dry or productive cough with blood-tinged sputum, fever, restlessness, and diaphoresis.

OTHER
Drugs
◆ Tachypnea may result from an overdose of salicylates.

Nursing considerations

◆ Evaluate cardiopulmonary status.
◆ Monitor vital signs, including oxygen saturation.
◆ Check for cyanosis, chest pain, dyspnea, tachycardia, and hypotension.
◆ Administer supplemental oxygen, and, if possible, place the patient in semi-Fowler's position.
◆ If respiratory failure occurs, endotracheal intubation and mechanical ventilation may be needed. Keep suction and emergency equipment nearby.
◆ Insert an I.V. catheter for fluid and drug administration and begin cardiac monitoring.

PATIENT TEACHING
◆ Teach about the underlying diagnosis and the treatment plan.
◆ Explain that slight increases in respiratory rate may be normal.
◆ Discuss the importance of compliance with drug therapy.

S & S

Tracheal deviation

Overview

Tracheal deviation, the displacement of the trachea to one side of the neck rather than its normal central position, can cause airway obstruction and impaired breathing. It signals an underlying condition that can compromise pulmonary function and possibly cause respiratory distress. It also occurs with disorders that produce mediastinal shift from asymmetrical thoracic volume or pressure.

Assessment

HISTORY

◆ Take a history of pulmonary or cardiac disorders, surgery, trauma, or infection.
◆ Ask about smoking habits.
◆ Find out about other signs and symptoms, such as breathing difficulty, pain, and cough.

PHYSICAL ASSESSMENT

◆ Obtain the patient's vital signs and pulse oximetry.
◆ Auscultate lung fields, noting decreased or absent breath sounds.
◆ Observe for signs and symptoms of respiratory distress.

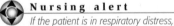 **Nursing alert**

If the patient is in respiratory distress, place him in semi-Fowler's position to aid chest expansion and improve oxygenation, if possible. Give supplemental oxygen, and intubate the patient if needed. Insert an I.V. catheter for fluid and drug administration. Palpate for subcutaneous crepitation in the neck and chest, a sign of tension pneumothorax.

◆ Perform a complete cardiopulmonary assessment.

Causes

MEDICAL

Atelectasis
◆ Extensive lung collapse may produce tracheal deviation toward the affected side.
◆ Other findings include dyspnea, tachypnea, pleuritic chest pain, dry cough, dullness on percussion, decreased vocal fremitus and breath sounds, inspiratory lag, and substernal or intercostal retractions.

Hiatal hernia
◆ Intrusion of abdominal viscera into the pleural space causes tracheal deviation toward the unaffected side.
◆ Other findings include pyrosis, regurgitation or vomiting, chest or abdominal pain, and respiratory distress.

Kyphoscoliosis
◆ Rib cage distortion and mediastinal shift produces tracheal deviation toward the compressed lung.
◆ Other findings include dry cough, dyspnea, asymmetrical chest expansion, possible asymmetrical breath sounds, backache, and fatigue.

Mediastinal tumor
◆ If large, a mediastinal tumor can press against the trachea and nearby structures, causing tracheal deviation and dysphagia.
◆ Other late findings include stridor, dyspnea, brassy cough, hoarseness, and stertorous respirations with suprasternal retraction.
◆ Shoulder, arm, or chest pain, and edema of the neck, face, or arm may develop.
◆ Jugular and chest wall veins may be dilated.

S & S

Pleural effusion

- If the effusion is large, the mediastinum can shift to the contralateral side, producing tracheal deviation.
- Other findings include dry cough, dyspnea, pleuritic pain, pleural friction rub, tachypnea, decreased chest motion, decreased or absent breath sounds, egophony, flatness on percussion, decreased tactile fremitus, fever, and weight loss.

Pulmonary fibrosis

- Tracheal deviation occurs as the mediastinum shifts toward the affected side.
- Other possible findings include dyspnea, cough, clubbing, malaise, and fever.

Pulmonary tuberculosis

- Tracheal deviation occurs toward the affected side along with asymmetrical chest excursion and inspiratory crackles.
- Insidious early findings include anorexia, weight loss, fever, chills, and night sweats.
- Productive cough, hemoptysis, pleuritic chest pain, and dyspnea occur as the disease progresses.

Tension pneumothorax

- Tracheal deviation occurs toward the unaffected side.
- Other findings include sudden onset of respiratory distress, sharp chest pain, dry cough, severe dyspnea, tachycardia, wheezing, cyanosis, accessory muscle use, nasal flaring, air hunger, asymmetrical chest movement, restlessness, anxiety, subcutaneous crepitation in the neck and upper chest, decreased or absent breath sounds on the affected side, jugular vein distention, and hypotension.

Thoracic aortic aneurysm

- The trachea usually deviates to the right.
- Other findings may include stridor; dyspnea; wheezing; brassy cough; hoarseness; dysphagia; edema of the face, neck, or arm; jugular vein distention; and substernal, neck, shoulder, or lower back pain.

Nursing considerations

- Monitor the patient's respiratory and cardiac status continually.
- Administer oxygen and monitor pulse oximetry.
- Monitor vital signs.
- Provide supportive measures, if indicated.
- Give analgesics for comfort, if needed.
- Provide emotional support.

PATIENT TEACHING

- Teach about the underlying diagnosis and the treatment plan.
- Teach the patient how to perform coughing and deep-breathing exercises.
- Explain the signs and symptoms of respiratory difficulty to report to the practitioner.

S & S

Tremors

Overview

Tremors are rhythmic, involuntary, oscillatory trembling that result from alternating contractions of opposing muscle groups. They are characterized by their location, amplitude, and frequency and are classified as resting (occurring in an extremity at rest but subsiding with movement), intention (occurring with movement and subsiding at rest), or postural (occurring when the extremity or trunk is actively held in a particular position).

Assessment

HISTORY

◆ Ask about the onset, duration, and progression of tremors.
◆ Determine what aggravates or alleviates tremors.
◆ Find out about other symptoms, such as behavioral changes or memory loss.
◆ Explore personal and family history of neurologic, endocrine, or metabolic disorders.
◆ Obtain a drug history, especially use of phenothiazines.
◆ Ask about alcohol use.

PHYSICAL ASSESSMENT

◆ Assess the patient's overall appearance and demeanor, noting mental condition.
◆ Test range of motion and strength in all major muscle groups while observing for chorea, athetosis, dystonia, and other involuntary movements.
◆ Check deep tendon reflexes (DTRs).
◆ Observe the patient's gait.

Causes

MEDICAL
Alcohol withdrawal syndrome
◆ Resting and intention tremors occur as soon as 7 hours after the last drink and progressively worsen.
◆ Early findings include diaphoresis, tachycardia, elevated blood pressure, anxiety, restlessness, irritability, insomnia, headache, nausea, and vomiting.
◆ With severe withdrawal, profound tremors, agitation, confusion, hallucinations, and seizures occur.

Alkalosis
◆ A severe intention tremor occurs with twitching, carpopedal spasms, agitation, diaphoresis, and hyperventilation.
◆ Other findings include dizziness, tinnitus, palpitations, and peripheral and circumoral cyanosis.

Cerebellar tumor
◆ An intention tremor is a classic sign.
◆ Related findings include ataxia, nystagmus, incoordination, muscle weakness and atrophy, and hypoactive or absent DTRs.

Graves' disease
◆ Fine hand tremors occur along with nervousness, weight loss, fatigue, palpitations, dyspnea, heat intolerance, an enlarged thyroid gland and, possibly, exophthalmos.

Hypercapnia
◆ A rapid, fine intention tremor occurs.
◆ Associated findings include headache, fatigue, blurred vision, weakness, lethargy, and decreased level of consciousness (LOC).

Hypoglycemia
◆ A rapid, fine intention tremor occurs along with confusion, weakness, tachycardia, diaphoresis, and cold, clammy skin.
◆ The tremor may disappear as hypoglycemia worsens and hypotonia and decreased LOC become evident.
◆ Early findings include headache, profound hunger, nervousness, and blurred or double vision.

Multiple sclerosis
◆ An intention tremor that waxes and wanes may be an early sign along with visual and sensory impairments.

◆ Other findings may include nystagmus, muscle weakness, paralysis, spasticity, hyperreflexia, ataxic gait, dysphagia, dysarthria, constipation, urinary frequency and urgency, incontinence, impotence, and emotional lability.

Parkinson's disease
◆ Tremors, a classic early sign, usually begin in the fingers and may eventually affect the foot, eyelids, jaw, lips, and tongue.
◆ Other characteristic findings include cogwheel rigidity, bradykinesia, propulsive gait with forward-leaning posture, monotone voice, masklike facies, drooling, dysphagia, dysarthria, and, occasionally, oculogyric crisis or blepharospasm.

Porphyria
◆ Resting tremor and rigidity with chorea and athetosis occur.
◆ As the disease progresses, generalized seizures with aphasia and hemiplegia occur.

Thalamic syndrome
◆ With central midbrain syndrome, contralateral ataxic tremors and other abnormal movements occur along with Weber's syndrome, paralysis of vertical gaze, and stupor or coma.
◆ With anteromedial-inferior syndrome, tremor, deep sensory loss, hemiataxia, and extrapyramidal dysfunction may occur.

Thyrotoxicosis
◆ A rapid, fine intention tremor of the hands and tongue, clonus, and hyperreflexia occur.
◆ Other findings include tachycardia, cardiac arrhythmias, palpitations, anxiety, dyspnea, diaphoresis, heat intolerance, weight loss despite increased appetite, diarrhea, an enlarged thyroid and, possibly, exophthalmos.

Wernicke's disease
◆ An intention tremor is an early sign of thiamine deficiency.

◆ Other findings include ocular abnormalities, ataxia, apathy, confusion, orthostatic hypotension, and tachycardia.

West Nile encephalitis
◆ With severe infections, headache, high fever, neck stiffness, stupor, disorientation, coma, tremors, occasional seizures, and paralysis occur.

OTHER
Drugs
◆ Antipsychotics, phenothiazines, metoclopramide hydrochloride (Reglan), and metyrosine (Demser) may cause resting and pill-rolling tremors.
◆ Amphetamines, lithium (Eskalith) toxicity, phenytoin (Dilantin), and sympathomimetics may cause tremors that disappear with dose reduction.

Manganese toxicity
◆ Early signs of manganese toxicity include resting tremor, chorea, propulsive gait, cogwheel rigidity, personality changes, amnesia, and masklike facies.

Mercury toxicity
◆ Mercury toxicity is characterized by irritability, copious amounts of saliva, loose teeth, gum disease, slurred speech, and tremors.

Nursing considerations
◆ Assist the patient with activities as needed.
◆ Monitor the patient's neurologic status.
◆ Take precautions against possible injury during activities.
◆ Encourage the patient to talk about changes in body image.

PATIENT TEACHING
◆ Teach about underlying diagnosis and the treatment plan.
◆ Reinforce the patient's independence.
◆ Instruct the patient in the use of assistive devices as needed.

Vaginal discharge

Overview

Normal vaginal discharge appears mucoid, clear or white, nonbloody, and odorless. A marked increase or change in color, odor, or consistency may signal disease.

 Age considerations
Female neonates may have a white, mucous, vaginal discharge for the first month after birth; a yellow mucous discharge indicates disease. With an older child, purulent, foul-smelling, and possibly bloody vaginal discharge commonly results from a foreign object placed in the vagina, possibly a sign of sexual abuse.

Assessment

HISTORY
◆ Ask about the onset and description of the discharge.
◆ Find out about other symptoms, such as dysuria and perineal pruritus and burning.
◆ Ask about recent changes in sexual habits or hygiene practices.
◆ Ask about previous discharge or infection and the treatment used.
◆ Obtain a drug history, including use of antibiotics, oral estrogens, and hormonal contraceptives.
◆ Ask about the possibility of pregnancy.

PHYSICAL ASSESSMENT
◆ Examine the external genitalia and note the character of the discharge.
◆ Observe vulvar and vaginal tissues for redness, edema, and excoriation.
◆ Palpate the inguinal nodes for tenderness or enlargement.
◆ Palpate the abdomen for tenderness.
◆ Obtain vaginal discharge specimens for testing.
◆ Assist with a pelvic examination, if needed.

Causes

MEDICAL
Atrophic vaginitis
◆ A thin, scant, and watery white vaginal discharge may be accompanied by pruritus, burning, and tenderness.
◆ Sparse pubic hair, a pale vagina with decreased rugae and small hemorrhagic spots, clitoral atrophy, and shrinking of the labia minora may occur.

Bacterial vaginosis
◆ Thin, foul-smelling, green or gray-white discharge that's easily wiped away adheres to the vaginal walls.
◆ Pruritus, redness, and other signs of vaginal irritation may occur.

Candidiasis
◆ A profuse, white, curdlike discharge with a yeasty, sweet odor is produced.
◆ Onset of discharge is abrupt, usually just before menses or during a course of antibiotics.
◆ Exudate may be lightly attached to the labia and vaginal walls and is commonly accompanied by vulvar redness and edema.
◆ The inner thighs may be covered with a fine, red dermatitis and weeping erosions.
◆ Intense labial itching and burning and external dysuria may occur.

Chlamydial infection
◆ A yellow, mucopurulent, odorless, or acrid vaginal discharge is produced.
◆ Other findings include dysuria, dyspareunia, and vaginal bleeding after douching or coitus, especially following menses.

Endometritis
◆ A scant, serosanguineous discharge with a foul odor may occur.
◆ Other findings include fever, lower back and abdominal pain, abdominal muscle spasm, malaise, dysmenorrhea, and an enlarged uterus.

Genital warts

◆ A profuse, mucopurulent vaginal discharge, which may be foul-smelling if the warts are infected, may be produced.
◆ Mosaic, papular vulvar lesions occur, commonly with burning or paresthesia around the vaginal opening.
◆ Genital warts may also appear around the anus or on the cervix.

Gonorrhea

◆ Occasionally, yellow or green, foul-smelling discharge can be expressed from Bartholin's or Skene's ducts, but 80% of women have no symptoms.
◆ Other findings include dysuria, urinary frequency and incontinence, bleeding, vaginal redness and swelling, fever, and severe pelvic and abdominal pain.

Gynecologic cancer

◆ Chronic, watery, bloody or purulent vaginal discharge may be foul-smelling.
◆ Other findings include abnormal vaginal bleeding and, later, weight loss; pelvic, back, and leg pain; fatigue; urinary frequency; and abdominal distention.

Herpes simplex, genital

◆ Copious mucoid discharge results, but the initial complaint is painful, indurated vesicles and ulcerations on the labia, vagina, cervix, anus, thighs, or mouth.
◆ Erythema, marked edema, and tender inguinal lymph nodes may occur with fever, malaise, and dysuria.

Trichomoniasis

◆ A foul-smelling discharge, which may be frothy, green-yellow, and profuse or thin, white, and scant, may be produced, although about 70% of patients are asymptomatic.
◆ Other findings include pruritus; a red, inflamed vagina with tiny petechiae; dysuria and urinary frequency; and dyspareunia, postcoital spotting, menorrhagia, or dysmenorrhea.

OTHER

Contraceptive creams and jellies

◆ Contraceptive creams and jellies may increase vaginal secretions.

Drugs

◆ Drugs that contain estrogen may cause increased mucoid vaginal discharge.
◆ Antibiotics may increase the risk of candidal vaginal infection and discharge.

Radiation therapy

◆ Irradiation of the reproductive tract may cause a watery, odorless, vaginal discharge.

Nursing considerations

◆ Obtain cultures of the discharge.
◆ Give antibiotics, antivirals, or other drugs, if ordered.
◆ Observe standard precautions to prevent the spread of infection.
◆ Report indications of sexual abuse to the proper authorities.

PATIENT TEACHING

◆ Explain the underlying cause and the treatment plan.
◆ Explain the importance of keeping the perineum clean and dry and avoiding tight-fitting clothing.
◆ Stress compliance with prescribed drugs.
◆ Instruct the patient to avoid intercourse until signs and symptoms of infection clear.
◆ Provide information on safer sex practices.

S & S

Weight gain, excessive

Overview

Excessive weight gain occurs when an individual's ingested calories exceed the body's requirements for energy, resulting in increased adipose tissue storage. It may also occur with fluid retention.

Assessment

HISTORY

◆ Ask about previous patterns of weight gain and loss.
◆ Find out about a family history of obesity, thyroid disease, or diabetes mellitus.
◆ Ask about eating and activity patterns.
◆ Determine exercise habits.
◆ Ask about vision disturbances, hoarseness, paresthesia, increased urination and thirst, impotence, or menstrual irregularities.
◆ Obtain a drug history.

PHYSICAL ASSESSMENT

◆ Assess the patient's mental status, memory, and response time.
◆ Measure skin-fold thickness.
◆ Note fat distribution and the presence of edema.
◆ Note overall nutritional status.
◆ Inspect for other abnormalities, such as abnormal body hair distribution or hair loss and dry skin.
◆ Take the patient's vital signs and obtain his weight.
◆ Determine the patient's body mass index and waist circumference.

Causes

MEDICAL
Acromegaly
◆ Moderate weight gain occurs with coarse facial features, a projecting jaw, enlarged hands and feet, increased sweating, oily skin, deep voice, back and joint pain, lethargy, sleepiness, and heat intolerance.
◆ Hirsutism may occur occasionally.

Diabetes mellitus
◆ Increased appetite may lead to weight gain, although weight loss may also occur.
◆ Other findings include fatigue, polydipsia, polyuria, polyphagia, nocturia, weakness, and somnolence.

Gestational hypertension
◆ Rapid weight gain with nausea and vomiting, epigastric pain, elevated blood pressure, and blurred or double vision occur.

Heart failure
◆ Weight gain results from edema.
◆ Associated findings include paroxysmal nocturnal dyspnea, tachypnea, nausea, orthopnea, and fatigue.

Hypercortisolism
◆ Excessive weight gain, usually over the trunk and the back of the neck (buffalo hump), occurs.
◆ Related findings include slender extremities, moon face, weakness, purple striae, emotional lability, and increased susceptibility to infection.
◆ In men, gynecomastia occurs.
◆ In women, hirsutism, acne, and menstrual irregularities occur.

Hyperinsulinism
◆ Increased appetite leads to weight gain.
◆ Emotional lability, indigestion, weakness, diaphoresis, tachycardia, vision disturbances, and syncope may occur.

Hypogonadism
◆ Weight gain is common.
◆ Prepubertal hypogonadism causes eunuchoid body proportions with relatively sparse facial and body hair and a high-pitched voice.
◆ Postpubertal hypogonadism causes loss of libido, impotence, and infertility.

Hypothyroidism
◆ Weight gain occurs despite anorexia.
◆ Other signs and symptoms include fatigue; cold intolerance; constipation; menorrhagia; slowed intellectual and motor activity; dry, pale, cool skin; dry, sparse hair; and thick, brittle nails.

Nephrotic syndrome
◆ Weight gain results from edema; in severe cases, anasarca develops, increasing body weight as much as 50%.
◆ Related findings include abdominal distention, orthostatic hypotension, and lethargy.

Pancreatic islet cell tumor
◆ Excessive hunger leads to weight gain.
◆ Other findings include emotional lability, weakness, malaise, fatigue, restlessness, diaphoresis, palpitations, tachycardia, vision disturbances, and syncope.

OTHER
Drugs
◆ Corticosteroids, phenothiazines, and tricyclic antidepressants from fluid retention and increased appetite may cause excessive weight gain.
◆ Cyproheptadine hydrochloride (Periactin) may cause increased appetite, leading to excessive weight gain.
◆ Hormonal contraceptives cause fluid retention, leading to excessive weight gain.
◆ Lithium (Eskalith) may cause hypothyroidism, leading to excessive weight gain.

Nursing considerations

◆ Assist with dietary choices and nutritional counseling.
◆ Encourage exercise and participation in physical therapy, if appropriate.
◆ Monitor daily weight, if weight gain is fluid-related.
◆ Prepare the patient for studies to rule out possible secondary causes, including serum thyroid function studies, lipid level, glucose level, and dexamethasone suppression testing.

PATIENT TEACHING
◆ Discuss the underlying disorder, if present.
◆ Emphasize the importance of weight control.
◆ Explain the importance of behavior modification and dietary compliance.
◆ Provide guidance in appropriate exercise.
◆ Teach about medications and possible adverse effects.

S & S

Weight loss, excessive

Overview

Excessive weight loss occurs with decreased food intake, decreased food absorption, increased metabolic requirements, or a combination of these factors.

 Age considerations

Weight loss in the elderly may be attributed to lack of teeth, social isolation, financial resources, or depression.

Assessment

HISTORY

◆ Take a diet history, noting use of diet pills and laxatives.

◆ Ask about the patient's previous weight and if weight loss is intentional.

◆ Note sources of anxiety or depression.

◆ Ask about bowel habits, nausea, vomiting, abdominal pain, excessive thirst, excessive urination, or heat intolerance.

◆ Ask about history of cancer or participation in cancer screening.

◆ Obtain a surgical history, especially noting abdominal procedures.

◆ Obtain a drug history.

◆ Ask about socioeconomic factors.

PHYSICAL ASSESSMENT

◆ Obtain the patient's height and weight.

◆ Obtain the patient's vital signs and observe his general appearance.

◆ Examine the skin for turgor and abnormal pigmentation.

◆ Look for signs of infection or irritation on the roof of the mouth; note hyperpigmentation of the buccal mucosa.

◆ Check the eyes for exophthalmos and the neck for swelling.

◆ Evaluate breath sounds.

◆ Inspect the abdomen for wasting; palpate for masses, tenderness, and an enlarged liver.

Causes

MEDICAL

Adrenal insufficiency

◆ Weight loss, anorexia, weakness, fatigue, irritability, syncope, nausea, vomiting, abdominal pain, and diarrhea or constipation occur.

◆ Other findings include hyperpigmentation at the joints, belt line, palmar creases, lips, gums, tongue, and buccal mucosa.

Anorexia nervosa

◆ Self-imposed weight loss of 10% to 50% of premorbid weight characterizes this disorder.

◆ Findings include a morbid fear of becoming fat, skeletal muscle atrophy, loss of fatty tissue, hypotension, constipation, dental caries, cold intolerance, hairiness on the face and body, dryness or loss of scalp hair, amenorrhea, and dehydration or metabolic acidosis or alkalosis.

Cancer

◆ Weight loss occurs with findings specific to the tumor, including fatigue, pain, nausea, vomiting, anorexia, abnormal bleeding, or a palpable mass.

Crohn's disease

◆ Weight loss occurs with chronic cramping, abdominal pain, and anorexia.

◆ Associated findings include diarrhea, nausea, fever, tachycardia, abdominal tenderness and guarding, hyperactive bowel sounds, and abdominal distention.

Depression

◆ Excessive weight loss or gain occurs with insomnia or hypersomnia, anorexia, apathy, fatigue, suicidal thoughts, and feelings of worthlessness.

Diabetes mellitus

◆ Weight loss occurs despite increased appetite.

◆ Other findings include polydipsia, polyuria, fatigue, and blurred vision.

S & S

Esophagitis
◆ Avoidance of eating and weight loss from painful inflammation of the esophagus occur.
◆ Associated findings include intense pain in the mouth and anterior chest with hypersalivation, dysphagia, tachypnea, and hematemesis.

Herpes simplex, type 1
◆ Painful fluid-filled blisters in and around mouth make eating painful, causing decreased food intake and weight loss.
◆ Fever and pharyngitis may also occur.

Leukemia
◆ The acute form causes progressive weight loss; severe prostration; high fever; swollen, bleeding gums; and bleeding tendencies.
◆ The chronic form causes progressive weight loss, malaise, fatigue, pallor, enlarged spleen, bleeding tendencies, anemia, skin eruptions, anorexia, and fever.

Lymphoma
◆ Gradual weight loss occurs along with fever, fatigue, night sweats, malaise, hepatosplenomegaly, and lymphadenopathy.

Pulmonary tuberculosis
◆ Weight loss occurs along with fatigue, weakness, anorexia, night sweats, and low-grade fever.
◆ A cough with bloody or mucopurulent sputum, dyspnea, and pleuritic chest pain may occur.

Stomatitis
◆ Weight loss results from the inability to eat because of inflamed oral mucosa.
◆ Related findings include fever, increased salivation, malaise, mouth pain, anorexia, and swollen, bleeding gums.

Thyrotoxicosis
◆ Increased metabolism causes weight loss.

◆ Other characteristic findings include nervousness, heat intolerance, diarrhea, increased appetite, palpitations, tachycardia, diaphoresis, fine tremor, an enlarged thyroid, and exophthalmos.

Ulcerative colitis
◆ Weight loss is a late sign.
◆ Bloody diarrhea with pus or mucus is an initial characteristic sign.
◆ Weakness, crampy lower abdominal pain, tenesmus, anorexia, low-grade fever, and nausea and vomiting may occur.

OTHER
Drugs
◆ Amphetamines and inappropriate dosage of thyroid preparations commonly lead to weight loss.
◆ Chemotherapeutics cause stomatitis, which, when severe, causes weight loss.

Surgery
◆ Intestinal and stomach surgeries that remove or bypass portions of the digestive tract may cause weight loss as a result of decreased absorption or intake capacity.

Nursing considerations
◆ Assess the patient's GI status.
◆ Take daily calorie counts and weigh the patient weekly.
◆ Assist with dietary choices and nutritional counseling.
◆ Administer hyperalimentation or tube feedings as ordered.

PATIENT TEACHING
◆ Explain the underlying disorder, if applicable, and treatment plan.
◆ Provide guidance in proper diet and keeping a food diary.
◆ Instruct the patient in good oral hygiene.
◆ Provide referrals to nutritional and psychological counseling, if appropriate.
◆ Refer the patient to social services, if appropriate.

VI   *Drugs*

acetaminophen

Abenol†, Acephen, Aceta, Acetaminophen, Actamin, Aminofen, Apacet, Apo-Acetaminophen†, Atasol†, Banesin, Dapa, Exdol†, FeverAll, Genapap, Genebs, Liquiprin, Neopap, Oraphen-PD, Panadol, Redutemp, Robigesic†, Rounox†, Snaplets-FR, St. Joseph Aspirin-Free Fever Reducer for Children, Suppap, Tapanol, Tempra, Tylenol, Valorin

Pregnancy risk category B

Indications and dosages

Mild pain or fever
P.O.
Adults: 325 to 650 mg P.O. q 4 to 6 hours; or 1 g P.O. t.i.d. or q.i.d., p.r.n. Or, two extended-release caplets P.O. q 8 hours. Maximum, 4 g daily. For long-term therapy, don't exceed 2.6 g daily unless prescribed and monitored closely by practitioner.
Children older than age 14: 650 mg P.O. q 4 to 6 hours, p.r.n.
Children ages 12 to 14: 640 mg P.O. q 4 to 6 hours, p.r.n.
Children age 11: 480 mg P.O. q 4 to 6 hours, p.r.n.
Children ages 9 to 10: 400 mg P.O. q 4 to 6 hours, p.r.n.
Children ages 6 to 8: 320 mg P.O. q 4 to 6 hours, p.r.n.
Children ages 4 to 5: 240 mg P.O. q 4 to 6 hours, p.r.n.
Children ages 2 to 3: 160 mg P.O. q 4 to 6 hours, p.r.n.
Children ages 12 to 23 months: 120 mg P.O. q 4 to 6 hours, p.r.n.
Children ages 4 to 11 months: 80 mg P.O. q 4 to 6 hours, p.r.n.
Children up to age 3 months: 40 mg P.O. q 4 to 6 hours, p.r.n. Or, 10 to 15 mg/kg/dose q 4 hours, p.r.n. Don't exceed five doses in 24 hours.
P.R.
Adults and children ages 12 and older: 650 mg P.R. q 4 to 6 hours, p.r.n. Maximum, 4 g daily.

Children ages 6 to 12: 325 mg P.R. q 4 to 6 hours, p.r.n.
Children ages 3 to 6: 120 to 125 mg P.R. q 4 to 6 hours, p.r.n.
Children ages 1 to 3: 80 mg P.R. q 4 to 6 hours, p.r.n.
Children ages 3 to 11 months: 80 mg P.R. q 6 hours, p.r.n.

Adverse reactions

Hemolytic anemia ◆ hepatic damage ◆ hypoglycemia ◆ jaundice ◆ leukopenia ◆ neutropenia ◆ pancytopenia ◆ rash ◆ urticaria

Nursing considerations

◆ Use cautiously with patients with long-term alcohol use because therapeutic dosages cause hepatotoxicity.

◆ Nursing alert
Many over-the-counter and prescription products contain acetaminophen; be aware of this factor when calculating total daily dose.

---

† indicates a Canadian trade name

acyclovir

Avirax†, Lovir†, Zovirax

acyclovir sodium

Avirax†, Zovirax

Pregnancy risk category C

Indications and dosages

First and recurrent episodes of mucocutaneous herpes simplex virus (HSV-1 and HSV-2) infections in immunocompromised patients; severe first episodes of genital herpes in patients who aren't immunocompromised

Adults and children ages 12 and older: 5 mg/kg given I.V. over 1 hour q 8 hours for 7 days. Give for 5 to 7 days for severe first episode of genital herpes.

Children younger than age 12: 10 mg/kg given I.V. over 1 hour q 8 hours for 7 days.

First genital herpes episode

Adults: 200 mg P.O. q 4 hours while awake, five times daily; or 400 mg P.O. q 8 hours. Continue for 7 to 10 days.

Intermittent therapy for recurrent genital herpes

Adults: 200 mg P.O. q 4 hours while awake, five times daily. Continue for 5 days. Begin therapy at first sign of recurrence.

Long-term suppressive therapy for recurrent genital herpes

Adults: 400 mg P.O. b.i.d. for up to 12 months. Or, 200 mg P.O. three to five times daily for up to 12 months.

Varicella (chickenpox) infections in immunocompromised patients

Adults and children ages 12 and older: 10 mg/kg I.V. over 1 hour q 8 hours for 7 days. Dosage for obese patients is 10 mg/kg based on ideal body weight q 8 hours for 7 days. Don't exceed maximum dosage equivalent of 20 mg/kg q 8 hours.

Children younger than age 12: 20 mg/kg I.V. over 1 hour q 8 hours for 7 days.

Varicella infection in immunocompetent patients

Adults and children weighing more than 40 kg (88 lb): 800 mg P.O. q.i.d. for 5 days.

Children ages 2 and older weighing less than 40 kg: 20 mg/kg (maximum 800 mg/dose) P.O. q.i.d. for 5 days. Start therapy as soon as symptoms appear.

Acute herpes zoster infection in immunocompetent patients

Adults and children ages 12 and older: 800 mg P.O. q 4 hours five times daily for 7 to 10 days.

Herpes simplex encephalitis

Adults and children ages 12 and older: 10 mg/kg I.V. over 1 hour q 8 hours for 10 days.

Children ages 3 months to 12 years: 20 mg/kg I.V. over 1 hour q 8 hours for 10 days.

Neonatal herpes simplex virus infection

Neonates to age 3 months: 10 mg/kg I.V. over 1 hour q 8 hours for 10 days.

Adverse reactions

Acute renal failure ◆ diarrhea ◆ encephalopathic changes ◆ headache ◆ hematuria ◆ inflammation or phlebitis at injection site ◆ itching ◆ urticaria ◆ rash ◆ leukopenia ◆ malaise ◆ nausea ◆ thrombocytopenia ◆ thrombocytosis ◆ vomiting

Nursing considerations

◆ Give I.V. infusion over at least 1 hour to prevent renal tubular damage. Don't give by bolus injection.

◆ Solutions concentrated at 7 mg/ml or more may increase the risk of phlebitis.

◆ Encourage fluid intake because the patient must be adequately hydrated during acyclovir infusion. Monitor intake and output, especially within the first 2 hours after I.V. administration.

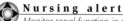 **Nursing alert**

Monitor renal function in patients with renal disease or dehydration and in those taking other nephrotoxic drugs.

Drugs

---

† indicates a Canadian trade name

adenosine

Adenocard
Pregnancy risk category C

Indications and dosages

**Conversion of paroxysmal supra-
ventricular tachycardia (PSVT) to
sinus rhythm**
*Adults and children weighing 50 kg (110 lb)
or more:* 6 mg I.V. by rapid bolus injection
over 1 to 2 seconds. If PSVT isn't eliminated in 1 to 2 minutes, give 12 mg by rapid
I.V. push and repeat, if needed.
Children weighing less than 50 kg: Initially,
0.05 to 0.1 mg/kg I.V. by rapid bolus injection, followed by a saline flush. If PSVT
isn't eliminated in 1 to 2 minutes, give additional bolus injections, increasing the
amount given by 0.05- to 0.1-mg/kg increments, followed by a saline flush. Continue, p.r.n., until conversion or a maximum
single dose of 0.3 mg/kg is given.

Adverse reactions

Chest pressure ◆ dizziness ◆ dyspnea ◆ facial flushing ◆ headache ◆ nausea ◆
numbness ◆ tingling in arms

Nursing considerations

◆ Drug is contraindicated in patients with
second- or third-degree heart block or sinus node disease, except those with pacemakers.
◆ Use cautiously in patients with asthma,
emphysema, or bronchitis because bronchospasm may occur.
◆ Flush the line immediately and rapidly
with normal saline solution to ensure that
the drug quickly reaches systemic circulation.
◆ Don't give single doses exceeding 12 mg.

⬥ **Nursing alert**
*Because heart block, prolonged asystole,
or other new arrhythmias may develop, monitor
the patient's cardiac rhythm and be prepared to
give appropriate therapy.*

---

† indicates a Canadian trade name

alprazolam

Apo-Alpraz†, Novo-Alprazol†, Nu-Alpraz†, Xanax, Xanax XR

Pregnancy risk category D

Indications and dosages

Anxiety

Adults: Usual first dose, 0.25 to 0.5 mg P.O. t.i.d. Maximum, 4 mg daily in divided doses.

Elderly patients: Usual first dose, 0.25 mg P.O. b.i.d. or t.i.d. Maximum, 4 mg daily in divided doses.

Panic disorders

Adults: 0.5 mg P.O. t.i.d., increased at intervals of 3 to 4 days in increments of no more than 1 mg. Maximum, 10 mg daily in divided doses. If using extended-release tablets, start with 0.5 to 1 mg P.O. once daily. Increase by no more than 1 mg q 3 to 4 days. Maximum daily dose, 10 mg.

Adverse reactions

Agitation ◆ anxiety ◆ allergic rhinitis ◆ arthralgia ◆ impaired coordination ◆ blurred vision ◆ chest pain ◆ palpitations ◆ confusion ◆ memory impairment ◆ constipation ◆ diarrhea ◆ depression ◆ suicide ◆ dermatitis ◆ difficulty speaking ◆ difficulty urinating ◆ dizziness ◆ syncope ◆ drowsiness ◆ fatigue ◆ nausea ◆ vomiting ◆ change in appetite

Nursing considerations

◆ Drug is contraindicated in patients with acute angle-closure glaucoma.

◆ Use cautiously in patients with hepatic, renal, or pulmonary disease.

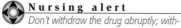 **Nursing alert**
Don't withdraw the drug abruptly; withdrawal symptoms, including seizures, may occur. Abuse or addiction is possible.

◆ Monitor hepatic, renal, and hematopoietic function periodically in patients receiving repeated or prolonged therapy.

amiodarone hydrochloride

Cordarone, Pacerone

Pregnancy risk category D

Indications and dosages

Life-threatening recurrent ventricular fibrillation, recurrent hemodynamically unstable ventricular tachycardia unresponsive to adequate doses of other antiarrhythmics, or when alternative drugs can't be tolerated
Adults: Loading dose of 800 to 1,600 mg P.O. daily divided b.i.d. for 1 to 3 weeks until first therapeutic response occurs; then 600 to 800 mg P.O. daily for 1 month, followed by maintenance dose of 200 to 600 mg P.O. daily. Or, loading dose of 150 mg I.V. over 10 minutes (15 mg/minute); then 360 mg I.V. over next 6 hours (1 mg/minute), followed by 540 mg I.V. over next 18 hours (0.5 mg/minute). After first 24 hours, continue with maintenance I.V. infusion of 720 mg/24 hours (0.5 mg/minute).

Adverse reactions

Abdominal pain ◆ abnormal smell or taste ◆ acute respiratory distress syndrome ◆ anorexia ◆ nausea ◆ vomiting ◆ arrhythmias ◆ heart block ◆ ataxia ◆ blue-gray skin ◆ coagulation abnormalities ◆ constipation ◆ edema ◆ fatigue ◆ malaise ◆ headache ◆ heart failure ◆ hepatic dysfunction or failure ◆ hypotension ◆ insomnia ◆ sleep disturbances ◆ paresthesia ◆ peripheral neuropathy ◆ photosensitivity ◆ visual disturbances ◆ thyroid dysfunction

Nursing considerations

◆ Drug is contraindicated in patients with cardiogenic shock, second- or third-degree atrioventricular block, severe sinoatrial node disease resulting in bradycardia (unless an artificial pacemaker is present), and in patients whose bradycardia has caused syncope.

◆ Drug is incompatible with normal saline solution. When giving over 2 hours or longer, mix infusions in glass or polyolefin bottles.

◆ Use an in-line filter with I.V. administration.

◆ Continuously monitor cardiac status and vital signs of the patient receiving the drug I.V. If hypotension occurs, reduce infusion rate.

◆ Be aware of the high risk of adverse reactions.

◆ Monitor prothrombin time and International Normalized Ratio if the patient takes warfarin (Coumadin) and digoxin (Lanoxin) level if he takes digoxin.

aspirin
(acetylsalicylic acid)

Artria S.R, ASA, Aspergum, Bayer Aspirin, Coryphen†, Easprin, Ecotrin, Empirin, Entrophen†, Halfprin, Norwich Extra-Strength, Novasen†, ZORprin

Pregnancy risk category D

Indications and dosages

Rheumatoid arthritis, osteoarthritis, or other polyarthritic or inflammatory conditions
Adults: Initially, 2.4 to 3.6 g P.O. daily in divided doses. Maintenance dosage, 3.2 to 6 g P.O. daily in divided doses.
Juvenile rheumatoid arthritis
Children who weigh more than 25 kg (55 lb): 2.4 to 3.6 g P.O. daily in divided doses.
Children who weigh 25 kg or less: 60 to 130 mg/kg daily P.O. in divided doses. Increased by 10 mg/kg daily at no more than weekly intervals. Maintenance doses usually range from 80 to 100 mg/kg daily; up to 130 mg daily.
Mild pain or fever
Adults and children older than age 11: 325 to 650 mg P.O. or P.R. q 4 hours, p.r.n.
Children ages 2 to 11: 10 to 15 mg/kg/dose P.O. or P.R. q 4 hours up to 80 mg/kg daily.
Thrombosis prevention
Adults: 1.3 g P.O. daily in two to four divided doses to reduce myocardial infarction (MI) risk in patients with previous MI or unstable angina.
Adults: 75 to 325 mg P.O. daily.
Kawasaki syndrome (mucocutaneous lymph node syndrome)
Adults: 80 to 100 mg/kg P.O. daily in four divided doses with immune globulin I.V. When fever subsides, decrease to 3 to 5 mg/kg once daily. Aspirin therapy usually continues for 6 to 8 weeks.

Acute rheumatic fever
Adults: 5 to 8 g P.O. daily.
Children: 100 mg/kg daily P.O. for 2 weeks; then 75 mg/kg daily P.O. for 4 to 6 weeks.
To reduce the risk of recurrent transient ischemic attacks and stroke or death in at-risk patients
Adults: 50 to 325 mg P.O. daily.
Acute ischemic stroke
Adults: 160 to 325 mg P.O. daily, started within 48 hours of stroke onset and continued for up to 2 to 4 weeks.
Acute pericarditis after MI
Adults: 160 to 325 mg P.O. daily. Higher doses (650 mg P.O. q 4 to 6 hours) may be needed.

Adverse reactions

Angioedema ◆ dyspepsia ◆ nausea ◆ GI bleeding ◆ hearing loss ◆ hepatitis ◆ hypersensitivity reactions ◆ prolonged bleeding time ◆ bruising ◆ rash ◆ urticaria ◆ Reye's syndrome ◆ thrombocytopenia ◆ tinnitus

Nursing considerations

◆ Drug is contraindicated in patients with G6PD deficiency; bleeding disorders, and nonsteroidal anti-inflammatory drug-induced sensitivity reactions.
◆ Febrile, dehydrated children can develop toxicity rapidly.
◆ Monitor salicylate level. Therapeutic salicylate level with arthritis is 150 to 300 mcg/ml.
◆ During prolonged therapy, assess hematocrit, hemoglobin, prothrombin time, International Normalized Ratio, and renal function periodically.
◆ Stop aspirin 5 to 7 days before elective surgery to allow time for production and release of new platelets.

Drugs

---

† indicates a Canadian trade name

atenolol

Apo-Atenolol[†], Tenormin

Pregnancy risk category D

Indications and dosages

Hypertension
Adults: Initially, 50 mg P.O. daily alone or with a diuretic as a single dose, increased to 100 mg once daily after 7 to 14 days. Dosages of more than 100 mg daily are unlikely to produce further benefit.

Angina pectoris
Adults: 50 mg P.O. once daily, increased, p.r.n. to 100 mg daily after 7 days for optimal effect. Maximum, 200 mg daily.

Acute myocardial infarction (MI)
Adults: 5 mg I.V. over 5 minutes; repeat in 10 minutes. After another 10 minutes, if the patient tolerates the full 10-mg I.V. dose, give 50 mg P.O.; then give another 50 mg P.O. in 12 hours. Subsequently, give 100 mg P.O. daily (as a single dose or 50 mg b.i.d.) for at least 6 to 9 days or until discharged.

Migraine prophylaxis
Adults: 100 mg P.O. daily.

Unstable angina, non-ST-segment elevation MI in patients at high risk for ischemic events
Adults: Initially, 5 mg I.V. over 2 to 5 minutes, repeat q 5 minutes to maximum of 10 mg. Initiate oral therapy 1 to 2 hours after last I.V. dose at 50 to 100 mg P.O. daily. Maintenance dose, 50 to 200 mg daily.

Adverse reactions

Bradycardia ◆ bronchospasm ◆ dyspnea ◆ diarrhea ◆ dizziness ◆ vertigo ◆ drowsiness ◆ fatigue ◆ fever ◆ heart failure ◆ hypotension ◆ intermittent claudication ◆ nausea ◆ rash

Nursing considerations

◆ Drug is contraindicated in patients with sinus bradycardia, heart block (greater than first degree), overt cardiac failure, or cardiogenic shock.

◆ Check the patient's apical pulse before giving drug; if slower than 60 beats/minute, withhold drug and call the practitioner.

◆ Monitor the patient's blood pressure.

◆ Monitor hemodialysis patients closely because of hypotension risk.

◆ Beta-adrenergic blockers such as atenolol may mask tachycardia caused by hyperthyroidism. In patients with suspected thyrotoxicosis, expect to withdraw the beta-adrenergic blocker gradually to avoid thyroid storm.

◆ Drug may mask signs and symptoms of hypoglycemia in patients with diabetes.

◈ Nursing alert
Expect to withdraw drug gradually over 2 weeks to avoid serious adverse reactions.

atropine sulfate

Sal-Tropine
Pregnancy risk category C

Indications and dosages

Symptomatic bradycardia or bradyarrhythmia (junctional or escape rhythm)
Adults: Usually, 0.5 to 1 mg I.V. push, repeated q 3 to 5 minutes to maximum of 2 mg, p.r.n.
Children and adolescents: 0.02 mg/kg I.V., with minimum dose of 0.1 mg and maximum single dose of 0.5 mg in children and 1 mg in adolescents. May repeat dose at 5-minute intervals to a maximum total dose of 1 mg in children and 2 mg in adolescents.

Antidote for anticholinesterase insecticide toxicity
Adults: Initially, 1 to 2 mg I.V.; may repeat with 2 mg I.M. or I.V. q 5 to 60 minutes until muscarinic signs and symptoms disappear or signs of atropine toxicity occur. Severe toxicity may require up to 6 mg hourly.
Children: 0.05 mg/kg I.M. or I.V. repeated q 10 to 30 minutes until muscarinic signs and symptoms disappear (may be repeated if they reappear) or until signs of atropine toxicity occur.

Preoperatively to diminish secretions and block cardiac vagal reflexes
Adults and children weighing 20 kg (44 lb) or more: 0.4 to 0.6 mg I.V., I.M., or subcutaneously 30 to 60 minutes before anesthesia.
Children weighing less than 20 kg: 0.01 mg/kg I.V., I.M., or subcutaneously up to maximum dose of 0.4 mg 30 to 60 minutes before anesthesia. May repeat q 4 to 6 hours, p.r.n.
Infants weighing more than 5 kg (11 lb): 0.03 mg/kg q 4 to 6 hours, p.r.n.
Infants weighing 5 kg or less: 0.04 mg/kg q 4 to 6 hours, p.r.n.

Adjunct treatment of peptic ulcer disease or functional GI disorders such as irritable bowel syndrome
Adults: 0.4 to 0.6 mg P.O. q 4 to 6 hours.

Adverse reactions

Agitation ◆ confusion ◆ restlessness ◆ anaphylaxis ◆ ataxia ◆ blurred vision ◆ cycloplegia ◆ mydriasis ◆ photophobia ◆ increased intraocular pressure ◆ bradycardia ◆ tachycardia ◆ palpitations ◆ constipation ◆ delirium ◆ disorientation ◆ hallucinations ◆ dizziness ◆ dry mouth ◆ thirst ◆ headache ◆ impotence ◆ insomnia ◆ nausea ◆ vomiting ◆ urine retention

Nursing considerations

◆ Drug is contraindicated in patients with acute angle-closure glaucoma, obstructive uropathy, obstructive disease of the GI tract, paralytic ileus, toxic megacolon, intestinal atony, unstable cerebrovascular status in acute hemorrhage, tachycardia, myocardial ischemia, asthma, or myasthenia gravis.
◆ In adults, avoid doses less than 0.5 mg because of the risk of paradoxical bradycardia.

◆ Nursing alert
Watch for tachycardia in patients with cardiac conditions because it may lead to ventricular fibrillation.

---

† indicates a Canadian trade name

Drugs

captopril

Capoten, Novo-Captoril[†]

Pregnancy risk category C; D in second and third trimesters

Indications and dosages

Hypertension
Adults: Initially, 25 mg P.O. b.i.d. or t.i.d. If blood pressure isn't controlled satisfactorily in 1 or 2 weeks, increase dosage to 50 mg b.i.d. or t.i.d. If that dosage doesn't control blood pressure satisfactorily after another 1 or 2 weeks, expect to add a diuretic. If the patient needs further blood pressure reduction, dosage may be raised to 150 mg t.i.d. while continuing diuretic. Maximum dosage, 450 mg daily.

Diabetic nephropathy
Adults: 25 mg P.O. t.i.d.

Heart failure
Adults: Initially, 25 mg P.O. t.i.d. Patients with normal or low blood pressure who have been vigorously treated with diuretics and who may be hyponatremic or hypovolemic may start with 6.25 mg or 12.5 mg P.O. t.i.d.; starting dosage may be adjusted over several days. Gradually increase dosage to 50 mg P.O. t.i.d.; delay further dosage increases for at least 2 weeks. Maximum, 450 mg daily.

Elderly patients: Initially, 6.25 mg P.O. b.i.d. Increase gradually, p.r.n.

Left ventricular dysfunction after acute myocardial infarction (MI)
Adults: Start therapy as early as 3 days after MI with 6.25 mg P.O. for one dose, followed by 12.5 mg P.O. t.i.d. Increase over several days to 25 mg P.O. t.i.d., then increase to 50 mg P.O. t.i.d. over several weeks.

Adverse reactions

Abdominal pain ◆ agranulocytosis ◆ alopecia ◆ anemia ◆ angina pectoris ◆ angioedema ◆ anorexia ◆ constipation ◆ diarrhea ◆ dizziness ◆ syncope ◆ dry mouth ◆ dry, persistent, nonproductive cough ◆ dysgeu-sia ◆ dyspnea ◆ fatigue, malaise ◆ fever ◆ headache ◆ hyperkalemia ◆ hypotension ◆ leukopenia ◆ pancytopenia ◆ thrombocytopenia ◆ nausea ◆ vomiting ◆ pruritus ◆ urticarial or maculopapular rash ◆ tachycardia

Nursing considerations

◆ Monitor the patient's blood pressure and pulse rate frequently.

Nursing alert
Elderly patients may be more sensitive to the drug's hypotensive effects.

◆ In patients with impaired renal function or collagen vascular disease, monitor white blood cell and differential counts before starting treatment, every 2 weeks for the first 3 months of therapy, and periodically thereafter.

Drugs

cefazolin sodium

Ancef

Pregnancy risk category B

Indications and dosages

Perioperative prevention in contaminated surgery
Adults: 1 g I.M. or I.V. 30 to 60 minutes before surgery; then 0.5 to 1 g I.M. or I.V. q 6 to 8 hours for 24 hours. In operations lasting longer than 2 hours, give another 0.5- to 1-g dose I.M. or I.V. intraoperatively. Continue treatment for 3 to 5 days if life-threatening infection is likely.

Infections of respiratory, biliary, and genitourinary tracts; skin, soft-tissue, bone, and joint infections; septicemia; endocarditis caused by *Escherichia coli,* Enterobacteriaceae organisms, gonococci, *Haemophilus influenzae,* Klebsiella species, *Proteus mirabilis, Staphylococcus aureus, Streptococcus pneumoniae,* and group A beta-hemolytic streptococci
Adults: 250 to 500 mg I.M. or I.V. q 8 hours for mild infections, or 500 mg to 1.5 g I.M. or I.V. q 6 to 8 hours for moderate to severe or life-threatening infections. Maximum, 12 g/day in life-threatening situations.
Children older than age 1 month: 25 to 50 mg/kg/day I.M. or I.V. in three or four divided doses. In severe infections, may increase dosage to 100 mg/kg/day.

Adverse reactions

Abdominal cramps ◆ anaphylaxis ◆ hypersensitivity reactions ◆ anorexia ◆ candidiasis ◆ confusion ◆ diarrhea ◆ drug fever ◆ dyspepsia ◆ eosinophilia ◆ glossitis ◆ headache ◆ maculopapular and erythematous rashes ◆ nausea ◆ vomiting ◆ neutropenia ◆ leukopenia ◆ thrombocytopenia ◆ pain ◆ phlebitis ◆ pruritus ◆ pseudomembranous colitis ◆ seizures ◆ serum sickness ◆ sterile abscesses ◆ Stevens-Johnson syndrome ◆ tissue sloughing at injection site ◆ urticaria ◆ vaginitis

Nursing considerations

◆ Before administration, ask the patient if he's allergic to penicillins or cephalosporins.
◆ Alternate injection sites if I.V. therapy lasts longer than 3 days. Use of small I.V. needles in larger available veins may be preferable.
◆ Obtain a specimen for culture and sensitivity testing before giving the first dose. Therapy may begin pending results.
◆ Give the injection deeply into a large muscle, such as the gluteus maximus.
◆ Monitor the patient for signs and symptoms of superinfection.

Drugs

---

† indicates a Canadian trade name

cefepime hydrochloride

Maxipime

Pregnancy risk category B

Indications and dosages

Mild to moderate urinary tract infections (UTIs) caused by *Escherichia coli, Klebsiella pneumoniae,* or *Proteus mirabilis,* including concurrent bacteremia with these microorganisms
Adults and children ages 12 and older: 0.5 to 1 g I.M. or I.V. infused over 30 minutes q 12 hours for 7 to 10 days. I.M. route used only for *E. coli* infections.

Severe UTIs, including pyelonephritis, caused by *E. coli* or *K. pneumoniae*
Adults and children ages 12 and older: 2 g I.V. infused over 30 minutes q 12 hours for 10 days.

Moderate to severe pneumonia caused by *Streptococcus pneumoniae, Pseudomonas aeruginosa, K. pneumoniae,* or Enterobacter species
Adults and children ages 12 and older: 1 to 2 g I.V. infused over 30 minutes q 12 hours for 10 days.

Moderate to severe skin infections, uncomplicated skin infections, and skin-structure infections caused by *Streptococcus pyogenes* or methicillin-susceptible strains of *Staphylococcus aureus*
Adults and children ages 12 and older: 2 g I.V. infused over 30 minutes q 12 hours for 10 days.

Complicated intra-abdominal infections caused by *E. coli,* viridans group streptococci, *P. aeruginosa, K. pneumoniae,* Enterobacter species, or *Bacteroides fragilis*
Adults: 2 g I.V. infused over 30 minutes q 12 hours for 7 to 10 days. Use with metronidazole (Flagyl).

Empiric therapy for febrile neutropenia
Adults: 2 g I.V. q 8 hours for 7 days or until neutropenia resolves.

Uncomplicated and complicated UTIs (including pyelonephritis), uncomplicated skin and skin-structure infections, pneumonia in children; as empiric therapy for febrile neutropenic children
Children ages 2 months to 16 years weighing up to 40 kg (88 lb): 50 mg/kg/dose I.V. infused over 30 minutes q 12 hours (q 8 hours for febrile neutropenia), for 7 to 10 days. Don't exceed 2 g/dose.

Adverse reactions

Anaphylaxis ◆ hypersensitivity reactions ◆ colitis ◆ diarrhea ◆ fever ◆ headache ◆ inflammation ◆ nausea ◆ vomiting ◆ oral candidiasis ◆ pain ◆ phlebitis ◆ pruritus ◆ rash ◆ urticaria ◆ vaginitis

Nursing considerations

◆ Before administration, ask the patient if he's allergic to penicillin or cephalosporins.
◆ Obtain a specimen for culture and sensitivity testing before giving first dose. Therapy may begin pending results.
◆ Monitor the patient for signs and symptoms of superinfection.
◆ Monitor prothrombin time and International Normalized Ratio in patients requiring prolonged therapy as ordered. Give exogenous vitamin K as indicated.

ciprofloxacin

Cipro, Cipro I.V, Cipro XR, Proquin XR
Pregnancy risk category C

Indications and dosages

Complicated intra-abdominal infection
Adults: 500 mg P.O. or 400 mg I.V. q 12 hours for 7 to 14 days. Give with metronidazole (Flagyl).
Severe or complicated bone or joint infection, severe respiratory tract infection, severe skin or skin-structure infection
Adults: 750 mg P.O. q 12 hours or 400 mg I.V. q 8 hours.
Mild to moderate urinary tract infection (UTI)
Adults: 250 mg P.O. or 200 mg I.V. q 12 hours.
Severe or complicated UTIs, mild to moderate bone or joint infection, mild to moderate respiratory infection, mild to moderate skin and skin-structure infection, infectious diarrhea, typhoid fever
Adults: 500 mg P.O. or 400 mg I.V. q 12 hours. Or, 1,000 mg extended-release tablets P.O. q 24 hours.
Complicated UTI or pyelonephritis
Children ages 1 to 17: 6 to 10 mg/kg I.V. q 8 hours for 10 to 21 days. Maximum I.V. dose, 400 mg. Or, 10 to 20 mg/kg P.O. q 12 hours. Maximum P.O. dose, 750 mg. Don't exceed maximum dose, even in patients who weigh more than 51 kg (112 lb).
Nosocomial pneumonia
Adults: 400 mg I.V. q 8 hours for 10 to 14 days.
Chronic bacterial prostatitis
Adults: 500 mg P.O. q 12 hours or 400 mg I.V. q 12 hours for 28 days.
Acute uncomplicated cystitis
Adults: 100 mg or 250 mg P.O. q 12 hours for 3 days.
Uncomplicated UTIs
Adults: 500 mg extended-release tablet P.O. once daily for 3 days.

Mild to moderate acute sinusitis
Adults: 500 mg P.O. or 400 mg I.V. q 12 hours for 10 days.
Empirical therapy in febrile neutropenic patients
Adults: 400 mg I.V. q 8 hours used with piperacillin (Zosyn) 50 mg/kg I.V. q 4 hours (not to exceed 24 g/day).
Inhalation anthrax (postexposure)
Adults: Initially, 400 mg I.V. q 12 hours until susceptibility test results are known; then 500 mg P.O. b.i.d.
Children: 10 mg/kg I.V. q 12 hours; then 15 mg/kg P.O. q 12 hours. Don't exceed 800 mg/day I.V. or 1,000 mg/day P.O.
For all patients: Give drug with one or two additional antimicrobials. Switch to oral therapy when appropriate. Treat for 60 days (I.V. and P.O. combined).
Cutaneous anthrax
Adults: 500 mg P.O. b.i.d. for 60 days.
Children: 10 to 15 mg/kg q 12 hours. Don't exceed 1,000 mg/day. Treat for 60 days.

Adverse reactions

Diarrhea ◆ leukopenia ◆ neutropenia ◆ thrombocytopenia ◆ pseudomembranous colitis ◆ seizure ◆ Stevens-Johnson syndrome ◆ toxic epidermal necrolysis

Nursing considerations

◆ Obtain a specimen for culture and sensitivity testing before giving the first dose. Therapy may begin while awaiting results.
◆ Be aware of drug interactions. It may be necessary to wait up to 6 hours after ciprofloxacin administration before giving another drug to avoid decreasing ciprofloxacin's effects.
◆ Monitor the patient's intake and output and observe for indicators of crystalluria.
◆ Follow current Centers for Disease Control and Prevention recommendations for anthrax.
◆ Pregnant women and immunocompromised patients should receive the usual doses and regimens for anthrax.

Drugs

† indicates a Canadian trade name

clindamycin hydrochloride

Cleocin HCl, Dalacin C†

clindamycin palmitate hydrochloride

Cleocin Pediatric, Dalacin C Flavored Granules†

clindamycin phosphate

Cleocin Phosphate, Dalacin C Phosphate Sterile Solution†

Pregnancy risk category B

Indications and dosages

Infections caused by sensitive staphylococci, streptococci, pneumococci, Bacteroides species, Fusobacterium species, *Clostridium perfringens,* and other sensitive aerobic and anaerobic organisms
Adults: 150 to 450 mg P.O. q 6 hours; or 300 to 600 mg I.M. or I.V. q 6, 8, or 12 hours.
Children older than age 1 month: 8 to 20 mg/kg P.O. daily in divided doses q 6 to 8 hours; or 15 to 40 mg/kg I.M. or I.V. daily in divided doses q 6 or 8 hours.
Pelvic inflammatory disease
Adults and adolescents: 900 mg I.V. q 8 hours, with gentamicin (Garamycin). Continue at least 48 hours after symptoms improve; then switch to oral clindamycin 450 mg q.i.d. for total of 10 to 14 days or doxycycline (Vibramycin) 100 mg P.O. q 12 hours for total of 10 to 14 days.
***Pneumocystis carinii* pneumonia**
Adults: 600 mg I.V. q 6 hours or 900 mg I.V. q 8 hours, with primaquine.
Central nervous system toxoplasmosis in patients with acquired immunodeficiency syndrome (as alternative to sulfonamides with pyrimethamine)
Adults: 1,200 to 2,400 mg/day in divided doses.

Adverse reactions

Abdominal pain ◆ anaphylaxis ◆ diarrhea ◆ eosinophilia ◆ transient leukopenia ◆ jaundice ◆ maculopapular rash ◆ nausea ◆ vomiting ◆ pseudomembranous colitis ◆ thrombocytopenia ◆ thrombophlebitis ◆ urticaria

Nursing considerations

 Nursing alert
Never give any form of this drug undiluted as a bolus.
◆ Obtain a specimen for culture and sensitivity testing before giving first dose. Therapy may begin pending results.
◆ For I.M. administration, inject the drug deeply. Rotate injection sites. Don't exceed 600 mg per injection.
◆ Drug is stable for 2 weeks at room temperature.
◆ Monitor renal, hepatic, and hematopoietic functions during prolonged therapy.
◆ Observe the patient for signs and symptoms of superinfection.

Drugs

clonidine

Catapres-TTS

clonidine hydrochloride

Catapres, Dixarit†, Duraclon
Pregnancy risk category C

Indications and dosages

Essential and renal hypertension
Adults and children age 12 and older: Initially, 0.1 mg P.O. b.i.d.; then increase by 0.1 to 0.2 mg daily on a weekly basis. Usual range is 0.2 to 0.6 mg daily in divided doses; infrequently, dosages as high as 2.4 mg daily are used. Or, apply the transdermal patch to nonhairy area of intact skin on the upper arm or torso once q 7 days, starting with 0.1-mg system and adjusted with another 0.1-mg or larger system.

Severe cancer pain unresponsive to epidural or spinal opiate analgesia or other more conventional methods of analgesia
Adults: Initially, 30 mcg/hour by continuous epidural infusion. Experience with rates greater than 40 mcg/hour is limited.
Children: Initially, 0.5 mcg/kg/hour by epidural infusion. Dosage should be cautiously adjusted based on response.

Pheochromocytoma diagnosis
Adults: 0.3 mg P.O. as a single dose.

Migraine prophylaxis
Adults: 0.025 mg P.O. two to four times daily, or up to 0.15 mg P.O. daily in divided doses.

Dysmenorrhea
Adults: 0.025 mg P.O. b.i.d. for 14 days before and during menses.

Vasomotor symptoms of menopause
Adults: 0.025 to 0.2 mg P.O. b.i.d or 0.1 mg/24-hour patch applied once q 7 days.

Opiate dependence
Adults: Initially, 0.005 or 0.006 mg/kg test dose, followed by 0.017 mg/kg P.O. daily in three or four divided doses for 10 days. Or, initially, 0.1 mg P.O. three or four times

daily, with dosage adjusted by 0.1 to 0.2 mg daily. Dosage range is 0.3 to 1.2 mg P.O. daily. Stop drug gradually. Follow protocols.

Alcohol dependence
Adults: 0.5 mg P.O. b.i.d. to t.i.d.

Smoking cessation
Adults: Initially, 0.1 mg P.O. b.i.d., beginning on or shortly before the day of smoking cessation. Increase dosage q 7 days by 0.1 mg daily, if needed. Or, 0.1 mg/24-hour transdermal patch applied q 7 days beginning on or shortly before the day of smoking cessation. Increase dosage by 0.1 mg/24 hour at weekly intervals, if needed.

Attention deficit hyperactivity disorder
Children: Initially, 0.05 mg P.O. at bedtime. May increase dosage cautiously over 2 to 4 weeks. Maintenance dosage, 0.05 to 0.4 mg P.O. daily.

Adverse reactions

Anorexia ◆ bradycardia ◆ constipation ◆ depression ◆ agitation ◆ dermatitis (with transdermal patch) ◆ dizziness ◆ drowsiness ◆ sedation ◆ dry mouth ◆ fatigue ◆ malaise ◆ weakness ◆ impotence ◆ loss of libido ◆ nausea ◆ vomiting ◆ orthostatic hypotension ◆ severe rebound hypertension ◆ pruritus ◆ rash ◆ urine retention ◆ weight gain

Nursing considerations

◆ Monitor the patient's blood pressure and pulse rate frequently.
◆ Noticeable antihypertensive effects of transdermal clonidine may take 2 to 3 days. Oral antihypertensive therapy may have to be continued in the interim.

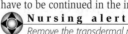 **Nursing alert**
Remove the transdermal patch before defibrillation to prevent arcing.

◆ When stopping therapy in patients receiving clonidine and a beta-adrenergic blocker, gradually withdraw the beta-adrenergic blocker first to minimize adverse reactions.

Drugs

---

† indicates a Canadian trade name

clopidogrel bisulfate

Plavix
Pregnancy risk category B

Indications and dosages

To reduce thrombotic events in patients with atherosclerosis documented by recent stroke, myocardial infarction (MI), or peripheral arterial disease
Adults: 75 mg P.O. daily.

To reduce thrombotic events in patients with acute coronary syndrome (unstable angina and non–Q-wave MI), including those receiving drugs and those having percutaneous coronary intervention (with or without stent) or coronary artery bypass graft
Adults: Initially, a single 300-mg P.O. loading dose; then 75 mg P.O. once daily. Start and continue aspirin (75 to 325 mg once daily) with clopidogrel.

ST-segment elevation acute MI
Adults: 75 mg P.O. once daily, with aspirin, with or without thrombolytics. A 300 mg loading dose is optional.

Adverse reactions

Abdominal pain ◆ arthralgia ◆ bronchitis ◆ dyspnea ◆ coughing ◆ constipation ◆ diarrhea ◆ depression ◆ dizziness ◆ dyspepsia ◆ edema ◆ epistaxis ◆ hemorrhage ◆ fatigue ◆ flulike syndrome ◆ gastritis ◆ ulcers ◆ headache ◆ hypertension ◆ pain ◆ pruritus ◆ rash ◆ purpura ◆ rhinitis ◆ upper respiratory infection ◆ urinary tract infection

Nursing considerations

◆ Drug is contraindicated in patients with pathologic bleeding, such as peptic ulcer disease or intracranial hemorrhage.
◆ Platelet aggregation won't return to normal for at least 5 days after the drug is stopped.

◆ Tell the patient to inform all health care providers, including dentists, that he's taking the drug before undergoing procedures or starting new drug therapy.

Drugs

---

† indicates a Canadian trade name

dexamethasone

Decadron, Dexameth, Dexone,
Hexadrol

dexamethasone acetate

Cortastat LA, Dalalone D.P., Decaject-
LA, Dexasone L.A., Dexone LA,
Solurex LA

dexamethasone sodium phosphate

Cortastat, Dalalone, Decadron
Phosphate, Decaject, Dexasone,
Hexadrol Phosphate, Solurex
Pregnancy risk category C

Indications and dosages

Cerebral edema
Adults: Initially, 10 mg phosphate I.V.; then
4 mg I.M. q 6 hours until symptoms subside (usually 2 to 4 days); then tapered
over 5 to 7 days. Oral therapy (1 to 3 mg
t.i.d.) should replace I.M. dosing as soon
as possible.
**Inflammatory conditions, allergic
reactions, neoplasias**
Adults: 0.75 to 9 mg/day P.O. or 0.5 to
9 mg/day phosphate I.M. depending on
size of affected area. Or, 8 to 16 mg acetate
I.M. into joint or soft tissue q 1 to 3 weeks.
Or, 0.8 to 1.6 mg acetate into lesions q 1 to
3 weeks.
Shock
Adults: 20 mg phosphate as single first
dose; then 3 mg/kg/24 hours via continuous I.V. infusion. Or, 1 to 6 mg/kg phosphate I.V. as single dose. Or, 40 mg phosphate I.V. q 2 to 6 hours, p.r.n., continued
only until patient is stabilized (usually not
longer than 48 to 72 hours).
**Dexamethasone suppression test for
Cushing's syndrome**
Adults: After determining baseline 24-hour
urine levels of 17-hydroxycorticosteroids,
0.5 mg P.O. q 6 hours for 48 hours. Repeat
24-hour urine collection to determine 17-

hydroxycorticosteroid excretion during second 24 hours of dexamethasone administration. Or, 1 mg P.O. as single dose at
11 p.m. with determination of plasma cortisol at 8 a.m. the next morning.
Adrenocortical insufficiency
Children: 0.024 to 0.34 mg/kg or 0.66 to
10 mg/m^2 dexamethasone P.O. daily, in
four divided doses.
Tuberculosis meningitis
Adults: 8 to 12 mg phosphate I.M. daily,
taper over 6 to 8 weeks.
**Adjunctive therapy in bacterial
meningitis**
Adults, children, infants: 0.15 mg/kg phosphate I.V. q.i.d. for the first 2 to 4 days of
anti-infective therapy.

Adverse reactions

Arrhythmias ◆ heart failure ◆ hyperglycemia ◆ insomnia ◆ osteoporosis ◆ pancreatitis ◆ peptic ulceration ◆ pseudotumor
cerebri ◆ seizures ◆ thromboembolism

Nursing considerations

◆ For better results and less toxicity, give
once-daily dose in morning.
◆ Give oral dose with food when possible.
Patient may need drugs to prevent GI irritation.
◆ Give I.M. injection deeply into gluteal
muscle. Rotate injection sites to prevent
muscle atrophy.
◆ Monitor the patient's weight, blood pressure, and electrolyte levels.
◆ Patients with diabetes may need increased insulin; monitor blood glucose levels.
◆ Drug may mask or worsen infections, including latent amebiasis.

Drugs

---

† indicates a Canadian trade name

diazepam

Apo-Diazepam†, Diastat, Diazemuls†,
Diazepam Intensol, Novo-Dipam†,
PMS-Diazepam†, Valium, Vivol†

Pregnancy risk category D

Indications and dosages

Anxiety
Adults: Depending on severity, 2 to 10 mg
P.O. b.i.d. to q.i.d. Or, 2 to 10 mg I.M. or
I.V. q 3 to 4 hours, p.r.n.
Children ages 6 months and older: 1 to
2.5 mg P.O. t.i.d. or q.i.d.; increase grad-
ually, as needed and tolerated.
Elderly patients: Initially, 2 to 2.5 mg once
daily or b.i.d.; increase gradually.

Acute alcohol withdrawal
Adults: 10 mg P.O. t.i.d. or q.i.d. during
first 24 hours; reduce to 5 mg P.O. t.i.d. or
q.i.d., p.r.n. Or, initially, 10 mg I.M. or I.V.;
then 5 to 10 mg I.M. or I.V. q 3 to 4 hours,
p.r.n.

Before endoscopic procedures
Adults: Adjust I.V. dosage to desired seda-
tive response (up to 20 mg). Or, 5 to 10 mg
I.M. 30 minutes before the procedure.

Muscle spasm
Adults: 2 to 10 mg P.O. b.i.d. to q.i.d. Or,
5 to 10 mg I.M. or I.V. initially; then 5 to 10
mg I.M. or I.V. q 3 to 4 hours, p.r.n. For
tetanus, larger doses, up to 20 mg q 2 to 8
hours, may be needed.
Children ages 5 and older: 5 to 10 mg I.M.
or I.V. q 3 to 4 hours, p.r.n.
Children ages 1 month to 5 years: 1 to 2 mg
I.M. or I.V. slowly; repeat q 3 to 4 hours,
p.r.n.

Preoperative sedation
Adults: 10 mg I.M. (preferred) or I.V. before
surgery.

Cardioversion
Adults: 5 to 15 mg I.V. 5 to 10 minutes before the procedure.

Adjunct treatment for
seizure disorders
Adults: 2 to 10 mg P.O. b.i.d. to q.i.d.
Children ages 6 months and older: Initially,
1 to 2.5 mg P.O. t.i.d. or q.i.d.; increase as
needed and tolerated.

Status epilepticus, severe
recurrent seizures
Adults: Initially, 5 to 10 mg I.V. or I.M. Use
I.M. route only if I.V. access is unavailable.
Repeat q 10 to 15 minutes, p.r.n., up to
maximum of 30 mg. Repeat q 2 to 4 hours,
if needed.
Children ages 5 and older: 1 mg I.V. q 2 to
5 minutes up to maximum of 10 mg. Repeat q 2 to 4 hours, if needed.
Children ages 1 month to 5 years: 0.2 to
0.5 mg I.V. slowly q 2 to 5 minutes up to
maximum of 5 mg. Repeat q 2 to 4 hours,
if needed.

Patients on stable regimens of
antiepileptic drugs who need
diazepam intermittently to control
bouts of increased seizure activity
Adults and children ages 12 and older:
0.2 mg/kg P.R., rounding up to the nearest
available dose form. A second dose may be
given 4 to 12 hours later.
Children ages 6 to 11: 0.3 mg/kg P.R.,
rounding up to the nearest available dose
form. A second dose may be given 4 to 12
hours later.
Children ages 2 to 5: 0.5 mg/kg P.R.,
rounding up to the nearest available dose
form. A second dose may be given 4 to 12
hours later.

Adverse reactions

Bradycardia ◆ cerebrovascular collapse ◆
drowsiness ◆ hypotension ◆ neutropenia ◆
respiratory depression

Nursing considerations

◆ Use Diastat rectal gel to treat no more
than five episodes per month and no more
than one episode every 5 days because tolerance may develop.
◆ When using oral concentrate solution, dilute the dose just before giving it.
◆ Monitor periodic hepatic, renal, and
hematopoietic function studies in patients
receiving repeated or prolonged therapy.

† indicates a Canadian trade name

digoxin

Digitek, Digoxin, Lanoxicaps, Lanoxin
Pregnancy risk category C

Indications and dosages

Heart failure, paroxysmal supra-ventricular tachycardia, atrial fibrillation and flutter
Tablets, elixir
Adults: For rapid digitalization, 0.75 to 1.25 mg P.O. over 24 hours in two or more divided doses q 6 to 8 hours. For slow digitalization, 0.125 to 0.5 mg daily for 5 to 7 days. Maintenance, 0.125 to 0.5 mg daily.
Children age 10 and older: 10 to 15 mcg/kg P.O. over 24 hours in two or more divided doses q 6 to 8 hours. Maintenance, 25% to 35% of total digitalizing dose.
Children ages 5 to 10: 20 to 35 mcg/kg P.O. over 24 hours in two or more divided doses q 6 to 8 hours. Maintenance, 25% to 35% of total digitalizing dose.
Children ages 2 to 5: 30 to 40 mcg/kg P.O. over 24 hours in two or more divided doses q 6 to 8 hours. Maintenance, 25% to 35% of total digitalizing dose.
Infants ages 1 month to 2 years: 35 to 60 mcg/kg P.O. over 24 hours in two or more divided doses q 6 to 8 hours. Maintenance, 25% to 35% of total digitalizing dose.
Neonates: 25 to 35 mcg/kg P.O. over 24 hours in two or more divided doses q 6 to 8 hours. Maintenance, 25% to 35% of total digitalizing dose.
Premature infants: 20 to 30 mcg/kg P.O. over 24 hours in two or more divided doses q 6 to 8 hours. Maintenance, 20% to 30% of total digitalizing dose.
Injection
Adults: For rapid digitalization, 0.4 to 0.6 mg I.V. initially, followed by 0.1 to 0.3 mg I.V. q 4 to 8 hours, p.r.n. and as tolerated, for 24 hours. For slow digitalization, appropriate daily maintenance dosage for 7 to 22 days p.r.n. until therapeutic levels are reached. Maintenance, 0.125 to 0.5 mg I.V. daily.
Children: Digitalizing dosage is based on the child's age and is given in three or more divided doses over the first 24 hours. First dose is 50% of total dose; subsequent doses are given q 4 to 8 hours p.r.n. and as tolerated.
Children age 10 and older: For rapid digitalization, 8 to 12 mcg/kg I.V. over 24 hours divided as above. Maintenance, 25% to 35% of total digitalizing dose, given daily as a single dose.
Children ages 5 to 10: For rapid digitalization, 15 to 30 mcg/kg I.V. over 24 hours, divided as above. Maintenance, 25% to 35% of total digitalizing dose, divided and given in two or three equal doses daily.
Children ages 2 to 5: For rapid digitalization, 25 to 35 mcg/kg I.V. over 24 hours, divided as above. Maintenance, 25% to 35% of total digitalizing dose, divided and given in two or three equal doses daily.
Infants ages 1 month to 2 years: For rapid digitalization, 30 to 50 mcg/kg I.V. over 24 hours, divided as above. Maintenance, 25% to 35% of total digitalizing dose, divided and given in two or three equal doses daily.
Neonates: For rapid digitalization, 20 to 30 mcg/kg I.V. over 24 hours, divided as above. Maintenance, 25% to 35% of total digitalizing dose, divided and given in two or three equal doses daily.
Premature neonates: For rapid digitalization, 15 to 25 mcg/kg I.V. over 24 hours, divided as above. Maintenance, 20% to 30% of total digitalizing dose, divided and given in two or three equal doses daily.

Adverse reactions

Nausea ◆ vomiting ◆ arrhythmias ◆ diarrhea ◆ dizziness ◆ generalized muscle weakness ◆ headache ◆ light flashes ◆ yellow-green halos around visual images

Nursing considerations

◆ Before giving the drug, take the patient's apical-radial pulse for 1 minute. Withhold the drug and notify the practitioner if the pulse rate is less than 60 beats/minute.
◆ Monitor digoxin level.

† indicates a Canadian trade name

diltiazem hydrochloride

Apo-Diltiaz†, Cardizem, Cardizem CD,
Cardizem LA, Cardizem SR, Cartia XT,
Dilacor XR, Diltia XT, Tiazac
Pregnancy risk category C

Indications and dosages

Management of Prinzmetal's or variant angina or chronic stable angina pectoris
Adults: 30 mg P.O. q.i.d. before meals and bedtime. Increase dose gradually to a maximum of 360 mg/day divided into three to four doses as indicated. Or, 120 or 180 mg (extended-release capsules) P.O. once daily. Adjust over a 7- to 14-day period as needed and tolerated up to a maximum of 360 mg/day (Cardizem LA), 480 mg/day (Cardizem CD, Cartia XT, Dilacor XR, Diltia XT), or 540 mg/day (Tiazac).

Hypertension
Adults: 180 to 240 mg extended-release capsules P.O. once daily. Based on the patient's response, adjust the dosage to a maximum of 480 mg/day. Or, 120 to 240 mg P.O. (Cardizem LA) once daily. Dosage may be adjusted about every 2 weeks to maximum of 540 mg daily.

Atrial fibrillation or flutter, paroxysmal supraventricular tachycardia
Adults: 0.25 mg/kg I.V. as a bolus injection over 2 minutes. If response isn't adequate after 15 minutes, 0.35 mg/kg I.V. over 2 minutes. Follow bolus with continuous I.V. infusion at 5 to 15 mg/hour (for up to 24 hours).

Adverse reactions

Abdominal discomfort ◆ arrhythmias ◆ constipation ◆ dizziness ◆ edema ◆ headache ◆ heart failure ◆ hypotension ◆ nausea ◆ rash ◆ somnolence

Nursing considerations

◆ Monitor the patient's blood pressure and heart rate at the start of therapy and during dosage adjustments.
◆ Maximum antihypertensive effect may not be seen for 14 days.
◆ If systolic blood pressure is less than 90 mm Hg or heart rate is less than 60 beats/minute, withhold dose and notify the practitioner.
◆ Don't crush or open extended-release capsules.

† indicates a Canadian trade name

diphenhydramine hydrochloride

Allerdryl†, AllerMax Allergy and Cough Formula, AllerMax Caplets, Aller-med, Banophen, Banophen Caplets, Benadryl, Benadryl Allergy, Benylin Cough, Bydramine Cough, Compoz, Diphen Cough, Diphenhist, Diphenhist Captabs, Dormarex 2, Genahist, Hydramine, Hydramine Cough, Nervine Nighttime Sleep-Aid, Nordryl Cough, Sleep-eze 3, Sominex, Tusstat, Twilite Caplets, Uni-Bent Cough

Pregnancy risk category B

Indications and dosages

Rhinitis, allergy symptoms, motion sickness, Parkinson's disease
Adults and children age 12 and older: 25 to 50 mg P.O. t.i.d. or q.i.d. Maximum, 300 mg P.O. daily. Or, 10 to 50 mg deep I.M. or I.V. Maximum by I.M. or I.V. route, 400 mg daily.
Children younger than age 12: 5 mg/kg/ day P.O., deep I.M. or I.V. in divided doses q.i.d. Maximum, 300 mg daily.
Sedation
Adults: 25 to 50 mg P.O. or deep I.M., p.r.n.
Nighttime sleep aid
Adults: 25 to 50 mg P.O. at bedtime.
Nonproductive cough (syrup only)
Adults and children age 12 and older: 25 mg P.O. q 4 to 6 hours. Don't exceed 150 mg daily.
Children ages 6 to 11: 12.5 mg P.O. q 4 to 6 hours. Don't exceed 75 mg daily.
Children ages 2 to 5: 6.25 mg P.O. q 4 to 6 hours. Don't exceed 25 mg daily.

Adverse reactions

Agranulocytosis ◆ anaphylactic shock ◆ dizziness ◆ drowsiness ◆ dry mouth ◆ epigastric distress ◆ incoordination ◆ nausea ◆ sedation ◆ seizures ◆ sleepiness ◆ thickening of bronchial secretions ◆ thrombocytopenia

Nursing considerations

◆ Don't exceed administering 25 mg/ minute I.V.
◆ Drug is contraindicated in patients having acute asthmatic attacks.
◆ Alternate injection sites to prevent irritation. Give I.M. injection deeply into large muscle.
◆ Infiltration causes tissue irritation.
◆ Expect to stop the drug 4 days before diagnostic skin testing because the drug may prevent, reduce, or mask a positive response to the test.

Drugs

dopamine hydrochloride

Intropin
Pregnancy risk category C

Indications and dosages

To treat shock and correct hemodynamic imbalances, to improve perfusion to vital organs, to increase cardiac output, or to correct hypotension
Adults: Initially, 2 to 5 mcg/kg/minute by I.V. infusion. Titrate dosage to desired hemodynamic or renal response. Infusion may be increased by 1 to 4 mcg/kg/minute at 10- to 30-minute intervals. In seriously ill patients, start with 5 mcg/kg/minute and increase gradually in increments of 5 to 10 mcg/kg/minute to a rate of 20 to 50 mcg/kg/minute, p.r.n.

Adverse reactions

Anaphylactic reactions ◆ angina ◆ palpitations ◆ asthmatic episodes ◆ dyspnea ◆ azotemia ◆ ectopic beats ◆ headache ◆ hyperglycemia ◆ hypotension ◆ nausea ◆ vomiting ◆ necrosis and tissue sloughing (with extravasation) ◆ piloerection ◆ tachycardia

Nursing considerations

◆ Drug is contraindicated in patients with uncorrected tachyarrhythmias, pheochromocytoma, or ventricular fibrillation.
◆ Dosages of 0.5 to 2 mcg/kg/minute predominantly stimulate dopamine receptors and produce vasodilation of the renal vasculature. Dosages of 2 to 10 mcg/kg/minute stimulate beta-adrenergic receptors for a positive inotropic effect. Higher dosages also stimulate alpha receptors, constricting blood vessels and increasing blood pressure. Most patients are satisfactorily maintained on dosages of less than 20 mcg/kg/minute.
◆ Use a central line or a large vein, such as in the antecubital fossa, to minimize the risk of extravasation. Watch the infusion site carefully for signs of extravasation; if it occurs, stop the infusion immediately and notify the practitioner. Extravasation may require infiltrating the area with 5 to 10 mg phentolamine (Regitine) in 10 to 15 ml normal saline solution.

◉ Nursing alert
Taper the dosage slowly to evaluate the stability of the patient's blood pressure. After the drug is stopped, watch closely for a sudden drop in blood pressure.

---

† indicates a Canadian trade name

Drugs

enalapril maleate

Vasotec

Pregnancy risk category C; D in second and third trimesters

Indications and dosages

Hypertension

Adults: In patients not taking diuretics, initially, 5 mg P.O. once daily; then adjusted based on response. Usual dosage range, 10 to 40 mg daily as a single dose or two divided doses. Or, 1.25 mg I.V. infusion over 5 minutes q 6 hours.

Children ages 1 month to 16 years: 0.08 mg/kg (up to 5 mg) P.O. once daily; dosage should be adjusted as needed up to 0.58 mg/kg (maximum 40 mg). Don't use if creatinine clearance is less than 30 ml/minute.

To convert from I.V. therapy to oral therapy

Adults: Initially, 2.5 mg P.O. once daily; if patient was receiving 0.625 mg I.V. q 6 hours, then 2.5 mg P.O. once daily. Adjust dosage based on the patient's response.

To convert from oral therapy to I.V. therapy

Adults: 1.25 mg I.V. over 5 minutes q 6 hours. Higher dosages aren't more effective.

To manage symptomatic heart failure

Adults: Initially, 2.5 mg P.O. daily or b.i.d., increased gradually over several weeks. Maintenance dosage, 5 to 20 mg daily in two divided doses. Maximum dosage, 40 mg daily in two divided doses.

Asymptomatic left ventricular dysfunction

Adults: Initially, 2.5 mg P.O. b.i.d. Increase as tolerated to target daily dosage of 20 mg P.O. in divided doses.

Adverse reactions

Abdominal pain ◆ angina pectoris ◆ angioedema ◆ asthenia ◆ bone marrow depression ◆ chest pain ◆ decreased renal function in patients with bilateral renal artery stenosis or heart failure ◆ diarrhea ◆ dizziness ◆ dry, persistent, tickling, nonproductive cough ◆ dyspnea ◆ fatigue ◆ headache ◆ hypotension ◆ nausea ◆ rash ◆ syncope ◆ vertigo ◆ vomiting

Nursing considerations

◆ Closely monitor the patient's blood pressure for therapeutic response.

Nursing alert

I.V. form and pancuronium, a paralyzing drug, have similar packaging and labeling, which could result in a fatal medication error. Check all labeling carefully.

◆ Monitor complete blood count before and during therapy.

◆ Patients with diabetes, impaired renal function, or heart failure and those receiving drugs that can increase potassium level may develop hyperkalemia. Monitor potassium intake and potassium level.

Drugs

enoxaparin sodium

Lovenox

Pregnancy risk category B

Indications and dosages

To prevent pulmonary embolism and deep vein thrombosis (DVT) after hip or knee replacement surgery

Adults: 30 mg subcutaneously q 12 hours for 7 to 10 days. Give initial dose 12 to 24 hours after surgery, if hemostasis is established. Continue treatment until risk of DVT has diminished. Hip replacement patients may receive 40 mg subcutaneously given 12 hours preoperatively. After initial phase of therapy, hip replacement patients should continue with 40 mg subcutaneously daily for 3 weeks.

To prevent pulmonary embolism and DVT after abdominal surgery

Adults: 40 mg subcutaneously daily with initial dose 2 hours before surgery. Give subsequent dose, if hemostasis is established, 24 hours after initial preoperative dose and continue once daily for 7 to 10 days. Continue treatment until risk of DVT has diminished.

To prevent pulmonary embolism and DVT in patients with acute illness who are at increased risk because of decreased mobility

Adults: 40 mg subcutaneously once daily for 6 to 11 days. Treatment for up to 14 days has been well tolerated.

To prevent ischemic complications of unstable angina and non-Q-wave myocardial infarction (with oral aspirin therapy)

Adults: 1 mg/kg subcutaneously q 12 hours until clinical stabilization (minimum 2 days) with aspirin 100 to 325 mg P.O. once daily.

Inpatient treatment of acute DVT with and without pulmonary embolism when given with warfarin (Coumadin)

Adults: 1 mg/kg subcutaneously q 12 hours or 1.5 mg/kg subcutaneously once daily (at same time each day) for 5 to 7 days until International Normalized Ratio (INR) of 2 to 3 is achieved. Warfarin therapy is usually started within 72 hours of initial enoxaparin dose.

Outpatient treatment of acute DVT without pulmonary embolism when given with warfarin

Adults: 1 mg/kg subcutaneously q 12 hours for 5 to 7 days until INR of 2 to 3 is achieved. Warfarin therapy is usually started within 72 hours of initial enoxaparin dose.

Adverse reactions

Anaphylaxis ◆ angioedema ◆ bleeding complications ◆ ecchymoses ◆ edema ◆ fever ◆ hemorrhage ◆ hypochromic anemia ◆ injection site irritation ◆ nausea ◆ peripheral edema ◆ rash ◆ thrombocytopenia ◆ urticaria

Nursing considerations

◆ Drug contraindicated in patients hypersensitive to pork products and in those with active major bleeding or thrombocytopenia.

◆ Drug isn't recommended for thromboprophylaxis in patients with prosthetic heart valves.

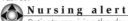 **Nursing alert**

Patients receiving the drug who also have epidural or spinal anesthesia or spinal puncture are at risk for developing epidural or spinal hematoma that can result in long-term paralysis.

◆ Monitor coagulation studies before and during therapy.

◆ Don't massage the injection site after subcutaneously injection. Watch for signs of bleeding at injection site. Document and rotate injection sites.

◆ To treat severe enoxaparin overdose, give protamine sulfate by slow I.V. infusion at a concentration of 1% to equal dose of drug injected.

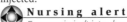 **Nursing alert**

Enoxaparin isn't interchangeable with heparin or other low-molecular-weight heparins.

---

† indicates a Canadian trade name

epinephrine (adrenaline)
Bronkaid Mistometer†, Primatene Mist

epinephrine bitartrate
AsthmaHaler Mist, Primatene Mist

epinephrine hydrochloride
Adrenalin Chloride, AsthmaNefrin, EpiPen, EpiPen Jr, microNefrin, Nephron, Vaponefrin
Pregnancy risk category C

Indications and dosages

Bronchospasm, hypersensitivity reactions, anaphylaxis
Adults: 0.1 to 0.5 ml of 1:1,000 solution subcutaneously or I.M. Repeat q 10 to 15 minutes, p.r.n. Or, 0.1 to 0.25 ml of 1:1,000 solution I.V. slowly over 5 to 10 minutes (1 to 2.5 ml of a 1:10,000 injection). May repeat q 5 to 15 minutes, p.r.n., or follow with a continuous I.V. infusion, starting at 1 mcg/minute and increasing to 4 mcg/minute, p.r.n.
Children: 0.01 ml/kg (10 mcg) of 1:1,000 solution subcutaneously; repeat q 20 minutes to 4 hours, p.r.n. Maximum single dose shouldn't exceed 0.5 mg.
Hemostasis
Adults: 1:50,000 to 1:1,000, sprayed or applied topically.
Acute asthma attacks
Adults and children ages 4 and older: 1 inhalation, repeated once if needed after at least 1 minute; don't give subsequent doses for at least 3 hours. Or, 1 to 3 deep inhalations using a hand-bulb nebulizer containing 1% (1:100) solution of epinephrine or 2.25% solution of racepinephrine, repeated q 3 hours, p.r.n.
To prolong local anesthetic effect
Adults and children: With local anesthetics, may be used in concentrations of 1:500,000 to 1:50,000; most common concentration, 1:200,000.

To restore cardiac rhythm in cardiac arrest
Adults: 0.5 to 1 mg I.V. repeated q 3 to 5 minutes, if needed. Higher-dose epinephrine may be used if 1-mg doses fail: give 3- to 5-mg (about 0.1 mg/kg) doses of epinephrine, repeated q 3 to 5 minutes.
Children: 0.01 mg/kg (0.1 ml/kg of a 1:10,000 injection) I.V. First endotracheal dose is 0.1 mg/kg (0.1 ml/kg of a 1:1,000 injection) diluted in 1 to 2 ml of normal or half-normal saline solution. Subsequent I.V. or intratracheal doses from 0.1 to 0.2 mg/kg (0.1 to 0.2 ml/kg of a 1:1,000 injection), repeated q 3 to 5 minutes, if necessary.

Adverse reactions

Agitation ◆ altered electrocardiogram ◆ anginal pain ◆ disorientation ◆ dizziness drowsiness ◆ dyspnea ◆ fear ◆ headache ◆ hemorrhage at injection site ◆ hypertension ◆ nausea ◆ nervousness ◆ pain ◆ pallor ◆ palpitations ◆ shock ◆ stroke ◆ tachycardia ◆ tissue necrosis ◆ tremor ◆ urticaria ◆ ventricular fibrillation ◆ vertigo ◆ vomiting ◆ weakness ◆ widened pulse pressure

Nursing considerations

◆ When treating the patient with reactions caused by other drugs that were given I.M. or subcutaneously, inject this drug into the site where the other drug was given to minimize further absorption.
◆ Note that 1 mg equals 1 ml of 1:1,000 solution or 10 ml of 1:10,000 solution.
◆ Discard epinephrine solution after 24 hours or if it's discolored or contains precipitate. Keep the solution in a light-resistant container until you're ready to use it.
◆ Massage the site after I.M. injection to counteract possible vasoconstriction.
◆ If blood pressure increases sharply, rapid-acting vasodilators, such as nitrates or alpha blockers, can be given to counteract the effect.

Drugs

---

† indicates a Canadian trade name

esomeprazole magnesium

Nexium

esomeprazole sodium

Nexium I.V.
Pregnancy risk category B

Indications and dosages

Gastroesophageal reflux disease (GERD) or to heal erosive esophagitis
Adults: 20 or 40 mg P.O. daily for 4 to 8 weeks. Maintenance dosage for healing erosive esophagitis is 20 mg P.O. for no longer than 6 months.
Children and adolescents ages 12 to 17 (GERD only): 20 or 40 mg P.O. once daily for up to 8 weeks.
Symptomatic GERD
Adults: 20 mg P.O. daily for 4 weeks. If symptoms are unresolved, treatment may be continued for 4 more weeks.
Short-term therapy (up to 10 days) of GERD in patients with a history or erosive gastritis who are unable to take drug orally
Adults: Reconstitute 20 or 40 mg with 5 ml of dextrose 5% in water, normal saline solution, or lactated Ringer injection and give by I.V. bolus over 3 minutes. Or, further dilute to a total volume of 50 ml and give I.V. over 10 to 30 minutes. Switch the patient to oral therapy as soon as he can tolerate it.
To reduce the risk of gastric ulcers in patients receiving continuous nonsteroidal anti-inflammatory drug therapy
Adults: 20 to 40 mg P.O. once daily for up to 6 months.
Long-term treatment of pathological hypersecretory conditions, including Zollinger-Ellison syndrome
Adults: 40 mg P.O. b.i.d. Adjust dosage based on the patient's response.
Helicobacter pylori **eradication**
Adults: 40 mg esomeprazole magnesium P.O. daily, 1,000 mg amoxicillin (Amoxil) P.O. b.i.d., and 500 mg clarithromycin (Biaxin) P.O. b.i.d., given together for 10 days to reduce duodenal ulcer recurrence.

Adverse reactions

Abdominal pain ◆ constipation ◆ diarrhea ◆ dry mouth ◆ flatulence ◆ headache ◆ nausea ◆ vomiting

Nursing considerations

◆ It's unknown if esomeprazole appears in breast milk. Because omeprazole does appear in breast milk, use esomeprazole cautiously in breast-feeding women.
◆ Give the drug at least 1 hour before meals. If patient has difficulty swallowing the capsule, contents of the capsule may be emptied and mixed with 1 tablespoon of applesauce and swallowed (without chewing the enteric-coated pellets).
◆ The patient may use antacids while taking esomeprazole, unless otherwise directed by the practitioner.
◆ Monitor liver function test results, especially in patients with preexisting hepatic disease.
◆ Long-term therapy may cause atrophic gastritis.

† indicates a Canadian trade name

famotidine

Pepcid, Pepcid AC

Pregnancy risk category B

Indications and dosages

Short-term treatment for duodenal ulcer

Adults: For acute therapy, 40 mg P.O. once daily at bedtime, or 20 mg P.O. b.i.d. Healing usually occurs within 4 weeks. For maintenance therapy, 20 mg P.O. once daily at bedtime.

Short-term treatment for benign gastric ulcer

Adults: 40 mg P.O. daily at bedtime for 8 weeks.

Children ages 1 to 16: 0.5 mg/kg P.O. daily at bedtime or divided b.i.d., up to 40 mg daily.

Pathologic hypersecretory conditions such as Zollinger-Ellison syndrome

Adults: 20 mg P.O. q 6 hours, up to 160 mg q 6 hours.

Hospitalized patients who can't take oral form or who have intractable ulcers or hypersecretory conditions

Adults: 20 mg I.V. q 12 hours.

Gastroesophageal reflux disease (GERD)

Adults: 20 mg P.O. b.i.d. for up to 6 weeks. For esophagitis caused by GERD, 20 to 40 mg b.i.d. for up to 12 weeks.

Children ages 1 to 16: 1 mg/kg/day P.O. in two divided doses, up to 40 mg b.i.d.

To prevent or treat heartburn

Adults: 10 mg Pepcid AC P.O. 1 hour before meals to prevent symptoms, or 10 mg Pepcid AC P.O. with water when symptoms occur. Maximum dosage, 20 mg daily. Drug shouldn't be taken daily for longer than 2 weeks.

Adverse reactions

Acne ◆ anorexia ◆ bone and muscle pain ◆ constipation ◆ diarrhea ◆ dizziness ◆ dry mouth ◆ dry skin ◆ fever ◆ flushing ◆ headache ◆ malaise ◆ orbital edema ◆ palpitations ◆ paresthesia ◆ taste perversion ◆ tinnitus ◆ transient irritation at I.V. site ◆ vertigo

Nursing considerations

◆ Oral suspension must be reconstituted and shaken before use.
◆ Store reconstituted oral suspension below 86° F (30° C). Discard after 30 days.
◆ Assess the patient for abdominal pain. Watch for and note blood in emesis, stool, or gastric aspirate.

fentanyl citrate
Sublimaze

fentanyl iontophoretic transdermal
Ionsys

fentanyl transdermal system
Duragesic

fentanyl transmucosal
Actiq, Fentora
Pregnancy risk category C

Indications and dosages

Adjunct to general anesthesia
Adults: For low-dosage therapy, 2 mcg/kg I.V. For moderate-dosage therapy, 2 to 20 mcg/kg I.V.; then 25 to 100 mcg I.V., p.r.n. For high-dosage therapy, 20 to 50 mcg/kg I.V.; then 25 mcg to one-half initial loading dose I.V., p.r.n.
Adjunct to regional anesthesia
Adults: 50 to 100 mcg I.M. or slowly I.V. over 1 to 2 minutes, p.r.n.
To induce and maintain anesthesia
Children ages 2 to 12: 2 to 3 mcg/kg I.V.
Postoperative pain, restlessness, tachypnea, and emergence delirium
Adults: 50 to 100 mcg I.M. q 1 to 2 hours, p.r.n.
Preoperative medication
Adults: 50 to 100 mcg I.M. 30 to 60 minutes before surgery.
Short-term management of acute postoperative pain in patients requiring opioid analgesia during hospitalization
Adults: First, use another form of opioid to make the patient comfortable. Apply the Ionsys system to intact, nonirritated skin on the chest or upper outer arm. To activate a dose, instruct the patient to firmly press the system's dose delivery button twice within 3 seconds. Each activation of

the system delivers 40 mcg of fentanyl. A maximum of six 40 mcg doses can be delivered each hour. Each system operates for 80 doses or up to 24 hours. A maximum of three systems can be used sequentially, applied to different skin sites, for a total of 72 hours of pain management.
To manage persistent, moderate to severe chronic pain in opioid-tolerant patients who require around-the-clock opioid analgesics for an extended time
Adults and children age 2 and older: When converting to the transdermal system, base the first dose on the daily dose, potency, and characteristics of the current opioid therapy; the reliability of the relative potency estimates used to calculate the needed dose; the degree of opioid tolerance; and the patient's condition. Each patch may be worn for 72 hours, although some patients may need a system applied q 48 hours. May increase dose q 3 days after first dose; thereafter, don't increase more often than q 6 days.
To manage breakthrough cancer pain in patients already receiving and tolerating an opioid
Adults: 200 mcg Actiq initially; may give second dose 15 minutes after completion of first dose (30 minutes after first lozenge has been placed in mouth). Maximum dosage, 2 lozenges per breakthrough episode. If several episodes of breakthrough pain requiring 2 lozenges occur, dosage may be increased to the next available strength. Once a successful dosage has been reached, the patient should limit use to no more than 4 lozenges daily. Or, initially 100 mcg Fentora between the upper cheek. May repeat same dose once per breakthrough episode after at least 30 minutes. Adjust in 100 mcg increments. Doses above 400 mcg may be increased by 200 mcg.
Switching from Actiq to Fentora to manage breakthrough cancer pain in opioid-tolerant patients
Adults: If current Actiq dose is 200 to 400 mcg, start with 100 mcg Fentora; if cur-

rent Actiq dose is 600 to 800 mcg, use 200 mcg Fentora; if current Actiq dose is 1,200 to 1,600 mcg, use 400 mcg Fentora.

 Nursing alert
Actiq and Fentora aren't bioequivalent.

Adverse reactions

Abdominal or chest pain ◆ anorexia ◆ anxiety ◆ apnea ◆ arrhythmias ◆ asthenia ◆ constipation or diarrhea ◆ depression ◆ diaphoresis ◆ dizziness ◆ clouded sensorium ◆ confusion ◆ hallucinations ◆ dry mouth ◆ dyspepsia ◆ dyspnea ◆ erythema at application site (with transdermal form) ◆ euphoria ◆ headache ◆ hypertension or hypotension ◆ hypoventilation ◆ ileus ◆ nausea and vomiting ◆ nervousness ◆ physical dependence ◆ pruritus ◆ respiratory depression ◆ sedation or somnolence ◆ seizures ◆ skeletal muscle rigidity (dose-related) ◆ urine retention

Nursing considerations

◆ For better analgesic effect, give the drug before the patient has intense pain.

 Nursing alert
High doses can produce muscle rigidity, which can be reversed with neuromuscular blockers; however, the patient must be artificially ventilated.

◆ Monitor the patient's circulatory and respiratory status and urinary function carefully. Drug may cause respiratory depression, hypotension, urine retention, nausea, vomiting, ileus, or altered level of consciousness.
◆ Dosage equivalent charts are available to calculate the fentanyl transdermal dose based on the daily morphine intake.
◆ When using the transdermal system, reaching steady-state level of a new dosage may take up to 6 days; expect to delay dosage adjustment until after at least two applications.
◆ Monitor the patient who develops adverse reactions to the transdermal system for at least 12 hours after removal. Fen-

tanyl level may take as long as 17 hours to decline by 50%.
◆ Because the fentanyl level rises for the first 24 hours after application, the analgesic effect can't be evaluated on the first day. Make sure the patient has adequate supplemental analgesia to prevent breakthrough pain.

Nursing alert
The Actiq lozenge shouldn't be chewed and should be consumed over about 15 minutes.

---

† indicates a Canadian trade name

fluconazole

Diflucan
Pregnancy risk category C

Indications and dosages

Oropharyngeal candidiasis
Adults: 200 mg P.O. or I.V. on first day; then 100 mg once daily for at least 2 weeks.
Children: 6 mg/kg P.O. or I.V. on first day; then 3 mg/kg daily for 2 weeks.

Esophageal candidiasis
Adults: 200 mg P.O. or I.V. on first day; then 100 mg once daily. Up to 400 mg daily has been used, depending on patient's condition and tolerance of treatment. Patients should receive the drug for at least 3 weeks and for 2 weeks after symptoms resolve.
Children: 6 mg/kg P.O. or I.V. on first day; then 3 mg/kg daily for at least 3 weeks and for at least 2 weeks after symptoms resolve. Maximum, 12 mg/kg daily.

Vulvovaginal candidiasis
Adults: 150 mg P.O. for one dose only.

Systemic candidiasis
Adults: 400 mg P.O. or I.V. on first day; then 200 mg once daily for at least 4 weeks and for 2 weeks after symptoms resolve. Doses up to 400 mg/day may be used.
Children: 6 to 12 mg/kg/day P.O. or I.V.

Cryptococcal meningitis
Adults: 400 mg P.O. or I.V. on first day; then 200 mg once daily for 10 to 12 weeks after cerebrospinal fluid (CSF) culture result is negative. Doses up to 400 mg/day may be used.
Children: 12 mg/kg/day P.O. or I.V. on first day; then 6 mg/kg/day for 10 to 12 weeks after CSF culture result is negative.

To prevent candidiasis in bone marrow transplant
Adults: 400 mg P.O. or I.V. once daily. Start treatment several days before anticipated agranulocytosis, and continue for 7 days after neutrophil count exceeds 1,000 cells/mm^3.

To suppress relapse of cryptococcal meningitis in patients with acquired immunodeficiency syndrome
Adults: 200 mg P.O. or I.V. daily.
Children: 3 to 6 mg/kg/day P.O. or I.V.

Adverse reactions

Abdominal pain ◆ anaphylaxis ◆ diarrhea ◆ dizziness ◆ dyspepsia ◆ headache ◆ leukopenia ◆ nausea ◆ vomiting ◆ rash ◆ taste perversion ◆ thrombocytopenia

Nursing considerations

◆ Serious hepatotoxicity has occurred in patients with underlying medical conditions; periodically monitor liver function during prolonged therapy.
◆ If the patient develops a mild rash, monitor him closely. Stop the drug and notify the practitioner if lesions progress.
◆ Risk of adverse reactions appears to be greater in patients infected with human immunodeficiency virus.

flumazenil

Romazicon
Pregnancy risk category C

Indications and dosages

Complete or partial reversal of sedative effects of benzodiazepines after anesthesia or conscious sedation

Adults: Initially, 0.2 mg I.V. over 15 seconds. If the patient doesn't reach desired level of consciousness after 45 seconds, repeat the dose. Repeat at 1-minute intervals, if needed, until a cumulative dose of 1 mg has been given (first dose plus four more doses). Most patients respond after 0.6 to 1 mg of drug. In case of resedation, dosage may be repeated after 20 minutes, but never give more than 1 mg at any one time or exceed 3 mg/hour.

Children ages 1 year and older: 0.01 mg/kg I.V. over 15 seconds. If the patient doesn't reach desired level of consciousness after 45 seconds, repeat the dose. Repeat at 1-minute intervals, if needed, until cumulative dose of 0.05 mg/kg or 1 mg, whichever is lower, has been given (first dose plus four more doses).

Suspected benzodiazepine overdose

Adults: Initially, 0.2 mg I.V. over 30 seconds. If the patient doesn't reach desired level of consciousness after 30 seconds, give 0.3 mg over 30 seconds. If the patient still doesn't respond adequately, give 0.5 mg over 30 seconds. Repeat 0.5-mg doses, p.r.n., at 1-minute intervals until a cumulative dose of 3 mg has been given. Most patients with benzodiazepine overdose respond to cumulative doses between 1 and 3 mg; rarely, patients who respond partially after 3 mg may need additional doses, up to 5 mg total. If the patient doesn't respond in 5 minutes after receiving 5 mg, sedation is unlikely to be caused by benzodiazepines. In case of resedation, dose may be repeated after 20 minutes, but never give more than 1 mg at any one time or exceed 3 mg/hour.

Adverse reactions

Abnormal or blurred vision ◆ agitation ◆ arrhythmias ◆ cutaneous vasodilation ◆ diaphoresis ◆ dizziness ◆ dyspnea ◆ emotional lability ◆ headache ◆ hyperventilation ◆ insomnia ◆ nausea and vomiting ◆ pain at injection site ◆ palpitations ◆ seizures ◆ tremor

Nursing considerations

◆ Drug is contraindicated in patients hypersensitive to benzodiazepines, patients who show evidence of serious tricyclic antidepressant overdose, and patients who received a benzodiazepine to treat a potentially life-threatening condition, such as status epilepticus or increased intracranial pressure.

◆ Monitor the patient closely for resedation that may occur after reversal of benzodiazepine effects because flumazenil's duration of action is shorter than all benzodiazepines.

furosemide

Apo-Furosemide[†], Furosemide
Special[†], Furoside[†], Lasix,
Novosemide[†], Uritol[†]
Pregnancy risk category C

Indications and dosages

Acute pulmonary edema
Adults: 40 mg I.V. injected slowly over 1 to
2 minutes; then 80 mg I.V. in 60 to 90 minutes if needed.

Edema
Adults: 20 to 80 mg P.O. daily in the morning, with second dose in 6 to 8 hours; carefully adjusted up to 600 mg daily if needed.
Or, 20 to 40 mg I.V. or I.M., increased by
20 mg q 2 hours until desired effect
achieved.
Infants and children: 2 mg/kg P.O. daily,
increased by 1 to 2 mg/kg in 6 to 8 hours if
needed; carefully adjusted up to 6 mg/kg
daily if needed.

Hypertension
Adults: 40 mg P.O. b.i.d. Dosage adjusted
based on response. Drug may be used as
adjunct to other antihypertensives if needed.
Children: 0.5 to 2 mg/kg P.O. once or twice
daily. Increase dose as needed up to 6 mg/
kg daily.

Adverse reactions

Abdominal discomfort ◆ agranulocytosis ◆
anorexia ◆ aplastic anemia ◆ azotemia ◆
blurred or yellowed vision ◆ constipation ◆
diarrhea ◆ dizziness ◆ fever ◆ gout ◆
headache ◆ hepatic dysfunction ◆ hyperglycemia ◆ hyperuricemia (asymptomatic)
◆ hypocalcemia ◆ hypokalemia ◆ hypomagnesemia ◆ dilutional hyponatremia ◆
hypochloremic alkalosis ◆ leukopenia ◆
muscle spasm ◆ nausea ◆ vomiting ◆ oliguria ◆ orthostatic hypotension ◆ pancreatitis ◆ paresthesia ◆ photosensitivity reactions ◆ purpura ◆ restlessness ◆ thrombocytopenia ◆ transient deafness ◆ vertigo ◆
weakness

Nursing considerations

◆ Drug is contraindicated in patients with
anuria, hepatic coma, or severe electrolyte
depletion.
◆ Give P.O. and I.M. preparations in the
morning to prevent nocturia. Give second
dose in early afternoon.
◆ Monitor weight, blood pressure, pulse
rate, intake and output, and electrolyte,
blood urea nitrogen, and carbon dioxide
levels frequently, especially during rapid
diuresis.
◆ Consult the practitioner and a dietitian
about a high-potassium diet.
◆ Monitor glucose level in patients with diabetes.
◆ Drug may need to be given I.V. in patients with severe heart failure.
◆ Monitor uric acid level, especially in patients with a history of gout.
◆ Store tablets in light-resistant container
to prevent discoloration (doesn't affect potency).
◆ Refrigerate oral furosemide solution to
ensure drug stability.

† indicates a Canadian trade name

Drugs

gentamicin sulfate

Cidomycin†, Garamycin
Pregnancy risk category D

ritus ♦ rash ♦ urticaria ♦ seizures ♦ thrombocytopenia ♦ tingling sensation ♦ tinnitus ♦ vertigo

Indications and dosages

Serious infections caused by sensitive strains of *Pseudomonas aeruginosa, Escherichia coli,* and Proteus, Klebsiella, or Staphylococcus species
Adults: 3 mg/kg I.M. or I.V. daily in three divided doses q 8 hours. For life-threatening infections, give up to 5 mg/kg I.M. or I.V. daily in three to four divided doses; reduce dose to 3 mg/kg I.M. or by I.V. infusion daily as soon as patient improves.
Children: 2 to 2.5 mg/kg I.M. or by I.V. infusion q 8 hours.
Neonates older than 1 week and infants: 2.5 mg/kg I.M. or by I.V. infusion q 8 hours.
Neonates younger than 1 week and preterm infants: 2.5 mg/kg I.M. or by I.V. infusion q 12 hours.
To prevent endocarditis caused by GI or genitourinary procedure or surgery
Adults: 1.5 mg/kg I.M. or I.V. 30 minutes before procedure or surgery. Maximum dose is 80 mg. Give with ampicillin (Principen) (vancomycin [Vancocin] in patients allergic to penicillin).
Children: 2 mg/kg I.M. or I.V. 30 minutes before procedure or surgery. Maximum, 80 mg. Give with ampicillin (vancomycin in patients allergic to penicillin).

Adverse reactions

Granulocytosis ♦ anaphylaxis ♦ anemia ♦ apnea ♦ ataxia ♦ blurred vision ♦ confusion ♦ dizziness ♦ encephalopathy ♦ eosinophilia ♦ fever ♦ headache ♦ hypotension ♦ injection site pain ♦ lethargy ♦ leukopenia ♦ myasthenia gravis–like syndrome ♦ muscle twitching ♦ nausea ♦ vomiting ♦ nephrotoxicity ♦ numbness ♦ ototoxicity ♦ peripheral neuropathy ♦ pru-

Nursing considerations

♦ Drug is contraindicated in patients with sensitivity to aminoglycosides.
♦ Obtain a specimen for culture and sensitivity testing before giving the first dose. Therapy may begin while awaiting results.
♦ Weigh the patient and review renal function study results before therapy begins.
♦ Evaluate the patient's hearing before and during therapy. Notify the practitioner of complaints of tinnitus, vertigo, or hearing loss.
♦ Obtain a blood sample to determine peak gentamicin level 1 hour after I.M. injection or 30 minutes after end of I.V. infusion; for trough levels, draw blood just before next dose.
♦ Maintain peak levels at 4 to 12 mcg/ml and trough levels at 1 to 2 mcg/ml. The maximum peak level is usually 8 mcg/ml, except in patients with cystic fibrosis, who need increased lung penetration.
♦ Monitor urine output, specific gravity, urinalysis, blood urea nitrogen and creatinine levels, and creatinine clearance.
♦ Watch for signs and symptoms of superinfection.

glipizide

Glucotrol, Glucotrol XL
Pregnancy risk category C

Indications and dosages

Adjunct to diet to lower glucose level in patients with type 2 diabetes mellitus
Immediate-release tablets
Patients older than age 65: Initially, 2.5 mg P.O. daily.
Adults: Initially, 5 mg P.O. daily 30 minutes before breakfast. Maximum once-daily dosage is 15 mg. Divide doses of more than 15 mg. Maximum dosage is 40 mg daily.
Extended-release tablets
Adults: Initially, 5 mg P.O. daily with breakfast. Increase by 5 mg q 3 months, depending on level of glycemic control. Maximum dosage is 20 mg daily.
To replace insulin therapy
Adults: If insulin dosage is more than 20 units daily, start patient at usual dosage in addition to 50% of insulin. If insulin dosage is 20 units or less daily, insulin may be stopped when glipizide starts.

Adverse reactions

Agranulocytosis ◆ aplastic anemia ◆ cholestatic jaundice ◆ constipation ◆ diarrhea ◆ dizziness ◆ drowsiness ◆ headache ◆ hemolytic anemia ◆ hypoglycemia ◆ leukopenia ◆ nausea ◆ photosensitivity reactions ◆ pruritus ◆ rash ◆ thrombocytopenia

Nursing considerations

◆ Give the immediate-release tablet 30 minutes before meals.
◆ Some patients may attain control on a once-daily regimen.
◆ The patient may switch from immediate-release to extended-release tablets at the nearest equivalent total daily dose as prescribed.
◆ During periods of stress, the patient may need insulin therapy.
◆ A patient who is switching from insulin therapy to an oral antidiabetic should check his glucose level before each meal.

---

† indicates a Canadian trade name

glyburide

DiaBeta, Euglucon†, Glynase PresTab, Micronase

Pregnancy risk category B

Indications and dosages

Adjunct to diet to lower glucose level in patients with type 2 diabetes mellitus
Nonmicronized form
Adults: Initially, 2.5 to 5 mg P.O. once daily with breakfast or first meal. Adjust to maintenance dose at no more than 2.5-mg increments at weekly intervals. Usual maintenance dosage is 1.25 to 20 mg daily as a single dose or divided doses. Maximum dosage is 20 mg P.O. daily.
Micronized form
Adults: Initially, 1.5 to 3 mg daily with breakfast or first meal. Adjust to maintenance dose at no more than 1.5-mg increments at weekly intervals. Usual maintenance dosage, 0.75 to 12 mg daily. Dosages exceeding 6 mg daily may have better response with b.i.d. dosing. Maximum dosage is 12 mg P.O. daily.
To replace insulin therapy
Adults: If insulin dosage is less than 20 units/day, initial dosage is 2.5 to 5 mg (1.5 to 3 mg micronized) P.O. daily. If insulin dosage is 20 to 40 units/day, initial dosage is 5 mg (3 mg micronized) P.O. daily. If insulin dosage is 40 or more units/day, initially may give 5-mg regular tablets or 3-mg micronized formulation P.O. once daily in addition to 50% of the insulin dosage.

Adverse reactions

Agranulocytosis ◆ angioedema ◆ aplastic anemia ◆ arthralgia ◆ blurred vision ◆ changes in accommodation ◆ cholestatic jaundice ◆ epigastric fullness ◆ heartburn ◆ hemolytic anemia ◆ hepatitis ◆ hypoglycemia ◆ leukopenia ◆ myalgia ◆ nausea ◆ pruritus, rash, or other allergic reactions ◆ thrombocytopenia

Nursing considerations

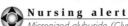 **Nursing alert**
Micronized glyburide (Glynase PresTab) isn't bioequivalent to regular glyburide tablets. Patients who have been taking Micronase or DiaBeta need dosage adjustment.
◆ Patients may need insulin therapy during periods of stress.
◆ Patients switching from insulin therapy to an oral antidiabetic should check their glucose level before each meal.

---

† indicates a Canadian trade name

haloperidol

Apo-Haloperidol†, Haldol, Novo-Peridol†, Peridol

haloperidol decanoate

Haldol Decanoate, Haldol LA†

haloperidol lactate

Haldol, Haldol Concentrate, Haloperidol Intensol
Pregnancy risk category C

Indications and dosages

Psychotic disorders
Adults and children older than age 12:
Dosage varies for each patient. Initially, 0.5 to 5 mg P.O. b.i.d. or t.i.d. Or, 2 to 5 mg I.M. lactate q 4 to 8 hours, although hourly administration may be needed until control is obtained. Maximum, 100 mg P.O. daily.
Children ages 3 to 12 who weigh 15 to 40 kg (33 to 88 lb): Initially, 0.5 mg P.O. divided b.i.d. or t.i.d. May increase dose by 0.5 mg at 5 to 7 day intervals, depending on therapeutic response and patient tolerance. Maintenance dose, 0.05mg/kg to 0.15 mg/kg P.O. daily given in two to three divided doses. Severely disturbed children may need higher doses.
Chronic psychosis requiring prolonged therapy
Adults: 50 to 100 mg I.M. decanoate q 4 weeks.
Nonpsychotic behavior disorders
Children ages 3 to 12: 0.05 to 0.075 mg/kg P.O. daily, in two to three divided doses. Maximum, 6 mg daily.
Tourette syndrome
Adults: 0.5 to 5 mg P.O. b.i.d. , t.i.d., or p.r.n.
Children ages 3 to 12: 0.05 to 0.075 mg/kg P.O. daily, in two to three divided doses.
Elderly patients: 0.5 to 2 mg P.O. b.i.d. or t.i.d.; increase gradually p.r.n.
Delirium
Adults: 1 to 2 mg I.V. lactate q 2 to 4 hours. Severely agitated patients may require higher doses.

Elderly patients: 0.25 to 0.5 mg I.V. q 4 hours.

Adverse reactions

Anorexia ◆ blood pressure changes ◆ blurred vision ◆ confusion ◆ diaphoresis ◆ diarrhea ◆ drowsiness ◆ electrocardiogram changes ◆ headache ◆ insomnia ◆ nausea and vomiting ◆ neuroleptic malignant syndrome ◆ sedation ◆ seizures ◆ severe extrapyramidal reactions ◆ tardive dyskinesia ◆ urine retention ◆ vertigo

Nursing considerations

◆ Protect the drug from light. Slight yellowing of injection or concentrate is common and doesn't affect potency. Discard markedly discolored solutions.
◆ When switching from tablets to decanoate injection, give 10 to 15 times the oral dose once per month (maximum 100 mg).
◆ Dilute oral dose with water or a beverage, such as orange juice, apple juice, tomato juice, or cola, immediately before administration.

 Nursing alert
Don't give decanoate form I.V.

◆ Monitor the patient for tardive dyskinesia, which may occur after prolonged use. It may not appear until months or years later and may disappear spontaneously or persist for life, despite discontinuing the drug.

 Nursing alert
Watch for signs and symptoms of neuroleptic malignant syndrome (extrapyramidal effects, hyperthermia, autonomic disturbance), which is rare but commonly fatal.

 Nursing alert
Don't withdraw the drug abruptly unless required by severe adverse reactions.

---

† indicates a Canadian trade name

heparin sodium

Hepalean†, Heparin Leo†, Heparin Lock Flush Solution (with Tubex), Heparin Sodium Injection, Hep-Lock, Hep-Pak

Pregnancy risk category C

Indications and dosages

Full-dose continuous I.V. infusion therapy for deep vein thrombosis (DVT), myocardial infarction (MI), and pulmonary embolism
Adults: Initially, 5,000 units by I.V. bolus; then 750 to 1,500 units/hour by I.V. infusion. Titrate hourly rate based on partial thromboplastin time (PTT) results (q 4 to 6 hours in the early stages of treatment).
Children: Initially, 50 units/kg I.V.; then 25 units/kg/hour or 20,000 units/m² daily by I.V. infusion. Titrate dosage based on PTT.
Full-dose subcutaneous therapy for DVT, MI, and pulmonary embolism
Adults: Initially, 5,000 units I.V. bolus and 10,000 to 20,000 units in a concentrated solution subcutaneously; then 8,000 to 10,000 units subcutaneously q 8 hours or 15,000 to 20,000 units subcutaneously in a concentrated solution q 12 hours.
Full-dose intermittent I.V. therapy for DVT, MI, and pulmonary embolism
Adults: Initially, 10,000 units by I.V. bolus; then titrate according to PTT, with 5,000 to 10,000 units I.V. q 4 to 6 hours.
Children: Initially, 100 units/kg by I.V. bolus; then 50 to 100 units/kg q 4 hours.
Fixed low-dose therapy for venous thrombosis, pulmonary embolism, atrial fibrillation with embolism, postoperative DVT, and prevention of embolism
Adults: 5,000 units subcutaneously q 12 hours. For surgical patients, give first dose 1 to 2 hours before procedure; then 5,000 units subcutaneously q 8 to 12 hours for 5 to 7 days or until the patient can walk.

Consumptive coagulopathy (such as disseminated intravascular coagulation)
Adults: 50 to 100 units/kg by I.V. bolus or continuous I.V. infusion q 4 hours.
Children: 25 to 50 units/kg by I.V. bolus or continuous I.V. infusion q 4 hours. If no improvement within 4 to 8 hours, stop heparin.
Open-heart surgery
Adults: For total body perfusion, 150 to 400 units/kg via continuous I.V. infusion.
To maintain patency of I.V. indwelling catheters
Adults: 10 to 100 units I.V. flush. Use sufficient volume to fill the device.

Adverse reactions

Anaphylactoid reactions ◆ cutaneous or subcutaneous necrosis ◆ fever ◆ hematoma ◆ hemorrhage ◆ hypersensitivity reactions ◆ overly prolonged clotting time ◆ thrombocytopenia ◆ urticaria ◆ white clot syndrome

Nursing considerations

◆ Draw blood to establish baseline coagulation parameters before initiating therapy.
◆ Inject subcutaneous drug slowly into fat pad. Leave needle in place for 10 seconds after injection, and then withdraw needle. Don't massage the area after injection, and watch for signs of bleeding at injection site. Alternate injection sites every 12 hours.
◆ Measure PTT carefully and regularly. Anticoagulation is present when PTT value is 1½ to 2 times the control value.
◆ Monitor platelet count regularly. When new thrombosis accompanies thrombocytopenia (white clot syndrome), expect to stop heparin.
◆ Regularly inspect the patient for signs of bleeding.

◆ Nursing alert
To treat severe heparin overdose, use protamine sulfate.

hydrochlorothiazide

Apo-Hydro†, Diuchlor H†, Esidrix, Ezide, HydroDIURIL, Hydro-Par, Microzide, Neo-Codema†, Novo-Hydrazide†, Oretic, Urozide†

Pregnancy risk category B

Indications and dosages

Edema
Adults: 25 to 100 mg P.O. daily as a single or divided dose; patient may respond to intermittent therapy on alternate days or 3 to 5 days/week.

Hypertension
Adults: 12.5 to 50 mg P.O. once daily. Increase or decrease daily dosage based on blood pressure.
Children ages 2 to 12: 2.2 mg/kg P.O. or 60 mg/m² P.O. daily in two divided doses. Usual dosage range is 37.5 to 100 mg daily.
Children ages 6 months to 2 years: 2.2 mg/kg P.O. or 60 mg/m² P.O. daily in two divided doses. Usual dosage range is 12.5 to 37.5 mg daily.
Children younger than age 6 months: Up to 3.3 mg/kg P.O. daily in two divided doses.

Adverse reactions

Agranulocytosis ◆ anaphylactic reaction ◆ aplastic anemia ◆ leukopenia ◆ pancreatitis ◆ renal failure ◆ respiratory distress ◆ thrombocytopenia

Nursing considerations

◆ Hydrochlorothiazide is contraindicated in patients with anuria, hepatic coma, or hypersensitivity to other thiazides or sulfonamide derivatives.
◆ To prevent nocturia, give drug in the morning.
◆ Monitor fluid intake and output, weight, blood pressure, and blood urea nitrogen, creatinine, and electrolyte levels.
◆ Monitor uric acid level, especially in patients with history of gout.
◆ Monitor glucose level, especially in patients with diabetes.
◆ Monitor elderly patients, who are especially susceptible to excessive diuresis.
◆ Expect to stop thiazides and thiazide-like diuretics before parathyroid function tests.
◆ In patients with hypertension, therapeutic response may be delayed several weeks.

† indicates a Canadian trade name

Drugs

hydrocortisone

Aquacort†, Cortef, Cortenema, Hydrocortone

hydrocortisone acetate

Anucort-HC, Anusol-HC, Cortifoam, Hydrocortone Acetate, Proctocort

hydrocortisone cypionate

Cortef

hydrocortisone sodium phosphate

Hydrocortone Phosphate

hydrocortisone sodium succinate

A-Hydrocort, Solu-Cortef
Pregnancy risk category C

Indications and dosages

Severe inflammation or adrenal insufficiency
Adults: 10 to 320 mg P.O. t.i.d., or q.i.d. Or, initially, 100 to 500 mg succinate I.M. or I.V.; repeat q 2 to 10 hours, as needed. Or, 15 to 240 mg phosphate I.M., subcutaneously, or I.V. daily in divided doses q 12 hours. Or, 5 to 75 mg acetate into joints or soft tissue, repeated at 3 to 5 days for bursae and 1 to 4 weeks for joints. Dosage varies with size of joint. Local anesthetics commonly are injected with dose.
Shock
Adults: Initially, 50 mg/kg succinate I.V., repeated in 4 hours; repeat dosage q 24 hours, p.r.n. Or, 0.5 to 2 g q 2 to 6 hours, continued until the patient is stabilized (usually not longer than 48 to 72 hours).
Children: 0.16 to 1 mg/kg or 6 to 30 mg/m² I.M. (phosphate or succinate) or I.V. (succinate) once or twice daily.
Adjunct treatment for ulcerative colitis and proctitis
Adults: 1 enema (100 mg) P.R. nightly for 21 days. Or, 1 applicatorful (90-mg foam)

P.R. daily or b.i.d. for 14 to 21 days. Or, 25 mg rectal suppository b.i.d. for 2 weeks. For severe proctitis, 25 mg P.R. t.i.d. or 50 mg P.R. b.i.d.

Adverse reactions

Adrenal insufficiency with increased stress or following abrupt withdrawal after long-term therapy ◆ delayed wound healing and easy bruising ◆ euphoria ◆ GI irritation ◆ heart failure ◆ hyperglycemia ◆ increased appetite ◆ increased urine calcium level ◆ insomnia ◆ menstrual irregularities ◆ muscle weakness ◆ nausea and vomiting ◆ osteoporosis ◆ pancreatitis ◆ peptic ulceration ◆ seizures ◆ susceptibility to infections ◆ thromboembolism ◆ thrombophlebitis ◆ vertigo

After abrupt withdrawal
Depression ◆ dizziness ◆ dyspnea ◆ fainting ◆ fatigue ◆ hypoglycemia ◆ lethargy ◆ orthostatic hypotension ◆ rebound inflammation ◆ weakness

Nursing considerations

◆ For better results and less toxicity, give a once-daily dose in the morning.
◆ Give oral dose with food when possible. The patient may need medication to prevent GI irritation.
◆ Give I.M. injection deeply into gluteal muscle. Rotate injection sites to prevent muscle atrophy. Avoid subcutaneous injection because atrophy and sterile abscesses may occur.
◆ Enema may produce systemic effects. If enema therapy must exceed 21 days, expect to stop therapy gradually.
◆ High-dose therapy usually isn't continued beyond 48 hours.
◆ Drug may mask or worsen infections, including latent amebiasis.
◆ Watch for depression or psychotic episodes, especially during high-dose therapy.
◆ Patients with diabetes may need increased insulin; monitor glucose level.

Drugs

† indicates a Canadian trade name

hydromorphone hydrochloride (dihydromorphinone hydrochloride)

Dilaudid, Dilaudid-5, Dilaudid-HP
Pregnancy risk category C

Indications and dosages

Moderate to severe pain
Adults: 2 to 4 mg P.O. q 4 to 6 hours, p.r.n. Or, 1 to 4 mg I.M., subcutaneously, or I.V. (slowly over at least 2 to 5 minutes) q 4 to 6 hours, p.r.n. Or, 3 mg P.R. suppository q 6 to 8 hours, p.r.n.
Cough
Adults and children older than age 12: 1 mg cough syrup P.O. q 3 to 4 hours, p.r.n.
Children ages 6 to 12: 0.5 mg cough syrup P.O. q 3 to 4 hours, p.r.n.

Adverse reactions

Blurred vision ◆ bradycardia ◆ bronchospasm ◆ clouded sensorium ◆ constipation ◆ diaphoresis ◆ diplopia ◆ dry mouth ◆ euphoria ◆ flushing ◆ ileus ◆ induration (with repeated subcutaneous injections) ◆ light-headedness ◆ nausea and vomiting ◆ nystagmus ◆ physical dependence ◆ pruritus ◆ respiratory depression ◆ sedation or somnolence ◆ urine retention

Nursing considerations

◆ Drug is contraindicated in patients with intracranial lesions caused by increased intracranial pressure and whenever ventilator function is depressed, such as in status asthmaticus, chronic obstructive pulmonary disease, cor pulmonale, and kyphoscoliosis.
◆ Reassess the patient's pain level 15 and 30 minutes after administration.
◆ Rotate injection sites to avoid induration.
◆ Monitor respiratory and circulatory status and bowel function.

◆ Keep the opioid antagonist naloxone (Narcan) available.

---

† indicates a Canadian trade name

ibuprofen

Advil, Apo-Ibuprofen†, Bayer Select
Ibuprofen Pain Relief Formula,
Children's Advil, Children's Motrin,
Excedrin IB, Genpril, Haltran, Ibu-Tab,
Medipren, Menadol, Midol IB, Motrin,
Novo-Profen†, Nuprin, Pamprin-IB,
Rufen, Saleto-200, Trendar
*Pregnancy risk category B; D in third
trimester*

Indications and dosages

**Rheumatoid arthritis, osteoarthritis,
and arthritis**
Adults: 300 to 800 mg P.O. t.i.d. or q.i.d.
Maximum dosage, 3.2 g daily.
**Mild to moderate pain or
dysmenorrhea**
Adults: 400 mg P.O. q 4 to 6 hours, p.r.n.
Fever
Adults: 200 to 400 mg P.O. q 4 to 6 hours,
for no longer than 3 days. Maximum
dosage is 1.2 g daily.
Children ages 6 months to 12 years: If
child's temperature is below 102.5° F
(39.2° C), give 5 mg/kg P.O. q 6 to 8 hours.
Treat higher temperatures with 10 mg/kg q
6 to 8 hours. Maximum, 40 mg/kg daily.
Juvenile arthritis
Children: 30 to 40 mg/kg P.O. daily in three
or four divided doses. Maximum, 50 mg/kg
daily.

Adverse reactions

Abdominal pain ◆ acute renal failure ◆
agranulocytosis ◆ anemia or aplastic anemia ◆ aseptic meningitis ◆ azotemia ◆
bloating ◆ bronchospasm ◆ constipation or
diarrhea ◆ cystitis ◆ decreased appetite ◆
dizziness ◆ dyspepsia ◆ edema ◆ epigastric distress ◆ flatulence ◆ fluid retention ◆
headache ◆ heartburn ◆ hematuria ◆ hyperkalemia ◆ hypoglycemia ◆ leukopenia
◆ neutropenia ◆ pancytopenia ◆ thrombocytopenia ◆ nausea ◆ nervousness ◆ occult
blood loss ◆ peptic ulceration ◆ peripheral
edema ◆ prolonged bleeding time ◆ pruri-

tus ◆ rash or urticaria ◆ Stevens-Johnson
syndrome ◆ tinnitus

Nursing considerations

◆ Drug is contraindicated in patients with
nasal polyps, angioedema, or bronchospas-
tic reaction to aspirin or other nonsteroidal
anti-inflammatory drugs (NSAIDs).
◆ Check renal and hepatic function periodically in patients on long-term therapy.
◆ NSAIDs such as ibuprofen may mask
signs and symptoms of infection.

 Nursing alert
*Serious GI toxicity can occur in patient
taking NSAIDs, despite a lack of symptoms.*
◆ It may take 1 or 2 weeks before full anti-
inflammatory effects are evident.
◆ If patient consumes three or more alcoholic drinks per day, use of ibuprofen may
lead to stomach bleeding.

---

† indicates a Canadian trade name

insulins

insulin (regular)

Humulin R, Humulin R Regular U-500 (concentrated), Novolin R, Novolin R PenFill, Novolin R Prefilled

insulin (rDNA) inhalation powder

Exubera

insulin (lispro)

Humalog

insulin lispro protamine and insulin lispro

Humalog Mix 75/25

isophane insulin suspension

Humulin N, Novolin N, Novolin N PenFill, Novolin N Prefilled

isophane insulin suspension and insulin injection combinations

Humulin 70/30, Novolin 70/30, Novolin 70/30 PenFill, Novolin 70/30 Prefilled, Humulin 50/50

Pregnancy risk category B

Indications and dosages

Moderate to severe diabetic ketoacidosis or hyperosmolar hyperglycemia (regular insulin)
Adults older than age 20: Give loading dose of 0.15 units/kg I.V. direct injection, followed by 0.1 unit/kg/hour as a continuous infusion. If glucose level doesn't fall by 50 mg/dl in the first hour, double the insulin infusion rate q hour until glucose level decreases steadily by 50 to 75 mg/dl. Decrease insulin infusion rate to 0.05 to 0.1 unit/kg/hour when glucose level reaches 250 to 300 mg/dl. Start infusion of dextrose 5% in water (D_5W) in half-normal saline solution separately from the insulin infusion when glucose level is 150 to 200 mg/dl in patients with diabetic ketoacidosis or 250 to 300 mg/dl in those with hyperosmolar hyperglycemia. Give dose of insulin subcutaneously 1 to 2 hours before stopping insulin infusion (intermediate-acting insulin is recommended).
Adults and children ages 20 and younger: Loading dose isn't recommended. Begin therapy at 0.1 unit/kg/hour by I.V. infusion. When the patient's condition improves, decrease insulin infusion rate to 0.05 unit/kg/hour. Start infusion of D_5W in half-normal saline solution separately from the insulin infusion when glucose level is 250 mg/dl.
Mild diabetic ketoacidosis (regular insulin)
Adults older than age 20: Give loading dose of 0.4 to 0.6 unit/kg divided in two equal parts, with half the dose given by direct I.V. injection and half given I.M. or subcutaneously. Subsequent doses can be based on 0.1 unit/kg/hour I.M. or subcutaneously.
Newly diagnosed diabetes mellitus (regular insulin)
Adults older than age 20: Individualize dosage. Initially, 0.5 to 1 unit/kg/day subcutaneously as part of a regimen with short-acting and long-acting insulin therapy.
Adults and children ages 20 and younger: Individualize dosage. Initially, 0.1 to 0.25 unit/kg subcutaneously q 6 to 8 hours for 24 hours; then adjust accordingly.
Control of hyperglycemia in patients with type 1 diabetes mellitus (Humalog and longer-acting insulin)
Adults: Dosage varies and must be determined by a practitioner who is familiar with the patient's metabolic needs, eating habits, and other lifestyle variables. Inject subcutaneously within 15 minutes before or after a meal.

---

† indicates a Canadian trade name

Control of hyperglycemia in patients with type 2 diabetes mellitus (Humalog and sulfonylureas)

Adults and children older than age 3: Dosage varies and must be determined by a practitioner familiar with the patient's metabolic needs, eating habits, and other lifestyle variables. Inject subcutaneously within 15 minutes before or after a meal.

For patients with type 1 or type 2 diabetes to control hyperglycemia with inhalation powder (Exubera)

Adults: Initially, 0.05 mg/kg oral inhalation per meal, rounded down to the nearest whole milligram. Give within 10 minutes of a meal. Adjust dosage based on the patient's need and glucose response.

Off-label use for hyperkalemia

Adults: 50 ml dextrose 50% given over 5 minutes, followed by 5 to 10 units of regular insulin by I.V. push.

♦ Lispro insulin may be mixed with Humulin N; give within 15 minutes before a meal to prevent a hypoglycemic reaction.
♦ For a patient using inhaled insulin, obtain baseline pulmonary function tests.
♦ Carefully monitor glucose levels when switching from subcutaneous to inhaled insulin.

Adverse reactions

Anaphylaxis ♦ hyperglycemia or hypoglycemia ♦ hypersensitivity reactions ♦ hypokalemia ♦ hypomagnesemia ♦ lipoatrophy ♦ lipohypertrophy ♦ pruritus ♦ rash or redness ♦ swelling, stinging, urticaria, warmth at injection site

Nursing considerations

♦ Insulin requirements increase in pregnant women with diabetes and then decline immediately postpartum. Monitor these patients closely.
♦ Use only syringes calibrated for the particular concentration of insulin given.
♦ To mix insulin suspension, swirl the vial gently or rotate it between the palms or between the palm and the thigh. Don't shake vigorously; doing so causes bubbling and air in the syringe.
♦ When mixing regular insulin with intermediate or long-acting insulin, always draw up regular insulin into syringe first.

Drugs

† indicates a Canadian trade name

isosorbide dinitrate
Apo-ISDN†, Cedocard SR†, Dilatrate-SR, Isordil, Isordil Titradose

isosorbide mononitrate
Imdur, ISMO, Monoket
Pregnancy risk category C

Indications and dosages

Acute anginal attacks (sublingual [S.L.] and chewable tablets of isosorbide dinitrate only)
Adults: 2.5 to 5 mg S.L. tablets for relief of angina, repeated q 5 to 10 minutes (maximum of three doses for each 30-minute period). For prevention, 2.5 to 10 mg q 2 to 3 hours.

For prevention in situations likely to cause anginal attacks
Adults: 5 to 40 mg isosorbide dinitrate P.O. b.i.d. or t.i.d. for prevention only (use smallest effective dose).
Adults: 30 to 60 mg isosorbide mononitrate (Imdur) P.O. once daily on arising; increase to 120 mg once daily after several days, if needed.
Adults: 20 mg isosorbide mononitrate (ISMO or Monoket) b.i.d. with the two doses given 7 hours apart.

Adverse reactions

Ankle edema ◆ cutaneous vasodilation ◆ dizziness ◆ fainting ◆ orthostatic hypotension ◆ flushing ◆ headache ◆ nausea ◆ vomiting ◆ palpitations ◆ rash ◆ S.L. burning ◆ tachycardia ◆ weakness

Nursing considerations

◆ Drug is contraindicated in patients with idiosyncratic reactions to nitrates and in those with severe hypotension, shock, or acute myocardial infarction with low left ventricular filling pressure.
◆ To prevent tolerance, a nitrate-free interval of 8 to 12 hours per day is recommended. The regimen for isosorbide mononitrate (1 tablet on awakening with the second dose in 7 hours, or 1 extended-release tablet daily) is intended to minimize nitrate tolerance by providing a substantial nitrate-free interval.
◆ Monitor the patient's blood pressure and the intensity and duration of drug response.
◆ Drug may cause headaches, especially at beginning of therapy. Dosage may be reduced temporarily, but tolerance usually develops. Treat headache with aspirin or acetaminophen (Tylenol).
◆ Methemoglobinemia has occurred with nitrate use. Signs and symptoms of methemoglobinemia are those of impaired oxygen delivery despite adequate cardiac output and adequate arterial partial pressure of oxygen.

---

† indicates a Canadian trade name

Drugs

lansoprazole

Prevacid, Prevacid IV, Prevacid SoluTab

Pregnancy risk category B

Indications and dosages

Short-term treatment of active duodenal ulcer
Adults: 15 mg P.O. daily before eating for 4 weeks.
Maintenance of healed duodenal ulcer
Adults: 15 mg P.O. daily.
Short-term treatment of active benign gastric ulcer
Adults: 30 mg P.O. once daily for up to 8 weeks.
Short-term I.V. therapy for erosive esophagitis when patient can't take oral drug
Adults: 30 mg I.V. daily over 30 minutes for up to 7 days. As soon as the patient can take the drug orally, switch to P.O. form and continue for 6 to 8 weeks.
Short-term treatment of erosive esophagitis
Adults: 30 mg P.O. daily before eating for up to 8 weeks. If healing doesn't occur, 8 more weeks of therapy may be given. Maintenance dosage for healing is 15 mg P.O. daily.
Children ages 12 to 17: 30 mg P.O. once daily for up to 8 weeks.
Children ages 1 to 11 weighing more than 30 kg (66 lb): 30 mg P.O. once daily for up to 12 weeks. Increase dosage up to 30 mg b.i.d. in patients who remain symptomatic after 2 weeks.
Children ages 1 to 11 weighing 30 kg or less: 15 mg P.O. once daily for up to 12 weeks. Increase dosage up to 30 mg b.i.d. in patients who remain symptomatic after 2 weeks.
Long-term treatment of pathologic hypersecretory conditions, including Zollinger-Ellison syndrome
Adults: Initially, 60 mg P.O. once daily. Increase dosage, p.r.n. Give daily amounts above 120 mg in evenly divided doses.

Helicobacter pylori **eradication to reduce risk of duodenal ulcer recurrence**
Adults: For patients receiving dual therapy, 30 mg P.O. lansoprazole with 1 g P.O. amoxicillin (Amoxil), each given t.i.d. for 14 days. For patients receiving triple therapy, 30 mg P.O. lansoprazole with 1 g P.O. amoxicillin and 500 mg P.O. clarithromycin (Biaxin), all given b.i.d. for 10 to 14 days.
Short-term treatment of symptomatic gastroesophageal reflux disease
Adults: 15 mg P.O. once daily for up to 8 weeks.
Children ages 12 to 17: 15 mg P.O. once daily for up to 8 weeks.
Children ages 1 to 11, weighing more than 30 kg (66 lb): 30 mg P.O. once daily for up to 12 weeks. Dosage may be increased up to 30 mg b.i.d. in patients who remain symptomatic after 2 weeks.
Children ages 1 to 11, weighing 30 kg or less: 15 mg P.O. once daily for up to 12 weeks. Dosage may be increased up to 30 mg b.i.d in patients who remain symptomatic after 2 weeks.
Nonsteroidal anti-inflammatory drug (NSAID)-related ulcer in patients who take NSAIDs
Adults: 30 mg P.O. daily for 8 weeks.
NSAID-related ulcer risk reduction in patients with history of gastric ulcer who need NSAIDs
Adults: 15 mg P.O. daily for up to 12 weeks.

Adverse reactions

Abdominal pain ◆ diarrhea ◆ nausea

Nursing considerations

◆ Capsule contents may be mixed with 40 ml of apple juice in a syringe and given within 3 to 5 minutes via a nasogastric (NG) tube. Flush the tube with additional apple juice to give the entire dose and maintain patency of the tube.

† indicates a Canadian trade name

Drugs

levothyroxine sodium (T₄, L-thyroxine sodium)

levothyroxine sodium (T_4, L-thyroxine sodium)

Eltroxin†, Levo-T, Levotec†, Levothroid, Levoxine, Levoxyl, Novothyrox, Synthroid, Thyro-Tabs, Unithroid
Pregnancy risk category A

Indications and dosages

Myxedema coma
♦ *Adults:* Give initial dose of 200 to 500 mcg I.V. An additional dose of 100 to 300 mcg may be given on the second day if there hasn't been any substantial or progressive improvement. Continue with lower daily I.V. dosages until the patient is stable and oral maintenance therapy can begin.

Thyroid hormone replacement
Adults younger than age 50 or those older than age 50 who have recently been treated for hyperthyroidism or who have been hypothyroid for a short period: Give 1.7 mcg/kg P.O. once daily. Monitor thyroid-stimulating hormone (TSH) level q 6 to 8 weeks, making dosage changes in 12.5 to 25 mcg increments until the patient is euthyroid and TSH level normalizes.
Adults age 50 or older or those younger than 50 with underlying cardiac disease: Give 25 to 50 mcg P.O. daily. Adjust dose q 6 to 8 weeks, if needed, until patient is euthyroid and TSH level normalizes.
Children older than age 12: More than 150 mcg or 2 to 3 mcg/kg P.O. daily.
Children ages 6 to 12: 100 to 150 mcg or 4 to 5 mcg/kg P.O. daily.
Children ages 1 to 5: 75 to 100 mcg or 5 to 6 mcg/kg P.O. daily.
Children ages 6 months to 1 year: 50 to 75 mcg or 6 to 8 mcg/kg P.O. daily.
Children ages 3 to 6 months: 25 to 50 mcg or 8 to 10 mcg/kg P.O. daily.
Infants and neonates from birth to 3 months: 10 to 15 mcg/kg P.O. daily. In neonates at risk for cardiac failure, use a lower initial dose and increase q 4 to 6 weeks, p.r.n.

Elderly patients with an underlying cardiovascular disease: 12.5 to 50 mcg P.O. daily; increase by 12.5 to 25 mcg q 6 to 8 weeks, depending on the patient's response.

Severe, long-standing hypothyroidism
Adults: 12.5 to 25 mcg P.O. daily. Increase in increments of 25 mcg q 2 to 4 weeks, p.r.n.
Children: 25 mcg P.O. daily. Increase in increments of 25 mcg q 2 to 4 weeks, p.r.n.

Adverse reactions

Allergic skin reactions ♦ angina pectoris ♦ arrhythmias ♦ cardiac arrest ♦ decreased bone density ♦ diaphoresis ♦ diarrhea ♦ fever ♦ headache ♦ heat intolerance ♦ insomnia ♦ menstrual irregularities ♦ nervousness ♦ palpitations ♦ tachycardia ♦ tremor ♦ vomiting ♦ weight loss

Nursing considerations

♦ Drug may be given I.V. or I.M. when P.O. route isn't available for long periods. The I.V. dose is about one-half the previously established oral dose.
♦ Patients with diabetes mellitus may need increased antidiabetic dosages when starting thyroid hormone replacement.
♦ In patients with coronary artery disease who must receive thyroid hormone, observe carefully for possible coronary insufficiency.
♦ Patients with adult hypothyroidism are unusually sensitive to thyroid hormone. Start at lowest dosage and adjust to higher dosages according to patient's symptoms and laboratory data.
♦ When changing from levothyroxine to liothyronine (Cytomel), stop levothyroxine and begin liothyronine. Increase dosage in small increments, as prescribed, after residual effects of levothyroxine have disappeared. When changing from liothyronine to levothyroxine, start levothyroxine several days before withdrawing liothyronine to avoid relapse. These drugs aren't interchangeable.

† indicates a Canadian trade name

Drugs

lisinopril

Prinivil, Zestril

Pregnancy risk category C; D in second and third trimesters

Indications and dosages

Hypertension

Adults: Initially, 10 mg P.O. daily for patients not taking a diuretic. Most patients are well controlled on 20 to 40 mg daily as a single dose. For patients taking a diuretic, initially, 5 mg P.O. daily.

Children age 6 and older: Initially, 0.07 mg/kg (up to 5 mg) P.O. once daily. Increase dosage based on the patient's response and tolerance. Maximum dosage is 0.61 mg/kg (don't exceed 40 mg). Don't use in children with creatinine clearance less than 30 ml/minute.

Adjunct treatment (with diuretics and cardiac glycosides) for heart failure

Adults: Initially, 5 mg P.O. daily; increased, p.r.n., to a maximum of 20 mg P.O. daily.

Hemodynamically stable patients within 24 hours of acute myocardial infarction to improve survival

Adults: Initially, 5 mg P.O.; then 5 mg after 24 hours, 10 mg after 48 hours, followed by 10 mg once daily for 6 weeks.

Adverse reactions

Chest pain ◆ diarrhea ◆ dizziness ◆ Dry, persistent, tickling, nonproductive cough ◆ dyspepsia ◆ dyspnea ◆ fatigue ◆ headache ◆ hyperkalemia ◆ hypotension ◆ impaired renal function ◆ impotence ◆ nasal congestion ◆ nausea ◆ orthostatic hypotension ◆ paresthesia ◆ rash

Nursing considerations

◆ Although angiotensin-converting enzyme (ACE) inhibitors such as lisinopril reduce blood pressure in all races, they reduce it less in black patients taking an ACE inhibitor alone. Black patients should take the drug with a thiazide diuretic for a more favorable response.

◆ Monitor blood pressure frequently. If the drug doesn't adequately control blood pressure, diuretics may be added.

◆ Monitor white blood cell with differential counts before therapy, every 2 weeks for first 3 months of therapy, and periodically thereafter.

Drugs

---

† indicates a Canadian trade name

lorazepam

Apo-Lorazepam†, Ativan, Lorazepam Intensol, Novo-Lorazem†, Nu-Loraz

Pregnancy risk category D

Indications and dosages

Anxiety
Adults: 2 to 6 mg P.O. daily in divided doses. Maximum, 10 mg daily.
Elderly patients: 1 to 2 mg P.O. daily in divided doses. Maximum, 10 mg daily.
Insomnia from anxiety
Adults: 2 to 4 mg P.O. at bedtime.
Preoperative sedation
Adults: 2 mg I.V. total or 0.044 mg/kg I.V., whichever is smaller. Larger doses up to 0.05 mg/kg I.V., to total of 4 mg, may be needed. Or, 0.05 mg/kg I.M. 2 hours before procedure. Total dose shouldn't exceed 4 mg.
Status epilepticus
Adults: 4 mg I.V. if seizures continue or recur after 10 to 15 minutes, then an additional 4 mg dose may be given. Drug may be given I.M. if I.V. access isn't available.
Children: 0.05 to 0.1 mg/kg (off-label use).
For nausea and vomiting caused by emetogenic cancer chemotherapy (off-label use)
Adults: 2.5 mg P.O. the evening before and just after starting chemotherapy. Or, 1.5 mg/m² (usually up to a maximum of 3 mg) I.V. over 5 minutes 45 minutes before starting chemotherapy.

Adverse reactions

Abdominal discomfort ◆ agitation ◆ amnesia ◆ change in appetite ◆ depression ◆ disorientation ◆ dizziness ◆ headache ◆ hypotension ◆ insomnia ◆ nausea ◆ sedation and drowsiness ◆ unsteadiness ◆ visual disturbances ◆ weakness

Nursing considerations

◆ Drug is contraindicated in patients with angle-closure glaucoma and in patients hypersensitive to benzodiazepines or the vehicle used in parenteral forms.

Nursing alert
Use of this drug may lead to abuse and addiction. Drug shouldn't be stopped abruptly after long-term use because withdrawal symptoms may occur.

◆ For I.V. use, dilute lorazepam with an equal volume of compatible diluent, such as dextrose 5% in water, sterile water for injection, or normal saline solution. The rate of I.V. injection shouldn't exceed 2 mg/minute. Keep emergency resuscitation equipment readily available.
◆ For I.M. administration, inject deeply into a muscle. Don't dilute.
◆ Monitor hepatic, renal, and hematopoietic function periodically in patients receiving repeated or prolonged therapy.

---

† indicates a Canadian trade name

magnesium sulfate

Pregnancy risk category A

Indications and dosages

To prevent or control seizures in preeclampsia or eclampsia

♦ *Women:* Initially, 4 g I.V. in 250 ml dextrose 5% in water (D$_5$W) or normal saline solution and 4 to 5 g deep I.M. into each buttock; then 4 to 5 g deep I.M. into alternate buttock q 4 hours, p.r.n. Or, 4 g I.V. loading dose; then 1 to 3 g hourly as I.V. infusion. Total dose shouldn't exceed 30 or 40 g daily.

Hypomagnesemia

Adults: For mild deficiency, 1 g I.M. q 6 hours for four doses; for severe deficiency, 5 g in 1,000 ml D$_5$W or normal saline solution infused over 3 hours.

Seizures, hypertension, and encephalopathy with acute nephritis in children

Children: 20 to 40 mg/kg I.M., p.r.n., to control seizures. Dilute 50% concentrate to a 20% solution and give 0.1 to 0.2 ml/kg of the 20% solution.

Management of paroxysmal atrial tachycardia

Adults: 3 to 4 g I.V. over 30 seconds, with extreme caution.

Management of life-threatening ventricular arrhythmias, such as sustained ventricular tachycardia or torsades de pointes (off-label use)

Adults: 1 to 6 g I.V. over several minutes; then continuous I.V. infusion of 3 to 20 mg/minute for 5 to 48 hours. Base dosage and duration of therapy on the patient's response and magnesium level.

Management of preterm labor (off-label use)

Women: 4 to 6 g I.V. over 20 minutes, followed by 2 to 4 g/hour I.V. infusion for 12 to 24 hours, as tolerated, after contractions have ceased.

Adverse reactions

Bradycardia ♦ circulatory collapse ♦ depressed cardiac function ♦ depressed reflexes ♦ diaphoresis ♦ diplopia ♦ drowsiness ♦ flaccid paralysis ♦ flushing ♦ hypocalcemia ♦ hypotension ♦ hypothermia ♦ respiratory paralysis

Nursing considerations

♦ Parenteral use is contraindicated in patients with heart block or myocardial damage.

♦ If drug is used to treat seizures, take appropriate seizure precautions.

 Nursing alert

Watch for respiratory depression and signs and symptoms of heart block.

♦ Give by I.V. infusion pump if possible; maximum infusion rate is 150 mg/minute.

♦ Keep I.V. calcium gluconate available to reverse magnesium toxicity, but use it cautiously in digitalized patients because of the danger of arrhythmias.

♦ Check magnesium level after repeated doses. Disappearance of knee-jerk and patellar reflexes is a sign of impending magnesium toxicity.

♦ Effective anticonvulsant level ranges from 2.5 to 7.5 mEq/L.

♦ Monitor fluid intake and output. Make sure urine output is 100 ml or more in 4-hour period before each dose.

♦ When giving I.V. form of the drug to a toxemic mother within 24 hours of delivery, plan to observe the neonate for signs and symptoms of magnesium toxicity, including neuromuscular or respiratory depression.

Drugs

---

† indicates a Canadian trade name

mannitol

Osmitrol

Pregnancy risk category C

Indications and dosages

Test dose for marked oliguria or suspected inadequate renal function
Adults and children older than age 12: 200 mg/kg or 12.5 g as a 15% to 20% I.V. solution over 3 to 5 minutes. Response is adequate if 30 to 50 ml of urine/hour is excreted over 2 to 3 hours; if response is inadequate, a second test dose is given. If still no response, stop the drug.

Oliguria
Adults and children older than age 12: 50 to 100 g I.V. as a 15% to 25% solution over 90 minutes to several hours.

To prevent oliguria or acute renal failure
Adults and children older than age 12: 50 to 100 g I.V. of a 5% to 25% solution. Determine exact concentration by fluid requirements.

To reduce intraocular or intracranial pressure
Adults and children older than age 12: 1.5 to 2 g/kg as a 15% to 20% I.V. solution over 30 to 60 minutes. For maximum intraocular pressure reduction before surgery, give 60 to 90 minutes preoperatively.

Diuresis in drug toxicity
Adults and children older than age 12: 5% to 10% solution continuously up to 200 g I.V., while maintaining 100 to 500 ml urine output/hour and a positive fluid balance.

Irrigating solution during transurethral resection of the prostate gland
Adults: 2.5% to 5% solution, p.r.n.

Adverse reactions

Angina-like chest pain ◆ blurred vision ◆ chills ◆ dehydration ◆ diarrhea ◆ dizziness ◆ dry mouth ◆ edema ◆ fever ◆ headache ◆ heart failure ◆ hypertension or hypotension ◆ local pain ◆ nausea and vomiting ◆ rhinitis ◆ seizures ◆ tachycardia ◆ thirst ◆ thrombophlebitis ◆ urine retention ◆ urticaria ◆ vascular overload

Nursing considerations

◆ Give the drug I.V. via an in-line filter. Monitor the I.V. site closely for signs of extravasation.
◆ Monitor vital signs, including central venous pressure and fluid intake and output, hourly. Report increasing oliguria. Check weight, renal function, fluid balance, and serum and urine sodium and potassium levels daily.
◆ Insert a urinary catheter in a comatose or an incontinent patient because therapy is based on strict evaluation of fluid intake and output.

† indicates a Canadian trade name

methylprednisolone

Medrol, Medrol Dosepak, Meprolone Unipak

methylprednisolone acetate

depMedalone 40, depMedalone 80, Depo-Medrol, Depopred-40, Depopred-80

methylprednisolone sodium succinate

A-Methapred, Solu-Medrol
Pregnancy risk category C

Indications and dosages

Severe inflammation or immunosuppression
Adults: 2 to 60 mg base P.O. usually in four divided doses. Or, initially, 24 mg (six 4-mg tablets) on the first day; taper by 4 mg per day until 21 tablets have been given. Or 10 to 80 mg acetate I.M. daily, or 10 to 250 mg succinate I.M. or I.V. up to six times daily. Or, 4 to 40 mg acetate into smaller joints or 20 to 80 mg acetate into larger joints. Intralesional use is usually 20 to 60 mg acetate. Intralesional and intra-articular injections may be repeated q 1 to 5 weeks.
Children: 0.117 to 1.66 mg/kg or 3.3 to 50 mg/m² P.O. daily in three or four divided doses. Or, 0.03 to 0.2 mg/kg or 1 to 6.25 mg/m² succinate I.M. once daily or b.i.d.

Congenital adrenogenital syndrome
Children: 40 mg acetate I.M. q 2 weeks.

Shock
Adults: 100 to 250 mg succinate I.V. at 2- to 6-hour intervals. Or, 30 mg/kg I.V. initially, repeated q 4 to 6 hours, p.r.n. Give over 3 to 15 minutes. Continue therapy for 2 to 3 days or until the patient is stable.

Adverse reactions

Acute adrenal insufficiency with increased stress or following abrupt withdrawal after long-term therapy ◆ arrhythmias ◆ cardiac arrest ◆ heart failure ◆ cataracts ◆ glaucoma ◆ circulatory collapse ◆ cushingoid state ◆ delayed wound healing ◆ edema ◆ euphoria ◆ GI irritation ◆ growth suppression in children ◆ hirsutism ◆ hypercholesterolemia ◆ hyperglycemia ◆ hypertension ◆ hypocalcemia ◆ hypokalemia ◆ increased appetite ◆ insomnia ◆ menstrual irregularities ◆ muscle weakness ◆ nausea ◆ vomiting ◆ osteoporosis ◆ seizures ◆ susceptibility to infections ◆ thromboembolism ◆ thrombophlebitis ◆ various skin eruptions

After abrupt withdrawal
Anorexia ◆ arthralgia ◆ depression ◆ dizziness ◆ fainting ◆ dyspnea ◆ fatigue ◆ lethargy ◆ fever ◆ hypoglycemia ◆ orthostatic hypotension ◆ rebound inflammation ◆ weakness

Nursing considerations

 Nursing alert
Sudden withdrawal after prolonged use may be fatal.

◆ For better results and less toxicity, give a once-daily dose in the morning.
◆ Give oral dose with food when possible. Critically ill patients may need to take drug with an antacid or a histamine-2 receptor antagonist.
◆ Give I.M. injection deeply into gluteal muscle. Avoid subcutaneous injection because atrophy and sterile abscesses may occur.
◆ When giving direct I.V. injection, inject over at least 1 minute.
◆ Discard reconstituted solution after 48 hours.
◆ Drug may mask or worsen infections, including latent amebiasis.
◆ Watch for depression or psychotic episodes, especially in high-dose therapy.
◆ Patients with diabetes may need increased insulin dosage; monitor blood glucose level.

Drugs

metoprolol succinate
Toprol XL

metoprolol tartrate
Apo-Metoprolol†, Apo-Metoprolol
(Type L)†, Betaloc Durules†, Lopresor†,
Lopresor SR†, Lopressor, Novo-
Metoprol†, Nu-Metop†
Pregnancy risk category C

Indications and dosages

Hypertension
Adults: Initially, 50 mg P.O. b.i.d. or 100 mg
P.O. once daily; then up to 100 to 450 mg
daily in two or three divided doses. Or, 50
to 100 mg extended-release tablets (tartrate
equivalent) once daily. Adjust dosage as
needed and tolerated at weekly intervals to
maximum of 400 mg daily.

Early intervention in acute myocardial infarction (MI)
Adults: 5 mg metoprolol tartrate I.V. bolus
q 2 minutes for three doses. Then, 15 minutes after the last I.V. dose, give 25 to
50 mg P.O. q 6 hours for 48 hours. Maintenance dosage, 100 mg P.O. b.i.d.

Angina pectoris
Adults: Initially, 100 mg P.O. daily as a single dose or in two equally divided doses;
increased weekly until adequate response
or a pronounced decrease in heart rate is
seen. Effects of daily dose beyond 400 mg
aren't known. Or, 100 mg extended-release
tablets (tartrate equivalent) once daily. Adjust dosage as needed and tolerated at
weekly intervals to maximum of 400 mg
daily.

Stable, symptomatic heart failure (New York Heart Association class II) resulting from ischemia, hypertension, or cardiomyopathy
Adults: 25 mg (succinate) P.O. once daily
for 2 weeks. Double the dosage q 2 weeks,
as tolerated, to a maximum of 200 mg daily.

Adverse reactions
Atrioventricular block ◆ bradycardia ◆ diarrhea ◆ depression ◆ dizziness ◆ fatigue
◆ dyspnea ◆ heart failure ◆ hypotension ◆
nausea ◆ rash ◆

Nursing considerations
◆ When used to treat hypertension or angina, drug is contraindicated in patients with
sinus bradycardia, greater than first-degree
heart block, cardiogenic shock, or overt
cardiac failure. When used to treat MI,
drug is contraindicated in patients with
heart rate less than 45 beats/minute,
greater than first-degree heart block, PR interval of 0.24 second or longer with first-
degree heart block, systolic blood pressure
less than 100 mm Hg, or moderate to severe cardiac failure.
◆ Check apical pulse before giving the
drug. Hold the drug and notify practitioner
if pulse is less than 60 beats/minute.
◆ Monitor blood glucose level in patients
with diabetes; this drug masks signs and
symptoms of hypoglycemia.
◆ Monitor blood pressure frequently; this
drug masks common signs and symptoms
of shock.
◆ Store the drug at room temperature and
protect from light. Discard the solution if
it's discolored or contains particles.

---

† indicates a Canadian trade name

morphine sulfate

Astramorph PF, Avinza, DepoDur, Duramorph, Epimorph†, Infumorph, Infumorph 500, Kadian, M-Eslon†, Morphine H.P.†, MS Contin, MSIR, Oramorph SR, RMS Uniserts, Roxanol, Statex

Controlled substance schedule II
Pregnancy risk category C

Indications and dosages

Severe pain
Adults: 5 to 20 mg subcutaneously or I.M. or 2.5 to 15 mg I.V. q 4 hours, p.r.n. Or, 5 to 30 mg P.O. or 10 to 20 mg P.R. q 4 hours, p.r.n. For continuous I.V. infusion, give loading dose of 15 mg I.V.; then continuous infusion of 0.8 to 10 mg/hour. May also give a 15- or 30-mg extended-release tablet P.O. q 8 to 12 hours. For sustained-release Kadian capsules used as a first opioid, give 20 mg P.O. q 12 hours or 40 mg P.O. once daily; increase conservatively in opioid-naive patients. For epidural injection, give 5 mg by epidural catheter; if pain isn't relieved in 1 hour, give supplementary doses of 1 to 2 mg at intervals sufficient to assess efficacy. Maximum total epidural dosage, 10 mg/24 hours. For intrathecal injection, a single dose of 0.2 to 1 mg may provide pain relief for 24 hours (only in the lumbar area). Don't repeat injections.
Children: 0.1 to 0.2 mg/kg subcutaneously or I.M. q 4 hours. Maximum single dose, 15 mg.

Moderate to severe pain requiring a continuous, around-the-clock opioid
Adults: Individualize dosage of Avinza. For patients with no tolerance to opioids, begin with 30 mg Avinza P.O. daily; adjust dosage by no more than 30 mg q 4 days. When converting from another oral morphine formulation, individualize the dosing schedule according to the patient's previous drug-dosing schedule.

Single-dose, epidural extended pain relief after major surgery
Adults: Inject 10 to 15 mg (maximum, 20 mg) DepoDur via lumbar epidural before surgery or after clamping of umbilical cord during cesarean section. Drug may be injected undiluted or may be diluted up to 5 ml total volume with preservative-free normal saline solution.

Adverse reactions

Anorexia ◆ apnea ◆ biliary tract spasms ◆ bradycardia ◆ cardiac arrest ◆ clouded sensorium ◆ hallucinations ◆ constipation ◆ decreased libido ◆ depression ◆ diaphoresis ◆ dizziness ◆ syncope ◆ dry mouth ◆ edema ◆ euphoria ◆ hypertension or hypotension ◆ ileus ◆ nausea ◆ vomiting ◆ nervousness ◆ nightmares ◆ physical dependence ◆ pruritus and skin flushing ◆ respiratory depression or arrest ◆ sedation or somnolence ◆ seizures ◆ shock ◆ tachycardia ◆ thrombocytopenia ◆ urine retention

Nursing considerations

◆ Reassess the patient's level of pain 15 and 30 minutes after giving parenterally and 30 minutes after giving orally.
◆ Keep the opioid antagonist naloxone (Narcan) and resuscitation equipment readily available.
◆ Oral capsules may be opened and the contents poured into cool, soft foods; the patient should consume the mixture immediately.
◆ When the drug has been given epidurally, monitor the patient closely for respiratory depression. Check respiratory rate and depth every 30 to 60 minutes for 24 hours after injection.
◆ Monitor circulatory, respiratory, bladder, and bowel functions carefully. Withhold the dose and notify the practitioner if respirations are below 12 breaths/minute.
◆ Constipation is commonly severe with maintenance dosage. Ensure that a stool softener or other laxative is prescribed.

Drugs

---

† indicates a Canadian trade name

naloxone hydrochloride

Narcan
Pregnancy risk category B

Indications and dosages

Known or suspected opioid-induced respiratory depression, including those caused by pentazocine and naloxone (Talwin NX) and propoxyphene (Darvon-N)
Adults: 0.4 to 2 mg I.V., I.M., or subcutaneously, repeated q 2 to 3 minutes, p.r.n. If there's no response after 10 mg has been given, question diagnosis of opioid-induced toxicity.
Children: 0.01 mg/kg I.V.; then second dose of 0.1 mg/kg I.V., if needed. If I.V. route isn't available, drug may be given I.M. or subcutaneously in divided doses.
Neonates: 0.01 mg/kg I.V., I.M., or subcutaneously. Repeat dose q 2 to 3 minutes, p.r.n.
Postoperative opioid depression
Adults: 0.1 to 0.2 mg I.V. q 2 to 3 minutes, p.r.n. Repeat dose within 1 to 2 hours if needed.
Children: 0.005 to 0.01 mg I.V. repeated q 2 to 3 minutes, p.r.n.
Neonates (asphyxia neonatorum): 0.01 mg/kg I.V. into the umbilical vein. Dose may be repeated q 2 to 3 minutes.

Adverse reactions

Diaphoresis ◆ hypertension (with higher-than-recommended doses) ◆ hypotension ◆ nausea and vomiting ◆ pulmonary edema ◆ seizures ◆ tachycardia ◆ tremor ◆ ventricular fibrillation ◆ withdrawal symptoms in opioid-dependent patients (with higher-than-recommended doses)

Nursing considerations

◆ Naloxone may be given by continous I.V. infusion; usual dosage is 2 mg in 500 ml of dextrose 5% in water or normal saline solution.

Nursing alert
The opioid's duration of action may exceed that of naloxone, and patients may relapse into respiratory depression.
◆ Monitor the patient's respiratory depth and rate. Be prepared to provide oxygen, ventilation, and other resuscitation measures.

---

† indicates a Canadian trade name

Drugs

naproxen

Apo-Naproxen†, EC-Naprosyn,
Naprosyn, Naprosyn-E†, Naprosyn-SR,
Naxen†, Novo-Naprox†, Nu-Naprox†

naproxen sodium

Aleve, Anaprox, Anaprox DS, Apo-
Napro-Na†, Naprelan, Novo-Naprox
Sodium†, Synflex†

*Pregnancy risk category B; D in third
trimester*

Indications and dosages

**Rheumatoid arthritis,
osteoarthritis, ankylosing
spondylitis, pain, dysmenorrhea,
tendinitis, and bursitis**
Adults: 250 to 500 mg naproxen b.i.d.;
maximum, 1.5 g daily for a limited time.
Or, 375 to 500 mg delayed-release EC-
Naprosyn b.i.d. Or, 750 to 1,000 mg controlled-release Naprelan daily. Or, 275 to
550 mg naproxen sodium b.i.d.
Juvenile arthritis
Children: 10 mg/kg P.O. in two divided
doses.
Acute gout
Adults: 750 mg naproxen P.O., then 250 mg
q 8 hours until the attack subsides. Or,
825 mg naproxen sodium; then 275 mg q 8
hours until attack subsides. Or, 1,000 to
1,500 mg daily controlled-release Naprelan
on first day; then 1,000 mg daily until the
attack subsides.
**Mild to moderate pain,
primary dysmenorrhea**
Adults: 500 mg naproxen P.O., then 250 mg
q 6 to 8 hours up to 1.25 g daily. Or, 550
mg naproxen sodium; then 275 mg q 6 to
8 hours up to 1,375 mg daily. Or, 1,000 mg
controlled-release Naprelan once daily.
Elderly patients: For patients older than age
65, don't exceed 400 mg daily.

Adverse reactions

Abdominal pain ◆ auditory and visual disturbances ◆ constipation or diarrhea ◆ diaphoresis ◆ dizziness ◆ drowsiness ◆ dyspepsia ◆ dyspnea ◆ ecchymoses ◆ edema
◆ epigastric pain ◆ headache ◆ heartburn
◆ hyperkalemia ◆ increased bleeding time
◆ occult blood loss ◆ nausea ◆ palpitations
◆ peptic ulceration ◆ pruritus, rash, purpura, or urticaria ◆ stomatitis ◆ thirst ◆ tinnitus ◆ vertigo

Nursing considerations

◆ Because nonsteroidal anti-inflammatory
drugs (NSAIDs) such as naproxen impair
synthesis of renal prostaglandins, they can
decrease renal blood flow and lead to reversible renal impairment, especially in patients with renal failure, heart failure, or
hepatic dysfunction; in elderly patients;
and in those taking diuretics. Monitor
these patients closely.
◆ Monitor complete blood count and renal
and hepatic function every 4 to 6 months
during long-term therapy.
◆ NSAIDs may mask signs and symptoms
of infection.
◆ Naproxen may have a heart benefit, similar to that of aspirin, in preventing blood
clotting.

Drugs

---

† indicates a Canadian trade name

nesiritide

Natrecor
Pregnancy risk category C

Indications and dosages

Acutely decompensated heart failure in patients with dyspnea at rest or with minimal activity
Adults: 2 mcg/kg by I.V. bolus over 60 seconds, followed by continuous infusion of 0.01 mcg/kg/minute.

Adverse reactions

Abdominal pain ◆ anemia ◆ angina ◆ anxiety ◆ apnea ◆ atrial fibrillation ◆ atrioventricular node conduction abnormalities ◆ back pain ◆ bradycardia ◆ confusion ◆ cough ◆ diaphoresis ◆ dizziness ◆ fever ◆ headache ◆ hypotension ◆ injection site reactions ◆ insomnia ◆ leg cramps ◆ nausea and vomiting ◆ pain at injection site ◆ paresthesia ◆ pruritus ◆ rash ◆ somnolence ◆ tremor ◆ ventricular extrasystoles ◆ tachycardia

Nursing considerations

◆ Contraindicated in patients with cardiogenic shock, systolic blood pressure below 90 mm Hg, low cardiac filling pressures, conditions in which cardiac output depends on venous return, or conditions that make vasodilators inappropriate, such as valvular stenosis, restrictive or obstructive cardiomyopathy, constrictive pericarditis, and pericardial tamponade.
◆ Reconstitute one 1.5-mg vial with 5 ml of diluent (such as dextrose 5% in water [D_5W], normal saline solution, D_5W and 0.2% saline solution injection, or D_5W and half-normal saline solution) from a prefilled 250-ml I.V. bag. Gently rock (don't shake) the vial until the solution becomes clear and colorless; withdraw contents of the vial and add contents back to the 250-ml I.V. bag to yield 6 mcg/ml. Invert the bag several times to ensure complete mixing, and use the solution within 24 hours.
◆ Use the formulas below to calculate bolus volume (2 mcg/kg) and infusion flow rate (0.01 mcg/kg/minute):
Bolus volume (ml) = 0.33 × patient weight (kg)
Infusion flow rate (ml/hr) = 0.1 × patient weight (kg)
◆ Before giving a bolus dose, prime the I.V. tubing. Withdraw the bolus and give over 60 seconds through an I.V. port in the tubing.
◆ Immediately after giving the bolus, infuse the drug at 0.1 ml/kg/hour to deliver 0.01 mcg/kg/minute.
◆ Store drug at 68° to 77° F (20° to 25° C).
◆ Don't start drug at higher-than-recommended dosage; doing so may cause hypotension and may increase creatinine level.
◆ Because hypotension may occur with nesiritide administration, monitor the patient's blood pressure closely, particularly if he's taking an angiotensin-converting enzyme inhibitor.

◆ Nursing alert

Nesiritide binds heparin and could bind the heparin lining of a heparin-coated catheter, decreasing the amount of nesiritide delivered. Don't give nesiritide through a central heparin-coated catheter. Additionally, nesiritide is incompatible with injectable forms of bumetanide (Bumex), enalaprilat (Vasotec), ethacrynate sodium (Edecrin), furosemide (Lasix), heparin, hydralazine, and insulins. Don't give these drugs through the same line as nesiritide.

nitroglycerin
(glyceryl trinitrate)

Deponit, Minitran, Nitrek, Nitro-Bid, Nitro-Bid IV, Nitrodisc, Nitro-Dur, Nitrogard, Nitroglyn, Nitrolingual, Nitrong, NitroQuick, Nitrostat, NitroTab, Nitro-Time, NTS, Transderm-Nitro, Tridil

Pregnancy risk category C

Indications and dosages

Prophylaxis against chronic anginal attacks
Adults: 2.5 or 2.6 mg sustained-release capsule or tablet q 8 to 12 hours, adjusted upward to an effective dose in 2.5- or 2.6-mg increments b.i.d. to q.i.d. Or, use 2% ointment: Start with ½-inch ointment, increasing by ½-inch increments until desired results are achieved. Ointment dosage range, ½ to 5 inches. Usual dosage, 1 to 2 inches q 6 to 8 hours. Or, transdermal disc or pad (Nitrodisc, Nitro-Dur, or Transderm-Nitro) 0.2 to 0.4 mg/hour once daily.

Acute angina pectoris or prophylaxis to prevent or minimize anginal attacks before stressful events
Adults: 1 sublingual (S.L.) tablet (¹⁄₄₀₀ grain, ¹⁄₂₀₀ grain, ¹⁄₁₅₀ grain, ¹⁄₁₀₀ grain) dissolved under the tongue or in the buccal pouch as soon as angina begins; repeat q 5 minutes, if needed, for 15 minutes. Or, one or two sprays (Nitrolingual) into mouth, preferably onto or under the tongue; repeat q 3 to 5 minutes, if needed, to maximum of three doses within a 15-minute period. Or, 1 to 3 mg transmucosally q 3 to 5 hours while awake.

Hypertension from surgery, heart failure after myocardial infarction (MI), angina pectoris in acute situations, or to produce controlled hypotension during surgery (by I.V. infusion)
Adults: Initially, infuse at 5 mcg/minute, increasing, p.r.n., by 5 mcg/minute q 3 to 5 minutes until response occurs. If a 20-mcg/minute rate doesn't produce a response, increase dosage by as much as 20 mcg/minute q 3 to 5 minutes. Up to 100 mcg/minute may be needed.

Adverse reactions

Contact dermatitis ◆ cutaneous vasodilation ◆ dizziness ◆ fainting ◆ flushing ◆ headache ◆ hypersensitivity reactions ◆ nausea ◆ vomiting ◆ orthostatic hypotension ◆ palpitations ◆ rash ◆ S.L. burning ◆ tachycardia ◆ weakness

Nursing considerations

◆ Always mix the drug in glass bottles. Avoid use of I.V. filters because the drug binds to plastic. Regular polyvinyl chloride tubing can bind up to 80% of drug, making it necessary to infuse higher dosages.
◆ When changing the concentration of infusion, flush the I.V. administration set with 15 to 20 ml of the new concentration before use to clear the line of the old drug solution.
◆ Closely monitor the patient's vital signs, particularly blood pressure, during infusion.
◆ To apply ointment, measure the prescribed amount onto the application paper; then place the paper on any nonhairy area. Don't rub in the drug. Cover with plastic film to aid absorption and protect clothing. Remove all excess ointment from the previous site before applying the next dose.
◆ Transdermal dosage forms may be applied to any nonhairy part of the skin except distal parts of the arms and legs.
◆ Remove the transdermal patch before defibrillation. Because of the aluminum backing on the patch, the electric current may cause arcing that can damage the paddles and burn the patient.
◆ Drug may cause headaches, especially at beginning of therapy. Dosage may be reduced temporarily, but tolerance usually develops.
◆ Tolerance to the drug may be minimized with a 10- to 12-hour nitrate-free interval.

Drugs

nitroprusside sodium

Nipride[†], Nitropress
Pregnancy risk category C

Indications and dosages

To lower blood pressure quickly in hypertensive emergencies, to produce controlled hypotension during anesthesia, to reduce preload and afterload in cardiac pump failure or cardiogenic shock (may be used with or without dopamine)
Adults and children: Begin infusion at 0.25 to 0.3 mcg/kg/minute I.V. and gradually titrate q few minutes to a maximum infusion rate of 10 mcg/kg/minute.

Adverse reactions

Abdominal pain ♦ acidosis ♦ apprehension ♦ bradycardia ♦ cyanide toxicity ♦ diaphoresis ♦ dizziness ♦ electrocardiogram changes ♦ flushing ♦ headache ♦ hypotension ♦ hypothyroidism ♦ ileus ♦ increased intracranial pressure ♦ irritation at infusion site ♦ loss of consciousness ♦ methemoglobinemia ♦ muscle twitching ♦ nausea ♦ palpitations ♦ rash ♦ restlessness ♦ tachycardia ♦ venous streaking

Nursing considerations

♦ Drug is contraindicated in patients with compensatory hypertension such as in arteriovenous shunt or coarctation of the aorta, inadequate cerebral circulation, acute heart failure with reduced peripheral vascular resistance, congenital optic atrophy, or tobacco-induced amblyopia.

Nursing alert
Excessive doses or infusing at a rate greater than 10 mcg/kg/minute may cause cyanide toxicity. If these factors are present, check thiocyanate level every 72 hours; a level higher than 100 mcg/ml may be toxic. If profound hypotension, metabolic acidosis, dyspnea, headache, loss of consciousness, ataxia, or vomiting occurs, stop the drug immediately and notify the practitioner.

♦ Prepare solution by dissolving 50 mg in 2 to 3 ml of dextrose 5% in water (D_5W) injection or according to manufacturer's instructions. Further dilute concentration in 250, 500, or 1,000 ml of D_5W to provide solutions with 200, 100, or 50 mcg/ml, respectively. Reconstitute ADD-Vantage vials labeled as containing 50 mg of the drug according to the manufacturer's directions.
♦ Because the drug is sensitive to light, wrap the I.V. solution in foil or other opaque material; it isn't necessary to wrap the tubing. Fresh solution should have faint brownish tint. Discard if highly discolored after 24 hours.
♦ Infuse with an infusion pump. Drug is best given via piggyback through a peripheral line with no other drug. Don't titrate rate of main I.V. line while drug is being infused. Even a small bolus of nitroprusside can cause severe hypotension.
♦ Check blood pressure every 5 minutes at start of infusion and every 15 minutes thereafter.
♦ If severe hypotension occurs, stop the nitroprusside infusion; effects of drug quickly reverse. If possible, start an arterial pressure line. Regulate drug flow to desired blood pressure response.

† indicates a Canadian trade name

norepinephrine bitartrate
Levophed
Pregnancy risk category C

Indications and dosages

To restore blood pressure in acute hypotensive states
Adults: Initially, 8 to 12 mcg/minute by I.V. infusion; then titrate to maintain systolic blood pressure at 80 to 100 mm Hg in previously normotensive patients and 30 to 40 mm Hg below preexisting systolic blood pressure in previously hypertensive patients. Average maintenance dosage, 2 to 4 mcg/minute.
Children: 2 mcg/minute or 2 mcg/m^2/minute by I.V. infusion; adjust dosage based on response.
Severe hypotension during cardiac arrest
Children: Initially, 0.1 mcg/kg/minute I.V. infusion. Titrate infusion rate based on response up to 2 mcg/kg/minute.

Adverse reactions

Anxiety ◆ anaphylaxis ◆ arrhythmias ◆ asthma attacks ◆ bradycardia ◆ dizziness ◆ headache ◆ insomnia ◆ irritation (with extravasation) ◆ necrosis and gangrene secondary to extravasation ◆ respiratory difficulties ◆ restlessness ◆ severe hypertension ◆ tremor ◆ weakness

Nursing considerations

◆ Use a central venous catheter or large vein, as in the antecubital fossa, to minimize risk of extravasation. Give in dextrose 5% in water in normal saline solution for injection. Use continuous infusion pump to regulate flow rate and a piggyback setup so I.V. line stays open if norepinephrine is stopped.
◆ Check the insertion site frequently for signs of extravasation. If they appear, stop the infusion immediately and notify the practitioner. Infiltrate area with 5 to 10 mg phentolamine (Regitine) in 10 to 15 ml of normal saline solution to counteract effect of extravasation. Also, check for blanching along course of infused vein, which may progress to superficial sloughing.
◆ Protect the drug from light. Discard discolored solutions or solutions that contain a precipitate. Norepinephrine solutions deteriorate after 24 hours.
◆ Drug isn't a substitute for blood or fluid replacement therapy. If the patient has a volume deficit, replace fluids before giving vasopressors.

◆ **Nursing alert**
Never leave the patient unattended during infusion. Check blood pressure every 2 minutes until stabilized; then check every 5 minutes. In previously hypertensive patients, blood pressure should increase no more than 40 mm Hg below baseline systolic blood pressure.

◆ Frequently monitor electrocardiograms, cardiac output, central venous pressure, pulmonary artery wedge pressure, pulse rate, urine output, and color and temperature of limbs. Titrate infusion rate based on findings and practitioner guidelines.
◆ Keep emergency drugs on hand to reverse effects of norepinephrine: atropine for reflex bradycardia, phentolamine to decrease vasopressor effects, and propranolol (Inderal) for arrhythmias.
◆ Notify the practitioner immediately of decreased urine output.
◆ When stopping the drug, gradually slow the infusion rate. Continue monitoring vital signs, watching for a possible severe drop in blood pressure.

Drugs

† indicates a Canadian trade name

pantoprazole sodium

Protonix, Protonix I.V.
Pregnancy risk category B

Indications and dosages

Erosive esophagitis with gastroesophageal reflux disease (GERD)
Adults: 40 mg P.O. once daily for up to 8 weeks. For patients who haven't healed after 8 weeks of treatment, another 8-week course may be considered.
Short-term treatment of GERD in patients who can't take delayed-release tablets orally
Adults: 40 mg I.V. daily for 7 to 10 days.
Short-term treatment of GERD linked to history of erosive esophagitis
Adults: 40 mg I.V. once daily for 7 to 10 days. Switch to P.O. form as soon as patient is able.
Long-term maintenance of healing erosive esophagitis and reduction in relapse rates of daytime and nighttime heartburn symptoms in patients with GERD
Adults: 40 mg P.O. once daily.
Short-term treatment of pathologic hypersecretion conditions caused by Zollinger-Ellison syndrome or other neoplastic conditions
Adults: Individualize dosage. Usual dosage is 80 mg I.V. q 12 hours for no more than 6 days. For those needing a higher dosage, 80 mg q 8 hours is expected to maintain acid output below 10 mEq/hour. Maximum dosage is 240 mg/day.
Long-term treatment of pathologic hypersecretory conditions, including Zollinger-Ellison syndrome
Adults: Individualize dosage. Usual starting dosage is 40 mg P.O. b.i.d. Adjust dosage to a maximum of 240 mg/day.

Adverse reactions

Abdominal pain ◆ anxiety ◆ arthralgia ◆ asthenia ◆ back, chest, or neck pain ◆ belching and flatulence ◆ bronchitis ◆ constipation ◆ diarrhea ◆ dizziness ◆ dyspepsia ◆ dyspnea ◆ flulike syndrome ◆ gastroenteritis ◆ GI and rectal disorders ◆ headache ◆ hyperglycemia ◆ hyperlipemia ◆ hypertonia ◆ increased cough ◆ infection ◆ insomnia ◆ migraine ◆ nausea and vomiting ◆ pharyngitis ◆ rash ◆ rhinitis and sinusitis ◆ upper respiratory tract infection ◆ urinary frequency ◆ urinary tract infection

Nursing considerations

◆ Reconstitute each vial with 10 ml normal saline solution; compatible diluents for infusion include normal saline solution, dextrose 5% in water, or lactated Ringer's solution for injection. For patients with GERD, further dilute with 100 ml of diluent to yield 0.4 mg/ml; for patients with hypersecretion conditions, combine two reconstituted vials and further dilute with 80 ml of diluent to a total volume of 100 ml to yield 0.8 mg/ml.
◆ Infuse diluted solutions I.V. over 15 minutes at a rate of about 7 ml/minute.
◆ For a 2-minute I.V. infusion, give the reconstituted vials (final yield of about 4 mg/ml) over at least 2 minutes.
◆ The reconstituted solution may be stored for up to 2 hours and the diluted solutions for up to 22 hours at room temperature.

Drugs

---

† indicates a Canadian trade name

penicillin V potassium (phenoxymethylpenicillin potassium)

Apo-Pen VK†, Nadopen-V 200†, Nadopen-V 400†, Novo-Pen-VK†, Nu-Pen-VK†, Pen-Vee†, PVF K†, Veetids

Pregnancy risk category B

Indications and dosages

Mild to moderate systemic infections
Adults and children ages 12 and older: 125 to 500 mg P.O. q 6 hours.
Children younger than age 12: 15 to 62.5 mg/kg P.O. daily in divided doses q 6 to 8 hours.
To prevent recurrent rheumatic fever
Adults and children: 250 mg P.O. b.i.d.
Erythema chronica migrans in Lyme disease (off-label use)
Adults: 250 to 500 mg P.O. q.i.d. for 10 to 20 days.
Children younger than age 2: 50 mg/kg/day (up to 2 g/day) P.O. in four divided doses for 10 to 20 days.
To prevent inhalation anthrax after possible exposure (off-label use)
Adults: 7.5 mg/kg P.O. q.i.d. Continue treatment until exposure is ruled out. If exposure is confirmed, anthrax vaccine may be indicated. Continue treatment for 60 days.
Children younger than age 9: 50 mg/kg P.O. daily given in four divided doses. Continue treatment until exposure is ruled out. If exposure is confirmed, anthrax vaccine may be indicated. Continue treatment for 60 days.

Adverse reactions

Anaphylaxis ◆ black, hairy tongue ◆ diarrhea ◆ eosinophilia ◆ epigastric distress ◆ hemolytic anemia ◆ hypersensitivity reactions ◆ leukopenia ◆ nausea ◆ vomiting ◆ nephropathy ◆ neuropathy ◆ overgrowth of nonsusceptible organisms ◆ thrombocytopenia

Nursing considerations

◆ Before giving the drug, ask the patient whether he has experienced allergic reactions to penicillins.
◆ Obtain a specimen for culture and sensitivity testing before giving the first dose. Therapy may begin pending results.
◆ Periodically assess renal and hematopoietic function in patients receiving long-term therapy.
◆ Watch for signs and symptoms of superinfection.
◆ The American Heart Association considers amoxicillin (Amoxil) the preferred drug to prevent endocarditis; however, penicillin V is considered an alternative drug.

Drugs

---

† indicates a Canadian trade name

phenytoin

Dilantin-125, Dilantin Infatab

phenytoin sodium (prompt)

Dilantin

phenytoin sodium (extended)

Dilantin Kapseals, Phenytek
Pregnancy risk category D

Indications and dosages

To control tonic-clonic (grand mal) and complex partial (temporal lobe) seizures
Adults: Dosage is highly individualized. Initially, 100 mg P.O. t.i.d., increasing by 100 mg P.O. q 2 to 4 weeks until desired response. Usual dosage range is 300 to 600 mg daily. If the patient is stabilized with extended-release capsules, once-daily dosing with 300-mg extended-release capsules is possible as an alternative.
Children: 5 mg/kg or 250 mg/m^2 P.O. divided b.i.d. or t.i.d. Usual dosage range is 4 to 8 mg/kg daily; maximum 300 mg daily.
For patients requiring a loading dose
Adults: Initially, 1 g P.O. daily divided into three doses and given at 2-hour intervals. Or, 10 to 15 mg/kg I.V. at a rate not exceeding 50 mg/minute. Normal maintenance dosage is started 24 hours after loading dose.
Children: 500 to 600 mg P.O. in divided doses, followed by maintenance dosage 24 hours after loading dose.
To prevent and treat seizures occurring during neurosurgery
Adults: 100 to 200 mg I.M. q 4 hours during and after surgery.
Status epilepticus
Adults: Loading dose of 10 to 15 mg/kg I.V. (1 to 1.5 g may be needed) at a rate not exceeding 50 mg/minute; then maintenance dosage of 100 mg P.O. or I.V. q 6 to 8 hours.

Children: Loading dose of 15 to 20 mg/kg I.V. at a rate not exceeding 1 to 3 mg/kg/minute; then highly individualized maintenance dosages.
Elderly patients: May need lower dosages.

Adverse reactions

Agranulocytosis ◆ ataxia ◆ blurred vision ◆ bullous, purpuric, or exfoliative dermatitis ◆ constipation ◆ decreased coordination ◆ dizziness ◆ diplopia ◆ headache ◆ hyperglycemia ◆ inflammation and necrosis at injection site ◆ insomnia ◆ leukopenia ◆ lymphadenopathy ◆ macrocythemia ◆ megaloblastic anemia ◆ mental confusion ◆ nausea ◆ vomiting ◆ nervousness ◆ nystagmus ◆ pain ◆ pancytopenia ◆ photosensitivity reactions ◆ scarlatiniform or morbilliform rash ◆ slurred speech ◆ Stevens-Johnson syndrome ◆ thrombocytopenia ◆ toxic hepatitis ◆ twitching

Nursing considerations

◆ Drug is contraindicated in patients with sinus bradycardia, sinoatrial block, second- or third-degree atrioventricular block, or Adams-Stokes syndrome.
◆ Give I.V. bolus slowly (50 mg/minute).
◆ Don't mix the drug with dextrose 5% in water because it will precipitate. Clear I.V. tubing first with normal saline solution.
◆ If possible, don't give phenytoin by I.V. push into the veins on the back of the hand to avoid discoloration (purple-glove syndrome). Inject the drug into larger veins or a central venous catheter, if available.
◆ Don't give the drug I.M. unless dosage adjustments are made; drug may precipitate at injection site, cause pain, and be absorbed erratically.
◆ Don't stop the drug suddenly; doing so may worsen seizures. Notify the practitioner at once if adverse reactions develop.
◆ Monitor drug levels. Therapeutic level is 10 to 20 mcg/ml.

† indicates a Canadian trade name

Drugs

potassium chloride

Apo-K†, Cena-K, Gen-K, K+8, K+10, Kaochlor, Kaochlor S-F, Kaon-Cl, Kaon Cl-10, Kaon-Cl 20%, Kay Ciel, K+ Care, K-Dur 20, K-Lease, K-Lor, Klor-Con, Klor-Con 8, Klor-Con 10, Klor-Con/25, Klorvess, Klotrix, K-Lyte/Cl, K-Norm, K-Tab, Micro-K, Micro-K 10, Micro-K LS, Potasalan, Rum-K, Slow-K, Ten-K

Pregnancy risk category C

Indications and dosages

To prevent hypokalemia
Adults and children: Initially, 20 mEq of potassium supplement P.O. daily in divided doses. Adjust dosage, p.r.n., based on potassium levels.
Hypokalemia
Adults and children: 40 to 100 mEq P.O. in two to four divided doses daily. Maximum dosage of diluted I.V. potassium chloride is 40 mEq/L at 10 mEq/hour. Don't exceed 150 mEq daily in adults and 3 mEq/kg daily in children. Further doses are based on potassium levels and blood pH. Give I.V. potassium replacement only with monitoring of electrocardiogram (ECG) and potassium level.
Severe hypokalemia
Adults and children: Dilute potassium chloride in a suitable I.V. solution of less than 80 mEq/L, and give at no more than 40 mEq/hour. Further doses are based on potassium level. Don't exceed 150 mEq I.V. daily in adults and 3 mEq/kg I.V. daily or 40 mEq/m^2 I.V. daily in children. Give I.V. potassium replacement only with monitoring of ECG and potassium level.
Acute myocardial infarction (off-label use)
Adults: For high dose, 80 mEq/L at 1.5 ml/kg/hour for 24 hours with an I.V. infusion of 25% dextrose and 50 units/L regular insulin. For low dose, 40 mEq/L at 1 ml/kg/hour for 24 hours, with an I.V. infusion of 10% dextrose and 20 units/L regular insulin.

Adverse reactions

Abdominal pain ◆ arrhythmias ◆ cardiac arrest ◆ confusion ◆ diarrhea ◆ ECG changes ◆ flaccid paralysis ◆ heart block ◆ hyperkalemia ◆ hypotension ◆ listlessness ◆ nausea ◆ vomiting ◆ paresthesia of limbs ◆ postinfusion phlebitis ◆ respiratory paralysis ◆ weakness or heaviness of limbs

Nursing considerations

◆ Use I.V. route only when oral replacement isn't feasible or when hypokalemia is life-threatening.

⬥ **Nursing alert**
When giving the drug parenterally, give by I.V. infusion only, never by I.V. push or I.M. Give slowly as a dilute solution; potentially fatal hyperkalemia may result from too-rapid infusion. Decrease the I.V. rate if burning occurs during infusion.

◆ Make sure powders are completely dissolved before giving the drug.
◆ Tablets in wax matrix sometimes lodge in the esophagus and cause ulceration in cardiac patients with esophageal compression from an enlarged left atrium. Use liquid form in such patients and in those with esophageal stasis or obstruction.
◆ Don't crush sustained-release forms of potassium.
◆ Monitor ECG and electrolyte levels during therapy.
◆ Monitor renal function. Potassium shouldn't be given during the immediate postoperative period until urine flow is established.

Drugs

prednisone

Apo-Prednisone†, Liquid Pred, Meticorten, Orasone, Panasol-S, Prednicen-M, Prednisone Intensol, Sterapred Unipak, Winpred†

Pregnancy risk category C

Indications and dosages

Severe inflammation, immunosuppression

Adults: 5 to 60 mg P.O. daily in single dose or as two to four divided doses. Maintenance dose given once daily or every other day; dosage must be individualized.
Children: 0.14 to 2 mg/kg or 4 to 60 mg/m² daily P.O. in four divided doses.

Contact dermatitis, poison ivy
Adults: Initially, 30 mg (six 5-mg tablets); taper by 5 mg daily until 21 tablets have been given.

Acute exacerbations of multiple sclerosis
Adults: 200 mg P.O. daily for 7 days; then 80 mg P.O. every other day for 1 month.

Advanced pulmonary tuberculosis
Adults: 40 to 60 mg P.O. daily; taper over 4 to 8 weeks.

Tuberculosis meningitis
Adults: 1 mg/kg P.O. daily for 30 days; taper over several weeks.

Adjunctive treatment in *Pneumocystis carinii* pneumonia in patients with acquired immunodeficiency syndrome. (off-label use)
Adults and children age 13 and older: 40 mg P.O. b.i.d. for 5 days; then 40 mg P.O. daily for 5 days; then 20 mg P.O. daily for 11 days or until completion of anti-infective therapy.

Adverse reactions

Acute adrenal insufficiency with increased stress or following abrupt withdrawal after long-term therapy ◆ arrhythmias ◆ cardiac arrest ◆ heart failure ◆ cataracts ◆ glaucoma ◆ circulatory collapse ◆ cushingoid state ◆ delayed wound healing ◆ edema ◆ euphoria ◆ GI irritation ◆ headache ◆ hirsutism ◆ hypercholesterolemia ◆ hyperglycemia ◆ hypertension ◆ hypocalcemia ◆ hypokalemia ◆ increased appetite ◆ insomnia ◆ menstrual irregularities ◆ muscle weakness ◆ nausea ◆ vomiting ◆ osteoporosis ◆ psychotic behavior ◆ seizures ◆ susceptibility to infections ◆ thromboembolism ◆ thrombophlebitis ◆ various skin eruptions ◆ vertigo

After abrupt withdrawal
Anorexia ◆ arthralgia ◆ depression ◆ dizziness ◆ fainting ◆ dyspnea ◆ fatigue ◆ lethargy ◆ fever ◆ hypoglycemia ◆ orthostatic hypotension ◆ rebound inflammation ◆ weakness ◆ death

Nursing considerations

◆ For better results and less toxicity, give a once-daily dose in the morning.
◆ Unless contraindicated, give oral doses with food when possible to reduce GI irritation. The patient may need medication to prevent GI irritation.
◆ The oral solution may be diluted in juice or other flavored diluent or semisolid food (such as applesauce) before using.
◆ Monitor the patient's blood pressure, sleep patterns, and potassium level.
◆ Weigh the patient daily; report sudden weight gain to the practitioner.
◆ Monitor the patient for cushingoid effects, including moon face, buffalo hump, central obesity, thinning hair, hypertension, and increased susceptibility to infection.
◆ Watch for depression or psychotic episodes, especially during high-dose therapy.
◆ Patients with diabetes may need an increase in insulin dosage; monitor blood glucose level.
◆ Drug may mask or worsen infections, including latent amebiasis.
◆ Unless contraindicated, give a low-sodium diet that's high in potassium and protein. Give potassium supplements, as needed.

† indicates a Canadian trade name

Drugs

propranolol hydrochloride

Apo-Propranolol†, Inderal, Inderal LA, InnoPran XL, Novopranol†, pms Propranolol†

Pregnancy risk category C

Indications and dosages

Angina pectoris
Adults: Total daily doses of 80 to 320 mg P.O. when given b.i.d., t.i.d., or q.i.d. Or, one 80-mg extended-release capsule daily. Dosage increased at 3- to 7-day intervals.

To decrease risk of death after myocardial infarction (MI)
Adults: 180 to 240 mg P.O. daily in divided doses, t.i.d or q.i.d., beginning 5 to 21 days after an MI.

Supraventricular, ventricular, and atrial arrhythmias; tachyarrhythmias caused by excessive catecholamine action during anesthesia, hyperthyroidism, or pheochromocytoma
Adults: 1 to 3 mg by slow I.V. push, not to exceed 1 mg/minute. After 3 mg has been given, another dose may be given in 2 minutes; give subsequent doses no sooner than q 4 hours. Usual maintenance dosage is 10 to 30 mg P.O. t.i.d. or q.i.d.

Hypertension
Adults: Initially, 80 mg P.O. daily in two divided doses or once daily for extended-release form. Increase at 3- to 7-day intervals to a maximum daily dosage of 640 mg. Usual maintenance dosage is 120 to 240 mg daily or 120 to 160 mg daily for extended-release. For InnoPran XL, dosage is 80 mg P.O. once daily at bedtime given consistently with or without food. Adjust to maximum of 120 mg daily if needed. Full effects are seen in about 2 to 3 weeks.
Children: 0.5 mg/kg (conventional tablets) P.O. b.i.d. Increase q 3 to 5 days to a maximum dosage of 16 mg/kg daily. Usual dosage, 2 to 4 mg/kg daily in two equally divided doses.

To prevent frequent, severe, uncontrollable, or disabling migraine or vascular headache
Adults: Initially, 80 mg P.O. daily in divided doses or one extended-release capsule daily. Usual maintenance dosage, 160 to 240 mg t.i.d. or q.i.d.

Essential tremor
Adults: 40 mg (tablets or oral solution) P.O. b.i.d. Usual maintenance dosage is 120 to 320 mg daily in three divided doses.

Hypertrophic subaortic stenosis
Adults: 20 to 40 mg P.O. t.i.d. or q.i.d.; or 80 to 160 mg extended-release capsules once daily.

Adjunct therapy in pheochromocytoma
Adults: 60 mg P.O. daily in divided doses with an alpha blocker 3 days before surgery.

Adverse reactions

Abdominal cramping ◆ agranulocytosis ◆ bradycardia ◆ bronchospasm ◆ constipation ◆ diarrhea ◆ depression ◆ dizziness ◆ fatigue ◆ lethargy ◆ fever ◆ hallucinations ◆ heart failure ◆ hypotension ◆ insomnia ◆ intensification of atrioventricular block ◆ intermittent claudication ◆ nausea and vomiting ◆ rash

Nursing considerations

◆ For direct injection, give into a large vessel or into the tubing of a free-flowing, compatible I.V. solution (dextrose 5% in water, half-normal saline solution, normal saline solution, or lactated Ringer's solution); don't give by continuous I.V. infusion.

◆ Always check the patient's apical pulse before giving the drug. If extremes in pulse rates occur, withhold the drug and notify the practitioner immediately.

◆ Give the drug consistently with meals. Food may increase absorption of propranolol.

◆ Drug masks common signs and symptoms of shock and hypoglycemia.

Drugs

† indicates a Canadian trade name

protamine sulfate
Pregnancy risk category C

Indications and dosages

Heparin overdose
Adults: Base dosage on venous blood coagulation studies, usually 1 mg for each 90 to 115 units of heparin. Give by slow I.V. injection over 10 minutes in doses not to exceed 50 mg.

Adverse reactions

Acute pulmonary hypertension ◆ anaphylactoid reactions ◆ anaphylaxis ◆ bradycardia ◆ circulatory collapse ◆ dyspnea ◆ fatigue ◆ feeling of warmth ◆ hypotension ◆ nausea and vomiting ◆ pulmonary edema ◆ transient flushing

Nursing considerations

◆ Have emergency equipment available to treat anaphylaxis or severe hypotension.

◆ Nursing alert
Give the drug slowly by direct I.V. injection. Excessively rapid I.V. administration may cause acute hypotension, bradycardia, pulmonary hypertension, dyspnea, transient flushing, and feeling of warmth.

◆ Base postoperative dose on coagulation studies, and repeat activated partial thromboplastin time 15 minutes after administration.

◆ Risk of hypersensitivity reaction increases in patients hypersensitive to fish; in vasectomized or infertile men; and in patients taking protamine-insulin products.

◆ Watch for spontaneous bleeding (heparin rebound), especially in dialysis patients and in those who have undergone cardiac surgery.

◆ Protamine may act as an anticoagulant in very high doses.

---

† indicates a Canadian trade name

ranitidine hydrochloride

Apo-Ranitidine†, Zantac, Zantac-C†, Zantac 75, Zantac 150, Zantac EFFERdose Tablets, Zantac 150 GELdose, Zantac 300, Zantac 300 GELdose

Pregnancy risk category B

Indications and dosages

Active duodenal and gastric ulcer
Adults: 150 mg P.O. b.i.d. or 300 mg daily at bedtime. Or, 50 mg I.V. or I.M. q 6 to 8 hours. Or, 150 mg by continuous infusion at 6.25 mg/hour over 24 hours. Maximum daily I.V. dose is 400 mg.
Children ages 1 month to 16 years: 2 to 4 mg/kg P.O. b.i.d., up to 300 mg/day.
Maintenance therapy for duodenal or gastric ulcer
Adults: 150 mg P.O. at bedtime.
Children ages 1 month to 16 years: 2 to 4 mg/kg P.O. daily, up to 150 mg daily.
Pathologic hypersecretory conditions such as Zollinger-Ellison syndrome
Adults: 150 mg P.O. b.i.d.; doses up to 6 g or more frequent intervals may be needed in patients with severe disease. Or, infuse continuously at 1 mg/kg/hour. After 4 hours, if patient remains symptomatic or gastric acid output is greater than 10 mEq/hour, increase dose in increments of 0.5 mg/kg/hour and recheck gastric acid output. Doses up to 2.5 mg/kg/hour and infusion rates up to 220 mg/hour have been used.
Gastroesophageal reflux disease
Adults: 150 mg P.O. b.i.d.
Children ages 1 month to 16 years: 5 to 10 mg/kg P.O. daily given as two divided doses.
Erosive esophagitis
Adults: 150 mg P.O. q.i.d. Maintenance dosage is 150 mg P.O. b.i.d.
Children ages 1 month to 16 years: 5 to 10 mg/kg P.O. daily given as two divided doses.

Heartburn
Adults and children ages 12 and older:
75 mg Zantac 75 P.O. as symptoms occur, up to 150 mg daily, not to exceed 2 weeks of continuous treatment.

Adverse reactions

Anaphylaxis ◆ angioedema ◆ blurred vision ◆ burning and itching at injection site ◆ headache ◆ jaundice ◆ malaise ◆ vertigo

Nursing considerations

◆ To prepare I.V. injection, dilute 2 ml (50 mg) ranitidine with compatible I.V. solution to a total volume of 20 ml, and inject over at least 5 minutes. Compatible solutions include sterile water for injection, normal saline solution for injection, dextrose 5% in water, and lactated Ringer's injection.
◆ To give drug by intermittent I.V. infusion, dilute 2 ml (50 mg) ranitidine in 100 ml compatible solution and infuse at a rate of 5 to 7 ml/minute. The premixed solution is 50 ml and doesn't need further dilution. Infuse over 15 to 20 minutes.
◆ Store I.V. injection at 39° to 86° F (4° to 30° C). Store premixed containers at 36° to 77° F (2° to 25° C).
◆ Assess the patient for abdominal pain. Report presence of blood in emesis, stool, or gastric aspirate to the practitioner.
◆ Ranitidine may be added to total parenteral nutrition solutions.

Drugs

---

† indicates a Canadian trade name

ranolazine

Ranexa
Pregnancy risk category C

Indications and dosages

Chronic angina; given with amlodipine (Norvasc), beta-adrenergic blockers, or nitrates in patients who haven't achieved an adequate response with other antianginals
Adults: Initially, 500 mg P.O. b.i.d. Increase as needed to maximum of 1,000 mg b.i.d.

Adverse reactions

Abdominal pain ◆ constipation ◆ dizziness ◆ dry mouth ◆ dyspnea ◆ headache ◆ nausea ◆ vomiting ◆ palpitations ◆ peripheral edema ◆ syncope ◆ tinnitus ◆ vertigo

Nursing considerations

Nursing alert
Ranolazine prolongs the QT interval in a dose-related manner. If ranolazine is given with other drugs that prolong the QTc interval, torsades de pointes or sudden death may occur. Don't exceed the maximum dosage.
◆ Monitor electrocardiogram for prolonged QT interval and measure the QTc interval regularly.
◆ If the patient has renal insufficiency, monitor blood pressure closely.
◆ Drug may be taken without regard to meals.
◆ Don't crush or cut tablets.

---

† indicates a Canadian trade name

risperidone

Risperdal, Risperdal Consta, Risperdal M-TAB

Pregnancy risk category C

Indications and dosages

Short-term (6 to 8 weeks) treatment of schizophrenia
Adults: Initially, 1 mg P.O. b.i.d. Increase by 1 mg b.i.d. on days 2 and 3 of treatment to a target dose of 3 mg b.i.d. Or, 1 mg P.O. on day 1; increase to 2 mg once daily on day 2, and 4 mg once daily on day 3. Wait at least 1 week before adjusting dosage further. Adjust dosages by 1 to 2 mg. Maximum dosage is 8 mg daily.

To delay relapse in schizophrenia therapy lasting 1 to 2 years
Adults: Initially, 1 mg P.O. on day 1; increase to 2 mg once daily on day 2, and 4 mg once daily on day 3. Dosage range is 2 to 8 mg daily.

Monotherapy or combination therapy with lithium (Lithobid) or valproate (Depakene) for 3-week treatment of acute manic or mixed episodes from bipolar I disorder
Adults: 2 to 3 mg P.O. once daily. Adjust dosage by 1 mg daily. Dosage range is 1 to 6 mg daily.

Irritability, including aggression, self-injury, and temper tantrums, associated with an autistic disorder
Adolescents and children age 5 and older who weigh 20 kg (44 lb) or more: Initially, 0.5 mg P.O. once daily or divided b.i.d. After 4 days, increase dose to 1 mg. Increase dosage further in 0.5 mg increments at intervals of at least 2 weeks.
Children age 5 and older who weigh less than 20 kg: Initially, 0.25 mg P.O. once daily or divided b.i.d. After 4 days, increase dosage further in 0.25 mg increments at intervals of at least 2 weeks. Increase cautiously in children who weigh less than 15 kg (33 lb).

Twelve-week schizophrenia therapy
Adults: Establish tolerance to oral risperidone before giving I.M. Give 25 mg deep I.M. gluteal injection q 2 weeks, alternating injections between each buttock. Adjust dose no sooner than q 4 weeks. Maximum, 50 mg I.M. q 2 weeks. Continue oral antipsychotic for 3 weeks after first I.M. injection, and then stop oral therapy.

Adverse reactions

Abnormal thinking and dreaming ◆ abnormal vision ◆ hallucinations ◆ aggressiveness ◆ agitation ◆ anxiety ◆ akathisia ◆ anemia ◆ anorexia ◆ arthralgia ◆ back, chest, abdominal, or leg pain ◆ constipation ◆ coughing ◆ depression ◆ dizziness ◆ syncope ◆ orthostatic hypotension ◆ dry mouth and skin ◆ dyspepsia ◆ fatigue ◆ fever ◆ headache ◆ hyperglycemia ◆ hypoesthesia ◆ increased saliva ◆ insomnia ◆ nausea ◆ vomiting ◆ neuroleptic malignant syndrome ◆ parkinsonism ◆ tremor ◆ peripheral edema ◆ pharyngitis ◆ photosensitivity reactions ◆ prolonged QT interval ◆ rash ◆ rhinitis or sinusitis ◆ somnolence ◆ suicide attempt ◆ tachycardia ◆ tardive dyskinesia ◆ transient ischemic attack or stroke ◆ toothache or tooth disorder ◆ upper respiratory tract infection ◆ weight gain

With I.M. form
Diarrhea ◆ ear disorders ◆ hypertension ◆ injection site pain ◆ myalgia ◆ nervousness ◆ weight loss

Nursing considerations

◆ Obtain baseline blood pressure measurements before starting therapy, and monitor pressure regularly. Watch for orthostatic hypotension, especially during first dosage adjustment.
◆ Monitor the patient for tardive dyskinesia, which may occur after prolonged use.
◆ Potentially severe or fatal hyperglycemia may occur; monitor patients with diabetes regularly.
◆ Give an oral antipsychotic for the first 3 weeks of I.M. injection therapy.

† indicates a Canadian trade name

sumatriptan succinate

Imitrex
Pregnancy risk category C

Indications and dosages

Acute migraine attacks (with or without aura)
Adults: For injection, 6 mg subcutaneously. Maximum is two 6-mg injections in 24 hours, separated by at least 1 hour. For tablets, 25 to 100 mg P.O., initially. If desired response isn't achieved in 2 hours, may give second dose of 25 to 100 mg. Additional doses may be used in at least 2-hour intervals. Maximum dosage is 200 mg daily. For nasal spray, 5 mg, 10 mg, or 20 mg once in one nostril; may repeat once after 2 hours, for maximum of 40 mg. A 10-mg dosage may be achieved by giving a 5-mg dose in each nostril.

Cluster headache
Adults: 6 mg subcutaneously. Maximum dosage is two 6-mg injections in 24 hours, separated by at least 1 hour.

Adverse reactions

Abdominal discomfort ◆ altered vision ◆ anxiety ◆ atrial or ventricular fibrillation or ventricular tachycardia ◆ cold sensation ◆ coronary artery vasospasm ◆ diaphoresis ◆ diarrhea ◆ discomfort of throat, nasal cavity or sinus, mouth, jaw, or tongue ◆ dizziness ◆ drowsiness ◆ dysphagia ◆ dyspnea (with P.O. route) ◆ fatigue ◆ flushing ◆ headache ◆ injection site reaction (with subcutaneous route) ◆ malaise ◆ muscle cramps ◆ myalgia ◆ myocardial infarction ◆ nausea ◆ vomiting ◆ neck pain ◆ numbness or tingling sensation ◆ pressure or tightness in chest ◆ tight feeling in head ◆ transient myocardial ischemia ◆ unusual or bad taste (with nasal spray) ◆ upper respiratory inflammation (with P.O. route) ◆ vertigo ◆ warm, hot, or burning sensation

Nursing considerations

◆ Drug is contraindicated within 24 hours of another 5-HT$_1$ agonist or a drug containing ergotamine and within 2 weeks of monoamine oxidase inhibitor therapy.
◆ Use cautiously in women who are or may become pregnant.

◆ Nursing alert
When giving sumatriptan succinate to a patient at risk for coronary artery disease, consider giving the first dose in presence of other medical personnel. Although rare, serious adverse cardiac effects may follow administration of drug.

◆ After subcutaneous injection, most patients experience relief in 1 to 2 hours.
◆ Redness or pain at the injection site should subside within 1 hour after injection.

Drugs

temazepam

Restoril
Controlled substance schedule IV
Pregnancy risk category X

Indications and dosages

Insomnia
Adults: 15 to 30 mg P.O. at bedtime.
Elderly or debilitated patients: 15 mg P.O.
at bedtime until individualized response is
determined.

Adverse reactions

Anxiety ◆ blurred vision ◆ confusion ◆
daytime sedation ◆ depression ◆ diarrhea
◆ disturbed coordination ◆ dizziness ◆
drowsiness ◆ dry mouth ◆ euphoria ◆ fatigue ◆ lethargy ◆ headache ◆ minor
changes in electrocardiogram pattern (usually low-voltage fast activity) ◆ nausea ◆
nervousness ◆ nightmares ◆ physical and
psychological dependence ◆ vertigo ◆
weakness

Nursing considerations

◆ Assess the patient's mental status before
starting therapy and expect to reduce
dosages in elderly patients; these patients
may be more sensitive to drug's adverse
central nervous system effects.
◆ Take precautions to prevent hoarding or
overdosing by patients who are depressed,
suicidal, or drug-dependent or who have a
history of drug abuse.

Drugs

† indicates a Canadian trade name

valproate sodium
Depacon, Depakene

valproic acid
Depakene

divalproex sodium
Depakote, Depakote ER, Depakote
Sprinkle, Epival†
Pregnancy risk category D

Indications and dosages

**Simple and complex absence
seizures, mixed seizure types
(including absence seizures)**
Adults and children: Initially, 15 mg/kg
P.O. or I.V. daily; then increase by 5 to
10 mg/kg daily at weekly intervals to maximum of 60 mg/kg daily.

 Age considerations
*Don't use Depakote ER in children
younger than age 10.*

Complex partial seizures
Adults and children ages 10 and older: 10
to 15 mg/kg Depakote or Depakote ER P.O.
or valproate sodium I.V. daily; then increase by 5 to 10 mg/kg daily at weekly intervals, up to 60 mg/kg daily.

Mania
Adults: Initially, 750 mg delayed-release divalproex sodium daily in divided doses.
Adjust dosage based on the patient's response. Maximum dosage, 60 mg/kg daily.

To prevent migraine
Adults: Initially, 250 mg delayed-release divalproex sodium P.O. b.i.d. Some patients
may need up to 1,000 mg daily. Or, 500 mg
Depakote ER P.O. daily for 1 week; then
1,000 mg P.O. daily.

Adverse reactions

Abnormal thinking and emotional upset ◆
alopecia ◆ amnesia ◆ anorexia ◆ ataxia ◆
back, neck, abdominal, or chest pain ◆
blurred vision ◆ diplopia ◆ bone marrow
suppression ◆ bruising ◆ petechiae ◆ constipation ◆ diarrhea ◆ depression ◆ dizziness ◆ dyspepsia ◆ dyspnea ◆ edema ◆
erythema multiforme ◆ fever ◆ headache ◆
hypertension or hypotension ◆ increased
appetite ◆ infection ◆ insomnia ◆ nausea
and vomiting ◆ nervousness ◆ nystagmus
◆ photosensitivity reactions ◆ pruritus ◆
rash ◆ rhinitis ◆ somnolence ◆ Stevens-
Johnson syndrome ◆ tachycardia ◆ tinnitus
◆ tremor ◆ weight gain or loss

Nursing considerations

◆ I.V. use is indicated only in patients who
can't take the drug orally. The patient
should be switched to the oral form as
soon as feasible; effects of using I.V.
dosage for longer than 14 days are unknown.
◆ Dilute valproate sodium injection with at
least 50 ml of a compatible diluent. It's
physically compatible and chemically stable in dextrose 5% in water, normal saline
solution, and lactated Ringer's solution for
24 hours.
◆ Infuse the drug I.V. over 60 minutes (at
no more than 20 mg/minute) with the
same frequency as oral dosage.
◆ Obtain liver function test results, platelet
count, and prothrombin and International
Normalized Ratio before starting therapy,
and monitor these values periodically.
◆ Don't give the syrup form to patients
who need sodium restriction. Check with
the practitioner.
◆ Adverse reactions may not be caused by
valproic acid alone because it's usually
used with other anticonvulsants.
◆ Notify the prescriber if tremors occur; a
dosage reduction may be needed.
◆ Monitor the drug level. Therapeutic level
is 50 to 100 mcg/ml.

Drugs

vancomycin hydrochloride

Vancocin, Vancoled

Pregnancy risk category C

Indications and dosages

Serious or severe infections when other antibiotics are ineffective or contraindicated, including those caused by methicillin-resistant *Staphylococcus aureus*, S. *epidermidis*, or diphtheroid organisms

Adults: 500 mg I.V q 6 hours or 1g I.V. q 12 hours.

Children: 10 mg/kg I.V. q 6 hours.

Neonates and young infants: 15 mg/kg I.V. loading dose; then 10 mg/kg I.V. q 12 hours if child is younger than age 1 week or 10 mg/kg I.V. q 8 hours if older than 1 week but younger than 1 month.

Elderly patients: 15 mg/kg I.V. loading dose. Subsequent doses are based on renal function and serum drug level.

Antibiotic-related pseudomembranous *Clostridium difficile* and S. *enterocolitis*

Adults: 125 to 500 mg P.O. q 6 hours for 7 to 10 days.

Children: 40 mg/kg P.O. daily in divided doses q 6 hours for 7 to 10 days. Maximum dosage is 2 g daily.

Endocarditis prophylaxis for dental procedures

Adults: 1 g I.V. slowly over 1 to 2 hours, completing infusion 30 minutes before procedure.

Children: 20 mg/kg I.V. over 1 to 2 hours, completing infusion 30 minutes before procedure.

Bacterial endocarditis from methicillin-resistant or methicillin-susceptible staphylococci in patients with native cardia valves

Adults: 30 mg/kg I.V. daily given in two divided doses for 4 to 6 weeks. Doses over 2 g require monitoring of drug level.

Adverse reactions

Anaphylaxis ◆ chills ◆ dyspnea ◆ eosinophilia ◆ fever ◆ hypotension ◆ leukopenia ◆ nausea ◆ nephrotoxicity ◆ neutropenia ◆ ototoxicity ◆ pain ◆ pseudomembranous colitis ◆ red-man syndrome (with rapid I.V. infusion) ◆ superinfection ◆ thrombophlebitis at injection site ◆ tinnitus ◆ wheezing

Nursing considerations

◆ Patients with renal dysfunction need dosage adjustment. Monitor blood levels to adjust I.V. dosage. Normal therapeutic levels of vancomycin are peak, 30 to 40 mg/L (drawn 1 hour after infusion ends) and trough, 5 to 10 mg/L (drawn just before next dose is given).

◆ Refrigerate the I.V. solution after reconstitution and use within 14 days.

◆ Obtain a specimen for culture and sensitivity testing before giving the first dose. Because of the emergence of vancomycin-resistant enterococci, reserve use of the drug for treatment of serious infections caused by gram-positive bacteria resistant to beta-lactam anti-infectives.

◆ Obtain a hearing evaluation and renal function studies before start of therapy.

◆ Monitor the patient's fluid balance and watch for oliguria and cloudy urine.

◆ Monitor the patient carefully for red-man syndrome, which can occur if drug is infused too rapidly. Signs and symptoms include maculopapular rash on face, neck, trunk, and limbs and pruritus and hypotension caused by histamine release. If wheezing, urticaria, or pain and muscle spasm of the chest and back occur, stop the infusion and notify the practitioner.

◆ Monitor renal function (blood urea nitrogen, creatinine and creatinine clearance levels, urinalysis, and urine output) during therapy.

◆ Have the patient's hearing evaluated during prolonged therapy.

Drugs

---

† indicates a Canadian trade name

vasopressin
Pitressin

Pregnancy risk category C

Indications and dosages

Nonnephrogenic, nonpsychogenic diabetes insipidus
Adults: 5 to 10 units I.M. or subcutaneously b.i.d. to q.i.d., p.r.n. Or, intranasally in individualized dosages, based on the patient's response.
Children: 2.5 to 10 units I.M. or subcutaneously b.i.d. to q.i.d., p.r.n. Or, intranasally in individualized dosages.

To prevent and treat abdominal distention
Adults: Initially, 5 units I.M.; give subsequent injections q 3 to 4 hours, increasing to 10 units if needed. Children may receive reduced dosages. Or, for adults, aqueous vasopressin 5 to 15 units subcutaneously at 2 hours before and again at 30 minutes before abdominal radiography or kidney biopsy.

Abdominal roentgenography
Adults: 2 injections of 10 units each I.M. or subcutaneously, given at 2 hours and at 30 minutes before abdominal radiography.

GI bleeding (off-label use)
Adults: Initially, 0.2 to 0.4 units/minute I.V.; increase to 0.9 units/minute as needed. For intra-arterial infusion, 0.1 to 0.5 units/minute. Aqueous vasopressin is diluted in normal saline solution or dextrose 5% in water to a concentration of 0.1 to 1 unit/ml.

Adverse reactions

Abdominal cramps ◆ angina (in patients with vascular disease) ◆ arrhythmias ◆ bronchoconstriction ◆ cardiac arrest ◆ circumoral pallor ◆ cutaneous gangrene ◆ decreased cardiac output ◆ diaphoresis ◆ flatulence ◆ headache ◆ hypersensitivity reactions ◆ myocardial ischemia ◆ nausea ◆ tremor ◆ urticaria ◆ uterine cramps ◆ vasoconstriction ◆ vertigo ◆ vomiting ◆ water intoxication

Nursing considerations

◆ Monitor the patient for hypersensitivity reactions, including urticaria, angioedema, bronchoconstriction, and anaphylaxis.
◆ Synthetic desmopressin is sometimes preferred because of its longer duration of action and less frequent adverse reactions. Desmopressin also is available commercially as a nasal solution.
◆ Drug may be used for transient polyuria resulting from antidiuretic hormone deficiency related to neurosurgery or head injury.
◆ Warm the vasopressin vial in your hands, and mix the solution well before administration.
◆ Give the drug with 1 to 2 glasses of water to reduce adverse reactions and improve therapeutic response.
◆ Monitor urine specific gravity and fluid intake and output to evaluate effectiveness.
◆ Monitor blood pressure of the patient taking vasopressin twice daily. Watch for excessively elevated blood pressure or lack of response to drug, which may be indicated by hypotension.
◆ Monitor weight daily.

† indicates a Canadian trade name

verapamil hydrochloride

Apo-Verap†, Calan, Calan SR, Covera-HS, Isoptin SR, Novo-Veramil†, Nu-Verap†, Verelan, Verelan PM

Pregnancy risk category C

Indications and dosages

Vasospastic angina (Prinzmetal's or variant angina); classic chronic, stable angina pectoris; chronic atrial fibrillation

Adults: Starting dose is 80 to 120 mg P.O. t.i.d. Increase dosage at daily or weekly intervals, p.r.n. Some patients may require up to 480 mg daily.

To prevent paroxysmal supraventricular tachycardia

Adults: 80 to 120 mg P.O. t.i.d. or q.i.d.

Supraventricular arrhythmias

Adults: 0.075 to 0.15 mg/kg (5 to 10 mg) by I.V. push over 2 minutes with electrocardiogram (ECG) and blood pressure monitoring. Repeat dose of 0.15 mg/kg (10 mg) in 30 minutes if no response occurs.

Children ages 1 to 15: 0.1 to 0.3 mg/kg as I.V. bolus over 2 minutes; not to exceed 5 mg. Repeat dose in 30 minutes if patient's response is inadequate.

Children younger than age 1: 0.1 to 0.2 mg/kg as I.V. bolus over 2 minutes with continuous ECG monitoring. Repeat dose in 30 minutes if no response occurs.

Digitalized patients with chronic atrial fibrillation or flutter

Adults: 240 to 320 mg P.O. daily, divided t.i.d. or q.i.d.

Hypertension

Adults: 240 mg extended-release tablet P.O. once daily in the morning. If response isn't adequate, give an additional 120 mg in the evening or 240 mg q 12 hours, or an 80-mg immediate-release tablet t.i.d. If using Verelan PM, give 200 mg P.O. daily at bedtime; may increase to 300 mg if response is inadequate. Maximum dose is 400 mg. If using Covera-HS, give 180 mg P.O. at bedtime; may increase to 240 mg daily if response is inadequate. Subsequent dosage adjust-ments may be made in 120-mg increments to a maximum of 420 mg at bedtime.

Adverse reactions

Asthenia ◆ atrioventricular (AV) block ◆ bradycardia ◆ constipation ◆ dizziness ◆ headache ◆ heart failure ◆ nausea ◆ peripheral and pulmonary edema ◆ rash ◆ transient hypotension ◆ ventricular asystole or fibrillation

Nursing considerations

◆ Drug is contraindicated in patients with severe left ventricular dysfunction, cardiogenic shock, second- or third-degree AV block or sick sinus syndrome (except in presence of functioning pacemaker), atrial flutter or fibrillation and accessory bypass tract syndrome, severe heart failure (unless secondary to verapamil therapy), and severe hypotension.

◆ I.V. verapamil is contraindicated in patients receiving I.V. beta-adrenergic blockers and in those with ventricular tachycardia.

◆ Give I.V. doses over at least 2 minutes (3 minutes in elderly patients) to minimize the risk of adverse reactions.

◆ Monitor ECG and blood pressure continuously in the patient receiving I.V. verapamil.

◆ Taking extended-release tablets with food may decrease rate and extent of absorption but allows smaller fluctuations of peak and trough blood levels.

◆ Pellet-filled capsules may be given by carefully opening the capsule and sprinkling the pellets on a spoonful of applesauce. This mixture should be swallowed immediately without chewing, followed by a glass of cool water to ensure all pellets are swallowed.

◆ Monitor blood pressure at the start of therapy and during dosage adjustments. Assist the patient with walking because dizziness may occur.

◆ Monitor liver function test results during prolonged treatment.

† indicates a Canadian trade name

warfarin sodium

Coumadin, Jantoven, Warfilone†

Pregnancy risk category X

Indications and dosages

Pulmonary embolism, deep vein thrombosis, myocardial infarction, rheumatic heart disease with heart valve damage, prosthetic heart valves, or chronic atrial fibrillation

Adults: 2 to 5 mg P.O. daily for 2 to 4 days; then dosage based on daily prothrombin time (PT) and International Normalized Ratio (INR). Usual maintenance dosage, 2 to 10 mg P.O. daily; I.V. dosage same as for P.O.

Adverse reactions

Alopecia ◆ anorexia ◆ cramps ◆ dermatitis ◆ diarrhea ◆ enhanced uric acid excretion ◆ excessive menstrual bleeding ◆ fever ◆ gangrene ◆ headache ◆ hematuria ◆ hemorrhage ◆ hepatitis ◆ jaundice ◆ melena ◆ mouth ulcerations ◆ nausea ◆ vomiting ◆ necrosis ◆ rash ◆ sore mouth ◆ urticaria

Nursing considerations

◆ Drug is contraindicated in patients with bleeding from the GI, genitourinary, or respiratory tracts; aneurysm; cerebrovascular hemorrhage; severe or malignant hypertension; severe renal or hepatic disease; subacute bacterial endocarditis, pericarditis, or pericardial effusion; or blood dyscrasias or hemorrhagic tendencies.

◆ Drug is contraindicated during pregnancy, threatened abortion, eclampsia, or preeclampsia, and after recent surgery involving large open areas, eye, brain, or spinal cord.

◆ I.V. form may be ordered in rare instances when oral therapy can't be given. Reconstitute powder with 2.7 ml sterile water, or as instructed in the manufacturer's guidelines. Give I.V. as a slow bolus injection over 1 to 2 minutes into a peripheral vein.

◆ Because onset of action is delayed, heparin sodium is usually given during the first few days of treatment.

◆ Draw blood samples for PT and INR before and during therapy.

◆ Give warfarin at the same time daily. INR range for chronic atrial fibrillation is usually 2 to 3.

◆ Regularly inspect the patient for bleeding gums, bruises on arms or legs, petechiae, nosebleeds, melena, tarry stools, hematuria, and hematemesis.

◆ Check for unexpected bleeding in breast-fed infants of women taking the drug.

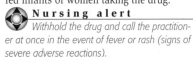 **Nursing alert**

Withhold the drug and call the practitioner at once in the event of fever or rash (signs of severe adverse reactions).

◆ The drug's effect can be neutralized by parenteral or oral vitamin K.

---

† indicates a Canadian trade name

Appendices, selected references, and index

Guide to laboratory test results

This chart provides normal values for common laboratory tests, including chemistry, hematology, and coagulation tests. Where indicated, conventional and SI units are given.

Comprehensive metabolic panel

Laboratory test	Conventional	SI Units
Albumin	3.5 to 5 g/dl	35 to 50 g/L
Alkaline phosphatase	45 to 115 units/L	45 to 115 units/L
Alanine aminotransferase	Male: 10 to 40 units/L	0.17 to 0.68 µkat/L
	Female: 7 to 35 units/L	0.12 to 0.60 µkat/L
Aspartate aminotransferase	12 to 31 units/L	0.21 to 0.53 µkat/L
Bilirubin, total	0.2 to 1 mg/dl	3.5 to 17 µmol/L
Blood urea nitrogen	8 to 20 mg/dl	2.9 to 7.5 mmol/L
Calcium	8.2 to 10.2 mg/dl	2.05 to 2.54 mmol/L
Carbon dioxide	22 to 26 mEq/L	22 to 26 mmol/L
Chloride	100 to 108 mEq/L	100 to 108 mmol/L
Creatinine	Male: 0.8 to 1.2 mg/dl	62 to 115 µmol/L
	Female: 0.6 to 0.9 mg/dl	53 to 97 µmol/L
Glucose	70 to 100 mg/dl	3.9 to 6.1 mmol/L
Potassium	3.5 to 5 mEq/L	3.5 to 5 mmol/L
Protein, total	6.3 to 8.3 g/dl	64 to 83 g/L
Sodium	135 to 145 mEq/L	135 to 145 mmol/L

Other chemistry tests

Laboratory test	Conventional	SI Units
Ammonia	< 50 ng/dl	< 36 µmol/L
Amylase	26 to 102 units/L	0.4 to 1.74 µkat/L
Anion gap	8 to 14 mEq/L	8 to 14 mmol/L
Bilirubin, direct	< 0.5 mg/dl	< 6.8 µmol/L
Calcium, ionized	4.65 to 5.28 mg/dl	1.1 to 1.25 mmol/L
C-reactive protein	< 0.8 mg/dl	< 8 mg/L
Ferritin	Male: 20 to 300 ng/ml	20 to 300 mcg/L
	Female: 20 to 120 ng/ml	20 to 120 mcg/L
Gamma-glutamyl transpeptidase	Male: 7 to 47 units/L	0.12 to 1.80 µkat/L
	Female: 5 to 25 units/L	0.08 to 0.42 µkat/L
Hb A_{1C}	4% to 7%	0.04 to 0.07
Iron	Male: 65 to 175 mcg/dl	11.6 to 31.3 µmol/L
	Female: 50 to 170 mcg/dl	9 to 30.4 µmol/L
Iron-binding capacity	250 to 400 mcg/dl	45 to 72 µmol/L
Lactic acid	0.5 to 2.2 mEq/L	0.5 to 2.2 mmol/L
Lipase	10 to 73 units/L	0.17 to 1.24 µkat/L
Magnesium	1.3 to 2.2 mg/dl	0.65 to 1.05 mmol/L
Phosphate	2.7 to 4.5 mg/dl	0.87 to 1.45 mmol/L
Prealbumin	19 to 38 mg/dl	190 to 380 mg/L

Lipid panel

Laboratory test	Conventional	SI Units
Total cholesterol	< 200 mg/dl	< 5.18 mmol/L
High-density lipoprotein cholesterol	≥ 60 mg/dl	≥ 1.55 mmol/L
Low-density lipoprotein cholesterol	< 130 mg/dl	< 3.36 mmol/L
Very-low-density lipoprotein cholesterol	< 130 mg/dl	< 3.4 mmol/L
Triglycerides	< 150 mg/dl	< 1.7 mmol/L

Coagulation tests

Laboratory test	Conventional	SI Units
Activated clotting time	107 sec ± 13 sec	107 sec ± 13 sec
Bleeding time	3 to 6 min	3 to 6 min
D-dimer	< 250 mcg/L	< 1.37 nmol/L
Fibrinogen	200 to 400 mg/dl	2 to 4 g/L
International Normalized Ratio (therapeutic target)	2.0 to 3.0	2.0 to 3.0
Partial thromboplastin time	21 to 35 sec	21 to 35 sec
Prothrombin time	10 to 14 sec	10 to 14 sec

Hematology tests

Laboratory test	Conventional	SI Units
Hemoglobin	Male: 14 to 17.4 g/dl	140 to 174 g/L
	Female: 12 to 16 g/dl	120 to 160 g/L
Hematocrit	Male: 42% to 52%	0.42 to 0.52
	Female: 36% to 48%	0.36 to 0.48
Red blood cells	Male: 4.5 to 5.5 million/µl	$4.5 \text{ to } 5.5 \times 10^{12}/L$
	Female: 4 to 5 million/µl	$4 \text{ to } 5 \times 10^{12}/L$
Leukocytes	4,000 to 10,000/µl	$4 \text{ to } 10 \times 10^{9}/L$
◆ Bands	0% to 5%	0.03 to 0.08
◆ Basophils	0% to 1%	0 to 0.01
◆ Eosinophils	1% to 4%	0.01 to 0.04
◆ Lymphocytes	25% to 40%	0.25 to 0.40
◆ B-Lymphocytes	270 to 640/µl	–
◆ T-Lymphocytes	1,400 to 2,700/µl	–
◆ Monocytes	2% to 8%	0.02 to 0.08
◆ Neutrophils	54% to 75%	0.54 to 0.75
Platelets	140,000 to 400,00/µl	$140 \text{ to } 400 \times 10^{9}/L$

Quick guide to arrhythmias

Use this guide to help you recognize various arrhythmias on a rhythm strip and to review their specific features.

Sinus arrhythmia

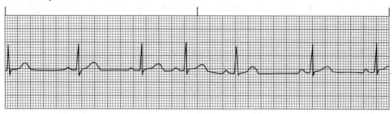

Features
- Rhythm irregular (varies with respiratory cycle)
- Normal P wave preceding each QRS complex
- P-P and R-R intervals shorter during inspiration and longer during expiration

Sinus tachycardia

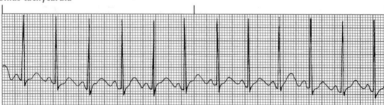

Features
- Rhythm regular
- Atrial and ventricular rates equal; rate > 100 beats/minute
- Normal P wave preceding each normal QRS complex

Sinus bradycardia

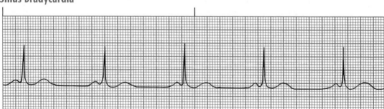

Features
- Rhythm regular
- Rate < 60 beats/minute
- Normal P wave preceding each normal QRS complex

Sinus arrest

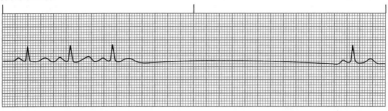

Features
- ◆ Rhythm regular, except for missing PQRST complexes (irregular as result of missing complexes)
- ◆ Normal P wave preceding each normal QRS complex

Premature atrial contractions (PACs)

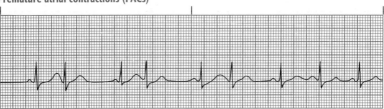

Features
- ◆ Premature, abnormal P waves (differ in configuration from normal P waves)
- ◆ QRS complexes after P waves, except in blocked PACs
- ◆ P wave commonly buried or identified in preceding T wave

Atrial tachycardia

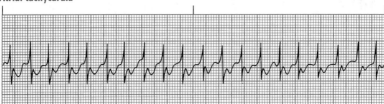

Features
- ◆ Rhythm regular if block is constant; irregular if not
- ◆ Rate 150 to 250 beats/minute
- ◆ P waves regular but hidden in preceding T wave; precede QRS complexes
- ◆ Sudden onset and termination of arrhythmia

Atrial flutter

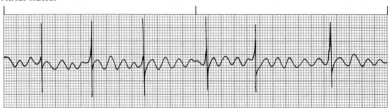

Features
- ◆ Atrial rhythm regular; ventricular rhythm variable, depending on degree of atrioventricular (AV) block
- ◆ Atrial rate 250 to 400 beats/minute; ventricular rate depends on degree of AV block
- ◆ Sawtooth P-wave configuration (known as flutter or F waves)
- ◆ QRS complexes uniform in shape

Atrial fibrillation

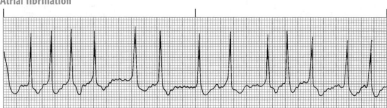

Features
- ◆ Atrial and ventricular rhythms grossly irregular
- ◆ Atrial rate > 400 beats/minute; ventricular rate varies
- ◆ No P waves; replaced by fine fibrillatory waves
- ◆ No PR interval
- ◆ QRS complexes uniform in configuration and duration

Junctional escape rhythm

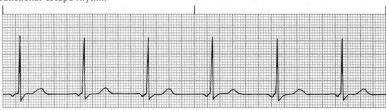

Features
- ◆ Rhythm regular
- ◆ Rate 40 to 60 beats/minute
- ◆ P waves before, hidden in, or after QRS complex; inverted if visible
- ◆ PR interval < 0.12 second (measurable only if P wave appears before QRS complex)
- ◆ QRS configuration and duration normal

Premature junctional contractions

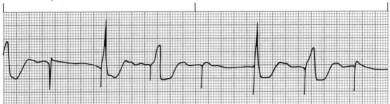

Features
- Rhythm irregular
- P waves before, hidden in, or after QRS complexes; inverted if visible
- PR interval < 0.12 second, if P wave preceding QRS complex
- QRS configuration and duration normal

Junctional tachycardia

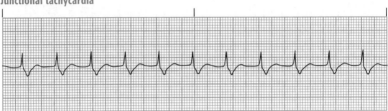

Features
- Rhythm regular
- Rate 100 to 200 beats/minute
- P wave before, hidden in, or after QRS complex; inverted if visible
- QRS configuration and duration normal

Wandering pacemaker

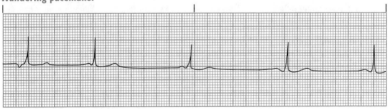

Features
- Rhythm irregular
- P waves change in configuration, indicating origin in sinoatrial node, atria, or AV junction
- *Hallmark:* At least three different P wave configurations
- PR interval varies
- QRS configuration and duration normal

Appendices

First-degree AV block

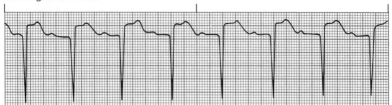

Features
- ◆ Rhythm regular
- ◆ P wave preceding each QRS complex; QRS complex normal
- ◆ PR interval > 0.20 second and constant

Second-degree AV block Type I (Mobitz I, Wenckebach)

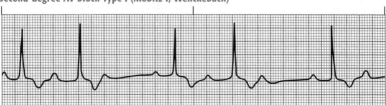

Features
- ◆ Atrial rhythm regular
- ◆ Ventricular rhythm irregular
- ◆ Atrial rate exceeds ventricular rate
- ◆ PR interval progressively, but only slightly, longer with each cycle until a P wave appears without a QRS complex

Second-degree AV block Type II (Mobitz Type II)

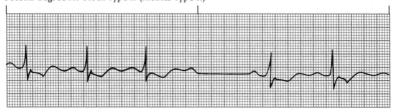

Features
- ◆ Atrial rhythm regular
- ◆ Ventricular rhythm possibly irregular, varying with degree of block
- ◆ P waves normal size, some not followed by a QRS complex
- ◆ PR interval is constant for conducted beats
- ◆ QRS complexes periodically absent

Third-degree AV block (complete heart block)

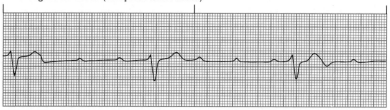

Features
- Atrial rhythm regular
- Ventricular rhythm regular and rate slow; if escape rhythm originates in AV node, rate is 40 to 60 beats/minute; if it originates in Purkinje system, rate is < 40 beats/minute
- No relationship between P waves and QRS complexes
- PR interval can't be measured
- QRS complex normal (originating in AV node) or wide and bizarre (originating in Purkinje system)

Premature ventricular contractions (PVCs)

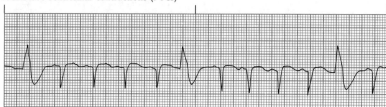

Features
- Atrial and ventricular rhythms may be regular in underlying rhythm; irregular during PVCs
- QRS premature
- QRS complex wide and bizarre, usually > than 0.12 second in premature beat
- T wave opposite direction to QRS complex
- PVCs may occur singly, in pairs, or in threes; alternating with normal beats; possibly unifocal or multifocal
- Most ominous when clustered, multifocal, and with R wave on T pattern
- PVC may be followed by full or incomplete compensatory pause

Ventricular tachycardia

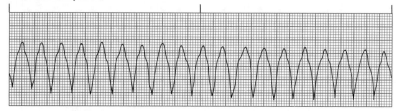

Features
- Atrial rhythm can't be determined; ventricular rhythm usually regular, may be slightly irregular
- Ventricular rate 100 to 250 beats/minute
- P waves indiscernible
- QRS complexes wide and bizarre; duration > 0.12 second
- May start and stop suddenly

Ventricular fibrillation

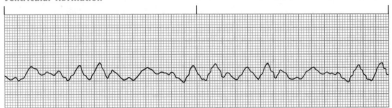

Features
◆ Ventricular rhythm rapid and chaotic
◆ No discernible P waves, QRS complexes, or T waves
◆ Fine or coarse fibrillatory waves

Asystole

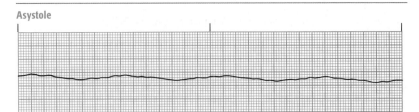

Features
◆ No atrial or ventricular rate or rhythm
◆ No discernible P waves, QRS complexes, or T waves

Selected references

American Association of Critical Care Nursing. *AACN's Quick Reference to Critical Care Nursing Procedures.* Philadelphia: Saunders Elsevier, 2007.

Bunting-Perry, L.K. "Palliative Care in Parkinson's Disease: Implications for Neuroscience Nursing," *The Journal of Neuroscience Nursing* 38(2):106-13, April, 2006.

Chair, S.Y., et al. "The Effect of Ambulation after Cardiac Catheterization on Patient Outcomes," *Journal of Clinical Nursing* 16(1):212-24, January 2006.

Conway, B., and Fuat, A. "Recent Advances in Angina Management: Implications for Nurses," *Nursing Standard* 21(38):49-56, May-June 2007.

Diseases, 4th ed. Philadelphia: Lippincott Williams & Wilkins, 2006.

Flanagan, J., et al. "Interpreting Laboratory Values in the Rehabilitation Setting," *Rehabilitation Nursing* 32(2):77-84, March-April 2007.

Gutierrez, K., and Peterson, P. *Saunders Nursing Survival Guide: Pathophysiology.* Philadelphia: Saunders Elsevier, 2007.

Honea, N., et al. "Treatment-Related Symptom Clusters," *Seminars in Oncology Nursing* 23(2):142-51, May 2007.

Kreiger, G. "A Basic Guide to Understanding Plasma B-type Natriuretic Peptide in the Diagnosis of Congestive Heart Failure," *Medsurg Nursing* 16(2):75-8; April, 2007.

Miller, J. "Keeping Your Patient Hemodynamically Stable," *Nursing2007* 37(5): 36-41, May 2007.

Nursing2008 Drug Handbook. Philadelphia: Lippincott Williams & Wilkins, 2008.

Nurse's 5-minute Clinical Consult: Signs & Symptoms. Philadelphia: Lippincott Williams & Wilkins, 2007.

Potter, P., and Perry, A. *Fundamentals of Nursing,* 7th ed. St. Louis: Mosby, 2008.

Portable ECG Interpretation. Philadelphia: Lippincott Williams & Wilkins, 2008.

Rhoads, J., and Meeker, B.J. *Davis's Guide to Clinical Nursing Skills.* Philadelphia: F.A. Davis Co., 2007.

Richards, N.M., and Stahl, M.A. "Ventricular Assist Devices in the Adult," *Critical Care Nursing Quarterly* 30(2):104-18, April-June 2007.

Suttner, S., et al. "Noninvasive Assessment of Cardiac Output Using Thoracic Electrical Bioimpedance in Hemodynamically Stable and Unstable Patients after Cardiac Surgery: A Comparison with Pulmonary Artery Thermodilution," *Intensive Care Medicine* 32(12):2053-58, December 2006.

Van Leeuwen, A.M., et al. *Davis's Comprehensive Handbook of Laboratory and Diagnostic Tests with Nursing Implications,* 2nd ed. Philadelphia: F.A. Davis Co., 2006.

Index

i refers to an illustration; t refers to a table.

i refers to an illustration; t refers to a table.

i refers to an illustration; t refers to a table.

Diltiazem hydrochloride, 682
Diphenhydramine hydrochloride, 683
Disseminated intravascular coagulation, 90-91
Divalproex sodium, 734
Diverticular disease, 92-93, 146, 514-515, 608
Dizziness, 558-559
Dopamine hydrochloride, 684
Double-lumen catheter, for hemodialysis, 294-295
Duodenal ulcer, 190, 515, 560
Dyspepsia, 560-561
Dyspnea, 562-563

E

Echocardiography, 474
Edema, generalized, 564-565
Electrocardiography, 286, 475
Electroencephalography, 476
Electromyography, 477
Electrophysiology studies, 478
Emphysema, 94-95, 562, 628, 631, 650-651
Enalapril maleate, 685
Encephalopathy, 596-597
  hypoglycemic, 554
  hypoxic, 554
Endocarditis, 96-97, 97i, 642
Endoscopic carpal tunnel release, 270
Endoscopic retrograde cholangiopancre-atography, 479
Endoscopic transnasal hypophysec-tomy, 297
Endoscopy, 480
Endotracheal intubation, insertion, 388-389
  manual ventilation and, 404-405
Enhanced external counterpulsation, 286-287, 287i
Enoxaparin sodium, 686
Epilepsy, 222
Epinephrine, 687
Epistaxis, 566
  nasal packing for, 408-409
Esomeprazole magnesium, 688
Esophageal spasm, 541

Esophageal varices, 10, 72, 582, 600
Esophagogastroduodenoscopy, 481
Essential tremor, deep vein stimulation for, 284-285
Evoked potential studies, 482
External counterpulsation, enhanced, 286-287, 287i
External ear canal tumor, 580
External radiation therapy, 320-321
Extracorporeal shock-wave litho-tripsy, 306

F

Famotidine, 689
Fatigue, 568-569
Feeding tube insertion and removal, 390-391
Femoral compression device, 392
Femoral popliteal bypass, 288-289
Fentanyl, 690-691
Fibrocystic breast disease, 532
Fibromyalgia syndrome, 98-99
Fine needle aspiration, 464
Flail chest, 538, 562, 629, 651
Flank pain, 570-571
Flesh-eating disease. *See* Necrotizing fasciitis.
Flat plate of the abdomen, 486
Fluconazole, 692
Flumazenil, 693
Foley catheter, 374
Food poisoning, 44
Fourth-degree burns, 50
Fractures, 523
  open reduction and internal fixation of, 310-311, 311i
Furosemide, 694

G

Gag reflex abnormalities, 572-573
Gallbladder attack, 70-71
Gallbladder disease, in obesity, 178
Gallop
  atrial, 574-575
  ventricular, 576-577
Gamma knife surgery, 330-331
Gas exchange impairment, 206

i refers to an illustration; t refers to a table.

Index

Gastric bypass, 290-291
Gastric cancer, 561, 583, 600
Gastric surgery, restrictive, 324-325, 325i
Gastric ulcer, 190, 232, 560
Gastritis, 100-102, 290, 324, 515, 560, 583, 601, 608
Gastroesophageal reflux disease, 102-103
Gentamicin sulfate, 695
Glaucoma, 104-105, 105i, 578, 626
Glipizide, 696
Glomerulonephritis, 106-107, 570, 584-585, 612, 624
Glyburide, 697
Graft rejection, 262, 326, 346, 348
Graft-versus-host disease, 226
Guided imagery, for pain management, 414
Guillain-Barré syndrome, 108-109, 124, 604, 606, 618, 620, 629

H
Haloperidol, 698
Headache, 110-111, 578-579
Hearing loss, 274, 580-581
Heart failure, 112-113
 left-sided, 80, 96, 112, 254, 552, 594, 614
 right-sided, 80, 112, 208, 552, 594
Heart transplantation, 348-349
Heart valve replacement, 292-293, 293i
Heat syndrome, 114-115
Heberden's nodes, 181i
Hematemesis, 582-583
Hematology tests, 741
Hematoma, after thoracentesis, 332-333
Hematuria, 584-585
Hemodialysis, 294-295
Hemolytic crisis, in sickle cell anemia, 20-21
Hemophilia, 116-117
Hemoptysis, 586-587
Hemorrhage
 intracerebral, 579, 597
 intracranial, 68, 282, 284
Hemothorax, 382, 538
 thoracentesis for, 332-333

Hemovac closed-wound drain management, 384
Heparin sodium, 699
Hepatic encephalopathy, 72, 118-119, 154, 554
Hepatitis, viral, 120-121, 561, 588, 591, 608, 642
Hepatomegaly, 80, 588-598
Hepatorenal syndrome, 72, 154
Herniated intervertebral disk, 122-123, 620
Herpes zoster, 124-125, 125i
Hiatal hernia, 541, 561
HIDA scan, 483
High-frequency ventilation, 308
Hip fracture, 126-127
Hip replacement, 302-303
Hodgkin's disease, 128-129, 598
 recognizing Reed-Sternberg cells in, 129i
Holter monitoring, 484
Hormonal antineoplastic agents, indications for, 274
Huntington's disease, 604-605
Hydrochlorothiazide, 700
Hydrocolloid dressing, for pressure ulcers, 420-421
Hydrogel dressing, for pressure ulcers, 421
Hydrocortisone, 701
Hydromorphone hydrochloride, 702
Hyperkalemia, 130-131, 260, 624
Hypertension, 132-133, 558, 566, 575, 578, 616
Hyperthermia-hypothermia blanket, 394-395
Hyperthyroidism, 134-135
Hypertrophic cardiomyopathy, 58-59
Hyperuricemia, 158
Hyperventilation syndrome, 558-559
Hypocalcemia, 136-137, 337t, 616, 645
Hypokalemia, 138-139
 clinical effects of, 139t
Hypomagnesemia, 140-141
 clinical effects of, 141t
Hypophysectomy, 296-297

Hypothermia, 530
 blanket for, 394-395
Hypothyroidism, 142-143
Hypovolemia, 86, 214, 559, 612-613
Hypovolemic shock, 230-231, 525,
    640-641
Hysteroscopy, 485

I

Ibuprofen, 703
Ileoanal reservoir, 263
Ileostomy, 264-265
Implantable cardioverter-defibrillator,
    298-299
 types of therapy with, 299t
Incentive spirometry, 396-397
Indwelling urinary catheter, 374-377
Inflammatory bowel disease, 26, 82
Infratentorial craniotomy, 282
Insulins, 88, 164, 704-705
Intermittent pulmonary artery wedge
    pressure, 424-427
Internal fixation, 310-311, 311i
Internal radiation therapy, 320-321
Interstitial fibrosis of the lungs, 548
Intervertebral disk rupture, 522
Intestinal obstruction, 82, 92, 144-145,
    515, 608-609
Intra-aortic balloon counterpulsation,
    300-301
Intra-arterial pressure monitoring, 360
Intracranial pressure, 527, 544
 monitoring of, 398-399
Intraductal papilloma, 532
Intrarenal failure, 214
Intravenous line insertion and removal,
    peripheral, 418-419
Intraventricular catheter, for intracranial
    pressure monitoring, 398
Iron deficiency anemia, 18-19
Iron overdose, 18-19
Irritable bowel syndrome, 146-147,
    515, 609
Isosorbide, 706

J

Jackson-Pratt closed drainage system, 384
Jaundice, 590-591
Jaw pain, 592-593
Joint replacement
 hip, 302-303, 303i
 knee, 304-305
Jugular vein distention, 594-595
Jugular venous oxygen saturation moni-
    toring, 400-401
Junctional escape rhythm, 744i
Junctional tachycardia, 745i

K

Ketoacidosis, 88, 534
Kidney-ureter-bladder radiography, 486
Knee replacement, 304-305

L

Laboratory test results, 740-741
Labyrinthitis, 609
Laënnec's cirrhosis, 72
Lansoprazole, 707
Laparoscopy, pelvic, 487
Laryngeal cancer, 586
Laser ablation, 257
Latex allergy, 148-149
 protocol for, 402-403
Lead placement, in deep brain stimula-
    tion, 284
Left-sided heart failure, 80, 96, 112, 254,
    552, 594, 614
Left ventricular hypertrophy, 132, 134
Leg venography, 508
Legionnaires' disease, 150-151, 548-549
Leukemia, acute, 152-153
Level of consciousness, decreased,
    596-597
Levin nasogastric tube, 410
Levothyroxine sodium, 708
Linear accelerator radiosurgery, 330-331
Lipid panel, 741
Lisinopril, 709
Lithotripsy, 306-307, 307t
Liver failure, 154-155
Liver-spleen scan, 488
Liver stent, 328-329

Index

Lobectomy, 334
Lorazepam, 710
Lou Gehrig disease, 14
Lumbar puncture, 489
Lumbosacral sprain, 522
Lung abscess, 549
Lung cancer, 156-157, 586
Lung perfusion and ventilation scan, 490
Lyme disease, 598
Lymphadenopathy, 598-599
Lymphoma, non-Hodgkin's, 158-159

M

Magnesium sulfate, 711
Magnetic resonance imaging, 491
Malignant lymphoma, 158
Mallory-Weiss syndrome, 583, 601
Mannitol, 712
Manual ventilation, 404-405, 405i
Marie-Strümpell disease, 26
Maxillofacial injury, 566
Maze procedure, 257
Mechanical obstruction, 144
Mechanical ventilation, 7, 308-309, 388
Meckel's diverticulum, 92
Melena, 600-601
Meningitis, 160-161, 520, 536, 579, 620-611
Menorrhagia, 602-603
Metabolic acidosis and alkalosis, 162-163
Metabolic syndrome, 164-165
Methicillin-resistant *staphylococcus aureus*, 166-168
Methylprednisolone, 713
Metoprolol succinate, 714
Microwave ablation, 257
Mitral insufficiency, 174, 575, 576
Mitral prolapse, 617
Mitral stenosis, 168-169, 169i, 617
Mitral valve prolapse, 170-171, 541
Mixed venous oxygen saturation, 406-407, 406i
Mobitz type atrioventricular blocks, 746i
Morphine sulfate, 715
Multiple-gated acquisition scan, 492
Multiple sclerosis, 172-173, 518-520

Muscle flaccidity, 604-605
Muscle weakness, 606-607
Myasthenia gravis, 134, 538, 569, 606, 618-619, 629
Myelography, 493
Myocardial infarction, 174-175
  ST segment monitoring for, 436-437

N

Naloxone hydrochloride, 716
Naproxen, 717
Nasal packing, 408-409
Nasogastric tube insertion and removal, 410-411
Nausea, 608-609
Necrotizing fasciitis, 176-177
Needle thoracentesis, 333
Negative-pressure ventilation, 308
Neurostimulator placement, in deep brain stimulation, 284
Nephrotic syndrome, 564-565
Nesiritide, 718
Nitroglycerin, 719
Nitroprusside sodium, 720
Non-Hodgkin's lymphoma, 158-159, 599
Norepinephrine bitartrate, 721
Nuchal rigidity, 610-611
Nuclear medicine scan, 494

O

Obesity, 178-179
Oliguria, 316, 612-613
Open biopsy, 464
Open reduction, 310-311
Optic disk, changes in, 105i
Optic neuritis, 160
Orbital fracture, 550
Oronasopharyngeal suction, 412-413
Orthopnea, 614-615
Osteoarthritis, 180-181, 181i
Osteomyelitis, 182-183, 592-593
Osteoporosis, 184-185, 523
Otitis externa, 580
Otitis media, 581
Otosclerosis, 581
Ovarian cysts, 513

i refers to an illustration; t refers to a table.

i refers to an illustration; t refers to a table.

Index

R

Radiation therapy, 320-321
Radiofrequency ablation, 257
  for tumors, 322-323, 323i
Range-of-motion exercises, passive,
  416-417
Ranson score, 187
Ranitidine hydrochloride, 729
Ranolazine, 730
Rectal tube, insertion and removal of,
  430-431
Reed-Sternberg cells, recognition of, 129i
Reflux esophagitis, 102
Reiter syndrome, 26
Renal abscess, 2
Renal artery occlusion, 546, 613
Renal calculi, 212-213, 306, 523, 546,
  571, 584
Renal cancer, 571, 585
Renal failure, 544, 565, 569
  acute, 214-215
  chronic, 216-217, 613, 637
Renal infarction, 571, 585
Renal parenchyma, 2, 212
Renal replacement therapy, continuous,
  278-279
Renal trauma, 571, 585
Renal vein occlusion, 546, 613
Renal vein thrombosis, 571
Respirations
  Cheyne-Stokes, 544-545
  shallow, 628-629
Respiratory acidosis and alkalosis, 4-5,
  218-219
Respiratory distress, prone positioning
  for, 422-423
Restrictive gastric surgeries, 324-325
Retavase, 336
Retention catheter, 374
Reticular dysgenesis, 226
Rh system, understanding of, 43
Rhabdomyolysis, 138, 607
Rhonchi, 630-631
Right-sided heart failure, 80, 112, 208,
  552, 594
Risperidone, 731
Roux-en-Y bypass, 290

Ruptured aneurysm, abdominal aortic,
  22-23, 25

S

Sacroiliac strain, 523
Saline gauze dressing, for pressure
  ulcers, 420
Salmonella infection, 220-221
Sarcoidosis, 549, 566-567, 599
Scratch testing, 17
Second-degree atrioventricular
  blocks, 746i
Segmental resection, 335
Seizure disorder, 222-223, 605, 621
Seizures
  absence, 632-633
  complex partial, 634-635
  generalized tonic-clonic, 636-637
  simple partial, 638-639
  vagus nerve stimulation for, 352-353
Sequential compression therapy, 432-433
Severe acute respiratory syndrome,
  224-225
Severe combined immunodeficiency dis-
  ease, 226-227
Shock, 16, 553, 563, 649
  cardiogenic, 228-230
  hypovolemic, 230-231
  neurogenic, 525
  septic, 232-233, 525, 565
Sickle cell anemia, 20-21, 542, 585,
  591, 625
Sigmoidoscopy, 502
Sinus arrest, 743i
Sinus arrhythmia, 742i
Sinus bradycardia, 742i
Sinus tachycardia, 742i
Skin, mottled, 640-641
Skin grafting, 326-327, 327i
  full-thickness, 326
  split-thickness, 326
Skin staple and clip removal,
  434-435, 435i
Slit-lamp examination, 503
Small-bowel obstruction, 513
Small-bowel tumors, 601
Spastic colon, 146

i refers to an illustration; t refers to a table.

Spinal cord tumor, 619, 621
Spinal stenosis, 523
Spinal trauma and disease, 607
Splenomegaly, 642-643
Staphylococcus aureus, methicillin-
     resistant, 166-168
Status asthmaticus, 36
Stent placement, 328-329
Stereotactic radiosurgery, 330-331
Stomatitis, 320, 661
  after chemotherapy, 274, 277t
Streptokinase, 336
Stroke, 234-235, 519, 521, 556, 597, 607,
     619, 621, 637, 639
ST segment monitoring, 436-437, 437i
Stridor, 644-645
Sumatriptan succinate, 732
Superior vena cava obstruction, 595
Surgical debridement, 326
Suture removal, 438-439
Swan-Ganz catheterization, 424, 498
Synchronized cardioversion, 268-269
Syncope, 646-647
Syndrome of inappropriate antidiuretic
     hormone, 236-237, 282, 296
Syphilis, 599
Systemic lupus erythematosus, 238-239,
     567, 569, 599, 641

T

Tachyarrhythmia, synchronized cardio-
     version for, 268-269
Tachycardia, 648-649
Tachypnea, 650-651
Telemetry monitoring, 370
Teletherapy, 320
Temazepam, 733
Tenecteplase, 336
Tension headache, 110
Tetany, after thyroidectomy, 338
Thermodilution, 372
Third-degree atrioventricular block, 747i
Thoracentesis, 332-333
Thoracic electrical bioimpedance moni-
     toring, 440-441
Thoracotomy, 334-335
Thrombocytopenia, 224, 240-241, 601

Thrombolytic therapy, 336-337
Thrombosis, deep vein, 84-85
Thyroidectomy, 338-339
Time-cycled ventilation, 308
Tonometry, 504
Total parenteral nutrition administration,
     442-443
Toxemia of pregnancy, 613
Toxic diffuse goiter, 134
Trachea
  deviation of, 652-653
  rupture of, 550
  suctioning, 444-445
Tracheostomy care, 446-449
Tracheotomy, 340-341, 341i
Transcranial Doppler
  monitoring, 450-451
  study, 505
Transcutaneous electrical nerve stimula-
     tion, 342-343
Transcutaneous pacemaker, 313
Transesophageal echocardiography, 506
Transfusion
  of blood and plasma products, 260-261
  reaction to, 42-43
Transplantation
  bone marrow, 344-345
  cerebral stem cell, 346-347
  heart, 348-349
Transsphenoidal hypophysectomy, 296
Transvenous pacemaker, 313
Tremors, 654-655
Tuberculosis, 242-243, 542, 563
Tube feeding, 452-453
Tubulin-interactive agents, indications
     for, 274
Tympanic membrane perforation, 581
Typhoid fever, 220

U

Ulcer, peptic, 190-191
Ulcerative colitis, 244-245, 515
Ultrasonography, 507
Ultrasound ablation, 257
Uremia, 561
Urethral stricture, 613
Urethral trauma, 585

i refers to an illustration; t refers to a table.

Index

i refers to an illustration; t refers to a table.